The Future of Post-Human Health Care

The Future of Post-Human Health Care

Towards a New Theory of Mind and Body

By

Peter Baofu

Nova Science Publishers, Inc.
New York

The Future of Post-Human Health Care: Towards a New Theory of Mind and Body, by Peter Baofu

Library of Congress Cataloging-in-Publication Data

ISBN 978-1-62948-236-1

Published by Nova Science Publishers, Inc. † New York

To Those in the Future World beyond Mind and Body

BOOKS ALSO BY PETER BAOFU

Category I: Social Sciences and Related Fields

- 58. *The Future of Post-Human Waste* (2012)
- 57. *The Future of Post-Human Migration* (2012)
- 56. *The Future of Post-Human Criminality* (2012)
- 55. *The Future of Post-Human Geography* (2011)
- 54. *The Future of Post-Human Gambling* (2011)
- 53. *The Future of Post-Human Education* (2011)
- 52. *The Future of Post-Human War and Peace* (2010)
- 51. *The Future of Post-Human Law* (2010)
- 50. *The Future of Post-Human Organization* (2009)
- 49. *The Future of Post-Human Mass Media* (2009)
- 48. *The Rise of Authoritarian Liberal Democracy* (2007)
- 47. *Beyond the World of Titans, and the Remaking of World Order* (2007)
- 46. *Beyond Capitalism to Post-Capitalism* (2005)
- 45. Volume 1: *Beyond Democracy to Post-Democracy* (2004)
- 44. Volume 2: *Beyond Democracy to Post-Democracy* (2004)
- 43. *The Future of Capitalism and Democracy* (2002)

Category II: Natural Sciences and Related Fields

- 42. *Beyond Natural Resources to Post-Human Resources* (2013)
- 41. *The Future of Post-Human Transportation* (2012)
- 40. *The Future of Post-Human Architecture* (2012)
- 39. *The Future of Post-Human Chemistry* (2011)
- 38. *The Future of Post-Human Acoustics* (2011)
- 37. *The Future of Post-Human Geology* (2010)
- 36. *Beyond Cosmology to Post-Cosmology* (2010)
- 35. *The Future of Post-Human Personality* (2010)
- 34. *The Future of Post-Human Sexuality* (2010)
- 33. *The Future of Post-Human Urban Planning* (2009)
- 32. *The Future of Post-Human Engineering* (2009)
- 31. *The Future of Post-Human Unconsciousness* (2008)
- 30. *The Future of Complexity* (2007)
- 29. *Beyond Nature and Nurture* (2006)
- 28. *The Future of Post-Human Space-Time* (2006)
- 27. *The Future of Post-Human Consciousness* (2004)

Category III: The Humanities and Related Fields

- 26. *The Future of Post-Human Thanatology* (2013)
- 25. *The Future of Post-Human Sports* (2013)
- 24. *The Future of Post-Human Culinary Art* (2012)
- 23. *The Future of Post-Human History* (2012)
- 22. *The Future of Post-Human Performing Arts* (2012)
- 21. *The Future of Post-Human Literature* (2011)
- 20. *The Future of Post-Human Humor* (2011)
- 19. *Beyond Ethics to Post-Ethics* (2011)
- 18. *The Future of Post-Human Religion* (2010)
- 17. *The Future of Post-Human Chess* (2010)
- 16. *The Future of Post-Human Martial Arts* (2009)
- 15. *The Future of Post-Human Creative Thinking* (2009)
- 14. *The Future of Post-Human Knowledge* (2008)
- 13. *The Future of Aesthetic Experience* (2007)
- 12. *Beyond Civilization to Post-Civilization* (2006)
- 11. Volume 1: *The Future of Human Civilization* (2000)
- 10. Volume 2: *The Future of Human Civilization* (2000)

Category IV: Formal Sciences and Related Fields

- 09. *The Future of Post-Human Morphology* (2013)
- 08. *The Future of Post-Human Semantics* (2012)
- 07. *The Future of Post-Human Data Analysis* (2011)
- 06. *The Future of Post-Human Computing* (2011)
- 05. *The Future of Post-Human Formal Science* (2010)
- 04. *The Future of Post-Human Language* (2009)
- 03. *The Future of Post-Human Geometry* (2009)
- 02. *The Future of Post-Human Mathematical Logic* (2008)
- 01. *The Future of Information Architecture* (2008)

CONTENTS

Part One: Introduction

Part Two: Mind

Part Three: Body

Part Four: Conclusion

Tables

Category I. The Theoretical Debate on Health Care

Category II: Visions on Nature

Category III: Visions on the Mind

Category IV: Visions on History

Category IX: Visions on Culture

ACKNOWLEDGMENTS

As is often the case, this book, like all other previous books of mine, is written to challenge conventional wisdom or, more precisely, in the current context, the one on health care—and to replace it with an original way of thinking about its future fate (in relation to mind and body, or more precisely, mental health and physical health).

For this reason, this book receives no external funding nor help from any formal organization or institution, because of its political incorrectness—as this is something that I often stressed (and repeated) in all my previous books.

My only reward is the joy of thinking something original in the intellectual history of health care.

In any event, I bear the sole responsibility for the ideas presented in this book.

ABBREVIATIONS

ALD = Peter Baofu. 2007. *The Rise of Authoritarian Liberal Democracy: A Preface to a New Theory of Comparative Political Systems*. Cambridge, England: Cambridge Scholars Publishing, Ltd.

BCIV = Peter Baofu. 2006. *Beyond Civilization to Post-Civilization: Conceiving a Better Model of Life Settlement to Supersede Civilization*. NY: Peter Lang Publishing, Inc.

BCPC = Peter Baofu. 2005. *Beyond Capitalism to Post-Capitalism: Conceiving a Better Model of Wealth Acquisition to Supersede Capitalism*. NY: The Edwin Mellen Press.

BCOS = Peter Baofu. 2010. *Beyond Cosmology to Post-Cosmology: A Preface to a New Theory of Different Worlds*. Cambridge, England: Cambridge International Science Publishing, Ltd.

BDPD1 = Peter Baofu. 2004. Volume 1. *Beyond Democracy to Post-Democracy: Conceiving a Better Model of Governance to Supersede Democracy*. NY: The Edwin Mellen Press.

BDPD2 = Peter Baofu. 2004. Volume 2. *Beyond Democracy to Post-Democracy: Conceiving a Better Model of Governance to Supersede Democracy*. NY: The Edwin Mellen Press.

BEPE = Peter Baofu. 2011. *Beyond Ethics to Post-Ethics: A Preface to a New Theory of Morality and Immorality*. Charlotte, NC: Infomration Age Publishing.

BNN = Peter Baofu. 2006. *Beyond Nature and Nurture: Conceivng a Better Way to Understand Genes and Memes*. Cambridge, England: Cambridge Scholars Publishing, Ltd.

BNR = Peter Baofu. 2013. *Beyond Natural Resources to Post-Human Resources: Towards a New Theory of Diversity and Discontinuity*. Cambridge, England: Cambridge Scholars Publishing, Ltd.

BWT = Peter Baofu. 2007. *Beyond the World of Titans, and the Renaking of World Order: A Preface to a New Logic of Empire-Building*. Cambridge, England: Cambridge Scholars Publishing, Ltd.

FAE = Peter Baofu. 2007. *The Future of Aesthetic Experience: Conceiving a Better Way to Understand Beauty, Ugliness and the Rest.* Cambridge, England: Cambridge Scholars Publishing, Ltd.

FC = Peter Baofu. 2007. *The Future of Complexity: Conceiving a Better Way to Understand Order and Chaos.* London, United Kingdom: World Scientific Publishing Co.

FCD = Peter Baofu. 2002. *The Future of Capitalism and Democracy.* MD: The University Press of America.

FHC1 = Peter Baofu. 2000. Volume 1. *The Future of Human Civilization.* NY: The Edwin Mellen Press.

FHC2 = Peter Baofu. 2000. Volume 2. *The Future of Human Civilization.* NY: The Edwin Mellen Press.

FIA = Peter Baofu. 2008. *The Future of Information Architecture: Conceiving a Better Way to Understand Taxonomy, Network, and Intelligence.* Oxford, England: Chandos Publishing (Oxford) Limited.

FPHA = Peter Baofu. 2011. *The Future of Post-Human Acoustics: A Preface to a New Theory of Sound and Silence.* Cambridge, England: Cambridge International Science Publishing, Ltd.

FPHARCH = Peter Baofu. 2012. *The Future of Post-Human Architecture: A Preface to a New Theory of Form and Function.* Cambridge, England: Cambridge International Science Publishing, Ltd.

FPHC = Peter Baofu. 2004. *The Future of Post-Human Consciousness.* NY: The Edwin Mellen Press.

FPHCA = Peter Baofu. 2012. *The Future of Post-Human Culinary Art: Towards a New Theory of Ingredients and Techniques.* England: Cambridge Scholars Publishing, Ltd.

FPHCHEM = Peter Baofu. 2011. *The Future of Post-Human Chemistry: A Preface to a New Theory of Substances and their Changes.* England: Cambridge Scholars Publishing, Ltd.

FPHCHESS = Peter Baofu. 2010. *The Future of Post-Human Chess: A Preface to a New Theory of Tactics and Strategy.* Cambridge, England: Cambridge International Science Publishing, Ltd.

FPHCOM = Peter Baofu. 2011. *The Future of Post-Human Computing: A Preface to a New Theory of Hardware and Software.* Cambridge, England: Cambridge International Science Publishing, Ltd.

FPHCRIM = Peter Baofu. 2012. *The Future of Post-Human Criminality: A Preface to a New Theory of Heroes and Villains.* Cambridge, England: Cambridge International Science Publishing, Ltd.

FPHCT = Peter Baofu. 2009. *The Future of Post-Human Creative Thinking: A Preface to a New Theory of Invention and Innovation.* Cambridge, England: Cambridge Scholars Publishing, Ltd.

FPHDA = Peter Baofu. 2011. *The Future of Post-Human Data Analysis: A Preface to a New Theory of Quantitative and Qualitative Research.* Cambridge, England: Cambridge International Science Publishing, Ltd.

FPHE = Peter Baofu. 2009. *The Future of Post-Human Engineering: A Preface to a New Theory of Technology.* Cambridge, England: Cambridge Scholars Publishing, Ltd.

FPHEDU = Peter Baofu. 2011. *The Future of Post-Human Education: A Preface to a New Theory of Teaching and Learning.* Cambridge, England: Cambridge International Science Publishing, Ltd.

FPHFS = Peter Baofu. 2010. *The Future of Post-Human Formal Science: A Preface to a New Theory of Abstraction and Application.* Cambridge, England: Cambridge Scholars Publishing, Ltd.

FPHG = Peter Baofu. 2009. *The Future of Post-Human Geometry: A Preface to a New Theory of Infinity, Symmetry, and Dimensionality.* Cambridge, England: Cambridge Scholars Publishing, Ltd.

FPHGAM = Peter Baofu. 2011. *The Future of Post-Human Gambling: A Preface to a New Theory of Risk and Caution.* Cambridge, England: Cambridge International Science Publishing, Ltd.

FPHGEOG = Peter Baofu. 2011. *The Future of Post-Human Geography: A Preface to a New Theory of Environments and their Interactions.* Cambridge, England: Cambridge International Science Publishing, Ltd.

FPHGEOL = Peter Baofu. 2010. *The Future of Post-Human Geology: A Preface to a New Theory of Statics and Dynamics.* Cambridge, England: Cambridge International Science Publishing, Ltd.

FPHH = Peter Baofu. 2011. *The Future of Post-Human Humor: A Preface to a New Theory of Joking and Laughing.* Cambridge, England: Cambridge International Science Publishing, Ltd.

FPHHC = Peter Baofu. 2013. *The Future of Post-Human Health Care: Towards a New Theory of Mind and Body.* Hauppauge, NY: Nova Science Publishers, Inc.

FPHHIST = Peter Baofu. 2012. *The Future of Post-Human History: A Preface to a New Theory of Universality and Relativity.* Cambridge, England: Cambridge Scholars Publishing, Ltd.

FPHK = Peter Baofu. 2008. *The Future of Post-Human Knowledge: A Preface to a New Theory of Methodology and Ontology.* Oxford, England: Chandos Publishing (Oxford) Limited.

FPHL = Peter Baofu. 2009. *The Future of Post-Human Language: A Preface to a New Theory of Structure, Context, and Learning.* Cambridge, England: Cambridge Scholars Publishing, Ltd.

FPHLAW = Peter Baofu. 2010. *The Future of Post-Human Law: A Preface to a New Theory of Necessity, Contingency, and Justice.* Cambridge, England: Cambridge Scholars Publishing, Ltd.

FPHLIT = Peter Baofu. 2011. *The Future of Post-Human Literature: A Preface to a New Theory of Fiction and Non-Fiction.* Cambridge, England: Cambridge International Science Publishing, Ltd.

FPHMA = Peter Baofu. 2009. *The Future of Post-Human Martial Arts: A Preface to a New Theory of the Body and Spirit of Warriors.* Cambridge, England: Cambridge Scholars Publishing, Ltd.

FPHMIG = Peter Baofu. 2012. *The Future of Post-Human Migration: A Preface to a New Theory of Sameness, Otherness, and Identity.* Cambridge, England: Cambridge Scholars Publishing, Ltd.

FPHML = Peter Baofu. 2008. *The Future of Post-Human Mathematical Logic: A Preface to a New Theory of Rationality.* Cambridge, England: Cambridge Scholars Publishing, Ltd.

FPHMM = Peter Baofu. 2009. *The Future of Post-Human Mass Media: A Preface to a New Theory of Technology.* Cambridge, England: Cambridge Scholars Publishing, Ltd.

FPHMORP = Peter Baofu. 2013. *The Future of Post-Human Morphology: Towards a New Theory of Typologies and Rules.* Hauppauge, NY: Nova Science Publishers, Inc.

FPHO = Peter Baofu. 2009. *The Future of Post-Human Organization: A Preface to a New Theory of Communication, Decision-Making, and Leadership.*.Cambridge, England: Cambridge Scholars Publishing, Ltd.

FPHP = Peter Baofu. 2010. *The Future of Post-Human Personality: A Preface to a New Theory of Normality and Abnormality.* Cambridge, England: Cambridge International Science Publishing, Ltd.

FPHPA = Peter Baofu. 2012. *The Future of Post-Human Performing Arts: A Preface to a New Theory of the Body and its Presence.* Cambridge, England: Cambridge Scholars Publishing, Ltd.

FPHR = Peter Baofu. 2010. *The Future of Post-Human Religion: A Preface to a New Theory of Spirituality.* Cambridge, England: Cambridge International Science Publishing, Ltd.

FPHS = Peter Baofu. 2010. *The Future of Post-Human Sexuality: A Preface to a New Theory of the Body and Spirit of Love-Makers.* Cambridge, England: Cambridge Scholars Publishing, Ltd.

FPHSEM = Peter Baofu. 2012. *The Future of Post-Human Semantics: A Preface to a New Theory of Internality and Externality.* Cambridge, England: Cambridge Scholars Publishing, Ltd.

FPHSPORT = Peter Baofu. 2013. *The Future of Post-Human Sports: Towards a New Theory of Training and Winning.* Cambridge, England: Cambridge Scholars Publishing, Ltd.

FPHST = Peter Baofu. 2006. *The Future of Post-Human Space-Time: Conceivng a Better Way to Understand Space and Time.* New York: Peter Lang Publishing, Inc.

FPHTHAN = Peter Baofu. 2013. *The Future of Post-Human Thanatology: Towards a New Theory of Death and After-Death.* Berlin, Germany: Logos Verlag Berlin.

FPHTRAN = Peter Baofu. 2012. *The Future of Post-Human Transportation: A Preface to a New Theory of Networks and Operations.* Cambridge, England: Cambridge Scholars Publishing, Ltd.

FPHU = Peter Baofu. 2008. *The Future of Post-Human Unconsciousness: A Preface to a New Theory of Anomalous Experience.* Cambridge, England: Cambridge Scholars Publishing, Ltd.

FPHUP = Peter Baofu. 2009. *The Future of Post-Human Urban Planning: A Preface to a New Theory of Density, Void, and Sustainability.* Cambridge, England: Cambridge Scholars Publishing, Ltd.

FPHW = Peter Baofu. 2012. *The Future of Post-Human Waste: Towards a New Theory of Uselessness and Usefulness.* Cambridge, England: Cambridge Scholars Publishing, Ltd.

FPHWP = Peter Baofu. 2010. *The Future of Post-Human War and Peace: A Preface to a New Theory of Aggression and Pacificity.* Cambridge, England: Cambridge Scholars Publishing, Ltd.

• PART ONE •

Introduction

CHAPTER 1
INTRODUCTION—THE VALUE OF HEALTH CARE

[A] psychology of positive human functioning will arise, which achieves a scientific understanding and effective interventions to build thriving individuals, families, and communities.
—Martin Seligman et al. (2000)

A Debate on a Fashionable Psychology

Is positive thinking really so healthy that, as Martin Seligman (2000) and Mihaly Csikszentmihalyi passionately thus argued, "we believe that a psychology of positive human functioning will arise, which achieves a scientific understanding and effective interventions to build thriving individuals, families, and communities"?

This optimistic view on positive thinking for health can be contrasted with an opposing view by Barbara Ehrenreich (2009), who "extensively critiqued 'positive psychology'" and showed "how obsessive positive thinking impedes productive action, causes delusional assessments of situations, and…people are then blamed for not visualizing hard enough and thus 'attracting' failure even in situations when 'masses of lives were lost.'" (WK 2013; R. Byrne 2006)

Contrary to these opposing views (and other ones as will be discussed in the book), health care (in relation to mental health and physical health in the context of mind and body) are neither possible (or impossible) nor desirable (or undesirable) to the extent that the respective ideologues (on different sides) would like us to believe.

Surely, this questioning of the opposing views on health care does not suggest that the study of health care is worthless, or that those fields (related to health care) like medicine, chiropractic, health system, dentistry, health info tech, nursing, palliative care, psychiatrics, clinical psychology, occupational therapy, pharmacy, allied health, and so on are unimportant. (WK 2013b) Needless to say, neither of these extreme views is reasonable.

Instead, this book offers an alternative (better) way to understand the future of health care, especially in regard to the dialectic relationshp between mental health and physical health in the context of mind and body—while learning from different approaches in the literature but without favoring any one of them (nor integrating them, since they are not necessarily compatible with each other).

More specifically, this book offers a new theory (that is, *the interconnected theory of health care*) to go beyond the existing approaches in a novel way.

If successful, this seminal project is to fundamentally change the way that we think about health care in relation to mental health and physical health (in the context of mind and body) from the combined perspectives of the mind, nature, society, and culture, with enormous implications for the human future and what I originally called its "post-human" fate.

Definition and History of Health Care

A good point of departure for the present inquiry is to provide a working definition of the term "health care" and its brief history.

Definition

The term "health care," according to the Merriam-Webster dictionary, refers to "efforts made to maintain or restore health especially by trained and licensed professionals." (MWD 2013)

More specifically, the term "health care" (or "healthcare") is "the diagnosis, treatment, and prevention of disease, illness, injury, and other physical and mental impairments in humans. Health care is delivered by practitioners in medicine, chiropractic, dentistry, nursing, pharmacy, allied health, and other care providers. It refers to the work done in providing primary care, secondary care and tertiary care, as well as in public health." (WK 2013b)

Of course, even though "the definitions of the various types of health care vary depending on the different cultural, political, organizational and disciplinary perspectives, there appears to be some consensus that primary care constitutes the first element of a continuing health care process, that may also include the provision of secondary and tertiary levels of care. Healthcare can be defined as either public or private healthcare." (WK 2013b; R. Thomas-MacLean 2011)

History

Historically, "access to health care varies across countries, groups and individuals, largely influenced by social and economic conditions as well as the health policies in place. Countries and jurisdictions have different policies and plans in relation to the personal and population-based health care goals within their societies." (WK 2013b)

This means that "the...exact configuration [of heath care] varies from country to country. In some countries and jurisdictions, health care planning is distributed among market participants, whereas in others planning is made more centrally among governments or other coordinating bodies." (WK 2013b)

Nonetheless, "in all cases, according to the World Health Organization (WHO), a well-functioning health care system requires a robust financing mechanism; a well-trained and adequately-paid workforce; reliable information on which to base decisions and policies; and well maintained facilities and logistics to deliver quality medicines and technologies." (WK 2013b; WHO 2013)

Nowadays, "health care can form a significant part of a country's economy. In 2008, the health care industry consumed an average of 9.0 percent of the gross domestic product (GDP) across the most developed OECD countries. The United States (16.0%), France (11.2%), and Switzerland (10.7%) were the top three spenders." (WK 2013b)

And the success of health care cannot be underestimated; after all, "an example of this is the worldwide eradication of smallpox in 1980—declared by the WHO as the first disease in human history to be completely eliminated by deliberate health care interventions." (WK 2013b)

Mind and Body in Health Care

With this definition and brief history of health care in mind—the two different main concerns in health care, as defined in the previous section, are about "physical and mental impairments in humans."

Thus, the purpose of this book to focus on the dialectic relationship between "mental health" and "physical health" in the context of *mind* and *body*, as explained below (and summarized in *Table 1.1*), with the ultimate goal to transcend both mental health and physical health for a different approach to health care altogether.

Mental Health

In accordance to the Merriam-Webster dictionary, the word "mind" refers to the "complex of elements in an individual that feels, perceives, thinks, wills, and especially reasons." (MWD 2013a)

More specifically in the context of health care, the term "mind" refers to "mental health," which "describes a level of psychological well-being, or an absence of a mental disorder"; from one perspective, "mental health may include an individual's ability to enjoy life, and create a balance between life activities and efforts to achieve psychological resilience. Mental health can also be defined as an expression of emotions, and as signifying a successful adaptation to a range of demands." (WK 2013c; ABO 2013)

For illustration, consider the following three main examples of mental health used in health care, namely, (a) problem-solving ability, (b) emotional expression, and (c) resilience.

Problem-Solving Ability

The first example to understand mental health in the study of health care has to do with problem-solving ability.

Problem-solving ability is important for mental health, because mental well-being requires the ability to cope with life's challenges, and problem-solving is useful here, because it "consists in using generic or ad hoc methods, in an orderly manner, for finding solutions to problems." (WK 2013c & 2013d)

Especially in psychology, "problem solving refers to a state of desire for reaching a definite goal from a present condition that either is not directly moving toward the goal, is far from it, or needs more complex logic for finding a missing description of conditions or steps toward the goal....Problem solving has two major domains: mathematical problem solving and personal problem solving where, in the second, some difficulty or barrier is encountered. Further problem solving occurs when moving from a given state to a desired goal state is needed for either living organisms or an artificial intelligence system." (WK 2013d; B. Zimmermann 2013; S. Robertson 2001)

In fact, "the nature of human problem solving processes and methods has been studied by psychologists over the past hundred years. Methods of studying problem solving include introspection, behaviorism, simulation, computer modeling, and experiment." (WK 2013d)

Emotional Expression

The second example to understand mental health in the study of health care has to do with emotional expression.

Emotional expression is important for mental health, because "researchers have focused on the role of emotions in problem solving, demonstrating that poor emotional control can disrupt focus on the target task and impede problem resolution." (WK 2013d; J. Rath 2004; T. D'Zurilla1982)

In fact, "emotional mental disorders are a leading cause of disabilities worldwide. Investigating the degree and severity of untreated emotional mental disorders throughout the world is a top priority of the World Mental Health (WMH) survey initiative, which was created in 1998 by the World Health Organization (WHO)"; for instance, "neuropsychiatric disorders are the leading causes of disability worldwide, accounting for 37% of all healthy life years lost through disease.These disorders are most destructive to low and middle-income countries due to their inability to provide their citizens with proper aid." (WK 2013c; G. Thornicroft 2007)

Resilience

And the third example to understand mental health in the study of health care has to do with resilience.

"Resilence" is important for mental health, because it refers to an individual's ability "to cope with stress and adversity. This coping may result in the individual 'bouncing back' to a previous state of normal functioning, or simply not showing negative effects. A third, more controversial form of resilience is sometimes referred to as 'posttraumatic growth' or 'steeling effects' where in the experience adversity leads to better functioning (much like an inoculation gives one the capacity to cope well with future exposure to disease)." (WK 2013e; A. Masten 2009)

Broadly speaking, "commonly used terms, which are closely related within psychology, are 'psychological resilience,'...'hardiness,' 'resourcefulness,' and 'mental toughness.'" (WK 2013e)

Physical Health

A different (second) concern in heatlh care concerns "physical health" in the context of the body.

In accordance to the Merriam-Webster dictionary, the word "body" refers to "the main part of a plant or animal body especially as distinguished from limbs and head" (or in the case of humans, "the material part or nature of a human being"). (MWD 2013b)

More specifically in the context of health care, the term "body" refers to "physical health" to mean the well-being of the body. For illustration, consider the following three main examples of physical health used in health care, namely, (a) fitness, (b) abuse control, and (c) violence regulation.

Fitness

The first example to understand physical health in the study of health care has to do with fitness.

Fitness is important for physical health, because it refers to good health as a result of exercise, in two major ways, that is, "general fitness (a state of health and well-being), and specific fitness (a task-oriented definition based on the ability to perform specific aspects of sports or occupations). Physical fitness is generally achieved through correct nutrition, exercise, and rest." (WK 2013f)

For example, "a comprehensive fitness program tailored to an individual typically focuses on one or more specific skills, and on age- or health-related needs such as bone health....Physical fitness can also prevent or treat many chronic health conditions brought on by unhealthy lifestyle or aging. Working out can also help people sleep better. To stay healthy it is important to engage in physical activity." (WK 2013f; G. Colfer 2006; R. Nied 2002; ASPE 2002; CDC 2013)

Abuse Control

The second example to understand physical health in the study of health care has to do with abuse control.

Abuse control is important for physical health, because it refers to the prevention of any practice, usage, or treatment which causes harm to the body, and good examples include "unsafe sex" (which can result in HIV infection and other diseases), "substance abuse" (which can result in addiction and other health problems), and so on.

For illustration, "substance abuse" (or "drug abuse") is "a patterned use of a substance (drug) in which the user consumes the substance in amounts or with methods neither approved nor supervised by medical professionals. Substance abuse/drug abuse is not limited to mood-altering or psycho-active drugs. If an activity is performed using the objects against the rules and policies of the matter (as in steroids for performance enhancement in sports), it is also called substance abuse....Using illicit drugs—narcotics, stimulants, depressants (sedatives), hallucinogens, cannabis, even glues and paints, are also considered to be classified as drug/substance abuse. Substance abuse often includes problems with impulse control and impulsive behaviour." (WK 2013g; O. Ray 2002)

Violence Regulation

And the first example to understand mental health in the study of health care has to do with violence regulation.

Violence regulation is important for physical health, because "violence," as defined by the World Health Organization, refers to "the intentional use of physical force or power, threatened or actual, against a person, or against a group or community, that either results in or has a high likelihood of resulting in injury, death, psychological harm, maldevelopment or deprivation. This definition associates intentionality with the committing of the act itself, irrespective of the outcome it produces." (WK 2013h)

At the global level, "violence takes the lives of more than 1.5 million people annually: just over 50% due to suicide, some 35% due to homicide, and just over 12% as a direct result of war or some other form of conflict. For each single death due to violence, there are dozens of hospitalizations, hundreds of emergency department visits, and thousands of doctors' appointments. Furthermore, violence often has lifelong consequences for victims' physical and mental health and social functioning and can slow economic and social development." (WK 2013h; WHO 2008)

Diverse Aspects of Health Care

This introduction to "mental health" and "physical health" in the context of mind and body thus shows the more complicated nature of health care.

To illustrate this more complicated nature of health care further, consider the diverse aspects of health care below (as summarized in *Table 1.1*).

Conceptual Distinctions

The first aspect of health care to be illustrated here in regard to its more complicated nature concerns some main conceptual distinctions. For illustration, consider three main examples below.

Illness vs. Disease

The first example to clarify some main conceptual distinctions in health care has to do with illness vs. disease.

On the one hand, the term "disease" refers to "any condition that impairs normal function, and is therefore associated with dysfunction of normal homeostasis. Commonly, term *disease* is used to refer specifically to infectious diseases, which are clinically evident diseases that result from the presence of pathogenic microbial agents, including viruses, bacteria, fungi, protozoa, multicellular organisms, and aberrant proteins known as prions. An infection that does not and will not produce clinically evident impairment of normal functioning, such as the presence of the normal bacteria and yeasts in the gut, or of a passenger virus, is not considered a disease....Non-infectious diseases are all other diseases, including most forms of cancer, heart disease, and genetic disease." (WK 2013i; OCSD 2012)

On the other hand, the term "illness" is "occasionally used to refer specifically to the patient's personal experience of their disease. In this model, it is possible for a person have a disease without being ill (to have an objectively definable, but asymptomatic, medical condition), and to be ill without being diseased (such as when a person perceives a normal experience as a medical condition, or medicalizes a non-disease situation their life). Illness is often not due to infection, but to a collection of evolved responses—sickness behavior by the body—that helps clear infection. Such aspects of illness can include lethargy, depression, anorexia, sleepiness, hyperalgesia, and inability to concentrate." (WK 2013i; H. Emson 1987; I. McWhinney 1987; B. Hart 1988; R. Johnson 2002; K. Kelley 2003)

Brain vs. Mind

The second example to clarify some main conceptual distinctions in health care has to do with the brain vs. the mind.

On the one hand, the term "brain" (or "encephalon" in Greek for "in the head") refers to "the control center of the central nervous system, responsible for thought. In most animals, the brain is located in the head, protected by the skull and close to the primary sensory apparatus of vision, hearing, equilibrioception, taste and olfaction. While all vertebrates have a brain, most invertebrates have either a centralized brain or collections of individual ganglia. Primitive animals such as sponges do not have a brain at all. Brains can be extremely complex. For example, the human brain contains more than 100 billion neurons, each linked to as many as 10,000 others." (WK 2013j; I. Whishaw 2010; L. Sherwood 2011)

On the other hand, the term "mind" refers to "the complex of cognitive faculties that enables consciousness, thinking, reasoning, perception, and judgement—a characteristic of human beings, but which also may apply to other life forms"—and "the most straightforward scientific evidence that there is a strong relationship between the physical brain matter and the mind is the impact physical alterations to the brain have on the mind, such as with traumatic brain injury and psychoactive drug use." (WK 2013j) In philosophy, "there are three major…schools of thought" concerning the relationship between the mind and the brain, namely, "dualism, materialism, and idealism. Dualism holds that the mind exists independently of the brain; materialism holds that mental phenomena are identical to neuronal phenomena; and idealism holds that only mental phenomena exist." (WK 2013j Hart, W. D. 1997)

Mind vs. Soul

The third example to clarify some main conceptual distinctions in health care has to do with the mind vs. the soul.

On the one hand, the term "mind," as already indicated in the previous sub-section, refers to "the complex of cognitive faculties that enables consciousness, thinking, reasoning, perception, and judgement—a characteristic of human beings, but which also may apply to other life forms." (WK 2013j)

On the other hand, the term "soul" is more spiritual, in that it refers to, "in many mythological, religious, philosophical, and psychological traditions,…the incorporeal and, in many conceptions, immortal essence of a person, living thing, or object. According to some religions (including the Abrahamic religions in most of their forms), souls—or at least immortal souls capable of union with the divine—belong only to human beings. For example, the Catholic theologian Thomas Aquinas attributed 'soul' (*anima*) to all organisms but taught that only human souls are immortal. Other religions (most notably Jainism) teach that all biological organisms have souls, and others further still that even non-biological entities (such as rivers and mountains) possess souls. This latter belief is called animism." (WK 2013k; P. Eardley 2010)

Private Health vs. Public Health

And the fourth example to clarify some main conceptual distinctions in health care has to do with private health vs. public health.

On the one hand, the term "public health" refers to "healthcare and medicine provided by…the government" and "is concerned with threats to health based on population health analysis. The population in question can be as small as a handful of people or as large as all the inhabitants of several continents (for instance, in the case of a pandemic). The dimensions of health can encompass 'a state of complete physical, mental and social well-being and not merely the absence of disease or infirmity,' as defined by the United Nations' World Health Organization"—and "promotion of hand washing and breastfeeding, delivery of vaccinations, and distribution of condoms to control the spread of sexually transmitted diseases are examples of common public health measures." (WK 2013s & 2013t)

On the other hand, the term "private health" (or "private healthcare") refers to "healthcare and medicine provided by entities other than the government. The term is generally used more in Europe and other countries which have publicly funded health care, to differentiate the arrangement from the usual system. Ethical issues relating to private healthcare primarily concerns the argument that the seriously ill be entitled to spend money on saving their lives. On the other hand, private healthcare can sometimes be more efficient than public sector provision. Private operators may be more innovative in areas such as telemedicine. Due to the profit motive, they can be more productive." (WK 2013s)

Types of Health Care

The second aspect of health care to be illustrated here in regard to its more complicated nature concerns different types of health care. For illustration, consider four main examples below.

Primary Care

The first type of health care to be described here has to do with primary care.

The term "primary care" refers to "the work of health care professionals who act as a first point of consultation for all patients within the health care system. Such a professional would usually be a primary care physician, such as a general practitioner or family physician, or a non-physician primary care provider, such as a physician assistant or nurse practitioner. Depending on the locality, health system organization, and sometimes at the patient's discretion, they may see another health care professional first, such as a pharmacist, a nurse (such as in the United Kingdom), a clinical officer (such as in parts of Africa), or an Ayurvedic or other traditional medicine professional (such as in parts of Asia)." (WK 2013b; R. Thomas-MacLean 2011)

Secondary Care

The second type of health care to be described here has to do with secondary care.

The term "secondary care" refers to "the health care services provided by medical specialists and other health professionals who generally do not have first contact with patients, for example, cardiologists, urologists and dermatologists. It includes acute care: necessary treatment for a short period of time for a brief but serious illness, injury or other health condition, such as in a hospital emergency department. It also includes skilled attendance during childbirth, intensive care, and medical imaging services." (WK 2013b)

Others, like "allied health professionals, such as physical therapists, respiratory therapists, occupational therapists, speech therapists, and dietitians, also generally work in secondary care, accessed through either patient self-referral or through physician referral." (WK 2013b)

Tertiary Care

The third type of health care to be described here has to do with tertiary care.

The term "tertiary care" refers to "specialized consultative health care, usually for inpatients and on referral from a primary or secondary health professional, in a facility that has personnel and facilities for advanced medical investigation and treatment, such as a tertiary referral hospital." (WK 2013b; JKM 2011)

Good examples of "tertiary care services are cancer management, neurosurgery, cardiac surgery, plastic surgery, treatment for severe burns, advanced neonatology services, palliative, and other complex medical and surgical interventions." (WK 2013b)

Quaternary Care

And the fourth type of health care to be described here has to do with quaternary care.

The term "quaternary care" is "used sometimes as an extension of tertiary care" and refers to "medicine of advanced levels which are highly specialized and not widely accessed. Experimental medicine and some types of uncommon diagnostic or surgical procedures are considered quaternary care. These services are usually only offered in a limited number of regional or national health care centres. This term is more prevalent in the United Kingdom, but just as applicable in the United States." (WK 2013b; ARPAP 2011)

The Theoretical Debate

These diverse aspects of health care, together with the introduction to "mental health" and "physical health" (in the context of mind and body) then lead us to a more important question concerning the theoretical debate on the very nature of health care. Indeed, this theoretical debate can also say much about the study of health care as a discipline over time.

Although there can be many different theoretical approaches in the debate—there are five main ones to be summarized hereafter, and they can be called, in the absence of better words, namely, (a) the *mental* argument, (b) the *natural* argument, (c) the *societal* argument, (d) the *cultural* argument, and (e) the *interconntected* argument (which is my original contribution to the debate), to be elabroated hereafter, respectively.

Lest misunderstanding occurs, three clarifications should be made here, as this is something that I regularly emphasize in my previous books, whenever a theoretical debate is summarized for a topic, *almost verbatim*.

Firstly, there can be other arguments besides the first four here, that is, the "mental," the "natural," the "societal," and the "cultural" arguments (as indicated above). The advantage to select these four here has to do with their illustrative representation of the diverse theories in the literature (which are deemed sufficient for the purpose at hand in this book).

Secondly, the examples (theories) given to illustrate each argument are also supposed to be illustrative, not exhaustive. After all, the arguments will be addressed again in the rest of the book, with other examples (theories) to be introduced.

And thirdly, the four arguments are not necessarily mutually exclusive. For instance, those who advocate the "mental" argument can also consider the "cultural" argument, although they do not focus on the latter.

And the reverse is also true, in that those who make the "cultural" argument can also consider the "mental" argument, although they do not focus on the latter.

In other words, their disagreement is often one in degree, not in kind.

The Mental Argument

With these three clarifications in mind—the first major theoretical approach is called, in the absence of better words, the *mental* argument, which focuses, relatively speaking of course, more on the biological and psychological aspects of health care.

Thus, the word "mental" in the title of the argument is suggestive, because it refers to the focus on the physiological, biological and psychological aspccts of health care so understood.

But the mental argument has different issues of concern, and different defenders of the argument offer their own distinctive stands on the issues, depending on their own interests.

For illustration, consider two major versions of the mental argument (with the first on mental health and the second on physical health), namely, (a) mental health, psychotherapy, and medicine, and (b) physical health, exercise, and effects—to be addressed below, in that order.

Mental Health, Psychotherapy, and Medicine

The first version of the mental argument has to do with mental health, psychotherapy, and medicine (in the context of mental health) in health care.

An argument in the literature is that psychotherapy can be used to treat mental health problems, as a form of modern medicine. (WK 2013c)

For example, "psychotherapists employ a range of techniques based on experiential relationship building, dialogue, communication and behavior change that are designed to improve the mental health of a client or patient, or to improve group relationships (such as in a family)." (WK 2013l)

However, for the critics, this argument on mental health, psychotherapy, and medicine has some major problems. Consider, for illustration, a few examples below.

Firstly, one main criticism of the argument on mental health, psychotherapy, and medicine is that "there is considerable controversy about which form of psychotherapy is most effective." (WK 2013l)

For instance, for the critics, there exists a "considerable controversy about which form of psychotherapy is most effective, and more specifically, which types of therapy are optimal for treating which sorts of problems. Furthermore, it is controversial whether the form of therapy or the presence of factors common to many psychotherapies best separates effective therapy from ineffective therapy." (WK 2013l; B. Casey 2004)

And secondly, another main criticism of the argument on mental health, psychotherapy, and medicine is that "the dropout rate" of psychotherapeutic patients is "quite high."

For example, for the critics, "the dropout level is quite high; one meta-analysis of 125 studies concluded that the mean dropout rate was 46.86%. The high level of dropout has raised some criticism about the relevance and efficacy of psychotherapy." (WK 2013l; M. Wierzbicki 1993)

Physical Health, Exercise, and Effects

And the second version of the mental argument has to do with physical health, exercise, and effects (in the context of physical health) in health care.

An argument in the literature is that "physical exercise is important for maintaining physical fitness and can contribute positively to maintaining a healthy weight, building and maintaining healthy bone density, muscle strength, and joint mobility, promoting physiological well-being, reducing surgical risks, and strengthening the immune system." (WK 2013a)

However, for the critics, the argument on physical health, exercise, and effects has some major problems. Consider, for illustration, a few examples below.

Firstly, one main criticism of the argument on physical health, exercise, and effects is that vigorous exercise can have its downside.

For instance, for the critics, "some studies have shown that vigorous exercise…for long periods of time, or without proper warmup beforehand and cooldown afterwards, can lead to an increased risk of injury and overtraining." (WK 2013a; P. Sparling 2003; A. Burfoot 2004)

And secondly, another main criticism of the argument on physical health, exercise, and effects is that some individuals can be exercise-resistant.

For instance, for the critics, "not everyone benefits equally from exercise. There is tremendous variation in individual response to training; where most people will see a moderate increase in endurance from aerobic exercise, some individuals will as much as double their oxygen uptake, while others can never augment endurance." (WK 2013a; C. Bouchard 1999; G. Kolata 2002)

The Natural Argument

The second theoretical approach is called, in the absence of better words, the *natural* argument, which focuses, relatively speaking of course, more on the natural aspects of health care, especially in relation to the state of nature.

Therefore, the word "natural" in the title of the argument is suggestive, because it refers to the focus on the natural aspects of health care so understood.

Like the mental argument—the natural argument has different issues of concern, and different defenders of the argument offer their own distinctive stands on the issues, depending on their own interests.

For illustration, consider two major versions of the natural argument (with the first on mental health and the second on physical health), namely, (a) mental health, evolutionary adaptedness, and the environment, and (b) physical health, infectious disease, and animals—to be summarized below, in that order.

Mental Health, Evolutionary Adaptedness, and the Environment

The first version of the natural argument has to do with mental health, evolutionary adaptedness, and the environment (in the context of mental health) in health care.

An argument in the literature is that "human psychological traits are evolved adaptations—that is, the functional products of natural selection or sexual selection," in that "the mind has a modular structure similar to that of the body, with different modular adaptations serving different functions. Evolutionary psychologists argue that much of human behavior is the output of psychological adaptations that evolved to solve recurrent problems in human ancestral environments." (WK 2013m; R. Durrant 2003; S. Pinker 2002; J. Tooby 2005).

However, for the critics, this argument on mental health, evolutionary adaptedness, and the environment has some major problems. Consider, for illustration, a few examples below.

Firstly, one main criticism of the argument on mental health, evolutionary adaptedness, and the environment is that there are "non-genetic and non-adaptive explanations" which are not adequately considered.

For instance, for the critics, there are non-adaptive "by-products" (of "an adaptive mechanism with no current or ancestral function," like "white color of bones" or "belly button") and "random noise" (i.e., "random variations in an adaptation or byproduct" like "bumps on the skull, convex or concave belly button shape"), which then led George C Williams (1996) to once suggest that an "adaptation is a special and onerous concept that should only be used where it is really necessary." (WK 2013m)

And secondly, another main criticism of the argument on mental health, evolutionary adaptedness, and the environment is that there is the controversial issues about testability and uncertainty.

For instance, for the critics, "controversies concerning EP involve questions of testability, cognitive and evolutionary assumptions (such as modular functioning of the brain, and large uncertainty about the ancestral environment)." (WK 2013m)

Physical Health, Infectious Disease, and Animals

And the second version of the natural argument has to do with physical health, infectious disease, and animals (in the context of physical health) in health care.

An argument in the literature is that there are certain "infectious diseases," like "zoonotic diseases," which can be "transmitted…from animals other than humans to humans," and "the emergence of a pathogen into a new host species is called *disease invasion* or 'disease emergence.'" (WK 2013n; L. Taylor 2001)

However, for the critics, this argument on physical health, infectious disease, and animals has some major problems. Consider, for illustration, a few examples below.

Firstly, one main criticism of the argument on physical health, infectious disease, and animals is that zoonotic diseases can be historically contingent.

For instance, for the critics, "most human prehistory was spent as groups of hunter-gatherers usually with fewer than 150 individuals that were not often in contact with other bands. Because of this, epidemic or pandemic diseases, which depend on a constant influx of humans who have not developed an immune response, tended to burn out after their first run through a population. To survive, a biological pathogen had to be a chronic infection, stay alive in the host for long periods, or have a non-human reservoir in which to live while waiting for new hosts to pass by. In fact, for many 'human' diseases, the human is actually an accidental victim and a dead-end host." (WK 2013n)

And secondly, another main criticism of the argument on physical health, infectious disease, and animals is that there are infectious diseases which can go in the opposite direction.

For instance, for the critics, "in a systematic review of 1,415 pathogens known to infect humans," 39% were not zoonotic at all and occurred in the opposite direction, that is, "from humans to other animals" instead, in what is now known as "reverse zoonosis or anthroponosis." (WK 2013n; L. Taylor 2001)

The Societal Argument

The third theoretical approach is called, in the absence of better words, the *societal* argument, which focuses, relatively speaking of course, more on the societal aspects of health care (e.g., organizational, institutional, structural, and technological issues).

In this sense, the word "societal" in the title of the argument is suggestive, because it refers to the societal aspects of health care so understood.

Like the mental and natural arguments—the societal argument has different issues of concern, and different defenders of the argument offer their own distinctive stands on the issues, depending on their own interests.

For illustration, consider two major versions of the societal argument (with the first on mental health and the second on physical health), namely, (a) mental health, illness, and income inequality, and (b) physical health, drug use, and the law—to be summarized in what follows, in that order.

Mental Health, Illness, and Income Inequality

The first version of the societal argument has to do with mental health, illness, and income inequality (in the context of mental health) in health care.

An argument in the literature is the one proposed by Richard G. Wilkinson (2009) and Kate Pickett, who argued that there are "pernicious effects that inequality has on societies: eroding trust, increasing anxiety and illness, (and) encouraging excessive consumption," especially in regard to "mental health" (and "physical health," for that matter). (WK 2013o; B. Jarvis 2010)

However, for the critics, this argument on mental health, illness, and income inequality has some major problems. Consider, for illustration, a few examples below.

Firstly, one main criticism of the argument on mental health, illness, and income inequality is that it constitutes a very narrow view of social stratification in relation to health care.

For instance, the critic like John Goldthorpe (2009) rebuked by saying that "the book relied too heavily on income inequality over other forms of inequality (including broader economic inequality), and demonstrated a one-dimensional understanding of social stratification, with social class being in effect treated as merely a marker for income. He concluded that much more research was needed to support either the Wilkinson and Pickett 'account of the psychosocial generation of the contextual effects of inequality on health or the rival neo-materialist account.'" (WK 2013o)

And secondly, another main criticism of the argument on mental health, illness, and income inequality is that it provides no verification of the claim.

For instance, the critic like "Richard Reeves [2009] in *The Guardian*...said there were problems with the book's approach. 'Drawing a line through a series of data points signals nothing concrete about statistical significance...since they do not provide any statistical analyses, this can't be verified,'" and another critic "John Kay [2009] in *The Financial Times* said that 'the evidence presented in the book is mostly a series of scatter diagrams, with a regression line drawn through them. No data is provided on the estimated equations, or on relevant statistical tests.'" (WK 2013o)

Physical Health, Drug Use, and the Law

And the second version of the societal argument has to do with physical health, drug use, and the law (in the context of physical health) in morphology.

An argument in the literature is that, as suggested by "advocates of drug prohibition,...particular drugs should be illegal because they are harmful. Drug Free Australia, for example, argues 'that illicit drugs are inherently harmful substances....' The U.S. government has argued that illegal drugs are 'far more deadly than alcohol' saying 'although alcohol is used by seven times as many people as drugs, the number of deaths induced by those substances is not far apart.'" (WK 2013p; DRA 2010)

However, for the critics, this argument on physical health, drug use, and the law has some major problems. Consider, for illustration, a few examples below.

Firstly, one main criticism of this argument on physical health, drug use, and the law is that its claims against illicit drugs are exaggerated.

For instance, for the critics, "there is evidence that many illicit drugs pose comparatively fewer health dangers than certain legal drugs. The health risks of MDMA (Ecstasy) have been exaggerated for instance, the risks from cannabis use also overstated, and health problems from the use of legal substances, particularly alcohol and tobacco, are even greater than from cocaine use for example (occasional cocaine use does not typically lead to severe or even minor physical or social problems)." (WK 2013p; D. Nutt 2007; R. Doblin 2004; B. Goldacre 2008 & 2007; P. Cohen 1994)

Secondly, another main criticism of this argument on physical health, drug use, and the law is that illicit drugs can be beneficial to health.

For instance, for the critics, "many trials have shown beneficial effects associated with psychoactive drug use. There is evidence that MDMA (ecstasy) can treat or cure post-traumatic stress disorder and anxiety in cases of terminal illness. LSD has been widely researched as a therapeutic agent, and has shown effectiveness against alcoholism, frigidity and various other disorders....A 2007 study by Santos et al. found that users of ayahuasca scored lower on tests measuring anxiety and hopelessness than people who did not use the drug." (WK 2013p)

The Cultural Argument

And the fourth theoretical approach is called, in the absence of better words, the *cultural* argument, which focuses, relatively speaking of course, more on the cultural aspects of health care (e.g., issues in relation to values and beliefs).

Therefore, the word "cultural" in the title of the argument is suggestive, because it refers to the focus on the cultural aspects of health care so understood.

Like the mental, natural, and societal arguments—the cultural argument has different issues of concern, and different defenders of the argument offer their own distinctive stands on the issues, depending on their own interests.

For illustration, consider two major versions of the cultural argument (with the first on mental health and the second on physical health), namely, (a) mental health, alternative medicine, and culture, and (b) physical health, torture, and culture—to be summarized in what follows, in that order.

Mental Health, Alternative Medicine, and Culture

The first version of the cultural argument has to do with mental health, alternative medicine, and culture (in the context of mental health) in health care.

An argument in the literature is that "alternative medicine" like "homeopathy, Ayurveda, chiropractic, and acupuncture" in different cultures (or subcultures) can be used to yield "the healing effects of medicine" but is "usually based on religion, tradition, superstition, belief in supernatural energies," and other "treatments…that are not part of the conventional, science-based healthcare system." (WK 2013q; NSF 2002; W. Sampson 1995; B. Beyerstein 2001; NCCAM 2005; USIM 2005)

However, for the critics, the argument on mental health, alternative medicine, and culture has some major problems. Consider, for illustration, a few examples below.

Firstly, one main criticism of the argument on mental health, alternative medicine, and culture is that it is not scientific.

For instance, "the United States' National Science Foundation has defined alternative medicine as 'all treatments that have not been proven effective using scientific methods,'" and "Edzard Ernst [2005], a professor of complementary medicine, characterizes the evidence for many alternative techniques as weak, nonexistent, or negative." (WK 2013q; NSF 2002)

And secondly, another main criticism of the argument on mental health, alternative medicine, and culture is that its misleading tendency is unethical.

For instance, "in November 2011 Edzard Ernst [2011] stated that the 'level of misinformation about alternative medicine has now reached the point where it has become dangerous and unethical. So far, alternative medicine has remained an ethics-free zone. It is time to change this.'" (WK 2013q)

Physical Health, Torture, and Culture

And the second version of the cultural argument has to do with physical health, torture, and culture (in the context of physical health) in health care.

An argument in the literature is that, as shown in many "national and international legal prohibitions on torture" in our time, as part of the global culture against torture, there is "a consensus that torture and similar ill-treatment are immoral, as well as impractical," since those who are physically violated are very unlikely to offer valuable information to the torturers. (WK 2013r; AMN 2005)

However, for the critics, this argument on physical health, torture, and culture has some major problems. Consider, for illustration, a few examples below.

Firstly, one main criticism of this argument on physical health, torture, and culture is that there is a divide among different countries on torture.

For instance, in a study, "there was a clear divide between those countries with strong rejection of torture (such as Italy, where only 14% supported torture) and nations where rejection was less strong. Often this lessened rejection is found in countries severely and frequently threatened by terrorist attacks. E.g., Israel, despite its Supreme Court outlawing torture in 1999, showed 43% supporting torture...." (WK 2013r; BBC 2006)

And secondly, another main criticism of this argument on physical health, torture, and culture is that there is a divide between the secularists and the religiously affiliated.

For instance, "in a 2005 U.S. survey 72% of American Catholics supported the use of torture in some circumstances compared to 51% of American secularists. A Pew survey in 2009 similarly found that the religiously unaffiliated are the least likely (40 percent) to support torture, and that the more a person *claims* to attend church, the more likely he or she is to condone torture; among racial/religious groups, white evangelical Protestants were far and away the most likely (62 percent) to support inflicting pain as a tool of interrogation." (WK 2013r; L. Pitts 2009; T. Carney 2006)

The Interconnected Argument

And fifthly, unlike the previous four arguments (viz., the mental, the natural, the societal, and the cultural)—the fifth one to be introduced here can be called, in the absence of better words again, the *interconnected* argument, which learns from all other theoretical approaches (which include the previous four arguments and also other examples as will be introduced in the rest of this book), without, however, favoring any of them, nor trying to integrate them (as they are not necessarily compatible with each other, as the introduction of the theoretical debate in the previous sub-sections has shown).

The Interconnected Theory of Health Care

My *interconnected* argument can be more precisely called *the interconnected theory of health care*, since it is to propose a new theory of mental health and physical health (in the context of mind and body) in health care.

My *interconnected theory of health care* has four major distinct features.

Firstly, my theory makes good use of all theoretical approaches to health care in relation to mental health and physical health (in the context of mind and body), be they about the mental argument, the natural argument, the societal argument, or the cultural argument—especially from the most comprehensive combined perspectives of the mind, nature, society, and culture (as will be dealt with in Chapter Two and Chapter Three).

Secondly, just like many other theories of mine in my previous books, my theory here does not heavily favor any specific theory over others in the literature, nor trying to integrate them (as they are not necessarily compatible with each other).

Thirdly, my theory treats the issue of health care in the distinctive dialectic context of no mental health without physical health, and vice versa—to be eventually transcended later.

And fourthly, it contains thirty-three major theses, namely, (a) the first thesis: the formalness-informalness principle, (b) the second thesis: the absoluteness-relativeness principle, (c) the third thesis: the partiality-totality principle, (d) the fourth thesis: the predictability-unpredictability principle, (e) the fifth thesis: the explicability-inexplicability principle, (f) the sixth thesis: the fiction-reality principle, (g) the seventh thesis: the cognitiveness-noncognitiveness principle, (h) the eighth thesis: the finiteness-transfiniteness principle, (i) the ninth thesis: the preciseness-vagueness principle, (j) the tenth thesis: the simpleness-complicatedness principle, (k) the eleventh thesis: the openness-hiddenness principle, (l) the twelfth thesis: the denseness-emptiness principle, (m) the thirteenth thesis: the prototypicality-variation principle, (n) the fourteenth thesis: the change-constancy principle, (o) the fifteenth thesis: the order-chaos principle, (p) the sixteenth thesis: the slowness-quickness principle, (q) the seventeenth thesis: the expansion-contraction principle, (r) the eighteenth thesis: the optimality-nonoptimality principle, (s) the nineteenth thesis: the theory-praxis principle, (t) the twentieth thesis: the convention-novelty principle, (u) the twenty-first thesis: the evolution-transformation principle, (v) the twenty-second thesis: the symmetry-asymmetry principle, (w) the twenty-third thesis: the softness-hardness principle, (x) the twenty-fourth thesis: the seriousness-playfulness principle, (y) the twenty-fifth thesis: the activeness-inactiveness principle, (z) the twenty-sixth thesis: the selfness-otherness principle, (aa) the twenty-seventh thesis: the regression-progression principle, (bb) the twenty-eighth thesis: the sameness-difference principle, (cc) the twenty-ninth thesis: the stability-reaction principle, (dd) the thirtieth thesis: the functionality-nonfunctionality principle, (ee) the thirty-first thesis: the intentionality-nonintentionality principle, (ff) the thirty-second thesis: the survivability-non-survivability principle, and (gg) the thirty-third thesis: the post-human interconnection—to be elaborated in the rest of the book, with a summary in the concluding chapter.

Because of the last thesis on "the post-human interconnection," the word "interconnective" in the title of my theory is suggestive, because it refers to the different relationships between mental health and physical health (in the context of mind and body) in health care, in the face of changing circumstances over time—which then require a multi-faceted inquiry of the dialectic relationship between mental health and physical health, as well as an understanding of the different views regarding the relationships in health care (together with other debates as will be discussed in the rest of the book)—and in the end it calls for a need to transcend mental health and physical health by future advanced humans and later post-humans in the context of the great transformations of health care in the future worlds (as will be discussed in the concluding chapter, Chapter Four).

With this clarification in mind—the seminal project here, if successful, will fundamentally change the way that we think about mental health and physical health (in the context of mind and body) in health care, together with other debates as will be discussed in the rest of the book, from the combined perspectives of the mind, nature, society, and culture, with enormous implications for the human future and what I originally called its "post-human" fate.

Theory and Meta-Theory

The *interconnected* argument, or *the interconnected theory of health care*, presupposes some kind of meta-theory, in special relation to methodology and ontology—just as all theories, either explicitly or implicitly, require their own versions of meta-theory.

Meta-Theory

As so often clarified in my previous books—theory and meta-theory, broadly speaking, can be further classified into different categories, as shown below:

- On Theory
  —Ex: in relation to the mind

—Ex: in relation to nature
—Ex: in relation to society
—Ex: in relation to culture

- On Meta-Theory
  —Ex: in relation to methodology
  —Ex: in relation to ontology

Each category, in its turn, can then be further sub-divided into different levels of analysis—which will be elaborated in the next two sections (and summarized in *Table 4.43*).

With this reminder in mind, I already proposed (in my previous books) my distinctive contribution to meta-theory, namely, methodology (like "theory of methodological holism," "complex theory of data analysis," "critical-dialectic theory of formal science," and "interpretivist theory of probability," for instance) and ontology (like "theory of existential dialectics" and "contrastive theory of rationality," for instance).

The next two sections are to introduce my meta-theory—especially, existential dialectics and sophisticated methodological holism, respectively—to be repeated, *often verbatim* (with only a few updated revisions), from my previous works, as this is something that I often do in each new book of mine as an introduction to some background information for the convenience of the readers.

In the process, I shall also introduce my numerous new theories (or to be exact, 67 of them in 59 books so far, as of February 28, 2013) in relation to the four categories of the mind, nature, society, and culture in the context of theory (as also summarized in *Table 4.43*).

A Unified Theory of Everything

In the end, my distinctive contribution to both meta-theory and theory serves as a foundation to unify all domains of knowledge (i.e., the social sciences, the formal sciences, the natural sciences, and the humanities) for an overarching understanding of all forms of reality (by way of some ontological principles at the meta-theoretical level and the comprehensive perspectives of the mind, nature, society, and culture at the theoretical level—as will be explained in the next two sections).

This is so, without commiting the sins of reductionism and reverse-reductionism (as often seen in many holistic approaches, with the fad of systems approach as a most recent notorious example, as already critically explained in *The Future of Post-Human Formal Science*, or *FPHFS*), since my distinctive contribution makes good use of different schools of thought without heavily favoring any of them nor trying to integrate them (as they are not necessarily compatible with each other), so as to include (or adjust for) heterogeneity, conflict, subjectivity, and complexity, for example.

In this sense, the word "unified" does not have to mean an integrative approach, in a narrow sense, nor a systems approach, in a broad one, both of which I have critically rebuked (in my previous books), while learning from them.

This overarching project (consisting of numerous theories of mine, as will be summarized in the next section), thus, constitutes my grand unifed theory of everything in the world and beyond.

The Logic of Existential Dialectics

To start, the ontology of existential dialectics can be summarized in this section—*often verbatim* (with only a few updated revisions), from my previous works, as this is something that I regularly do in each new book of mine as an introduction to some background information for the convenience of the readers.

After all, this book, like all others of mine, is in conversation with all previous ones of mine, for the final aim to converge all of them into a larger grand project on the future of intelligent life, both here on earth and there in deep space unto multiverses.

The summary can be organized in relation to (a) the conception of existential dialectics (or its ontics), (b) the syntax of existential dialectics (or its ontomethodology and ontologic), (c) the semantics of existential dialectics (or its ontosemantics), and (d) the pragmatics of existential dialectics (or its ontopragmatics), respectively hereafter—again *often verbatim*.

This means that, for those readers who had read some of my previous books, the summary below is really not much new (*almost verbatim*, with only some updated revisions).

But for those who have never read my previous books, it is a good review of them.

The Conception of Existential Dialectics (or Its Ontics)

This ontology was originally designated as "existential dialectics" in *Beyond Capitalism to Post-Capitalism* (herein abbreviated as *BCPC*), although it was already analyzed in other books of mine like the 2 volumes of *The Future of Human Civilization* (*FHC*), *The Future of Capitalism and Democracy* (*FCD*), *The Future of Post-Human Consciousness* (*FPHC*), and the 2 volumes of *Beyond Democracy to Post-Democracy* (*BDPD*).

Lest any confusion occurs, it is important to stress at the outset that the word 'existential' in "existential dialectics" has nothing to do with Existentialism, which I rebuked in *FHC*, *FCD*, and also *FPHC*. Instead, the word here merely refers to the existence of intelligent life (both primitive and advanced) in a broad sense.

Some Basic Concepts

The conception of existential dialectics (or its ontics) makes use of different concepts (like "sets," "elements," "relations," "operations," "functions," "truth values," "axioms," "postulates," and "principles"—as shown in *Table 4.3*), which are important for the understanding of any logic of ontology.

That clarified—existential dialectics, as a language of ontology, can be analyzed in different ways that a language, as an analogy, is often analyzed, namely, in relation to phonology ("the study of patterns of a language's sounds"), phonetics ("the study of the physical aspects of sounds of human language"), morphonology ("the study of the internal structure of words"), syntax ("the study of how words combine to form grammatical sentences"), semantics ("the study of the meaning of words [lexical semantics] and fixed word combinations [phraseology]"), and pragmatics ("the study of how utterances are used…literally, figuratively, or otherwise…in communicative acts"). (WK 2007)

But since my theory of existential dialectics makes use of the English language for communication here, it does not propose a new way to make the patterns of a language's sounds (as in phonology), to study the physical aspects of sounds (as in phonetics), or even to strive for a new organization of the internal structure of words for the English language (as in morphonology).

For this reason, the language of existential dialectics to be analyzed hereafter is not concerned with the phonological, phonetic, and morphonological aspects of the English language. Instead, the analysis will explore the syntax, semantics, and pragmatics of existential dialectics as a language of ontology to improve our understanding of reality.

The Ontic Dispute

But first, there is an ontic dispute to be addressed, which is related to what I called "the dilemma of ontology" as introduced earlier in *Sec. 1.4* of *The Future of Post-Human Knowledge* (*FPHK*).

A good point of departure concerns what I want to call *the ontic dispute*, on how to understand the very nature of ontology.

Traditionally, scholars in the field used to study the conception of ontology in terms of its entities (e.g., material objects, abstract numbers), properties (e.g., duration, plurality), and relationships (e.g., causation).

This is a good starting point, but it suffers from different problems. Consider three examples of bias below, which are quite common in the literature, and the recent version (of treating concepts and principles in ontology on the basis of "plurality," "dynamism," "duration," "interaction," "life," "consciousness," and "volition") by Reginald Firehammer (2005) only constitutes a latest addition to this old (impoverishing) tradition.

Firstly, the classification of entities, properties, and relationships is too material-centric, in often focusing more on the existence of material entities than on non-material ones.

Secondly, the classification is too anthropo-centric, in often favoring the factor of human agency in depicting reality.

And lastly, the classification is too confused among the three categories relating to each other, in often lumping them together without adequate consideration of their intricated interrelationships (both in relation to each and in relation to all).

A good alternative is precisely what I want to offer in this debate, that is, a new classification of ontological entities, properties, and their relationships in terms of *method*, *structure*, *process*, *agency*, and *outcome* instead. Let me explicate what these words mean below.

In relation to "method"—it concerns how ontology is to be studied. In this sense, the word 'method' here should not be confused with the different usage of the same term 'method' as a technique of investigation in the context of methodology (as already introduced in *Sec. 1.2* of *FPHK*).

In relation to "structure"—it concerns what the general patterns of entities, properties, and relationships are.

In relation to "process"—it concerns how these general patterns change over time.

In relation to "agency"—it concerns how agency affects any change of these general patterns over time (without putting, however, too much emphasis on the role of human agency).

And in relation to "outcome"—it concerns what the outputs of this change over time are.

The Syntax of Existential Dialectics (or Its Ontomethodology and Ontologic)

The syntax of existential dialectics, analogously speaking, refers here to the structure of an ontology which can be studied by way of combining ideas into complex relationships like ontological principles to depict reality in the world—and can be analyzed in seven sub-sections, namely, (a) the selection criteria, (b) further clarifications on classification, (c) ontomethodology, (d) ontologic, (e) the principles as short cuts, (f) the principles as family resemblances, and (g) the dialectic constraints imposed by the principles, respectively hereafter.

The Selection Criteria

To start, not any pair of relationship can be chosen as an ontological principle in existential dialectics; otherwise, there could be billions of them under the sky.

Six illustrations below suffice to clarify this point.

(a) Firstly, an ontological principle cannot *overlap* with other principles, in that it is too closely related with other ones.

Of course, one cannot totally rule out any relationship between two entities, especially in a complex world of everything being linked to everything else—but the comparison here is relative, not absolute.

In this sense, the flexibility-inflexibility pair cannot be an ontological principle, since it has something closely in common with other ones (like the simpleness-complicatedness principle, for instance).

As an illustration, something which is flexible in interpretation is more likely to allow multiple viewpoints and thus makes the overall picture more complicated than otherwise (simple).

(b) Secondly, an ontological principle cannot be *redundant* in relation to other principles, in that it somehow duplicates other principles.

In this sense, for instance, the directness-indirectness pair cannot be an ontological principle, because it somehow duplicates other ontological principles (like the preciseness-vagueness principle, for instance).

As an illustration, something which is direct means to be right to the point and does not need to go to an unnecessarily long loop—so it is less vague, in being clearer about the thing in question.

(c) Thirdly, an ontological principle cannot be *derived* from other ones—as if it is a child-parent relationship.

In this sense, the convenience-inconvenience pair cannot be an ontological principle, because it can be derived from other ones (like the slowness-quickness principle, for instance).

For instance, something which is convenient already implies that it can be obtained quickly (rather than slowly)—all things considered.

(d) Fourthly, an ontological principle cannot be *trivial* (or *parochial*)—as if it is only one component competing with other ones for inclusion in a set.

In this sense, the consistency-inconsistency pair cannot be an ontological principle, because its validity is limited (or parochial), as it can be easily challenged and replaced by opposing major (not minor) theories (e.g., the correspondence theory of truth, the pragmatic theory of truth, the semantic theory of truth, the disclosedness theory of truth, and whatnot), not just in accordance to the consistency (or coherence) theory of truth (for consistency).

Thus, the consistency argument is only one among different opposing arguments in relation to the logic of what constitutes "truth."

(e) Fifthly, an ontological principle cannot be *one-sided*, that is, part of one side (category) of a dialectic pair.

In this sense, the extroversion-introversion pair cannot be an ontological principle, since it is part of the side (category) of "normality" in the normality-abnormaltiy pair (because both extroversion and introversion are two different "normal" personality traits in psychology).

In addition, the normality-abnormality pair is already related to the symmetry-asymmetry principle, the density-emptiness principle, the convention-novelty principle, and the same-difference principle (as will be explained in the section on "the principles as family resemblances" later).

(f) And sixthly, an ontological principle cannot be *misleading*, in that the two apparent opposites are not really opposites at all, upon closer examination.

In this sense, the east-west pair cannot be an ontological principle, since east and west are not really opposites, as there are also north, south, and center to form a set of five opposing elements.

By the same logic, the left-right pair cannot be an ontological principle, since left and right (width) are not really opposites, as there are also top and bottom (height), back and front (depth), and center to form a set of seven elements in four categories. In the field of visual design, this set of seven elements is known as "form" (as opposed to "function"), as addressed in *FPHARCH*. (WK 2011nn)

Although these six examples (criteria) are not exhaustive, they illustrative the selectiveness of any ontological principle to be existentially dialectic.

Further Clarifications on Classification

Lest any misunderstanding carelessly occurs, some further clarifications on classification should be made here (and summarized in *Table 4.8*).

(a) Firstly, the total number of ontological principles is unknown, to be discovered later, as our knowledge of the world becomes more advanced.

Consequently, the principles as introduced in my books are not exhaustive, with new ones being added, whenever more of them are discovered in later research.

At least, future generations can pick up where I leave off and continue the discovery.

In this sense, my work should be treated as a pioneering effort for the development of a systematic, comprehensive analysis of a new general ontology for the future of knowledge.

(b) Secondly, the principles are not rigidly classified, as they can be reclassified in a different way.

For instance, the preciseness-vagueness principle is classified under the category of "structure" but can be reclassified under the category of "method," although in so doing, it has a different meaning in the context of method.

The same logic applies to the same-difference principle under the category of "outcome," which can be reclassified under the category of "structure," although in so doing, once more, it has a different meaning in the context of structure.

(c) Thirdly, the principles are to be understood together, not that each prinicple is to be treated independently of others. After all, the principles are mutually constraining, in that they work together as a whole.

(d) Fourthly, the principles are relevant to all subject matters, but some principles are, relatively speaking of course, more useful to some subject matters than others under certain conditions—as implied in the symmetry-asymmetry principle.

(e) And fifthly, the principles constitute only two levels of analysis, this time, at the ontological and methodological levels—while other levels of analysis (from the perspectives of the mind, nature, society, and culture) are also needed, in order to understand reality in its totality (as explained in the section on "sophisticated methodological holism," so as to avoid the dual dangers of reductionism and reverse-reductionism).

Ontomethodology

With these selection criteria and clarifications in mind—the syntax of existential dialectics can be divided into two main smaller sections for analysis, since they are related to each other in the context of some fundamental principles, that is, (a) ontomethodology and (b) ontologic, to be addressed hereafter, respectively.

In the context of ontomethodology, some ontological principles are proposed here in relation to the nature of methodology, which however is tied up with the general issue of ontology in the context of knowledge.

In this sense, ontomethodology (in the context of these ontological principles in the category of method) are related with ontologic in general (in the context of ontological principles in general).

Some good instances of ontological principles involving ontomethodology include the formalness-informalness principle, the absoluteness-relativeness principle, the partiality-totality principle, the predictability-unpredictability principle, the explicability-inexplicability principle, the fiction-reality principle, and the cognitiveness-noncognitiveness principle, which will be introduced in conjunction with ontological principles in the ontologic of existential dialectics in general hereafter.

Ontologic

With this clarification of the relationship between ontomethodology and ontologic in mind (which is comparable to the relationship between methodology and ontology as described in *Sec. 1.3* of *FPHK*)—the first three principles in existential dialectics were introduced in *BCPC*. And more principles were later added to the logic in my subsequent books (like *FC*, *FAE*, and others), as explained below.

More specifically, in *BCPC*, I proposed three principles (based on previous works of mine, not just something out of the blue) for the ontological logic, namely, (a) the regression-progression principle on the direction of history, (b) the symmetry-asymmetry principle on the relationships among existents, and (c) the change-constancy principle on the alteration of things—or in a more elegant term, the dynamics of space-time (in *FC*).

In *The Future of Complexity* (*FC*), I added three more principles, on top of the three aforementioned, namely, (d) the partiality-totality principle on the relationships between parts and whole, (e) the order-chaos principle on the pattern of things, and (f) the predictability-unpredictability principle on the occurrence of things—as part of the ontological logic of existential dialectics.

In *The Future of Aesthetic Experience* (or simply *FAE*), another principle is added, namely, (g) the evolution-transformation principle (on the multiple kinds of agency).

Also in *FAE*, I then reclassified the 7 principles into four categories, namely, (i) in relation to method, for the partiality-totality principle and the predictability-unpredictability principle, (ii) in relation to process, for the change-constancy principle and the order-chaos principle, (iii) in relation to agency, for the symmetry-asymmetry principle and the evolution-transformation principle, and (iv) in relation to outcome, for the regression-progression principle.

In *The Rise of Authoritarian Liberal Democracy* (*ALD*), I added two more principles, namely, (h) the softness-hardness principle on the force of agency (which is to be classified under the category about agency) and (i) the same-difference principle on the metamorphosis of change (which is to be classified under the category about outcome).

In *The Future of Information Architecture* (*FIA*), I introduce three additional principles, that is, (j) the simpleness-complicadness principle on the interconnection among things, (k) the preciseness-vagueness principle on the refinement of things, and (l) the slowness-quickness principle on the speed of change—with the first two in relation to structure and the third in relation to process.

In *The Future of Post-Human Unconsciousness* (*FPHU*), I added three more principles, that is, (m) the openness-hidden principle on the detection of things, in relation to structure, (n) the explicability-inexplicability principle on the underlying mechanisms of things, in relation to method, and (o) the expansion-contraction principle on the growth of things, in relation to process.

In *The Future of Post-Human Knowledge* (*FPHK*), I added one more principle, that is, (p) the absoluteness-relativeness principle on the multiplicity of entities, in relation to method.

In *The Future of Post-Human Mathematical Logic* (*FPHML*), I added one more principle, that is, (q) the formalness-informalness principle on the formal requirements of systems, in relation to method.

In *The Future of Post-Human Engineering* (*FPHE*), I added one more principle, that is, (r) the theory-praxis principle on the duality of knowledge, in relation to agency.

In *The Future of Post-Human Creative Thinking* (*FPHCT*), I added one more principle, that is, (s) the convention-novelty principle on the nature of creative thinking, in relation to agency.

In *The Future of Post-Human Geometry* (*FPHG*) here, I added one more principle, that is, (t) the finiteness-transfiniteness principle on the nature of numbers, in relation to structure.

In *The Future of Post-Human Urban Planning* (*FPHUP*), I added one more principle, that is, (u) the denseness-emptiness principle on the distribution of entities in space, in relation to structure.

In *The Future of Post-Human Humor* (*FPHH*), I added one more principle, that is, (v) the seriousness-playfulness principle on the extent of seriousness, in relation to agency.

In *The Future of Post-Human Literature* (*FPHLIT*), I added one more principle, that is, (w) the fiction-reality principle on the different faces of reality, in relation to method.

In *The Future of Post-Human Chemistry* (*FPHCHEM*), I added one more principle, that is, (x) the stability-reaction principle on the feedback mechanism for further changes, in relation to outcome.

In *The Future of Post-Human Transportation* (*FPHTRAN*), I added one more principle, that is, (y) the activeness-inactiveness principle on the extent of activeness, in relation to agency.

In *The Future of Post-Human Culinary Art* (*FPHCA*), I added two more principles, that is, (z) the selfness-otherness principle on the magnitude of self-centeredness in relation to agency and (aa) the functionality-nonfunctionality principle on the presence of function in relation to outcome.

In *The Future of Post-Human Waste* (*FPHW*), I added one more principle, that is, (bb) the intentionality-nonintentionality principle on the planning for outcomes in relation to outcome.

In *Beyond Natural Resources to Post-Human Resources* (*BNR*), I added one more principle, that is, (cc) the cognitiveness-noncognitiveness principle on the understanding of meaning in relation to method.

In *The Future of Post-Human Probability* (*FPHPROB*),), I added one more principle, that is, (dd) the survivability-nonsurvivability principle on the survival of things in relation to outcome.

And in *The Future of Post-Human Morphology* (*FPHMORP*),), I added two more principles, that is, (ee) the prototypicality-variation principle on the nature of duplication in relation to process, and (ff) the optimality-nonoptimality principle on the nature of highly favorable options in relation to process.

With this update, there are thirty-two principles so far in existential dialectics, that is:

- seven principles in the category of "method"—viz., the formalness-informalness principle, the absoluteness-relativeness principle, the partiality-totality principle, the predictability-unpredictability principle, the explicability-inexplicability principle, the fiction-reality principle, and the cognitiveness-noncognitiveness principle
- five principles in the category of "structure"—viz., the finiteness-transfiniteness principle, the simpleness-complicatedness principle, the preciseness-vagueness principle, the openness-hiddenness principle, and the denseness-emptiness principle
- six principles in the category of "process"—viz., the prototypicality-variation principle, the change-constancy principle, the slowness-quickness principle, the order-chaos principle, the expansion-contraction principle, and the optimality-nonoptimality principle
- eight principles in the category of "agency"—viz., the theory-praxis principle, the convention-novelty principle, the symmetry-asymmetry principle, the evolution-transformation principle, the softness-hardness principle, the seriousness-playfulness principle, the activeness-inactiveness principle, and the selfness-otherness principle
- six principles in the category of "outcome"—viz., the regression-progression principle, the same-difference principle, the stability-reaction principle, the functionality-nonfunctionality principle, the intentionality-nonintentionality principle, and the survivability-nonsurvivability principle

There can be more than thirty-two principles in existential dialectics, but they are what I have discovered so far (as summarized in *Table 4.4*).

The Principles as Short Cuts

Yet, these principles should be treated with caution, lest misunderstanding occurs, since they do not constitute rigid dualities (or dichotomies).

The reason is that each pair in an ontological principle consists of two opposites, which are, however, merely short cuts both for multiple variations and degrees, as well as for different interactions with multiple other entities unlike them.

In this light, each pair can end up having hundred (or even thousand, if not more) different versions, which interact with hundred (or even thousand, if not more) other entities—as summarized in *Table 4.5*.

There are two clarifications here.

Firstly, this conception of shortcuts is not mutually exclusive nor absolute, in that the opposites can come in all shapes and sizes, with different degrees. For instance, by analogy, just as there are different degrees of the two colors "white" and "black"—there are likewise different degrees of the opposites in each ontological pair, to the extent that there can be multiple entities (not only two) interacting with each other in each pair.

And secondly, this conception of shortcuts do not ignore other possible entities in interacting with the two opposites (with their different versions) in each pair. For instance, by analogy, there are not only the two colors "white" and "black" as opposites, since there are other colors too besides them like "yellow," "green," "purple," or else. The same logic can be applied to each ontological pair, in that they also interact with other entities, not with only two of them (with their different versions).

Therefore, with these two clarifications in mind—each pair in an ontological principle serves only as an abbreviation for something more complicated and, therefore, although it contains two opposites, it should not be confused as a duality (dualism).

Existential dialectics rejects any dualism (or dichotomy) as too rigid and instead allows the multiplicity of entities, to the extent that between the two opposites in each pair exist many other alternatives to choose from. They are named in that short form for aesthetic elegance only, instead of listing all possible entities between the two opposites in the title (which would be too cumbersome and sound extremely awkward).

To be dialectic is to go beyond any rigid dichotomy and transcend into something different altogether in the long haul. One may be tempted to call the dialectic logic here with a different name like existential "multilectics" (instead of "dialectics"), but this naming is incorrect (or even misleading), for the two reasons aforestated.

After all, all the possible entities between any two opposites in an ontological pair are still about the two opposites, although each ontological pair come in all shapes and sizes (with different degrees) and do not exist by themselves but also interact with other entities unlike them. The virtue of revealing an ontological pair is to show how they relate within themselves (in multiple versions) and also interact with others unlike them (also in multiple versions).

This will be clear in a later sub-section titled "the dialectic constraints imposed by the principles."

The Principles as Family Resemblances

In addition, each ontological principle is generic, with some other comparable ontological pairs to be put in the same family (like a *family resemblance*)—as summarized in *Table 4.6*.

Ludwig Wittgenstein (1953) once suggested the idea of "family resemblance" in explaining different games classified under the same family called *games*.

Why should, for instance, playing football and chess as playing "games," when it is well understood that football is not the same as chess? The answer is that, although each game is different and has different rules, many of them (though not all) share, more or less, some commonalites (e.g., scoring as necessary for winning).

And this is so, even though some games share more than some others in any given selection of critieria, and no two games are exactly identical. So, Wittgenstein's point here is that there is no essential core which is common to all games, and the best that one can look for is some characteristics which are common to many (but not all) games. (A. Biletzki 2006)

(a) Appropriate Family Resemblances

In the context of existential dialectics, I want to distinguish two types of family resemblances, and, in the absence of better words, let me call them (a) *appropriate* family resemblances and (b) *inappropriate* family resemblances.

In regard to appropriate family resemblances—good examples include some of the pairs as already explained in an earlier section on selection criteria, like the flexibility-inflexibility pair, which can be put in the family resemblance of the simpleness-complicatedness principle, although the two pairs are not exactly identical. Likewise, the directness-indirectness pair can be put in the family resemblance of the preciseness-vagueness principle, although, again, the two pairs are not exactly identical.

In this sense, which specific pair in a family should be used to designate the name of the family can be at times a bit arbitrary, but with good reason.

For illustration, in the context of method, the partiality-totality principle can take the different form like individualisticness-holisticness, just as the explicability-inexplicability principle can take the different form like underlyingness-regularness—although each two pairs are not exactly identical and have slightly different meanings and usages.

A more comprehensive listing of this family resemblance for all other principles is shown in *Table 4.6* on the syntax of existential dialectics.

In fact, this section on family resemblances overlaps with the semantics of existential dialectics, which will be introduced later in the next section (and summarized in *Table 4.11*).

(b) Inappropriate Family Resemblances

However, there are some family resemblances which are not appropriate, and let me distinugish them by calling them, in the absence of better words, (b1) *inadequate* family resemblances, (b2) *compound* family resemblances, (b3) *one-sided* family resemblances, and (b4) *vague* family resemblances (as summarized in *Table 4.10*).

(b1) In regard to "inadequate" family resemblances—there are some pairs which are not adequate, because they fail the test of selection criteria (as already pointed out in an earlier section), especially in relation to the criterion of not being *trivial* (or *parochial*)—as if it is only one component competing with other ones for inclusion in a set.

For instance, the *consistency-inconsistency* pair is inadequate, because it is only one component competing with other ones for inclusion in the larger set of the formalness-informalenss principle (like the *completeness-incompleteness* pair and the *soundness-unsoundness* pair, as discussed in my book titled *The Future of Post-Human Mathematical Logic*, or *FPHML* in short).

The same is true for the *cognition-noncognition* pair, which is related with both the completeness-incompleteness pair and the soundness-unsoundness pair in the larger set of the formalness-informalenss principle.

(b2) In regard to "compound" (or non-atomic) family resemblances—there are some pairs which are not appropriate for a different reason, because they fail the test of selection criteria (as already pointed out in an earlier section), especially in relation to the criterion of not *overlapping* with other principles, in that it is too closely related with other ones.

For instance, the *normality-abnormality* pair is compound (and thus inappropriate), because it overlaps with several other principles, like the symmetry-asymmetry principle, the density-emptiness principle, the convention-novelty principle, and the same-difference principle, for instance (as already discussed in *FPHP*).

The normality-abnormality pair overlaps with the symmetry-asymmetry principle, because being "abnormal" (say, for those with mental illnesses) is often treated not equally by others who are "normal." So, the relationship reveals the symmetry-asymmetry principle.

The normality-abnormality pair also overlaps with the density-emptiness principle, because being "abnormal" (say, for those with mental illnesses) is often not as dense in the overall (not local) distribution of a population as those who are "normal." So, the relationship reveals the density-emptiness principle.

The normality-abnormality pair also overlaps with the convention-novelty principle, because being "abnormal" (say, for those with mental illnesses) often exhibits non-conventional (non-conformist) ideas and behaviors when contrasted with those who are "normal." So, the relationship reveals the convention-novelty principle.

The normality-abnormality pair also overlaps with the same-difference principle, because being "abnormal" (say, for those with mental illnesses) shares some similarities in outcome when compared with those who are "normal" (in that both contribute to the control and regulation of human thoughts and behaviors in society, albeit in different ways). Yet, being "abnormal" also has something different from being "normal," in that abnormal thoughts and behaviors follow a different pattern when contrasted with those which are normal. So, the relationship reveals the same-difference principle.

(b2.1) There is a special case of compound family resemblances (as summarized in *Table 4.10*), which can be called, in the absence of better words, *one-sided and compound* family resemblances.

For instance, the extroversion-introversion pair is a good example of *one-sided and compound* family resemblances, because, firstly, it is "one-sided," in being part of the side (category) of "normality" in the normality-abnormality pair—and, secondly, the normality-abnormality pair is in turn "compounded," because it is related to the symmetry-asymmetry principle, the density-emptiness principle, the convention-novelty principle, and the same-difference principle, as already explained above.

(b3) In regard to "one-sided" family resemblances—there are some pairs which are not appropriate for another different reason, because they fail the test of selection criteria (as already pointed out in an earlier section), especially in relation to the criterion of not being *one-sided*, that is, part of one side (category) of a dialectic pair.

For instance, the extroversion-introversion pair cannot be an ontological principle, since it is part of the side (category) of "normality" in the normality-abnormaltiy pair (because both extroversion and introversion are two different "normal" personality traits in psychology).

By the same logic, the vision-blindness pair and the sound-silence pair cannot be ontological principles, because the pairs are part of the side (category) of "asymmetry" in the symmetry-asymmetry principle (since being able to see and hear for some individuals and being unable to see or hear for others are two contrastive abilities in the world of animals and humans, for instance).

These illustrations of indequate, compound, and one-sided family resemblances show how difficult it is to come up with an ontological principle in existential dialectics out of the bluc, bccause many of them violate the selection criteria in one way or the other. It is all too easy to join two opposing words and simply make them into a pair, but it is all too difficult to pass the test of the selection criteria to be qualified as an ontological principle in existential dialectics.

(b4) And in regard to "vague" family resemblances—there are some pairs which are not appropriate for still another different reason, because the terms in the pairs are vague in meaning, so that they are inappropriate family resemblances if defined in some particular ways, although they can be appropriate family resemblances if defined in other particular ways.

For instance, such pairs like shortness-longness, narrowness-broadness, smallness-largeness, smallness-greatness, microness-macroness, and littleness-muchness can be understood in at least three different meanings and thus have three different possibilities. The first possibility is that they are one-sided as part of finiteness (in the finiteness-transfiniteness principle), if both opposites are defined on a finite scale. The second possibility is that they are one-sided as part of transfiniteness (in the finiteness-transfiniteness principle) if both opposites are defined on a transfinite scale. And the third possibility is that they are appropriate family resemblances in relation to the finiteness-transfiniteness principle if one opposite is defined on a finite scale and the other opposite is defined on a transfinite scale.

Other examples of inappropriate family resemblances are shown in *Table 4.10* on "The Syntax of Existential Dialectics VII: Types of Inappropriate Family Resemblances."

The Dialectic Constraints Imposed by the Principles

The principles, as they constitute the syntax of existential dialectics, are dialectic in character, such that, when they are applied, they impose dialectic constraints on how reality is to be understood.

Consider, say, the symmetry-asymmetry principle as an illustration here, in order to summarize two main characters of the dialectic constraints in question (as summarized in *Table 4.7*).

Firstly, to be dialectic here is to go beyond the narrow dichotomies (and, for that matter, any rigid multi-dimensional classificatory scheme), be they about "self" vs. "world," "freedom" vs. "unfreedom," "barbarity" vs. "civilization," "individuality" vs. "communality," and so on.

One way to do so (to go beyond) is to consider them all in terms of co-existence (without heavily favoring one over the rest). For instance, my theory of "post-civilization" (to be summarized later in the section on the pragmatics of existential dialectics) is to go beyond barbarity and civilization in terms of understanding barbarity and civilization as being co-existent.

And the same logic can be said in relation to my theories of "post-democracy," "post-capitalsm," and others (also to be introduced later in the section on the pragmatics of existential dialectics), in regard to freedom vs. unfreedom, equality vs. inequality, communality vs. individuality, spirituality vs. materiality, and so on.

But to consider them all (in the dichotomies—and, for that matter, in any rigid multi-dimensional classifactory scheme) as co-existent is not the same as to imply that the opposing categories in any classificatory scheme are all equal, since, in accordance to the symmetry-asymmetry principle (as an illustration here), if they are equal in terms of being considered as co-existent, they are asymmetric in terms of being unequal in dialectic interaction (e.g., X can be more dominant than Y in case A, or Y is more dominant than X in case B), although in some special cases, they can be relatively equal (e.g., X and Y are relatively equal in case C).

For this reason, there are different versions of "post-democracy" and "post-capitalism" in my theories. As an illustration, in version I of the theory of post-democracy, freedom is more dominant than equality, whereas in version II of the theory of post-democracy, equality is more so than freedom.

But this "X more than Y" has to be understood in the context of dialectic logic (not in symbolic logic, as conventionally understood), in that both "X" and "Y" are important in post-democracy (in the context of dialectic logic), but in an asymmetry way.

By contrast, in symbolic logic, it often favors one over the other—be it in regard to privileging freedom over equality (in Fascism), favoring freedom relatively more than equality (in Liberal Democracy), or favoring equality relatively more than freedom (in Socialist Democracy). In regard to the latter two cases (about Liberal Democracy and Socialist Democracy), the difference between dialectic logic and symbolic logic can be one in degree, not in kind—in this sense, albeit not in other senses.

The same reasoning can be said about the relatonships between individuality and communality, between spirituality and materiality, and between formal legalism and informal legalism in the different versions of my theory of "post-capitalism."

Secondly, to be dialectic is to go beyond the narrow dichotomies (and, for that matter, any rigid multi-dimensional classificatory scheme) in another way, this time, in a transcendent way, that is, in exploring other possibilities or even other issues not considered within the narrow confines of narrow dichotomies (and, for that matter, any rigid multi-dimensional classificatory scheme).

As an analogy, in this second meaning, to go beyond the narrow dichotomy of "black" vs. "white" is not just to choose both "black" and "white" (as in the first meaning) but also to explore other options (e.g., "green," "purple," "blue," etc.—and, alternatively, "shade," "line," "curve," etc.).

By the same reasoning, to go beyond "democracy" is to transcend democracy (as in version III of my theory of "post-democracy") and to explore other possibilties of lifeforms (e.g., "floating consciousness," "hyper-spatial consciousness," etc., to live beyond the narrow obsession with freedom and equality).

This dialectic character of the principles in existential dialectics has important implications for the pragmatics of existential dialectics (as will be clear shortly, in the section on the pragmatics of existential dialectics).

The Semantics of Existential Dialectics (or Its Ontosemantics)

The syntax of existential dialectics so understood in terms of ontological principles only gives us the structure of ontology in the world, in an abstract (general) sense. These principles by themselves do not tell us the specific meanings in a given context.

In order to grasp the specific meanings of the principles in a given context, it is necessary to study the semantics of existential dialectics (as summarized in *Table 4.11*).

And the analysis of the ontological principles as family resemblances in the previous section on syntax is only a starting point (and thus overlaps a bit with the semantics of existential dialectics here).

For this reason, I have often gone to great lengths in my previous books on different subjects to explain the specific meanings of the principles when applied in different contexts.

Consider two examples below for illustration, which are not exhaustive.

In *FPHST*, for instance, I used the first three principles (i.e., the change-constancy principle, the regression-progression principle, and the symmetry-asymmetry principle) to propose "the perspectival theory of space-time," for a better way to understand space and time—especially, though not exclusively, in relation to future post-human history (as summarized in *Table 1.3*, *Table 1.4*, *Table 1.5*, and *Table 1.6*).

In so doing, I had to introduce concepts and theories specific to the field of physics and other related fields (e.g., "absolute space" and "absolute time" in "classical mechanics" and "relative space-time" in "the theory of relativity").

And in *BNN*, I also exploited the three principles to propose the "transcendent" approach to the study of genes and memes as a new way to understand the interaction between nature and nurture.

In so doing, I had to explore concepts and theories in the world of evolutionary biology (e.g., "mutation," "variation," "adaptation," "selection," and "inheritance" in classical evolutionary theory) and neural biology (e.g., "chromosome," "gene," "DNA," "RNA," "protein," "neuron," "neural network," and "behavior").

Other examples, besides these two here, are given in other books of mine on different topics.

Therefore, this semantic dimension of existential dialectics is important, since, in each of my books when the ontological principles are used, each principle becomes relevant in a different meaning when contextualized within a given case study in question.

In this book, for instance, the principles are relevant in relation to a different subject matter (as summarized in the concluding chapter), and they can be shown in all shapes and sizes (since they are also to be treated as "short cuts," as indicated before), without, however, being reduced to "specific ontology" (as opposed to "general ontology"), as explained in *Table 4.9*.

In the technical jargons of semantics, these exercises perform two essential functions of translation (or interpretation), namely, (a) "intensive" interpretation (about the properties or relations of the principles in existential dialectics), and (b) "extensive" interpretation (about the classes or cases to which the properties and relations of the principles in existential dialectics are applied). (WK 2011oo)

But there are limits of translation (or interpretation), and an excellent example is that "there is a problem with the 'objectivity' of translation, as it is relative to different cultural (or sub-cultural) contexts. For instance, one of the still unresolved problems in linguistics is: 'Is there an objective gauge for the quality of translation?'" (*FPHCOM* & WK 2011pp) And the problems of "radical translation" by W. V. Quine and "radical interpretation" by Donald Davidson are another well-known examples, as already discussed in *FPHSEM.*

This is one serious problem about the logic of translation and interpretation that I already addressed in *Sec. 2.5.2* of *FPHSEM, Sec. 3.5.1* of *FPHCOM* (and also, for that matter, in *FHC,* in the context of hermeneutics).

The Pragmatics of Existential Dialectics (or Its Ontopragmatics)

Even the semantics of existential dialectics is not enough to understand reality, since semantics by itself does not tell us the nature of intentionality and interests in relation to the matrix of power formations and conflicting interests when existential dialectics as an ontology is applied.

Surely, one cannot completely separate the pragmatics of existential dialectics from its semantics (and for that matter, its syntax), but the point here is to give each a more elaborated analysis.

For this reason, the pragmatics of existential dialectics needs to be studied too, in special relation to the inclusion of power formation and conflicting interests in the application of the principles of existential dialectics (as summarized in *Table 4.12*).

It is thus no wonder that all my previous books have shown in different ways how and why these ontological principles and their theoretical applications can reveal the future world to come in a way that humans have never known, in a totally different battleground for competing human (and later post-human) interests by myriad groups fighting for their own versions of hegemony.

Perhaps a summary of my previous works in relation to existential dialectics and their contributions to my new theories as proposed over the years is deemed revealing here, for the further understanding of the pragmatics of existential dialectics (in close relation to the semantics of existential dialectics too).

That stressed—the following summary in four sub-sections is something that I often do in my previous books too, as a way to introduce the intellectual background of my ideas.

So, for those readers who had read my previous works, the following sub-sections serve as a reminder, as they are repeated hereafter *often verbatim* (with only some updated changes, with the rest kept intact).

These sub-sections are, namely, (a) the two-way street connecting theory with meta-theory, (b) the theoretical application of existential dialectics, (c) direct and indirect applications of existential dialectics, and (d) multiple applications of existential dialectics—to be summaried herefafter, respectively.

The Two-Way Street Connecting Theory and Meta-Theory

However, lest any misunderstanding occurs, it is important to remember that the pragmatics of existential dialectics is not a one-way street (that is, using the ontological principles for theoretical insights in praxis) but a two-way one, namely, (a) from meta-theory to theory, and (b) from theory to meta-theory.

(a) On one side of the street, the ontological principles can inspire some theoretical insights in praxis, that is, in relation to some specific fields.

(b) On the other (opposing) side of the street, however, the study of a subject matter in the specific fields in turn reveals some more hitherto unknown ontological principles to be discovered and identified.

For this reason, three new principles were added in *FC*, one in *FAE*, two in *ALD*, and three in *FIA*, on top of the original three in *BCPC*, for example (as there are more)—after some research on the specific subject matters.

Both theory and meta-theory enrich each other in all my works over the years.

The Theoretical Application of Existential Dialectics

This two-way street connecting theory and meta-theory has contributed to my original construction of many theories in numerous books of mine on numerous fields in all domains of knowledge, which can be classified in terms of specific "meta-theories" (about epistemology, methodology, logic, ontology, etc.) and specific "theories" (about the mind, nature, culture, society, and the rest—as will be further explained later in the sub-section on "the holistic organization of an inquiry" in the section about "sophisticated methodological holism").

The final aim of my numerous new specific theories (on both theory and meta-theory) is to converge all of them (as proposed in my numerous books) into a grand project about the future of intelligent life, both here on earth and in deep space.

In this sense, all these theories of mine serve as a foundation to unify all domains of knowledge for an overarching understanding of all forms of reality (by way of some ontological principles and the comprehensive perspectives of the mind, nature, society, and culture), while allowing for heterogeneity, conflict, subjectivity, and complexity, for example.

With this grand project in mind—the summary of my specific theories on meta-theory are given in this section (on "existential dialectics") and the next (on "sophisticated methodological holism"), whereas the specific theories on theory will be summarized in the following categories of (a) society, (b) culture, (c) the mind, (d) nature, and (e) the rest, as shown below, in that order.

(a) Society

The category of "society" here can be divided into four sub-categories, i.e., (a1) social organizations, (a2) social institutions, (a3) social structure, and (a4) social systems (or trends).

(a1) Social Organizations

In relation to social organizations, I proposed a new thesis on the ambivalent nature of virtual organizations in the future, known as "the theory of e-civic alienation" in *FCD* (and summarized in *Table 4.19*).

And in *FPHO*, another theory called "the combinational theory of organization" was worked out, although it was first proposed in Ch.6 of *ALD*.

(a2) Social Institutions

There are different social institutions, be they about (a2.1) politics, (a2.2) economics, (a2.3) military affairs, (a2.4) mass media, (a2.5) law, (a2.6) education, and (a.7) gambling, for instance.

(a2.1) In relation to politics, I offered different visions on (a2.1.1) political theory, (a2.1.2) comparative politics, and (a2.1.3) international relations, to cite three main ones.

(a2.1.1) In the context of political theory, my vision of a path-breaking political system in future times concerns the different forms of "post-democracy" to supersede democracy unto the post-human age.

My vision of post-democracy was called "the theory of post-democracy" (as summarized in *Table 4.22*, *Table 4.23*, and *Table 4.24*), whereas *Table 4.25* explains the distinctions among democracy, non-democracy, and post-democracy.

And *Table 4.26* stresses the multiple causes of the emergence of post-democracy, while *Table 4.27* clarifies some possible misunderstandings in regard to post-capitalism and post-democracy.

(a2.1.2) In the context of comparative politics, I also showed, in *ALD*, how and why authoritarianism can be an advanced form of liberal democracy (just as it has its own counterpart in non-liberal democracy), or what I originally called "authoritarian liberal democracy" (as summarized in *Table 4.21*), before it is to be superceded by "post-democracy."

(a2.1.3) In the context of international relations (both at the institutional and structural levels), I provided, in *BWT*, "the theory of cyclical progression of empire-building," for a better way to understand the logic of empire-building on earth and beyond—with the rise of what I originally envisioned as "hyper-empires" (like "the Chinese Union" and "the Indian Union"), "meso-empires" (like "the European Union" and "the North American Union") and "micro-empires" (like "the Middle Eastern Union" and "the Latin American Union") in the coming "post-post-Cold War era" as a visionary illustration, as summarized in *Table 4.20*.

This is also related to the issues of "social structure" in (a3), "migration" in (a4,6), "identity" in (b11), and "geography" in (d4), for instance.

In addition, in *FPHWP*, I proposed "the multifaceted theory of war and peace" to understand war and peace, in a small sense—or aggression and pacificity, in a broad sense.

(a2.2) In relation to economics, I also offered another vision, this time to understand the future forms of economic systems, that is, the different forms of "post-capitalism" to supersede capitalism unto the post-human age.

My vision of post-capitalism was referred to (in *FCD*, *BDPD* and *BCPC*) as "the theory of post-capitalism" (as summarized in *Table 4.28*, *Table 4.29*, *Table 4.30*, *Table 4.31*, and *Table 4.32*). And *Table 4.33* clarifies the differences among capitalism, non-capitalism, and post-capitalism, whereas *Table 4.34* shows multiple causes of the emergence of post-capitalism.

This vision on "post-capitalism" constitutes the third theoretical application of existential dialectics, this time, in that there is no wealth without poverty (or the wealth/poverty dialectics).

(a2.3) In relation to military affairs, I also proposed "the multifaceted theory of war and peace" (in *FCD*, although it was first so labeled in *FPHK*) for a new way to understand the causes of war—and, for that matter, the rise and fall of different forms of warfare over time.

This theory was further expanded in *FPHWP*, where I suggested a new way to understand war and peace, in a small sense—or aggression and pacificity, in a broad sense.

(a2.4) In relation to mass media, I also proposed "the totalistic theory of communication" in *The Future of Post-Human Mass Media* (or in short, *FPHMM*).

(a2.5) In relation to law, I also proposed "the reconstruction theory of law" in *The Future of Post-Human Law* (or in short, *FPHLAW*). And in relation to criminality, I proposed "the reflective theory of criminality" in *FPHCRIM* for a different way to understand heroes and villains.

(a2.6) In relation to education, I proposed "the heterodox theory of education" in *The Future of Post-Human Education* (or in short, *FPHEDU*).

(a2.7) And in relation to gambling, I proposed "the detached theory of gambling" in *The Future of Post-Human Gambling* (or in short, *FPHGAM*).

(a3) Social Structure

In relation to social structure, I first proposed two additional theories, that is, "the theory of the cyclical progression of hegemony" in *FCD* (and also in *FPHC* and *BDPD*), and "the theory of the cyclical progression of empire-building" (in *BWT*, as already indicated above)—with important implications for the symmetry-asymmetry princple in existential dialectics, just to cite one example.

In addition, this is also related to the issues of "migration" in (a4,6), "identity" in (b11), and "geography" in (d4), for instance.

Then, in *BNN*, I proposed another theory, namely, "the theory of contrastive advantages" to understand the persistence of social structure by gender, race, ethnicity, or any other groupings.

(a4) Social Systems (or Trends)

In relation to social systems, there are several sub-categories for illustration, which can be about (a4.1) urbanization, (a4.2) technology, (a4.3) demography, (a4.4) the environment, (a4.5) social trends as a whole (which also include the current phenomenon of globalization), (a4.6) migration, and (a4.7) resources.

(a4.1) In relation to urbanization, I proposed "the contingent theory of urban planning" in *FPHUP* for a new way to understand density and void—which is also related to the issues of "social trends" (especially in relation to globalization) in (a4.5), "migration" in (a4.6), and "identity" in (b11).

(a4.2) In relation to technology, I worked out "the ambivalent theory of technology" in *FPHE* for a new way to understand the nature of technology.

Some other books (like *FPHMM*, *FAE*, *FCD*, and *FHC*) also deal with technology, and a good example concerns "the synthetic theory of information architecture" in *FIA* on taxonomy, network, and intelligence, in conjunction with the rise of technology.

(a4.3) In relation to demography, I proposed, first in *FHC* (and later in other books like *FCD*, *FPHC*, *FPHU*, etc.), "the theory of post-humanity," in relation to the "post-human" age at some distant point of "after-postmodernity," long after human extinction, to be eventually superseded by "post-humans" of various forms.

Some good candidates of the post-human lifeforms include, for instance, "thinking robots," "thinking machines," "cyborgs," "genetically altered superior beings," "floating consciousness," "hyper-spatial consciousness," "unfolding unconsciousness," "the hyper-sexual body," and "the hyper-martial body." This post-human vision of mine was first originally worked out in *FHC* and further elaborated in both *FCD*, *FPHC*, *FPHU*, *FPHS*, and *FPHMA*, for instance.

Lest any confusion occurs, I need to emphasize two clarifications here about the term "post-human" as a neologism in my works.

Firstly, the word "post-human" here should *not* be confused with another term which looks similar but has a totally different meaning in the literature of postmodernism, namely, "post-humanism"—which constitutes a critique of "humanism" as tradionally understood (especially, though not exclusively, in relation to the idea of progress in science and reason in the Enlightenment project). (WK 2008)

And secondly, the word "post-human" here should also *not* be confused with a similar term which is used to champion the ideology of technology for the future co-existence between humans and cyborgs in "trans-humanism." (WK 2008a)

Instead, my term "post-human" in relation to "posthuman-ism" also rejects "transhumanism" (especially, though not exclusively, in relation to the promises of technology) and refers to something else altogether, that is, the future extinction of humans and its post-human successors in deep space and beyond unto multiverses.

Later, in *BEPE*, I went further and provided a more comprehensive critique of "transhumanism," together with other issues.

With these two clarifications in mind (as summarized in *Table 1.31*)—in the end, a most fundamental question about intelligent life now has an answer, in that, if asked, "What is the future of human civilization?"—my answer in *FCD* (89) is thus: "As addressed in Ch.7 of *FHC*, a later epoch of the age of after-postmodernity (that is, at some point further away from after-postmodernity) will begin, as what I called the 'post-human' history (with the term 'post-human' originally used in my doctoral dissertation at M.I.T., which was finished in November 1995, under the title *After Postmodernity*, still available at M.I.T. library, and was later revised and published as *FHC*). The post-human history will be such that humans are nothing in the end, other than what culture, society, and nature (with some luck) have shaped them into, to be eventually superseded by post-humans (e.g., cyborgs, thinking machines, genetically altered superior beings, and others), if humans are not destroyed long before then."

(a4.4) In relation to the environment, I also addressed the issue of sustainability, especially in *FHC*, *FCD*, and *FPHUP*. For instance, in *FPHUP*, I specifically proposed a new theory, "the contingent theory of urban planning," on the need to go beyond the contemporoary obsession with sustainability, in the context of not only the environment but also other issues.

I also proposed "the interventive-reshaping theory of geography" in *FPHGEOG*—which is related to the issues of "migration" in (a4.6), "geography" in (d4), and "geology" in (d5).

In addition, I proposed "the transfigurative theory of waste" in *FPHW*.

(a4.5) In relation to social trends as a whole, I proposed in Ch.9 of *FCD* (367-8), that "civilizational history will continue into the following cyclical progression of expansion, before it is to be superseded (solely as a high probability, since humans might be destroyed sooner either by themselves or in a gigantic natural calamity) by posthumans at some distant point in after-postmodernity (which I already discussed in *FHC*)" unto multiverses (different constellations of universes):

Local → Regional → Global →Solar →
Galactic → Clustery...→ Multiversal

The current phenomeon of "globalization" lies in the third category on the line above and was extensively analyzed in *FCD*, in close connection with "globalism" at the cultural level—in the context of "postmodernity" (which will be introduced later in the section on history).

In *BDPD*, this thesis of mine was referred to as "the theory of the cyclical progression of system integration and fragmentation," at the systemic level—in close relation to another thesis analyzed in Ch.9 of *FCD*, which was called, in the absence of better words, "the multifaceted theory of war and peace" in *FPHK* (as already indicated above).

In *FC*, I also proposed "the dialectic theory of complexity" to account for the factor of uncertainty, which can have a major role to play in the world.

All this is also related to the issues of "urbanization" in (a4.1), "the environment" in (a4.4), "migration" in (a4,6), "identity" in (b11), "geography" in (d4), and "geology" in (d5).

(a4.6) In relation to migration, I proposed "the resettlement theory of geology" in *FPHGEOL* and "the theory of the cyclical progression of migration" in *FPHMIG*—which are also related to the issues of "social structure" in (a3), "urbanization" in (a4.1), "the environment" in (a4.4), "social trends" in (a4.5), "identity" in (b11), "geography" in (d4), and "geology" in (d5).

(a4.7) And in relation to resources, I proposed "the resilient theory of natural resources" in *BNR* —which is also related to the issue of "natural resources" in (d10).

(b) Culture

The category of "culture" here can also be divided into different sub-categories like (b1) aesthetics, (b2) religion, (b3) popular (mass) culture, (b4) logic, (b5) civilization as a whole, (b6) ethics, (b7) epistemology (methodology), (b8) metaphysics (ontology), (b9) ideology, (b10) language, and (b11) identity.

(b1) Aesthetics

In relation to aesthetics, I proposed "the transformative theory of aesthetic experience" in *FAE* about some great transformations of aesthetic experience in future history.

In *FPHLIT*, I further proposed "the comparative-impartial theory of literature" for a new way to understand fiction and non-fiction.

In *FPHPA*, I further proposed "the transdisciplinary theory of performing arts" for a new way to understand the body and its presence—which is also related to the issues of "popular (mass) culture" in (b3) and of "the human body" in (c1.2). And the aesthetic issue also overlaps with (d8) on architecture.

And in *FPHCA*, I further proposed "the inquisitive theory of culinary art" for a new way to understand ingredients and techniques.

(b2) Religion

In relation to religion, I proposed "the comparative theory of religion" in *FHC* (and also in *FCD*, although it was first so labeled in *FPHK*).

And in *FPHR*, I provided a solid foundation of this theory with a better name, that is, "the comparative-substitutive theory of religion" for a new way to understand spirituality.

(b3) Popular (Mass) Culture

In relation to popular (mass) culture, there are some sub-categories for illustration, which can be, for example, (b3.1) mass culture in general and (b3.2) sports—both of which are also related to the issues of "aesthetics" in (b1) and of "the human body" in (c1.2).

(b3.1) In relation to mass culture in general, I proposed, in *FHC*, a new way to understand mass culture in terms of some fundamental dilemmas, which is called, in the absence of better words, "the dualistic theory of mass culture" in *FPHO*.

(b3.2) In relation to sports (like chess), I proposed, in *FPHCHESS*, "the mediative-variative theory of chess" for a new way to understand tactics and strategy (in different traditions).

And in *FPHSPORT*, I proposed "the modificative theory of sports" for a new way to understand training and winning.

(b4) Logic

In relation to logic, I also worked out, in *FPHML*, "the contrastive theory of rationality" for a new way to understand rationality and knowledge (in the context of mathematical logic).

And in *FPHPROB*, I proposed "the interpretivist theory of probability" for a different way to understand objectivity and subjectivity—which is related to the issue of logic.

(b5) Civilization as a Whole

In relation to civilization as a whole, I also argued, in *FHC*, no freedom without unfreedom (as shown in *Table 4.13*) and no equality without inequality (as shown in *Table 4.14*), especially in relation to the seven dimensions of life existence first worked out in *FHC* (i.e., the technological, the everyday, the true, the holy, the sublime/beautiful, the good, and the just).

Even more interestingly, in *BDPD* and later in *BCIV*, I further revealed a theoretical refinement of existential dialectics, this time, in arguing that there is no civilization without barbarity, with human civilization to be eventually superseded by what I originally analyzed as "post-human post-civilization" (which should not be confused with "post-human civilization"), in the context of the freedom/unfreedom and equality/inequality dialectics.

In the final analysis, civilization cannot live without barbarity and has to learn to co-exist with it in ever new ways. Preposteorus as this may seem to many contemporaries—it is no more imperative to preserve civilization than necessary to destroy barbarity, and the ideal of civilization is essentially bankrupt, to be eventually superseded by "post-civilization" (as summarized in *Tables 4.35-4.43*).

This freedom/unfreedom and equality/inequality dialectics holds in pre-moderny, modernity, postmodernity, and what I orignally called "after-postmodernity" in *FHC* and *FCD*—especially, though not exclusively, in the context of the emergence of "post-humans."

There are two specific theories about "after-postmodernity" here. The first theory about "after-postmodernity" is about the trinity of pre-modernity, modernity, postmodernity, and after-postmodernity at the cultural level—and was called, in *BDPD*, "the theory of the trinity of modernity to its after-postmodern counterpart," although it was first analyzed in *FHC* and later in *FCD* and also *BCIV* (as summarized in *Table 1.34*, *Table 1.35*, *Table 1.36*, and *Table 1.37* and will be elaborated further in the later sub-section on "the rest" about future history).

The second theory about "after-postmodernity" is about pre-modernity, modernity, postmodernity, and after-postmodernity at the historical level. For instance, a conclusion in *FHC*, which is shocking indeed for many contemporaries, is none other than that "[t]he post-human history will therefore mark the end of human history as we know it and, for that matter, the end of human dominance and, practically speaking, the end of humans as well. The entire history of human civilization, from its beginning to the end, can be summarized by four words, linked by three arrows (as already discussed in *FHC*)":

Pre-Modernity → Modernity →
Post-Modernity → After-Postmodernity

In *BDPD*, this thesis of mine was specifically called "the theory of the evolution from pre-modernity to after-postmodernity," at the historical level—as shown in *Table 1.34*, *Table 1.35*, *Table 1.36*, and *Table 1.37* (and will be elaborated further in the later sub-section on "the rest" about future history).

Therefore, "[t]he end of humanity in the coming human extinction is the beginning of post-humanity. To say an untimely farewell to humanity is to foretell the future welcome of post-humanity." (P. Baofu 2002: 89) This thesis of mine was known in *BDPD* as "the theory of post-humanity," at the systemic level—as already indicated in (a4.3) above.

(b6) Ethics

In relation to ethics, I proposed, in *BEPE*, "the theory of post-ethics" for a new way to understand morality and immorality.

(b7) Epistemology (Methodology)

In relation to epistemology (methodology), I proposed "the complex theory of data analysis" in *FPHDA* for a different way to understand quantitative and qualitative research.

In addition, I already proposed "the critical-dialectic theory of formal science" in *FPHFS* and "the theory of methodological holism" in several books (like Ch.1 *FCD*, Ch.1of *FPHC*, *Sec.2.1* and *Sec.2.5* of *BCPC*, *FC*, *FPHK*, etc.) for a different way to do methodology.

In *FPHPROB*, I proposed "the interpretivist theory of probability" for a different way to understand objectivity and subjectivity.

(b8) Metaphysics (Ontology)

I proposed "the theory of existential dialectics" in several books (like *FHC*, *FCD*, *FPHC*, *BDPD*, *FC*, *FAE*, *ALD*, *FIA*, *FPHK*, etc,) and "the contrastive theory of rationality" in *FPHML* for a different way to understand ontology.

(b9) Ideology

The issue about ideology was already discussed under the categories of "social institutions" and of "civilization as a whole," especially in relation to my theories of "post-democracy," "post-capitalism," "post-civilization," and so on.

(b10) Language

I already proposed "the multilogical theory of learning" in *FPHL* for a new way to understand the nature of language structure and context.

I also worked out, in *FPHSEM*, "the interactive theory of semantics" for a new way to understand internality and externality (in the context of semantics).

In *FPHFS*, I proposed "the critical-dialectic theory of formal science," which is also related to pragmatics in regard to theory and application.

And in *FPHMORP*, I proposed "the fusional theory of morphology" for a different way to understand typologies and rules.

(b11) Identity

I proposed "the theory of the cyclical progression of migration" in *FPHMIG* for a new way to understand the nature of sameness, otherness, and identity—which is also related to the issues of "social structure" in (a3), "urbanization" in (a4.1), "social trends" (especially in relation to globalization) in (a4.5), "migration" in (a4.6), religion in (b2), and ideology in (b9).

(c) The Mind

The important vision about "post-humans" (as summarized earlier) brings us to the category of "the mind" here, which, as is often understood in everyday's usage, refers to the "brain" and the "body" (together with their interactions) and has different levels of consciousness which can be both "spiritual" and non-spiritual.

Therefore, the "mind" already presupposes the "brain," "body," and "spirit" (or "soul"), so that one does not fall into the intellectual trap of the "mind-body dualism" as debunked in modern (and especially, postmodern) philosophy (which I already went to great lengths to explain in *The Future of Human Civilization*).

That said—the category of "the mind" can be divided into two sub-categories, namely, in relation to (c1) biology and (c2) psychology

(c1) Biology

In relation to biology (which also overlaps with psychology too, however), there are three concerns here, namely, (c1.1) genes and intelligence, (c1.2) the human body, and (c1.3) health.

(c1.1) In relation to genes and intelligence, I worked out "the theory of contrastive advantages" (which was originally proposed in *FCD* and further worked out in *BNN*, as summarized in *Table 1.24*), to show the nature-nurture interactions of multiple levels in action (e.g., the biological, the psychological, the structural, the systemic, the cultural, and others) for humans and post-humans on earth and beyond, to the extent that different groups, be they on the basis of race, gender, ethnicity, class, age, or else, are not equal, on average, and have not been, nor will they be, even if there can be exceptions.

(c1.2) In relation to the human body, for instance, in *FPHMA*, I suggested "the expansive-contractive theory of martial arts," in which two great future transformations of the martial body were envisioned, that is, both "with the hyper-martial body" and "without the body" (as summarized in *Table 1.32*)—although this issue can also be classified under the category of "culture."

In *FPHS*, I proposed "the theory of virtual sexuality," in which three great future transformations of the sexual body were envisioned, that is, "virtual pleasure," "the hyper-sexual body," and "the post-sexual floating mind" (as summarized in *Table 1.33*).

And in *FPHPA*, I further proposed "the transdisciplinary theory of performing arts" for a new way to understand the body and its presence, with seven great future transformations of the body in performing arts—which is also related to the issues of "aesthetics" in (b1) and "popular (mass) culture" in (b3).

(c1.3) And in relation to health, for instance, in *FPHHC*, I suggest "the interconnected theory of health care" for a new way to understand mental health and physical health (in the context of mind and body)—which is also related to psychology in the category of "the mind" (as well as the issues in the categories of "culture" and "society").

(c2) Psychology

In relation to psypchology (which also overlaps with biology too, however), I also proposed some greater transformations of the mind to come in the future, especially though not exclusively in the post-human age.

These greater transformations of the mind in psychology can be further sub-divided into different categories, namely, (c2.1) consciousness, (c2.2) unconsciousness (together with subconsciousness), (c2.3) creativity, (c2.4) learning, (c2.5) aggression and pacificity, (c2.6) personality, (c2.7) humor, and (c2.8) artificial intelligence.

(c2.1) In relation to consciousness, I analyzed, in *FPHC*, the nature of consciousness in relation to the conceptual dimensions of consciousness (as shown in *Table 1.12*), the theoretical levels of consciousness (as shown in *Table 1.13*), the thematic issues of consciousness (as shown in *Table 1.14*), and the different dimensions of human existence (viz., having-ness, belonging-ness, and being-ness) in relation to consciousness (as shown in *Table 1.15*, *Table 1.16*, *Table 1.17*, and *Table 1.18*).

In *BCPC*, the nature of consciousness was further explored in relation to cognition, emotion, and behavior, which can be in consciousness and other mental states (e.g., subconsciousness and unconsciousness), in the context of existential dialectics, as shown in *Table 1.19*, *Table 1.20*, *Table 1.21*, *Table 1.22,* and *Table 1.23*.

In fact, in *FCD*, I already proposed three different theories in relation to the limits of cognition, emotion, and behavior, namely, "the theory of cognitive partiality," "the theory of emotional non-neutrality," and "the theory of behavioral alteration."

Then, I argued that the existence of human consciousness will be superseded one day with "floating consciousness" (as first proposed in *FCD*) and "hyper-spatial consciousness" (as first proposed in *FPHC*) as a climax of evolution in consciousness, after the future extinction of human consciousness (as shown below):

Primordial consciousness → Human consciousness →
Post-human consciousness (with floating consciousness and hyper-spatial consciousness as a climax in the evolution of consciousness)

In *BDPD*, these latest theses of mine were called "the theory of floating consciousness" and "the theory of hyper-spatial consciousness," both at the cosmological and psychological levels (as summarized in *Table 1.26* and *Table 1.25*).

(c2.2) In relation to unconsciousness, for instance, in *FPHU*, the unconsious mind will undergo tremendous change, to the rise of what I originally called "unfolding unconsciousess" in relation to anomalous experience, as a climax of evolution in unconsciousness, in conjunction with the conscious mind (both human now and post-human later), especially at the psychological level, as shown below:

Primordial unconsciousness → Human unconsciousness → Post-human unconsciousness (with unfolding unconsciousness as a climax in the evolution of unconsciousness)

In *FPHU*, this thesis of mine is called "the theory of unfolding unconsciousness" in a small sense, or "the unfolding theory of anomalous experience," in a larger one, as shown in *Table 1.27* and *Table 1.28*.

(c2.3) In relation to creativity, for instance, in *FPHCT*, I also proposed "the comprehensive theory of creative thinking" to explore the role of creative thinking, in relation to technology and other factors, together with my original proposal of important creative techniques and traits (as shown in *Table 1.29*) and its double nature of desirability and undesirability (as shown in *Table 1.30*).

(c2.4) In relation to learning, for instance, in *FPHL*, I worked out "the multilogical theory of learning" for a new way to understand the nature of structure and context in language, in relation to learning and its future development in the context of the mind.

(c2.5) In relation to aggression (and pacificity), I proposed "the multifaceted theory of war and peace" in *FPHWP* (as mentioned above).

(c2.6) In relation to personality, I worked out "the contrarian theory of personality" in *FPHP* for a new way to understand normality and abnormality.

(c2.7) In relation to humor, I worked out "the metamorphic theory of humor" in *FPHH* for a new way to understand joking and laughing.

(c2.8) And in relation to artificial intelligence, I proposed "the supersession theory of computing" in *FPHCOM* for a new way to understand hardware, software, and the mind.

In addition, I also proposed "the complex theory of data analysis" in *FPHDA* for a different way to understand quantitative and qualitative research in the context of the evolution of new minds.

(d) Nature

The category of "nature" here refers to the state of nature, which can be divided into some sub-categories like (d1) physics, (d2) cosmology, (d3) biology, (d4) geography, (d5) geology, (d6) acoustics, (d7) chemistry, (d8) architecture, (d9) transportation, and (d10) natural resources.

But since biology in (d3) overlaps with biology in (c1)—only the rest of the categories are addressed hereafter.

(d1) Physics

In relation to physics, I also proposed "the perspectival theory of space-time" in *FPHST* (based on *FPHC*) for a new way to understand space and time, as shown in *Table 1.3*, *Table 1.4*, *Table 1.5*, and *Table 1.7*.

In *FPHG* (based on *FPHC* and *FPHST*), I proposed "the selective theory of geometry" for a new way to understand geometry, with implications for the understanding of space-time in the context of infinity, symmetry, and dimensionality for future lifeforms that our world has never known (as shown in *Table 1.6*, *Table 1.7*, *Table 1.8; Table 1.9*, *Table 1.10,* and *Table 1.11*).

And in *FC*, I proposed "the dialectic theory of complexity" for a new way to understand order and chaos in the state of nature and beyond.

(d2) Cosmology

In relation to cosmology, my theories on physics (as indicated above) already have important implications for understanding the nature and the future of the universe (which was also addressed in *FHC*, among other works aforcited).

I also proposed "the theory of hyper-spatial consciousness" in *FPHC* (and also in *FPHG*) for a new way to understand the future evolution of the mind to enter into different dimensions of space-time that our current world has never known.

In addition, in *BCOS*, I proposed "the theory of post-cosmology" for a new way to understand the beginnings and ends of the cosmos and beyond.

(d4) Geography

In relation to geography, I proposed "the theory of the geopower of nature" in *ALD* for a different way to understand the relationships between geography and other entities (like the mind, culture, and society).

I further refined this issue of geography by proposing "the interventive-reshaping theory of geography" in *FPHGEOG*—which is related to the issues of "the environment" in (a4.4), "migration" in (a4.6), and "geology" in (d5).

(d5) Geology

In relation to geology, I proposed "the resettlement theory of geology" in *FPHGEOL* for a different way to understand the relationships between statics and dynamics—which is related to the issues of "the environment" in (a4.4), "migration" in (a4.6), and "geography" in (d4).

(d6) Acoustics

In relation to acoustics, I proposed "the multilateral theory of acoustics" in *FPHA* for a different way to understand the relationships between sound and silence.

(d7) Chemistry

In relation to chemistry, I proposed "the creational theory of chemistry" in *FPHCHEM* for a different way to understand substances and their changes.

(d8) Architecture

In relation to architecture, I proposed "the transcendent theory of architecture" in *FPHARCH* for a different way to understand form and function.

(d9) Transportation

In relation to transportation, I proposed "the panoramic theory of transportation" in *FPHTRAN* for a different way to understand networks and operations.

(d10) Natural Resources

And in relation to natural resources, I proposed "the resilient theory of natural resources" in *BNR*—which is also related to the issue of "resources" in (a4.7).

(e) The Rest

The category of "the rest" here refers to what cannot be strictly classified in any of the previous categories (i.e., society, culture, the mind, and nature). A good illustration of "the rest" refers to (e1) history.

(e1) History

The category of history can be divided into some sub-categories like (e1.1) empirical history and (e.1.2) meta-history.

(e1.1) In relation to empirical history, I proposed "the theory of the evolution from pre-modernity to after-postmodernity" (as first worked out in *FHC* and later in *FCD* and *FPHC*), which overlaps—as a reminder from (b5)—with the issue concerning "civilization as a whole" in (b5).

For instance, in both *FCD* and *FPHC*, I worked out the structure of "post-human civilization" in terms of the trinity of after-postmodernity (i.e., "free-spirited after-postmodernity," "post-capitalist after-postmodernity," and "hegemonic after-postmodernity").

Both conceptually and theoretically, the trinity of after-postmodernity is a sequential extension of the trinity of modernity (i.e., "free-spirited modernity," "capitalist modernity,"and "hegemonic modernity") and the trinity of postmodernity (i.e., "free-spirited postmodernity," "capitalist postmodernity," and "hegemonic postmodernity") as first proposed in *FHC*.

And the trinity of pre-modernity (i.e., "pre-free-spirited pre-modernity," "pre-capitalist pre-modernity" and "hegemonic pre-modernity") was later conceived in *BCIV* to complete the historical set from pre-modernity to after-postmodernity.

In *BDPD*, this thesis about the trinity of pre-modernity, modernity, postmodernity, and after-postmodernity was collectively known as "the theory of the trinity of modernity to its after-postmodern counterpart," at the cultural level—as already so mentioned in (b5) earlier, and summarized in *Table 1.34*, *Table 1.35*, *Table 1.36*, and *Table 1.37*.

At the structural level, all these trinities are subject to the existential constraints (e.g., the freedom/unfreedom and equality/inequality dialectics in the context of "the cyclical progression of hegemony"), be the historical epoch in pre-modernity, modernity, postmodernity, or after-postmodernity in future times. Each of the historical epochs has its ever new ways of coming to terms with the ever new (different) mixtures of freedom/unfreedom and equality/inequality.

This is importantly so, not because, as is falsely assumed in conventional wisdom, one certain way is superior (or better) than another in terms of achieving more freedom and less unfreedom, or more equality with less inequality.

On the contrary, indeed, in each of the historical epochs, each increase of unfreedom greets each freedom achieved, just as each increase of inequality welcomes each equality achieved, albeit in ever new (different) ways. In *BDPD*, this thesis of mine was labeled as "the theory of the cyclical progression of hegemony," at the structural level, though it was first analyzed in *FCD*.

In *BDPD*, more theoretical applications of existential dialectics were further examined, in relation to five main features, in the context of the duality of oppression, namely, (a) that each freedom/equality achieved is also each unfreedom/inequality created, (b) that the subsequent oppressiveness is dualistic, both by the Same against the Others and itself and by the Others against the Same and themselves, (c) that both oppression and self-oppression can be achieved by way of downgrading differences (between the Same and the Others) and of accentuating them, (d) that the relationships are relatively asymmetric among them but relatively symmetric within them, even when the Same can be relatively asymmetric towards itself in self-oppression, and the Others can be likewise towards themselves, and (e) that symmetry and asymmetry change over time, with ever new players, new causes, and new forms, be the locality here on Earth or in deep space unto multiverses—as summarized in *Table.4.13*, *Table 4.14*, *Table 4.15*, and *Table 4.16*.

The same logic also holds both in relation to wealth and poverty (as addressed in *BCPC* and summarized in *Table 4.17* on the wealth/poverty dialectics) and in relation to civilization and barbarity (as addressed in

BCIV and summarized in *Table 4.18* on the civilization/barbarity dialectics).

In *BDPD*, this thesis on existential dialectics was labeled as "the theory of existential dialectics."

(e.1.2) And in relation to meta-history, I proposed "the multifold theory of history" in *FPHHIST* for a different way to understand universality and relativity (together with other debates).

Direct and Indirect Applications of Existential Dialectics

A different way to appreciate the usefulness of existential dialectics is by way of the analysis of its (a) direct and (b) indirect applications.

(a) In direct applications, on the one hand, the logic of existential dialectics can shed some theoretical insights on diverse phenomena in the world, and good instances are the usage of the principles of existential dialectics for the theoretical insights on the freedom/unfreedom dialectics, the equality/inequality dialectics, and the wealth/poverty dialectics—as introduced earlier in (b5) and (e) in the previous sub-section.

For instance, my books like *FPHST*, *BNN*, *FAE*, *FC*, *FIA*, *FPHU*, *FPHK*, *FPHML*, *FPHE*, *FPHMM*, *FPHCT*, *FPHG*, *FPHUP*, *FPHL*, *FPHO*, *FPHMA*, *FPHS*, *FPHLAW*, *FPHFS*, *FPHWP*, *FPHP*, *BEPE*, *BCOS*, *FPHGEOL*, *FPHCHESS*, *FPHR*, *FPHEDU*, *FPHH*, *FPHA*, *FPHGAM*, *FPHCOM*, *FPHLIT*, *FPHCHEM*, *FPHDA*, *FPHGEOG*, *FPHPA*, *FPHSEM*, *FPHARCH*, *FPHCRIM*, *FPHHIST*, *FPHMIG*, *FPHTRAN*, *FPHCA*, *FPHW*, *BNR*, *FPHSPORT*, *FPHPROB*, *FPHMORP*, and *FPHHC* use the principles to reveal some theoretical insights on the perspectives of space and time (as in *FPHST*), of nature and nurture (as in *BNN*), of beauty and ugliness (as in *FAE*), of order and chaos (as in *FC*), of taxonomy and network (as in *FIA*), of the unconscious mind (as in *FPHU*), of the nature of knowledge (as in *FPHK*), of mathematical logic (as in *FPHML*), of engineering (as in *FPHE*), of mass media (as in *FPHMM*), of creative thinking (as in *FPHCT*), of geometry (as in *FPHG*), of urban planning (as in *FPHUP*), of language (as in *FPHL*), of organization (as in *FPHO*), of martial arts (as in *FPHMA*), of sexuality (as in *FPHS*), of law (as in *FPHLAW*), of formal science (as in *FPHFS*), of aggression and pacificity (as in *FPHWP*), of normality and abnormality (as in *FPHP*). of morality and immorality (as in *BEPE*), of the beginnings and ends of the universe (as in *BOCS*), of statics and dynamics (as in *FPHGEOL*), of tactics and strategy (as in *FPHCHESS*), of secularness and sacredness (as in *FPHR*), of teaching and learning (as in *FPHEDU*), of joking and laughing (as in *FPHH*), of sound and silence (as in *FPHA*), of risk and caution (as in *FPHGAM*), of hardware and software (as in

FPHCOM), of fiction and non-fiction (as in *FPHLIT*), of substances and their changes (as in *FPHCHEM*), of quantitative and qualitative research (as in *FPHDA*), of environments and their interactions (as in *FPHGEOG*), of the body and its presence (as in *FPHPA*), of internality and externality (as in *FPHSEM*). of form and function (as in *FPHARCH*), of heroes and villains (as in *FPHCRIM*), of universality and relativity (as in *FPHHIST*), of Sameness and Otherness (as in *FPHMIG*), of networks and operations (as in *FPHTRAN*), of ingredients and techniques (as in *FPHCA*), of uselessness and usefulness (as in *FPHW*), of diversity and discontinuity (as in *BNR*), of training and winning (as in *FPHSPORT*), of objectivity and subjectivity (as in *FPHPROB*), of typologies and rules (as in *FPHMORP*), and of mental health and physical health (as in *FPHHC*).

(b) In indirect applications, on the other hand, the theoretical insights can further be used to reveal other phenomena directly from them (viz., the theoretical insights) and therefore indirectly from the principles themselves.

A good illustration is of course the use of the theoretical insights on the freedom/unfreedom and equality/inequality dialectics for the understanding of the civilization/barbarity dialectics.

This distinction between direct and indirect applications may sound a bit academic, since even in indirect applications, the phenomena under study can still be directly related back to the principles themselves.

In the previous example, as an illustration, the civilization/barbarity dialectics can be directly related to the principles of existential dialectics without the intermediate role of the freedom/unfreedom and equality/inequality dialectics.

Multiple Levels of Application

There is another issue to be clarified, however. In other words, the theoretical insights can be applied to multiple levels of analysis—even though, in a given example, it may refer to one level or a few only.

For instance, in the example concerning the freedom/unfreedom dialectics, it can be used at the structural level (e.g., in relation to the theory of the cyclical progression of hegemony), but it can also be exploited for other levels (e.g., the theory of post-capitalism at the institutional level).

All these levels of application should not be misleadingly construed, as I stress this before, as a one-way street (that is, to use the ontological principles for theoretical application at multiple levels of specific analysis) but a two-way one, in which theoretical insights in praxis, when studied in more specific contexts, can in turn refine the nature of existential dialectics (for example, with the addition of new principles).

Sophisticated Methodological Holism

The summary of my original meta-theory on methodology is provided below, again, to be repeated *often verbatim* from my previous works—as this is something I regularly do in each new book to introduce my past works, which are in conversation with this current one.

This means that, for those readers who have not read any of my previous books, the summary below is helpful.

That clarified—this original contribution of mine to the study of methodology takes the form of an approach known as "the theory of methodological holism" or "methodological holism" in short, as already worked out in *FPHC* (2004).

I have made good use of this methodological approach of mine for all of my previous works.

The Confusion of Holism with Systems Approach

Yet, it is imperative to stress at the outset, as I often emphasized this in all my previous books, that my approach of "methodological holism" does not oppose or exclude "methodological individualism" (as some readers may be tempted to assume, as is conventionally understood) but actually includes it.

The confusion here has to do with equating holism with systems approach in general (be it about systems theory, chaos theory, complexity theory, or else), which I debunked, while learning something from it, as already elaborated in *The Future of Complexity* (2007)—and *The Future of Post-Human Formal Science* (2010) is another addition to this critique of the intellectual fad of systems approach.

In other words, my meta-theory of holism, or sophisticated methodological holism in short, makes a distinction between doing holistic work and doing systems work, for two reasons.

The first reason is that holism, in my theory, does not imply systems approach, since it rejects systems approach because of the myriad problems that the literature on systems approach has been unable to resolve, while learning something from it.

And the second reason is that my theory is related to the other theory of mine, that is, existential dialectics, which does not exclude methodological individualism (but includes it, because it simply goes beyond both reductionism and reverse-reductionism in a dialectic way).

For these reasons (and others too, as summarized in *Table 4.1*), my version of methodological holism is *sophisticated*—not *vulgar* as sometimes used by inapt scholars employing the same term.

The Ontological Constraints

Sophisticated methodological holism is subject to some ontological constraints, and some good examples include "the formalness-informalness principle," "the absoluteness-relativeness principle," "the partiality-totality principle," "the predictability-unpredictability principle," "the explicability-inexplicability principle," and "the fiction-reallity principle" in existential dialectics.

Of course, there can be more than six ontological principles in relation to method, but the examples here are sufficient to illustrate the point in question.

With this caveat in mind—the first two were already analyzed in previous books of mine like *FC* and *FAE*, whereas the third one was addressed in *FPHU*, the fourth and fifth ones were accounted for in *FPHK* and *FPHML*, respectively, and the last one was addressed in *FPHLIT*.

For now, it suffices to show that sophisticted methodological holism, because of these ontological constraints on methodology, targets two major sins of methodology, namely, what I call, in the absence of better words, (a) *reductionism* and (b) *reverse-reductionism*—both of which come in all shapes and sizes, to be summarized below (and also shown in *Table 4.2*).

Against the Varieties of Reductionism

There are four versions of reductionism to be summarized here, which sophisticated methodological holism rejects, namely, (a1) conceptual, (a2) theoretical, (a3) methodological, and (a4) ontological forms of reductionism.

(a1) In conceptual reductionism, a good case in point concerns myriad dualities like mind vs. body, self vs. world, democracy vs non-democracy, and the like (as already addressed in *FHC*, *FPHC*, and *BDPD*, for instance).

(a2) In theoretical reductionism, an illuminating case study is best exemplified by what I originally called "the foundation fallacy" in *FPHST*, in any attempt to naively understand space-time from the physical perspective as the foundation and, consequently, to dangerously dismiss (or belittle) other perspectives.

In *FAE*, I elaborated further these versions of reductionism in the literature on aesthetics (e.g., form vs. content, representation vs. expression, critics vs. artists, and externalism vs. internalism).

In *FIA*, I revealed other forms of reductionism in the literature on information architecture (e.g., the constructivist argument and the representational argument).

In *FPHU*, I showed the persistent legacy of reductionism, this time, in the literature on anomalous experience (e.g., the obsession with physics, chemistry, and biology for explaining anomalous experience).

In *FPHE*, I examined another case of reductionism in action, in the context of engineering (e.g., technical constraints vs. normative constraints).

In *FPHMM*, I elaborated one more version of reductionism, in relation to the three domains of communication (e.g., the competing views on sending, connecting, and receiving).

In *FPHCT*, I explored another version of reductionism, in relation to invention and innovation (e.g., the bio-psychological argument vs. the socio-cultural arguments).

In *FPHG*, I identified another version of reductionism, in relation to infinity, symmetry, and dimensionality (e.g., the Euclidean argument vs. the non-Euclidean arguments).

In *FPHUP*, I analyzed another version of reductionism, in relation to density and void (e.g., the engineering argument and the ecology argument).

In *PFHL*, I examined another version of reductionism, in relation to structure and context (e.g., the structuralist argument and the contextualist argument).

In *PFHO*, I explored another version of reductionism, in relation to communcation, decision-making, and leadership (e.g., the rational-system argument vs. the natural-system argument vs. the open-system argument).

In *PFHMA*, I revealed another version of reductionism, in relation to the martial body and spirit (e.g., the spiritual argument vs. the materialist argument vs. the defensive argument).

In *PFHS*, I analyzed another version of reductionism, in relation to the sexual body and spirit (e.g., the naturalist argument vs. the constructivist argument).

In *PFHLAW*, I examined another version of reductionism, in relation to law (e.g., the necessity argument vs. the contengency argument).

In *FPHWP*, I show another version of reductionism, in relation to war and peace (e.g., the aggressivist argument vs. the pacifist argument).

In *BEPE*, I analyzed another version of reductionism, in relation to morality and immorality (e.g., the objectivist argument vs. the non-objectivist argument vs. the skeptical argument).

In *BCOS*, I examined another version of reductionism, in relation to the contested beginnings and speculative ends of the universe (e.g., the scientific argument vs. the religious argument vs. the esoteric argument vs. the metaphysical argument).

In *FPHP*, I showed another version of reductionism, in relation to normality and abnormality (e.g., the natural argument vs. the social argument vs. the cultural argument vs. the mental argument).

In *FPHGEOL*, I scrutinized another version of reductionism, in relation to statics and dynamics (e.g., the catastrophe argument vs. the uniformity argument vs. the revision argument).

In *FPHCHESS*, I showed another version of reductionism, in relation to tactics and strategy (e.g., the natural argument vs. the social argument vs. the cultural argument vs. the mental argument).

In *FPHR*, I revealed another version of reductionism, in relation to secularness and sacredness (e.g., the critical argument vs. the skeptical argument vs. the theist argument).

In *FPHEDU*, I examined another version of reductionism, in relation to teaching and learning (e.g., the teacher-centered argument vs. the student-centered argument vs. the balanced argument).

In *FPHH*, I explored another version of reductionism, in relation to joking and laughing (e.g., the natural argument vs. the social argument vs. the cultural argument vs. the mental argument).

In *FPHA*, I revealed another version of reductionism, in relation to sound and silence (e.g., the natural argument vs. the social argument vs. the cultural argument vs. the mental argument).

In *FPHGAM*, I revealed another version of reductionism, in relation to risk and caution (e.g., the natural argument vs. the social argument vs. the cultural argument vs. the mental argument).

In *FPHCOM*, I showed another version of reductionism, in relation to hardware and software (e.g., the natural argument vs. the social argument vs. the cultural argument vs. the mental argument).

In *FPHLIT*, I proposed another version of reductionism, in relation to fiction and non-fiction (e.g., the natural argument vs. the social argument vs. the cultural argument vs. the mental argument).

In *FPHCHEM*, I proposed another version of reductionism, in relation to substances and their changes (e.g., the natural argument vs. the social argument vs. the cultural argument vs. the mental argument).

In *FPHDA*, I proposed another version of reductionism, in relation to quantitative and qualitative research (e.g., the natural argument vs. the social argument vs. the cultural argument vs. the mental argument).

In *FPHGEOG*, I proposed another version of reductionism, in relation to environments and their interactions (e.g., the natural argument vs. the social argument vs. the cultural argument vs. the mental argument).

In *FPHPA*, I proposed another version of reductionism, in relation to the body and its presence (e.g., the natural argument vs. the social argument vs. the cultural argument vs. the mental argument).

In *FPHSEM*, I proposed another version of reductionism, in relation to internality and externality (e.g., the natural argument vs. the social argument vs. the cultural argument vs. the mental argument).

In *FPHARCH*, I proposed another version of reductionism, in relation to form and function (e.g., the natural argument vs. the social argument vs. the cultural argument vs. the mental argument).

In *FPHCRIM*, I proposed another version of reductionism, in relation to heroes and villains (e.g., the natural argument vs. the social argument vs. the cultural argument vs. the mental argument).

In *FPHHIST*, I proposed another version of reductionism, in relation to universality and relativity (e.g., the natural argument vs. the social argument vs. the cultural argument vs. the mental argument).

In *FPHMIG*, I proposed another version of reductionism, in relation to Sameness and Otherness (e.g., the natural argument vs. the social argument vs. the cultural argument vs. the mental argument).

In *FPHTRAN*, I proposed another version of reductionism, in relation to networks and operations (e.g., the natural argument vs. the social argument vs. the cultural argument vs. the mental argument).

In *FPHCA*, I proposed another version of reductionism, in relation to ingredients and techniques (e.g., the natural argument vs. the social argument vs. the cultural argument vs. the mental argument).

In *FPHW*, I proposed another version of reductionism, in relation to uselessness and usefulness (e.g., the natural argument vs. the social argument vs. the cultural argument vs. the mental argument).

In *BNR*, I proposed another version of reductionism, in relation to diversity and discontinuity (e.g., the natural argument vs. the social argument vs. the cultural argument vs. the mental argument).

In *FPHSPORT*, I proposed another version of reductionism, in relation to training and winning (e.g., the natural argument vs. the social argument vs. the cultural argument vs. the mental argument).

In *FPHPROB*, I proposed another version of reductionism, in relation to objectivity and subjectivity (e.g., the natural argument vs. the social argument vs. the cultural argument vs. the mental argument).

In *FPHMORP*, I proposed another version of reductionism, in relation to typologies and rules (e.g., the natural argument vs. the social argument vs. the cultural argument vs. the mental argument).

And in *FPHHC*, I propose another version of reductionism, in relation to mental health and physical health (e.g., the natural argument vs. the social argument vs. the cultural argument vs. the mental argument).

(a3) In methodological reductionism, a good illustration can be the debate between different versions of qualitative and quantitative methods (as already analyzed in *FC* and also *FHC*).

In *FPHML*, I examined similar reductionism, this time, in the literature on mathematical logic (e.g., the obsession with consistency, soundness, and completeness).

And in *FPHFS*, I explored the problems of reductionism in the context of formal science (e.g., the analytical argument, as opposed to the synthetic argument).

(a4) In ontological reductionism, an excellent instance involves another debate, this time between emergentism and reductionism in complexity theory (as addressed in *FC*) and also in psychology (as elaborated in *FPHC*, in the context of Being and Belonging).

But to target against the varieties of reductionism constitutes only a side of the same coin, and the other side concerns the varieties of reverse-reductionism.

Against the Varieties of Reverse-Reductionism

The other side of the same coin is the reverse version of reductionism, which is what I want to call, in the absence of better words, *reverse-reductionism.*

My sophisticated version of methodological holism targets against the varieties of reverse-reductionism (just as it also rejects the ones of reductionism).

Perhaps nothing expresses better the popularity of reverse-reductionim than the "anything-goes" mentality in postmodernism of our time, as shown in the following four versions.

(b1) In conceptual reverse-reductionism, any concept of "art" (e.g., fine art, applied art, outsider art, junk art) is welcome in postmodernism (as already analyzed in Ch.4 of *FHC*—and also in *FAE*).

(b2) In theoretical reverse-reductionism, a variety of art and literary theories co-exist. Take the case of literary studies, as there are now Literary Structuralism, Marxist Literary Criticism, New Criticism, Phenomenology, Hermeneutics, Language-Game Literary Criticism, Feminist Literary Criticism, Reception Theory, Reader Response Criticism, Poststructuralism, Semiotics, Pyschoanalytic Literary Criticism, just to cite some well-known ones, with no one being said to be better than any others (as detailedly analyzed in Ch.4 of *FHC*). (S. Raman 1997)

In *BNN*, I even introduced "the compromise fallacy" as another good illustration of theoretical reverse-reductionism, in misleadingly treating both genetic and environmental approaches as equally valid.

(b3) In methodological reverse-reductionism, multiple methodologies are deemed as acceptable in postmodernism (e.g., doing art without praxis, doing art with praxis, and doing art by sublation), as analyzed in Ch.4 of *FHC*.

And in *FPHFS*, I exposed the problems of reverse-reductionism in the context of formal science in relation to systems theory (e.g., the synthetic argument).

(b4) In ontological reverse-reductionism, no privileged ontology is allowed, and the door is open practically for anything in postmodernism (e.g., the equal status of the ontology of Being vs. that of Becoming, as already addressed in Ch.4 of *FHC*—and also in *FPHC*).

In *FAE*, I also introduced another version of reverse-reductionism, that is, "the pluralist fallacy," in the context of understanding aesthetic experience, for instance—although this fallacy has been committed not exclusively in relation to the ontological level (but also at the conceptual, theoretical, and methodological ones).

These dual dangers against reverse-reductionism (in this sub-section) and reductionism (in the previous sub-section) are something that sophisticated methodological holism rejects. And in *FPHFS*, I addressed these two problems further.

This point about the dual dangers is important enough, since many scholars often favor one against the other, but it is vital to target both.

The Holistic Organization of an Inquiry

With these dual dangers against reductionism and reverse-reductionism in mind—sophisticated methodological holism suggests that an inquiry of any given phenomenon is more complete, if treated in the context of a comprehensive analysis at all relevant levels, which challengingly encompass all the fields of human knowledge, ranging from the natural sciences and formal sciences through the social sciences to the humanities.

This section is something that I had already stressed in all my previous books and repeat (*often verbatim*) hereafter. But, for those readers who had read my previous books, this serves as a reminder.

With this reminder in mind—there are multiple ways to engage in a holistic inquiry with all relevent levels of analysis. Over the years, I have proposed different ways to fulfill this holistic methodological requirement, as repeated in my previous books.

Hereafter is a summary of four major ways, namely, (a) by discipline, (b) by domain, (c) by subject, and (d) by meta-analysis—all of which fulfill the holistic requirement of sophisticated methodological holism on a given issue.

(a) In a holistic organization by discipline, a good illustration is the multiple levels of analysis, namely, (a1) the micro-physical, (a2) the chemical, (a3) the biological, (a4) the psychological, (a5) the organizational, (a6) the institutional, (a7) the structural, (a8) the systemic, (a9) the cultural, (a10) the macro-physical (cosmological), and (a11) other relevant levels, which are either a combination of all these levels or the practical applications with a combination of them.

This holistic organization by discipline is used in *FCD* and *BCPC*, for instance.

(b) In a holistic organization by domain, some good candidates include the classification of different perspectives of analysis in relation to (b1) nature, (b2) the mind, (b3) society, and (b4) culture, as already worked out in *BCIV*, *FPHST*, *FC*, *FAE*, *FPHU*, *FPHK*, *FPHE*, and *FPHFS*, just to cite some examples.

Culture in (b4), in this re-classification, is the same as culture in (a9) and can be further divided into different sub-categories, with good examples like (a9i) epistemology (methodology), (a9ii) aesthetics, (a9iii) ethics, (a9iv) metaphysics (ontology), and (a9v) religion. For clarification, epistemology (methodology) in (a9i) and metaphysics (ontology) in (a9iv) overlap with the category of "meta-theory."

Society in (b3) includes the organizational in (a5), the institutional in (a6), the structural in (a7), and the systemic in (a8).

The mind (b2) has more to do with the chemical in (a2), the biological in (a3), and the psychological in (a4), although it can overlap with (a1), (b3) and (b4), for instance.

It should be stressed that the "mind" here also includes the categories like the "brain," "body," and the "spirit" (or the "soul")—whenever needed in a given context, so that one does not fall into the intellectual trap of the "mind-body dualism" in the history of modern (and especially, postmodern) philosophy, which I already went to great lengths to explain in *The Future of Human Civilization*. After all, in everyday's usage, the "mind" already implies the "brain" and the "body" (together with their interactions) and has different levels of consciousness which can be both "spiritual" and non-spiritual.

And nature in (b1) refers to the micro-physical in (a1) and the macro-physical (cosmological) in (a10), although it can also overlap with (a2), (a3) and (a4).

(c) In a holistic organization by subject, some excellent examples concern the analysis of consciousness in *FPHC* (i.e., on Having, Belonging, and Being); of civilization in *FHC* (i.e., the True, the Holy, the Everyday, the Technological, the Beautiful/Sublime, the Good, and the Just); of international politics in *BWT* (i.e., Hyper-Empires, Meso-Empires, and Micro-Empires); of nature and nurture in *BNN* (i.e., genes and memes); of information architecture in *FIA* (i.e., taxonomy and network); of mathematical logic in *FPHML* (i.e., consistency, soundness, and completeness); of communication in *FPHMM* (i.e., sending, connecting, and receiving); of creative thinking in *FPHCT* (i.e., invention and innovation); of geometry in *FPHG* (i.e., infinity, symmetry, and dimensionality); of urban planning in *FPHUP* (i.e., density and void), of language in *FPHL* (i.e., structure and context), of organization in *FPHO* (i.e., communication, decision-making, and leadership), of martial arts in *FPHMA* (i.e., the martial body and the martial spirit), of sexuality in *FPHS* (i.e., the sexual body and the sexual spirit), of law in *FPHLAW* (i.e., necessity and contingency), of war and peace in *FPHWP* (i.e., aggression and pacificity), of personality in *FPHP* (i.e., normality and abnormality), of ethics in *BEPE* (i.e., morality and immorality), of cosmology in *BCOS* (i.e., the beginnings and ends of the universe), of geology in *FPHGEOL* (i.e., statics and dynamics), of chess in *FPHCHESS* (i.e., tactics and strategy), of religion in *FPHR* (i.e., secularness and sacredness), of education in *FPHEDU* (i.e., teaching and learning), of humor in *FPHH* (i.e., laughing and joking), of acoustics in *FPHA* (i.e., sound and silence), of gambling in *FPHGAM* (i.e., risk and caution), of computing in *FPHCOM* (i.e., hardware and software), of literature in *FPHLIT* (i.e., fiction and non-fiction), of chemistry in *FPHCHEM* (i.e., substances and their changes), of data analysis in *FPHDA* (i.e., quantitative and qualitative research), of geography in *FPHGEOG* (i.e., environments and their interactions), of performing arts in *FPHPA* (i.e., the body and its presence), of semantics in *FPHSEM* (i.e., internality and externality), of architecture in *FPHARCH* (i.e., form and function), of criminality in *FPHCRIM* (i.e., heroes and villains), of history in *FPHHIST* (i.e., universality and relativity), of migration in *FPHMIG* (i.e., Sameness and Otherness), of transportation in *FPHTRAN* (i.e., networks and operations), of culinary art in *FPHCA* (i.e., ingredients and techniques), of waste in *FPHW* (i.e., uselessness and usefulness), of natural resources in *BNR* (i.e., diversity and discontinuity), of sports in *FPHSPORT* (i.e., training and winning), of probability in *FPHPROB* (i.e., objectivity and subjectivity), of morphology in *FPHMORP* (i.e., typologies and rules), and of health care in *FPHHC* (i.e., mental health and physical health)—by incorporating all the relevent levels of analysis as cited above in each.

(d) And in a holistic organization by meta-analysis, two good cases in point involve the works on post-capitalism in *BCPC* and on authoritarian liberal democracy in *ALD*, with the classification of analysis in theory and meta-theory.

The essential point to remember here, as I thus stress in all my previous books, is that the multiple levels of analysis can be reorganized in many different ways, insofar as none of the levels (if relevant to an inquiry in question) is ignored or dismissed, to avoid the danger of reductionism (and for that matter, the one of reverse-reductionism, in the opposite direction).

Three Clarifications

Three clarifications are needed here, however, to avoid any hasty misunderstanding.

Firstly, the entities in each classification are not mutually exclusive. For instance, in the holisitc organization by domain, nature in (b1) can also be linked to the chemical in (a2), the biological in (a3), and the systemic in (a8). And the mind (b3) can alternatively be related to the micro-physical in (a1) and the chemical in (a2), for example.

Secondly, there is also the important factor of luck (or uncertainty in conventional usage), but it is already implied or allowed in each of the organizations of an inquiry—especially in relation to the predictability-unpredictability principle and the order-chaos principle in existential dialectics. This topic about uncertainty was already addressed in *FHC*—and more extensively, in *FC*, in the context of order and chaos (and later, to an extent, in *FPHK*, *FPHFS*, and *FPHGAM*, for example).

And lastly, the comparison in a classification is not absolute, but relative, as there are often some shades of gray, not exactly black or white (figuratively speaking).

Some further clarifications and qualifications of sophisticated methodological holism are shown in *Table 4.2*.

Some Distinctive Usefulness

In the end, sophisticated methodological holism—when applied, especially though not exclusively, as illustrated in my numerous works—can enrich the understanding of reality in some distinctive ways. Here are four examples (as revealed in each of my books).

Firstly, it provides a comprehensive analysis of a subject matter, from which much can be learned about reality, both in relation to the perspectives of the mind, nature, society, and culture.

Secondly, it offers a new classification of the subject matter.

Thirdly, it suggests some visions of the future in relation to the subject matter in question.

And fourthly, it proposes some insights on meta-theory (e.g., methodology and ontology) in general—with the clear understanding, however, of the dilemma of specific vs. general ontology (as shown in *Table 4.9* on the syntax of existential dialectics in the context of the dilemma of ontology).

For this very reason, all of these ways are important, without reducing one into the analysis of another. (*FPHCT*)

Chapter Outline

With this summary of my two original meta-theories (on methodology and ontology, *almost verbatim* from my previous works) in mind—this book is organized in four main parts, namely, (a) Part I on the introduction to this book, (b) Part II on mental health, (c) Part III on physical health, and (d) Part IV on the conclusion of the book.

The book is thus organized in four chapters.

The introductory chapter, that is, Chapter One titled "Introduction—The Value of Health Care," begins with a debate on a fashionable psychology, provides a definition and history of health care, and then introduces mental health and physical health in health care, as well as the diverse aspects of health care—together with the theoretical debate on health care, my interconnected theory of health care, the relationship between theory and meta-theory, existential dialectics, sophisticated methodological holism, and some further clarifications.

Chapter Two titled "Mental Health and its Duality" explores the nature of mental health in health care from the four perspectives of the mind, nature, society, and culture, with a constructive evaluation of each.

Chapter Three titled "Physical Health and its Ambivalence" examines the nature of physical health in health care from the four perspectives of the mind, nature, society, and culture, with a deconstructive assessment of each.

The last chapter titled "Conclusion—The Future of Health Care" summarizes the analysis in the book in the dialectic context of mental health and physical health in health care (together with the need to transcend them) with thirty-three major theses, namely, (a) the first thesis: the formalness-informalness principle, (b) the second thesis: the absoluteness-relativeness principle, (c) the third thesis: the partiality-totality principle, (d) the fourth thesis: the predictability-unpredictability principle, (e) the fifth thesis: the explicability-inexplicability principle, (f) the sixth thesis: the fiction-reality principle, (g) the seventh thesis: the cognitiveness-noncognitiveness principle, (h) the eighth thesis: the finiteness-transfiniteness principle, (i) the ninth thesis: the preciseness-vagueness principle, (j) the tenth thesis: the simpleness-complicatedness principle, (k) the eleventh thesis: the openness-hiddenness principle, (l) the twelfth thesis: the denseness-emptiness principle, (m) the thirteenth thesis: the prototypicality-variation principle, (n) the fourteenth thesis: the change-constancy principle, (o) the fifteenth thesis: the order-chaos principle, (p) the sixteenth thesis: the slowness-quickness principle, (q) the seventeenth thesis: the expansion-contraction principle, (r) the eighteenth thesis: the optimality-nonoptimality principle, (s) the nineteenth thesis: the theory-praxis principle, (t) the twentieth thesis: the convention-novelty principle, (u) the twenty-first thesis: the evolution-transformation principle, (v) the twenty-second thesis: the symmetry-asymmetry principle, (w) the twenty-third thesis: the softness-hardness principle, (x) the twenty-fourth thesis: the seriousness-playfulness principle, (y) the twenty-fifth thesis: the activeness-inactiveness principle, (z) the twenty-sixth thesis: the selfness-otherness principle, (aa) the twenty-seventh thesis: the regression-progression principle, (bb) the twenty-eighth thesis: the sameness-difference principle, (cc) the twenty-ninth thesis: the stability-reaction principle, (dd) the thirtieth thesis: the functionality-nonfunctionality principle, (ee) the thirty-first thesis: the intentionality-nonintentionality principle, (ff) the thirty-second thesis: the survivability-non-survivability principle, and (gg) the thirty-third thesis: the post-human interconnection—to be elaborated in the rest of the book, with a summary in the concluding chapter.

This seminal project here, if successful, will fundamentally change the way that we think about mental health and physical health in health care (together with other debates as will be discussed in the rest of the book), from the combined perspectives of the mind, nature, society, and culture, with enormous implications for the human future and what I originally called its "post-human" fate.

Some Clarifications

However, some additional (last) clarifications are needed.

These clarifications, lest any potential misunderstanding by the readers occurs, refer to (a) the conversation with my previous books, (b) the illustrative selection of case studies and examples, (c) detailed analysis versus overall analysis, (d) three distinctive features of using quotations, (e) two difficulties with understanding, (f) repetition, (g) chapter organization to counter conventional wisdom, (h) the political correctness of mainstream publishing, and (i) the use of neologisms.

These clarifications are something that I also regularly repeat in my previous books too, so these points are repeated hereafter, *often verbatim*—albeit in a different context this time.

In Conversation with My Previous Books

Firstly, my theory in this book is constructed on the theoretical foundation of my previous books (i.e., *FHC, FCD, FPHC, BDPD, BCPC, BCIV, FPHST, BNN, BWT, FC, FAE, ALD, FIA, FPHU, FPHK, FPHML, FPHE, FPHMM, FPHCT, FPHG, FPHUP, FPHL, FPHO, FPHMA, FPHS, FPHLAW, FPHFS, FPHWP, FPHP, BCOS, BEPE, FPHGEOL, FPHCHESS, FPHR, FPHEDU, FPHH, FPHA, FPHGAM, FPHCOM, FPHLIT, FPHCHEM, FPHDA, FPHGEOG, FPHPA, FPHSEM, FPHARCH, FPHCRIM, FPHHIST, FPHMIG, FPHTRAN, FPHCA, FPHW, BNR, FPHSPORT, FPHPROB,* and *FPHMORP*—as explicated in "The List of Abbreviations").

For this reason, many of my books have some familiar words in their titles like "The Future of Post-Human ____" or "Beyond ____to ____," as well as some tables for background information—as they constitute a series of books with the final aim to converge all of my original theories on numerous fields into a unified theory of everything (as already summarized in the section on theory and meta-theory in Chapter One).

Just consider the following two illustrations, namely, (a) in relation to other related theoretical debates and (b) in relation to different visions as worked out in my previous books.

(a) The first illustration is that the theoretical debate here also involves a few other related theoretical issues.

These other related theoretical issues have to do with some deeply contested theoretical debates, which, however, I had already gone to great lengths to analyze in my numerous (previous) books, as summarized below. It should also be stressed, lest misunderstanding occurs, that each of the theoretical debates (as listed below) does not exhaust the issues covered in the books, as each book covers more issues than what is listed below (for illustration only).

- On the Body
  - –Ex: *The Future of Post-Human Martial Arts*
  - –Ex: *The Future of Post-Human Performing Arts*
  - –Ex: *The Future of Post-Human Sexuality*
- On the Mind
  - –Ex: *The Future of Post-Human Consciousness*
  - –Ex: *The Future of Post-Human Unconsciousness*
  - –Ex: *The Future of Post-Human Personality*
  - –Ex: *The Future of Post-Human Computing*
  - –Ex: *The Future of Post-Human Data Analysis*
  - –Ex: *The Future of Post-Human Humor*
  - –Ex: *The Future of Post-Human Creative Thinking*
  - –Ex: *Beyond Nature and Nurture*
- On Fitness
  - –Ex: *The Future of Post-Human Sports*
- On Genetics
  - –Ex: *Beyond Nature and Nurture*
  - –Ex: *The Future of Post-Human Personality*
- On Evolution
  - –Ex: *Beyond Nature and Nurture*
  - –Ex: *Beyond Civilization to Post-Civilization*
  - –Ex: 2 volumes, *The Future of Human Civilization*
- On Complexity
  - –Ex: *The Future of Complexity*
- On Technology
  - –Ex: *The Future of Post-Human Computing*
  - –Ex: *The Future of Post-Human Engineering*
  - –Ex: *The Future of Post-Human Mass Media*

- On Decision-Making
  - –Ex: *The Future of Post-Human Organization*
- On Memory
  - –Ex: *The Future of Post-Human Data Analysis*
  - –Ex: *The Future of Post-Human Semantics*
  - –Ex: *The Future of Post-Human Consciousness*
- On Learning
  - –Ex: *The Future of Post-Human Language*
  - –Ex: *The Future of Post-Human Education*
- On Cognition
  - –Ex: *The Future of Post-Human Unconsciousness*
  - –Ex: *The Future of Post-Human Consciousness*
  - –Ex: *The Future of Capitalism and Democracy*
  - –Ex: *The Future of Post-Human Creative Thinking*
  - –Ex: *The Future of Post-Human Personality*
- On Intuition
  - –Ex: *The Future of Post-Human Unconsciousness*
  - –Ex: *The Future of Post-Human Consciousness*
  - –Ex: *Beyond Capitalism to Post-Capitalism*
  - –Ex: *The Future of Capitalism and Democracy*
- On Emotion
  - –Ex: *The Future of Post-Human Unconsciousness*
  - –Ex: *The Future of Post-Human Consciousness*
  - –Ex: *The Future of Aesthetic Experience*
  - –Ex: *Beyond Capitalism to Post-Capitalism*
  - –Ex: *The Future of Capitalism and Democracy*
  - –Ex: *The Future of Post-Human Personality*
- On Behavior
  - –Ex: *The Future of Post-Human Language*
  - –Ex: *The Future of Post-Human Unconsciousness*
  - –Ex: *The Future of Post-Human Consciousness*
  - –Ex: *Beyond Capitalism to Post-Capitalism*
  - –Ex: *The Future of Capitalism and Democracy*
  - –Ex: *The Future of Post-Human Sexuality*
  - –Ex: *The Future of Post-Human Personality*
  - –Ex: *The Future of Post-Human Martial Arts*
- On Spirituality
  - –Ex: 2 volumes, *The Future of Human Civilization*
  - –Ex: *The Future of Capitalism and Democracy*
  - –Ex: *The Future of Post-Human Religion*
  - –Ex: *Beyond Civilization to Post-Civilization*

–Ex: *The Future of Post-Human Sexuality*
–Ex: *The Future of Post-Human Martial Arts*
–Ex: *The Future of Post-Human Unconsciousness*
–Ex: *The Future of Post-Human Consciousness*
–Ex: *Beyond Ethics to Post-Ethics*

- On History
  –Ex: *The Future of Post-Human History*
- On Civilization
  –Ex: *Beyond Civilization to Post-Civilization*
  –Ex: 2 volumes, *The Future of Human Civilization*
- On Freedom
  –Ex: 2 volumes, *The Future of Human Civilization*
  –Ex: *The Future of Capitalism and Democracy*
  –Ex: *Beyond Capitalism to Post-Capitalism*
  –Ex: 2 volumes, *Beyond Democracy to Post-Democracy*
  –Ex: *Beyond Civilization to Post-Civilization*
- On Being and Belonging
  –Ex: *The Future of Post-Human Consciousness*
  –Ex: 2 volumes, *The Future of Human Civilization*
- On Different Dimensions of Human Existence
  –Ex: 2 volumes, *The Future of Human Civilization*
- On Modernity, Post-Modernity, and After-Postmodernity
  –Ex: 2 volumes, *The Future of Human Civilization*
  –Ex: *Beyond Civilization to Post-Civilization*
- On Pre-Modernity
  –Ex: *Beyond Civilization to Post-Civilization*

Therefore, those who are interested in these other theoretical issues (and debates) which are related to the current context can consult these other books of mine for more details.

(b) And the second illustration is that one of the major theses of this book concerns the future, be it human and later post-human, which is closely linked with the different visions that I had worked out in my previous books, in relation to the mind, nature, society, and culture.

Of course, for the convenience of the readers, a summary of some of these visions will be provided whenever necessary, as shown in the two sections on meta-theory above (*often verbatim*) and in different tables at the end of this chapter and the concluding chapter, for instance.

Yet, I still expect the readers to read my previous books directly for more details—as this book is written in conversation with my previous ones.

Case Studies and Examples

Secondly, the case studies and examples in the chapters are not exhaustive but solely illustrative. Nor are they necessarily mutually exclusive, as they can be reclassified in a different way. And exceptions are allowed.

One is tempted to assume, however, that, since the case studies and their examples are not exhaustive, more case studies and examples are needed. But the problem here is that just adding more of them does not necessarily change the conclusions to be drawn and may even lead to redundancy.

After all, the case studies and examples used in this book are chosen with care and deemed sufficient for the purpose at hand, even though they are solely illustrative.

Detailed Analysis versus Overall Synthesis

Thirdly, there is a distinction between detailed analysis and overall synthesis, in that the former is, especially though not exclusively, more for the specialized viewpoint of a specific discipline, whereas the latter is, especially though not exclusively, more for the broad horizon of an interdisciplinary approach—relatively speaking, of course.

Or, by analogy, there is a distinction between depicting a "tree" (with tiny details) in a "forest" and viewing the entire "forest" itself (with the broader horizon).

This book, like all previous ones of mine, tries to strike a balance between the two forms of understanding, although this does not imply that the two forms should be exactly equally offered, in an exact 50-50 balance.

Instead, the book, more often than not, does not allow the tiny details to obscure the larger picture in a given case study, because the entire book is inter-disciplinary in nature and tries to look at the entire "forest," not being bogged down with the detailed analysis of an individual "tree" in the forest, by analogy.

In this sense, although detailed analysis can be provided whenever needed for a given case study, the important point to remember is the overall horizon with its broadness of scope.

Three Distinctive Features of Using Quotations

Fourthly, the way that quotes are used in this book (and others of mine) has three distinctive features, as explained below.

The first distinctive feature is that, at the end of each quotation, sometimes there are more than one reference—in which case the first reference is for the original citation, and the rest of the references are for the convenience of the reader for more information about the issue(s) under quotation.

The second distinctive feature is that quotations are used as often as possible, so as to let others speak for themselves, without the nuisance of putting my own words into their mouths. Even more importantly, this allows me to use the original text as an evidence for critical analysis at the end of each section.

And the third distinctive feature is that all these quotations are used for my own purposes, in that I often creatively (or originally) re-organize them for a new way of analyzing the issue(s) in question.

Two Difficulties with Understanding

Fifthly, to understand this book (or any other book of mine) is difficult for two main reasons.

In regard to the first difficulty, this book, just like many other books of mine, is in conceptual and theoretical conversation with other books of mine (59 books, as of February 28, 2013), so this requires a vast background information on numerous subject matters.

And in regard to the second difficulty, this book also analyzes the subject matter in a way very different from the expectation of a conventional specialist reader, since it examines reality outside the specialist's interest (or outside his or her "comfort zone"), from the four broad perspectives of the mind, nature, society, and culture, such that it covers all domains of knowledge (in the social sciences, the natural sciences, the formal sciences, and the humanities). In other words, those who are truly interested in my project for a unified theory of everything would find many books of mine highly stimulating, but those who are specialists in a subject matter (like physics, geography, chess, and so on, in a strictly specialist sense) will not find them suitable to their specialist taste (or expectation).

Not surprisingly, a conventional specialist reader would find these two difficulties (with understanding) almost practically impossible to overcome, as they almost require the mind of a polymath. Even then, the best advice is that one should still try one's best to understand it.

Repetition

Sixthly, many of my books have something in common, and the reason is to show "the unified theory of everything" in all domains of knowledge.

For this reason, there is certain repetition in all books (especially in regard to the background information, together with the tables, in the introductory chapter and the concluding chapter). Therefore, these books are all titled "The Future of Post-Human ____" (or at times "Beyond ____ to ____") and constitute the "post-human" series.

Chapter Organization to Counter Conventional Wisdom

Seventhly, all of my books aim to deconstruct conventional wisdom and to replace it with new thinking, and the chapters in my books are often organized in two distinctive ways for this purpose

The first distinctive way is to show the polarized thinking in conventional wisdom by devoting two main chapters on opposites and then deconstructing them later. For example, in *Beyond Ethics to Post-Ethics* (2011), Chapter Two first introduces the conventional wisdom for morality but then shows that morality has its negative side often unsaid—and Chapter Three does just the opposite, that is, first introduces the conventional wisdom against immorality but then shows that immorality has its bright side often unspoken of.

And the second distinctive way is to show the opposites (embedded in conventional wisdom) in a dialectic way. For instance, in the above example, the task here is to show how and why the analysis of morality (in Chapter Two) is inadequate without the inclusion of its immorality, just as the examination of immorality (in Chapter Three) is insufficient without the consideration of its morality—to the extent that there is no morality without immorality, and vice versa.

But there are two qualifications.

The first qualification is that the opposites do not have to be always mutually exclusive in the conventional meaning (like morality vs. immorality in *BEPE* and heroes vs. villains in *FPHCRIM*)—but are simply disproportional in focus in other cases (in that some thinkers focus more on one than on the other), and good examples are networks vs. operations (in *FPHTRAN*), ingredients vs. techniques (in *FPHCA*), and form vs.

function (in *FPHARCH*). In other words, there are multiple meanings of the opposites.

And the second qualification is that some books (like the 2 volumes of *The Future of Human Civilization*, the 2 volumes of *Beyond Democracy to Post-Democracy*, and *The Future of Capitalism and Democracy*) are very lengthy and analyze many issues in more than two main chapters. Yet, there is a general pattern of introducing and then deconstructing conventional wisdom in my works.

The Political Correctness of Mainstream Publishing

Eighthly, all my books are politically incorrect—and consequently, they are not suitable for publication by major mainstream publishers, for three main reasons.

The first reason is that major mainstream publishers (in the U.S. as a prime example) have their own ideological agenda. For instance, any book which is perceived, either rightly or wrongly, as too "critical" to the U.S. (or to the West) is most unlikely to be accepted for publication by a top publishing house in the U.S. (as a prime example).

The second reason is that major mainstream publishers have their own methodological bias. For instance, any book which is truly interdisciplinary (with an analysis of almost everything, with no focus on a specific discipline or a few) is most unlikely to be accepted for publication by a top publishing house in the U.S. (as a prime example).

And the third reason is that major mainstream publishers have their own preference for visions. For instance, any book which envisions the future in the most distant horizon (with no practical relevance to the present) is most unlikely to be accepted for publication by a top publishing house in the U.S. (as a prime example).

These three reasons (or a combination of them) then add up to their argument that there is no "profitable market" for a book of such political incorrectness in a capitalist society (like the U.S. as a prime example).

The Use of Neologisms

And finally, I use different neologisms in my books, mostly to introduce my original concepts and theories, and good instances include those here or elsewhere in my previous books (e.g., "the interconnected theory of health care," "post-democracy," "hyper-spatial consciousness," "post-capitalism," and whatnot). Needless to say, they are used here solely for our current intellectual convenience, as they will be renamed differently in different ways in future history.

As I thus wrote in *FCD* (508-9), “all these terms 'post-capitalism,' 'post-democracy'...and other ones as introduced in...[the] project (e.g.,...'posthuman elitists,' and 'posthuman counter-elitists,' just to cite a few of them) are more for our current intellectual convenience than to the liking of future humans and post-humans, who will surely invent more tasteful neologisms to call their own eras, entities, and everything else, for that matter. But the didactic point here is to use the terms to foretell what the future might be like, not that its eras and entities must be called so exactly and permanently. After all, William Shakespeare (1995: Act II, Scene II, Line 47) well said long ago: 'What is in a name? That which we call a rose by any other name would smell as sweet.'”

As I had also stressed time and again before, each of the neologisms can be re-written as a different “X,” only to be re-named differently by the powers that be in different eras of future history.

With these clarifications for thought in mind—I now proceed to Chapter Two on mental health and its duality.

Table 1.1. Diverse Aspects of Health Care

- **Mental Health and Physical Health**
  - —Mental Health
    - Ex: problem-solving ability
    - Ex: emotional expression
    - Ex: resilience
  - —Physical Health
    - Ex: fitness
    - Ex: abuse control
    - Ex: violence regulation

- **Main Distinctions**
  - —Ex: conceptual distinctions
    - Ex: illness vs. disease
    - Ex: brain vs. mind
    - Ex: mind vs. soul
    - Ex: private health vs. public health
  - —Ex: types of health care
    - Ex: primary care
    - Ex: secondary care
    - Ex: tertiary care
    - Ex: quaternary care

Notes: The categories are solely illustrative (not exhaustive), and the comparison is relative (not absolute), nor are they necessarily mutually exclusive. And some can be easily re-classified elsewhere. As generalities, they allow exceptions.
Source: From *Sec. 1.3* & *Sec. 1.4* of *FPHHC*. See book for citations.

Table 1.2. Nine Great Future Transformations of Health Care (Part I)

- **In Relation to the Mind**
  - *—New Goals*
    - This search search for "new goals" will give future advanced humans and later their successors, namely, the post-humans, different motivations to provide health care in a way that current humans cannot—in relation to my previous visions on the future "post-human" supersession of the human mind like "supersession computing," "metamorphic humor," "contrarian personality," "hyper-martial body," "hyper-sexual body," "floating consciousness," "hyper-spatial consciousness," "thinking machines," "unfolding unconsciousness," "thinking robots," "genetically altered superior beings," "cyborgs," etc.
  - *—New Means*
    - This quest for "new means" will give future advanced humans and later their successors, namely, the post-humans, the capacity to find novel options to achieve the goals in regard to health care in a way that current humans cannot.

- **In Relation to Nature**
  - *—New Comparisons*
    - This search for "new comparisons" will give future advanced humans and later their successors, namely, the post-humans, the ability to learn from animals, plants, and the universe, through comparison and contrast, about health care in a way that current humans cannot.

(continued on next page)

Table 1.2. Nine Great Future Transformations of Health Care (Part II)

- **In Relation to Nature (*cont'd*)**

  —*New Integrations*

  - This search for "new integrations" will give future advanced humans and later their successors, namely, the post-humans, the ability to live and interact with nature for health care in a way that current humans cannot. This is especially so, in the context of the great future transformations of geology (in *FPHGEOL*), of geography (in *FPHGEOG*), of migration (in *FPHMIG*), and of transportation (in *FPHTRAN*)—in relation to my previous visions on the future "post-human" adventures into different dimensions of space-time unto multiverses like "the alteration of space-time" (*Table 1.3* & *Table 1.4*), "multiverses" (*Table 1.7* & *Table 1.8*), "hyperspace" (*Table 1.9* & *Table 1.25*), "time travel" (*Table 1.10* & *Table 1.11*), and others.

    This extension is consistent with my other theory, namely, "the theory of the cyclical progression of system integration and fragmentation" in *FCD* (2002)—at the social-systemic level (as already clarified in *Sec. 1.8* and shown below):

    Local → Regional → Global →Solar →
    Galactic → Clustery…→ Multiversal

(continued on next page)

Table 1.2. Nine Great Future Transformations of Health Care (Part III)

- **In Relation to Society**
  —*New Praxes*
    - This search for "new praxes" will give future advanced humans and later their successors, namely, the post-humans, the ability to engage in practice (like activism, politics, personal experience, etc.) for the future of health care in a way that current humans cannot.

  —*New Technologies*
    - This search for "new technologies" will give future advanced humans and later their successors, namely, the post-humans, the ability to come up with different techniques, materials, and experiments for heath care in a way that current humans cannot.

  —*New Stratifications*
    - This emergence of "new stratifications" will lead future advanced humans and later their successors, namely, the post-humans, to face new inequalities in the context of health care in a way that current humans cannot.

- **In Relation to Culture**
  —*New Sub-Fields*
    - This search for "new sub-fields" will give future advanced humans and later their successors, namely, the post-humans, the ability to explore new specialties for heatlh care in a way that current humans cannot.

  —*New Interpretations*
    - This search for "new interpretations" will give future advanced humans and later their successors, namely, the post-humans, the ability to come up with different evaluations and views about health care in a way that current humans cannot.

Notes: The categories and examples are solely illustrative (not exhaustive), and the comparison is relative (not absolute), nor are they necessarily mutually exclusive. And some can be easily re-classified elsewhere. As generalities, they allow exceptions.
Source: From *Ch.4* of *FPHHC*. See text for citations.

Table 1.3. The Theoretical Debate on Space-Time (Part I)

- **Isaac Newton's Absolutist (Substantivist) Theory of Space-Time**
  —space and time are independent from each other. The structure of space-time is $E3 \times E1$ (with the structure of space, *P*, as the set of spatial locations in a three-dimensional Euclidean space, *E3*, and the structure of time as the set of temporal moments, *T*, in the one-dimensional real time, *E1*).
  —space and time are also independent from the effects of matter and events. The existence of space and time is possible even in a world absent of matter (and, for that matter, even in a world absent of events), as if they were material objects but with their total unchangingness thorough time.

- **Albert Einstein's Relativist Theory of Space-Time**
  —space and time are interchangeable (not absolute), just as matter and energy are equivalent (not independent) with the famous equation, $E = mc^2$ (as in the special theory of relativity in 1905).
  —space-time and matter-energy are also relative in a grand union (as in the general theory of relativity in 1915). Thus, each pair affects the other pair, as "matter 'tells' spacetime how to curve [in a non-Euclidean geometry] and curved spacetime 'tells' matter how to behave....Space contracts near mass and dilates away from it. Time dilates near mass and contracts away from it. Clocks positioned farther away from the mass of the earth run faster than clocks closer to the earth." (L. Shlain 1991: 328-330)

(continued on next page)

Table 1.3. The Theoretical Debate on Space-Time (Part II)

- **Peter Baofu's Perspectival Theory of Space-Time**
  —space and time can be understood from multiple perspectives, be they in relation to culture, society, nature, and the mind, with each perspective revealing something about the nature of space-time and simultaneously delimiting its view. This is subject to "the regression-progression principle" in existential dialectics.
  —each perspective of space and time exists in society and culture with good reasons, with some being more successful and hegemonic (dominant) than others. This is subject to "the symmetry-asymmetry principle" in existential dialectics.
  —space and time will not last, to be eventually superseded (altered) by post-humans in different forms (e.g.,stretching/shrinking space-time, engineering more dimensions of space-time, and manipulating multiverses), be they here in this universe or in multiverses. Thus, even the physical existence of space-time cannot last forever, with ever more transformations in the process. This is subject to "the change-constancy principle" in existential dialectics.
  —the conventional wisdom (especially by physicists) of treating the physical perspective of space and time as the foundation of all other perspectives (of space and time) and of regarding them as much less important is a form of reductionism,committing what I call *the foundation fallacy*, in misleadingly dismissing the multiple perspectives of space and time in relation to culture, society, nature, and the mind.

Notes: The examples in each category are solely illustrative (not exhaustive), and the comparison is relative (not absolute), nor are they necessarily mutually exclusive. Some can be easily re-classified elsewhere. As generalities, they allow exceptions.
Source: A summary of *Sec.1.1*, *Sec.1.2*, and *Sec.1.3* of *FPHST*—and, for that matter, the rest of *FPHST*

Table 1.4. Main Reasons for Altering Space-Time

- **The Need to Make New Energy-Matter**
  —Ex: manipulating molecular bonds for new materials
  —Ex: creating nanotechnologies on the atomic scale
  —Ex: engineering the atomic nucleus
  —Ex: restructuring most elementary particles
  —Ex: inventing new forms of matter and energy

- **The Need to Create New Space-Time**
  —Ex: creating "warp drive" (as in science fiction) for space travel
  —Ex: creating "pocket universes"

- **The Need to Conquer the Cosmos unto Multiverses**
  —Ex: spreading floating consciousness and hyper-spatial consciousness, besides other forms that humans have never known, in the cosmos and beyond unto multiverses for ultimate conquest

Notes: The examples in each category are solely illustrative (not exhaustive) nor necessarily mutually exclusive, and the comparison is relative (not absolute). As generalities, they allow exceptions. Also, it should be stressed that the three reasons are all related, in that they all contribute to the evolution of intelligent life in the cosmos unto multiverses in the most distant future beyond our current knowledge.
Sources: A summary of *Sec.6.2* of *FPHST*. See also *FHC*, *FCD*, *FPHC*, *FC*, *FPHU*, and *FPHG*, for example.

Table 1.5. The Technological Frontiers of the Micro-World

- **Type I-Minus**
  —Ex: building structures and mining

- **Type II-Minus**
  —Ex: playing with the genetic makeups of living things

- **Type III-Minus**
  —Ex: manipulating molecular bonds for new materials

- **Type IV-Minus**
  —Ex: creating nanotechnologies on the atomic scale

- **Type V-Minus**
  —Ex: engineering the atomic nucleus

- **Type VI-Minus**
  —Ex: restructuring most elementary particles

- **Type Ω-Minus**
  —Ex: altering the structure of space-time

Notes: As already indicated in *Sec.4.4.2.2* of *FPHC*, the problem with this micro-classification (from Barrow's work) is that the civilization types (with the exception of Type Ω-Minus, for example) are not quite distinct, since many of them can be achieved more or less in a civilization, to the extent that Type II-minus and Type III-minus, just to cite two plausible types, can be historically contemporaneous, relatively speaking, unlike the vast historical distance between, say, Type O and Type I (or Type I and Type II) civilizations. In other words, the micro-classification here is not very useful to understand civilization types but is revealing to see the technological frontiers of the micro-world.
Sources: A reconstruction from J.Barrow (1998:133), as originally shown in *Table 4.7* of *FPHC*. See *FPHC* for more info.

Table 1.6. Finity, Transfinity, and Infinity (Part I)

- **Infinity**
  - —The term "infinity," which is "symbolically represented with ∞," derives from the Latin *infinitas* (or "unboundedness"), to refer to "several distinct concepts—usually linked to the idea of 'without end'—which arise in philosophy, mathematics, and theology." (WK 2008c)
  - —In the context of mathematics, "infinity" is often "treated as if it were a number (i.e., it counts or measures things: 'an infinite number of terms') but it is a different type of 'number' from the real numbers. Infinity is related to limits,...large cardinals,...projective geometry, extended real numbers and the absolute Infinite," for instance. (WK 2008c)

- **Transfinity**
  - —To avoid confusion, my usage of the word "transfinite" (as used here in the ontological principle) is not the same as the one which was originally coined by Georg Cantor to refer to "cardinal numbers or ordinal numbers that are larger than all finite numbers, yet not necessarily absolutely infinite" (in the mind of God), as opposed to "relative" infinity (in the mind of Man). (WK 2008d) In other words, for Cantor, there are two kinds of infinity, "absolute" and "relative"—with "relative" infinity or "transfinity" (in the mind of Man) being dependent on "absolute" infinity (in the mind of God) for its existence.
  - —By contrast, my usage of the word "transfinite" here differs radically from the one used by Cantor (and other mathematicians) and is more limited, in light of the problems confronting any attempt to understand the idea of infinity, be it by intuition, imagination, and conception (as already shown in the prevous three sub-sections).
  - —With this clarification in mind, I allow numbers which can be many times larger—or smaller, for that matter—than the finite things that we encounter in daily life, but they do not have to be related to the idea of infinity at all (which may not exist).

(continued on next page)

Table 1.6. Finity, Transfinity, and Infinity (Part II)

- **Transfinity *(cont'd)***
  —Of course, there may be some *borderline* cases, in which it is not clear whether the number in question is transfinite (in my usage) or simply a mathematical convenience. A good example of a borderline case is the Planck unit of length for "the smallest space possibly measured in nature," which is "less than billionths of trillionths of trillionths of an inch" (or something like 1.6×10^{-35} meters). (P. Baofu 2006a; N. McAleer 1987: 219; WKV 2008; D. Corbett 2008)
  —The ideas concerning symmetry and dimensions in the examples above were addressed in Chapter Three and Chapter Four of *FPHG*. For now, it suffices to further add that it is mind-boggling to even conceive or imagine extreme numbers like the Planck unit of length (or others). Does it really exist at all? Or is it merely a mathematical convenience to describe a physical situation that the human mind does not understand properly?
  —In any event, "transfinity" (in my usage) can be used as a further extension (of number) to the finite numbers in daily life—albeit with some borderline cases in mind.

- **Finity**
  —It refers to numbers which are bounded (that is, with an end), especially (though not exclusively) in relation to things in everyday life.

Source: From *Sec. 1.4* and *Sec. 2.2.3* of *FPHG*

Table 1.7. Theoretical Speculations of Multiverses

- **"Baby Universes" (Ex: Andre Linde and others)**
  —Ex: In a flat universe theory, "even if our part of it eventually collapses,...some spots in the cosmos would suddenly start inflating on their own, creating brand-new 'baby universes.'" (P. Baofu 2000: 623)

- **"Parallel Universes" (Ex: Stephen Hawking and others)**
  —Ex: In quantum cosmology, there allows the existence of infinite numbers of parallel universes, with tunneling among them. (M. Kaku 1994: 256) Hawking later revised his views on this.

- **"Pocket Universes" (Ex: Alan Guth)**
  —Ex: "As the pocket universes live out their lives and recollapse or dwindle away, new universes are generated to take their place....While life in our pocket universe will presumably die out, life in the universe as a whole will thrive for eternity." (A. Guth 1997: 248; P. Baofu 2002: 482)

- **"Brane Worlds" (Ex: Warren Siegel, Lisa Randall, and others)**
  —Ex: Our universe is stuck on a membrane of space-time embedded in a larger cosmos, with different brane worlds connecting and/or colliding with each other.

Notes: These examples are solely illustrative (not exhaustive), and some of the items can be reclassified somewhere else. Nor are they always mutually exclusive. Since they are generalities, exceptions are expected.
Source: From *Table 4.8* of *FPHC*

Table 1.8. The Confusion between "Many Worlds" and "Multiverse" (Part I)

- **First Problem**

—The first problem in this second confusion concerns a debate between the "many-worlds" interpretation of quantum mechanics by Hugh Everett (1957) and others, and the Copenhagen interpretation by Niels Bohr and Werner Heisenberg on the effects of quantum states after interacting with an external environment (e.g., by a measuring observer).

—On the one hand, the Copenhagen interpretation of quantum mechanics is more indeterministic in its concern with the probabilities of the outcomes of a wave function after interacting with an external environment (e.g., by a measuring observer using light to detect, for example, "an electron in a particular region around the nucleus at a particular time." (WK 2008e) Each wave function for the state of a particle refers to "a mathematical representation used to calculate the probability for it to be found in a location, or state of motion." (WK 2008f) And the "wavefunction collapse" means that "the act of measurement causes the calculated set of probabilities to 'collapse' to the value defined by the measurement." (WK 2008f)

—On the other hand, the Everett's interrpetation is more deterministic, in rejecting "the objective reality of wavefunction collapse" and "instead explaining the subjective appearance of wavefunction collapse with the mechanism of quantum decoherence." (WK 2008g) The words "quantum decoherence" here refers to "the mechanism by which quantum systems interact with their environments to exhibit probabilistically additive behavior," in such a way that "the quantum nature of the system is simply 'leaked' into the environment." (WK 2008g) For example, "[a]s a result of an interaction, the wave functions of the system and the measuring device become entangled with each other. Decoherence happens when different portions of the system's wavefunction become entangled *in different ways* [italic added] with the measuring device...." (WK 2008g) Thus, for Everett, the appearance of "wavefunction collapse" can be explained by "quantum decoherence" for quantum states to branch out in different independent worlds after interacting with an external environment.

(continued on next page)

Table 1.8. The Confusion between "Many Worlds" and "Multiverse" (Part II)

• **First Problem** ***(cont'd)***

—Yet, a major criticism against Everett's interpretation is that these different independent worlds in Everett's sense "will never be accessible to us," because of the interference by the measuring observer in an external environment. (WK 2008g)

—For illustration, "once a measurement is done, the measured system becomes entangled with both the physicist who measured it and a huge number of other particles, some of which are photons flying away towards the other end of the universe; in order to prove that the wave function did not collapse one would have to bring all these particles back and measure them again, together with the system that was measured originally. This is completely impractical, but even if one can theoretically do this, it would destroy any evidence that the original measurement took place (including the physicist's memory)." (WK 2008g)

—But then, the critics ask, If these independent worlds in Everett's sense are inaccessible to us, how do we know much of anything really about them?

• **Second Problem**

—What is relevant at the quantum mechanical level may not necessarily apply to the world at the physicsl level.

—In fact, the persistent inability among contemporoary physicists to unifiy the theory of relativity for large objects at the physical level and quantum mechanics for tiny objects at the quantum mechanical level should warn us about the danger of reductionism, by reducing the understanding of different universes ("parallel universes") at the physical level from a generalization of "many worlds" at the quantum mechanical level.

• **Third Problem**

—There is no empirical evidence to suggest that there are infinite (or extremely many) possible worlds in the cosmos as the many-worlds model by Everett would have us to believe.

Source: From *Sec.4.4.1* of *FPHG*

Table 1.9. Hyperspace and Its Challenge (Part I)

- **First Problem**
  —Hyperspace for intra- and inter-universal travel is assumed to be possible, on the basis of four main assumptions; although there may be others, these are the often cited ones.
  —The first assumption concerns the existence of "entry" and "exit" points in hyperspace, which is easier said than done to enter, go through, and then exit hyperspace.
  —For instance, using hyperspace "requires complex calculations...of single or multiple hyperspace jumps and the control of the jump....Peturbations such as those experienced by ship in space from the gravitional field around an object such as a planet or even a star are exacerbated in hyperspatial travel, since mass in real space distorts hyperspace in an equal measure. 'Jumping' near to a gravitational mass is likely to make resulting exit from hyperspace to be highly uncertain, with the level of improbability *i* increasing with the square of the distance to the nearest gravitional 'well.'" (WK 2008h)
  —Besides, "[o]nly spaceships equipped with a special force field can enter hyperspace, because exposure to hyperspace even for short period of time is hazardous to unprotected humans." (WK 2008h)

- **Second Problem**
  —The second assumption concerns the faster-than-light speed. It is well known that Einstein argued for the speed of light as the ultimate limit, but nowadays phyiscists do allow the violation of this limit under certain conditions (like the hypothetical existence of tachyons, as will be explained further in a later sub-section on time travel).
  —Even then, there is a challenge to explain in science fiction "why ships can travel faster than light in hyperspace," and two good arguments are that "hyperspace may be smaller than real space and therefore a star ship's propulsion seems to be greatly multiplied, or else the speed of light in hyperspace is not a barrier as it is in real space. Whatever the reasoning, the general effect is that ships traveling in hyperspace seem to have broken the speed of light, appearing at their destinations much more quickly and without the shift in time that the Theory of Relativity would suggest." (WK 2008h)

(continued on next page)

Table 1.9. Hyperspace and Its Challenge (Part II)

- **Third Problem**
  —The third assumption concerns the speed of time (to be measured, say, by a clock), but this is elaborated in a different section on the related issue of "time travel" (as shown in a different table on time travel).

- **Fourth Problem**
  —The fourth assumption concerns spatial shortcut, as it is possible, because of the curvature of space, in that "the manifold of ordinary three-dimensional space is curved in four or more 'higher' spacial dimensions (a 'hyperspace' in the geometric sense...). This curvature causes certain widely separated points in three-dimensional space to nonetheless be 'adjacent' to each other four-dimensionally. Creating an aperture in 4D space (a wormhole) between these locations can allow instantaneous transit between the two locations; a common comparison is that of a folded piece of paper, where a hole punched through two folded sections is more direct than a line drawn between them on the sheet. This idea probably arose out of certain popular descriptions of General Relativity and/or Riemannian manifolds, and may be the original form from which later concepts of hyperspace arose." (WK 2008h)
  —But this does not mean that hyperpsace is always safe. In fact, "in some science fiction, the danger of hyperspace travel is due to the chance that the route through hyperspace may take a ship too close to a celestial body with a large gravitational field, such as a star. In such scenarios, if a starship passes too close to a large gravitational field while in hyperspace, the ship is forcibly pulled out of hyperspace and reverts to normal space. Therefore, certain hyperspace 'routes' may be mapped out that are safe, not passing too close to stars or other dangers." (WJ 2008h)

Source: From *Sec.4.4.1* of *FPHG*

Table 1.10. The Problems of Time Travel into the Future (Part I)

- **First Problem**
  - —The first problem concerns "time dilation under the Theory of Special Relativity" (which separates space-time from mass-energy as special cases). Suppose you are on a moving train and an observer outside the train is watching you along the tracks. As your train moves along at the speed of light (or something close to it), "time, as measured by your watch, ticked along at a slower pace than time measured by the observer. Not only that, distance changed, too. For the observer, a one-foot ruler whizzing by on the train would have measured less than a foot." (NO 2000)
  - —In fact, you may not even notice that this slower clicking of the clock; in fact, everything looks normal to you inside the train as it was before: "The weird thing is that, for you on the train, time wouldn't seem to be moving slower and your ruler wouldn't be shorter—all would appear normal." (NO 2008) By contrast, you instead think that "time on the rest of the Earth would appear to be ticking along slower and its rulers would be shorter." (NO 2000) So, both of you insist that the other clock (not his) is clicking more slowly—assuming, of course, an inertial frame of reference.
  - —Now, change the story a bit, in that, this time, instead of an "inertial reference frame," acceleration is allowed, and you are on your way to board a spaceship. As an illustration, suppose "[y]ou board a spaceship and take off for deep space. The ship approaches the speed of light. Time for you seems to pass as it always has. It takes you about five seconds to tie your shoe. But to an observer on Earth (assuming he or she could watch you), you are moving at a snail's pace. It takes hours to tie your shoe." (NO 2000) In any event, "you continue on your journey. You slow down, stop, and accelerate back to Earth. You arrive home. You have aged two years during your flight. Two hundred years have passed on Earth. You have successfully travelled forward through time." (NO 2000) In this case, both the observer (if he is still alive) and you agree that you have aged less.

(continued on next page)

Table 1.10. The Problems of Time Travel into the Future (Part II)

- **First Problem *(cont'd)***
  —In other words, when you are back to Earth, a lot of things have changed since, and you may find rather strange to be in a new environment which you hardly recognize, when compared with what you used to think as your city, or the Earth (two years ago, well, in accordance to your time of measurement). This means that you are in the future (two hundred years later), even though you are still relatively young (only two years older). But, can you go back? Well, no. The reason is that "[a]ccording to relativity, you can only move through time in one direction." (NO 2000)

- **Second Problem**
  —The second problem concerns "time dilation under the Theory of General Relativity" (which unifies space-time with mass-energy in a general theory), the same result of time dilation occurs.
  —For instance, when "one clock is deeper in a gravity well than the other," a result is that "the clock deeper in the well" will "tick…more slowly; this effect must be taken into account when calibrating the clocks on the satellites of the Global Positioning System, and it could lead to significant differences in rates of aging for observers at different distances from a black hole." (WK 2008i)
  —More precisely, by way of another example, "it has been calculated that, under general relativity, a person could travel forward in time at a rate four times that of distant observers by residing inside a spherical shell with a diameter of 5 meters and the mass of Jupiter. For such a person, every one second of their 'personal' time would correspond to four seconds for distant observers. Of course, squeezing the mass of a large planet into such a structure is not expected to be within our technological capabilities in the near future." (WK 2008i; R. Gott 2002)
  —The point here, however, is that time travel into the future, in this sense, is allowed, theoretically speaking, but in a very limited way, from the theory of relativity. But one can also ask, What if the theory of relativity were wrong? Well, in that case, there would be a need to find a better theory to explain time travel into the future.

Source: From *Sec.4.4.2* of *FPHG*

Table 1.11. The Problems of Time Travel into the Past (Part I)

- **First Problem**
  - —The first problem concerns the faster-than-light-speed, since, in accordance to the theory of special relativity, when an object goes faster than the speed of light, something weird can happen, in that, instead of having the clock clicking more slowly, it is moving backward, in relation to some inertial frame of reference—which then raisies the issue of whether time travel into the past is possible at all.
  - —But the problem here is about the violation of the law of casuality. In everyday language, an excellent illustration of causality violation is that, suppose you travel back into the past and then kill your parents, this then means that you could not have been born. But this is not true, since you are alive.
  - —Yet, "in the case of a hypothetical signal moving faster than light, there would always be some frames in which the signal was received before it was sent, so that the signal could be said to have moved backwards in time." The violation of casuality exists in this case.
  - —The first part of the problem is that, in accordance to the theory of special relativity, "it would take an infinite amount of energy to accelerate a slower-than-light object to the speed of light"—let alone the energy needed to propel an object to go faster than the speed of light. (WK 2008i) Although some suggest the possibility of "negative energy," it remains to be seen to what extent this is true.
  - —And the second part of the problem is that, "although relativity does not forbid the theoretical possibility of tachyons which move faster than light at all times, when analyzed using quantum field theory it seems that it would not actually be possible to use them to transmit information faster than light and there is no evidence for their existence." (WK 2008i; S. Chase 1993)

(continued on next page)

Table 1.11. The Problems of Time Travel into the Past (Part II)

- **Second Problem**

—The second problem concerns cosmic string and black holes, since it is the theory of general relativity which "extends the special theory to cover gravity, illustrating it in terms of curvature in spacetime caused by mass-energy and the flow of momentum." (WK 2008i)

—On the other hand, "[g]eneral relativity describes the universe under a system of field equations...and there exist solutions to these equations that permit what are called 'closed time-like curves,' and hence time travel into the past....The first of these was proposed by Kurt Gödel, a solution known as the Gödel metric, but his (and many others') example requires the universe to have physical characteristics that it does not appear to have." (WK 2008i; K. Thorne 1994)

—But then, the problem now becomes: "Whether general relativity forbids closed time-like curves for all realistic conditions is unknown." (WK 2008i)

- **Third Problem**

—The third problem concerns wormholes and related ones, and "[w]ormholes are a hypothetical warped spacetime which are also permitted by the Einstein field equations of general relativity, although it would be impossible to travel through a wormhole unless it was what is known as a traversable wormhole." (WK 2008i; M. Visser 1995) In other words, "a wormhole is a hypothetical topological feature of spacetime that is fundamentally a 'shortcut' through space and time. Spacetime can be viewed as a 2D surface, and when 'folded' over, a wormhole bridge can be formed. A wormhole has at least two mouths which are connected to a single throat or tube. If the wormhole is traversable, matter can 'travel' from one mouth to the other by passing through the throat." (WK 2008j)

—But the problem here is three-fold, as shown in what follows.

(continued on next page)

Table 1.11. The Problems of Time Travel into the Past (Part III)

- **Third Problem *(cont'd)***
  —The first part of the problem is that "there is no observational evidence for wormholes." (WK 2008j)
  —The second part of the problem is that it is not clear how exactly wormholes (and black holes, for that matter) could allow time travel into the past at all.
  —And the third part of the problem is that if using wormholes (and black holes, for that matter) to travel into the past requires something to go faster than light too, then this raises another issue concerning the two problems as previously indicated in the sub-section on the faster-than-light-speed.

- **Fourth Problem**
  —The fourth problem is that some physicists have argued that, even should time travel into the past be possible, by way of these three methods, the person still would not return to the same past history that he exactly experienced before, but in a different one. (WK 2008i)
  —In other words, "strictly speaking," time travel into the past is not "really" possible, in light of these criticisms, so there is no need to worry that one could travel into the past and kill one's parent, as a way to violate the law of casuality.

Source: From *Sec.4.4.2* of *FPHG*

Table 1.12. The Conceptual Dimensions of Consciousness (and Other Mental States)

- **On Heredity and Time**
  —Heredity and the Environment
  —The Past and the Present

- **On Layers of Mental States and Abnormality**
  —Consciousness, Unconsciousness, and Preconsciousness
  —Normality and Paranormality

- **On Organicity and Motivation**
  —Mechanicity and Organicity
  —Primary Motivations and Multiple Motivations

- **On Other (Mostly Epistemic) Considerations**
  —Synthesis and Analysis
  —Situation and the Subject
  —Process and Outcome
  —Reasoning and Other Modes of Thinking
  —Meta-Conceptual Nominalism and Realism

Notes:: These examples are solely illustrative (not exhaustive), and some of the items can be reclassified somewhere else. Nor are they always mutually exclusive. Since they are generalities, exceptions are expected.
Sources: From *FPHC*. A re-construction, but with my own contribution, originally from G.Lindzey & C.Hall, *Introduction to Theories of Personality* (NY: John Wiley & Sons, 1985).

Table 1.13. The Theoretical Levels of Consciousness (and Other Mental States) (Part I)

- **At the Micro-Physical Theoretical Level**
  —Quantum-Mechanics
  —Electromagnetism

- **At the Chemical Theoretical Level**
  —Biochemistry

- **At the Biological Theoretical Level**
  —Evolutionary Biology
  —Neuroscience
  —Artificial Intelligence

- **At the Psychological Theoretical Level**
  —Psychodynamic Psychology
    - Psychoanalytical Psychology
    - Analytical Psychology
    - Socially Oriented Psychology

  —Experimental (Behavioral) Psychology
    - Operant Reinforcement Theory
    - Stimulus-Response Theory
    - Social Learning Theory

  —Cognitive (Gestalt) Psychology
    - Humanist Psychology
    - Existential Psychology
    - Field Theory

  —Psychometric Psychology
    - Idiographics
    - Constitutional Psychology

  —Social Psychology
    - Symbolic Interactive Theory
    - Social Exchange Theory

(continued on next page)

Table 1.13. The Theoretical Levels of Consciousness (and Other Mental States) (Part II)

- **At the Organizational Theoretical Level**
  - —Managerial-Bureaucratic Theory
  - —Oligarchic Theory
  - —Network Theory

- **At the Institutional Theoretical Level**
  - —Functionalist Theory
  - —Anomic Theory

- **At the Structural Theoretical Level**
  - —Conflict Theory
    - Marxian Theory
    - Critical Theory
    - Weberian Theory
  - —Games Theory (in Formal Theory)
  - —Feminist Theory
    - Feminist Concerns
    - Feminist Hopes

- **At the Systemic Theoretical Level**
  - —Equilibrium Theory
  - —System Theory
  - —Chaos Theory

- **At the Cosmological Theoretical Level**
  - —Superluminal Model
  - —The Theory of Floating Consciousness

(continued on next page)

Table 1.13. The Theoretical Levels of Consciousness (and Other Mental States) (Part III)

- **At the Cultural Theoretical Level**
  - —Substantive Theories
    - Structuralist Theory
    - Post-Structuralist Theory (in Postmodernism)
  - —Meta-Theories
    - Epistemic Objectivism vs. Epistemic Historicism
    - Epistemic Subjectivism vs. Epistemic Non-Subjectivism
      - –Phenomenology
      - –Ethnomethodology
      - –Hermeneutics
    - Epistemic Relativism vs. Epistemic Absolutism
    - Epistemic Reductionism vs. Epistemic Emergencism

- **At Other Levels**
  - —Structuration Theory
  - —Reflexive Socioanalysis

Notes: These examples are solely illustrative (not exhaustive), and some of the items can be reclassified somewhere else. Nor are they always mutually exclusive. Since they are generalities, exceptions are expected.
Source: From many different sources as indicated in *FPHC*

Table 1.14. The Thematic Issues of Consciousness (and Other Mental States)

- **The Factor of History**
  - —Pre-Modernity
  - —Modernity
  - —Postmodernity
  - —After-Postmodernity

- **The Importance of Needs**
  - —Having (e.g., the everyday, the technological)
  - —Belonging (e.g., the just and the good)
  - —Being (e.g., the true, the holy, the sublime/beautiful, and the good)

Notes: These examples are solely illustrative (not exhaustive). Nor are they always mutually exclusive. Since they are generalities, exceptions are expected. Also, some categories overlap with others; for instance, the good is also related with being-ness, just as the everyday can be connected with belong-ness.
Sources: From *FPHC*, based on *FHC* and *FCD*

Table 1.15. Having, Belonging, and Being in Consciousness

- **Having (e.g., About the Everyday and Technological)**
  —Ex: Physiological needs (e.g., thirst, hunger, sex)
  —Ex: Safety (e.g., stability, freedom from fear and anxiety)

- **Belonging (e.g., About the Good and Just)**
  —Ex: Social interaction
  —Ex: Friendship, acquaintance
  —Ex: Love, family
  —Ex: Self-respect, respect from others

- **Being (e.g., About the True, Holy, Beautiful/Sublime, and Good)**
  —Ex: Understanding of reality about self and world
  —Ex: Spiritual quest for holiness, beauty, sublimity, and goodness

Notes: These examples are solely illustrative (not exhaustive), and some of the items can be reclassified somewhere else. Nor are they always mutually exclusive. Since they are generalities, exceptions are expected.
Sources: From *FPHC*, based on *FHC* and *FCD*

Table 1.16. The Having-Ness of Consciousness (and Other Mental States)

- **At the Micro-Physical Level**
  —Ex: The finer physics of nutrition

- **At the Chemical Level**
  —Ex: Food guide pyramid

- **At the Bio-Psychological Level**
  —Ex: The hierarchy of needs

- **At the Institutional Level**
  —Ex: The production of commodity fetishism

- **At the Organizational Level**
  —Ex: Mass standardization (and customization); bureaucratic rationality

- **At the Structural Level**
  —Ex: The divide between the haves and the have-nots

- **At the Cultural Level**
  —Ex: The bondage of greater expectations

- **At the Systemic Level**
  —Ex: The technological transformation of poverty with transvaluations

- **At the Cosmological Level**
  —Ex: Floating consciousness in deep space without the human physiological needs

Notes: These examples are solely illustrative (not exhaustive), and some of the items can be reclassified somewhere else. Nor are they always mutually exclusive. Since they are generalities, exceptions are expected.
Sources: From *FPHC*. See also *FCD* and *FHC*.

Table 1.17. The Belonging-Ness of Consciousness (and Other Mental States)

- **At the Micro-Physical Level**
  —Ex: Statistical physics and social networks

- **At the Chemical Level**
  —Ex: Olfaction and social relations

- **At the Bio-Psychological Level**
  —Ex: Dual human nature on relationships

- **At the Institutional Level**
  —Ex: Private property and social cleavage

- **At the Organizational Level**
  —Ex: Legal formalism and iron cage

- **At the Structural Level**
  —Ex: Class conflicts and social alienation

- **At the Cultural Level**
  —Ex: Ruthless society and the culture of law

- **At the Systemic Level**
  —Ex: Human extinction and post-human relations

- **At the Cosmological Level**
  —Ex: The transcendence of equality in the cosmos and beyond

Notes: These examples are solely illustrative (not exhaustive), and some of the items can be reclassified somewhere else. Nor are they always mutually exclusive. Since they are generalities, exceptions are expected.
Sources: From *FPHC*. See also *FCD* and *FHC*.

Table 1.18. The Being-Ness of Consciousness (and Other Mental States) (Part I)

- **At the Micro-Physical Level**
  —Ex: Space-time and matter-energy in classical mechanics, quantum mechanics, and the theory of relativity

- **At the Chemical Level**
  —Ex: Drugs and well being

- **At the Biological Level**
  —Ex: Neuroscience and mystical experiences

- **At the Psychological Level**
  —Ex: Reductionism and emergencism

- **At the Institutional Level**
  —Ex: The proliferation of cults and sects, and the corporate-art industry

- **At the Organizational Level**
  —Ex: The organization of ideas in the scheme of things

- **At the Structural Level**
  —Ex: Disciplinary power and control in the order of things

- **At the Systemic Level**
  —Ex: Mutualism and ecological psychology

- **At the Cultural Level**
  —Ex: The recurrence of competing spirits, and floating consciousness as a climax of evolution

(continued on next page)

Table 1.18. The Being-Ness of Consciousness (and Other Mental States) (Part II)

- **At the Cosmological Level**
  —Ex: The search for elsewherewhen, and the evolution of other consciousnesses (e.g., the hyper-spatial consciousness)

Notes: These examples are solely illustrative (not exhaustive), and some of the items can be reclassified somewhere else. Nor are they always mutually exclusive. Since they are generalities, exceptions are expected.
Sources: From *FPHC*. See also *FCD* and *FHC*.

Table 1.19. Cognitive Partiality in Different Mental States

- **The Conscious**
  - —*Biased*
    - Ex: Self-overratingness
    - Ex: Self-modesty
    - Ex: Self-fulfilling prophesy
  - —*Shallow*
    - Ex: Attribution error
    - Ex: Heuristics
    - Ex: Illusory thinking
  - —*Short-term*
    - Ex: Deindividuation
  - —*Materialistic*
    - Ex: Hierarchy of needs

- **The Subconscious**
  - Ex: mental reconstruction
  - Ex: stereotyping

- **The Unconscious**
  - Ex: automatic processing
  - Ex: cognitive intuition

Notes: These examples are solely illustrative (not exhaustive), and some of the items can be reclassified somewhere else. Nor are they always mutually exclusive. Since they are generalities, exceptions are expected. And the comparison is relative, not absolute.
Source: From *BCPC*

Table 1.20. Emotional Non-Neutrality and Behavioral Alteration in Different Mental States

- **The Emotional**
  - —*Conscious*
    - Ex: Feelings
  - —*Subconscious*
    - Ex: Moods
  - —*Unconscious*
    - Ex: Empathy
    - Ex: Instincts

- **The Behavioral**
  - —*Conscious*
    - Ex: Foot-in-the-door
    - Ex: Role playing
    - Ex: Saying-is-believing
  - —*Subconscious*
    - Ex: Discrimination
  - —*Unconscious*
    - Ex: Non-Verbal Communication

Notes: These examples are solely illustrative (not exhaustive), and some of the items can be reclassified somewhere else. Nor are they always mutually exclusive. Since they are generalities, exceptions are expected. And the comparison is relative, not absolute.
Source: From *BCPC*

Table 1.21. The Limits of Intuition in Unconsciousness

- **Cognitive Intuition (or Intuitive Thinking)**
  - —*Features*
    - Ex: mental schemas
    - Ex: expertise
    - Ex: blindsight
  - —*Problems*
    - Ex: inaccurate
    - Ex: non-explanatory

- **Emotional Intuition**
  - —*Features*
    - Ex: empathy
    - Ex: instincts
  - —*Problems*
    - Ex: over-generalized
    - Ex: non-explanatory

- **Behavioral Intuition**
  - —*Features*
    - Ex: prosemics
    - Ex: kinesics
  - —*Problems*
    - Ex: unreliable
    - Ex: non-explanatory

Notes: These examples are solely illustrative (not exhaustive), and some of the items can be reclassified somewhere else. Nor are they always mutually exclusive. Since they are generalities, exceptions are expected. And the comparison is relative, not absolute.
Source: From *BCPC*

Table 1.22. The Wealth/Poverty Dialectics in Different Mental States: The Case of Cognition

- **The Conscious**
  - —*Biased*
    - Ex: If richer in self-serving bias, then poorer in understanding others
  - —*Shallow*
    - Ex: If richer in heuristic thinking, then poorer in comprehending reality
  - —*Short-term*
    - Ex: If richer in short-term tendency, then poorer in long-term planning
  - —*Materialistic*
    - Ex: If richer in physiological obsession, then poorer in spiritual enlightenment

- **The Subconscious**
  - Ex: If richer in mental reconstruction, then poorer in accuracy of recall
  - Ex: If richer in stereotyping, then poorer in understanding groups

- **The Unconscious**
  - Ex: If richer in automatic processing, then poorer in depth of analysis
  - Ex: If richer in cognitive intuition, then poorer in reliability of judgments

Notes: These examples are solely illustrative (not exhaustive), and some of the items can be reclassified somewhere else. Nor are they always mutually exclusive. Since they are generalities, exceptions are expected. And the comparison is relative, not absolute.
Source: From *BCPC*

Table 1.23. The Wealth/Poverty Dialectics in Different Mental States: The Case of Emotion and Behavior

- **Emotion**
  - —*Conscious*
    - Ex: If richer in relying on familiarity and similarity for social attraction, then poorer in having diverse social relations
  - —*Subconscious*
    - Ex: If richer in moodiness, then poorer in sober thinking
  - —*Unconscious*
    - Ex: If richer in empathy, then poorer in task-oriented efficiency
    - Ex: If richer in instincts, then poorer in critical thinking

- **Behavior**
  - —*Conscious*
    - Ex: If richer in foot-in-the-door technique, then poorer in instant Gratification
    - Ex: If richer in role playing, then poorer in identity stability
  - —*Subconscious*
    - Ex: If richer in discriminating, then poorer in social harmony
  - —*Unconscious*
    - Ex: If richer in kinesics and proxemics, then poorer in verbal skills, relatively speaking.

Notes: These examples are solely illustrative (not exhaustive), and some of the items can be reclassified somewhere else. Nor are they always mutually exclusive. Since they are generalities, exceptions are expected. And the comparison is relative, not absolute.
Source: From *BCPC*

Table 1.24. The Theoretical Debate on Nature vs. Nurture (Part I)

- **The Environmental Approach**
  —*Thesis*: It focuses, relatively speaking, more on the environment (culture and society) in explaining the achievement gap among individuals and for that matter, countries or regions, when contrasted with the natural factors.
  —*Discourse*: Examples include Jose Ortega y Gasset ("Man has no nature; what he has is history"), Ashley Montagu ("Man is man because he has no instincts, because everything he is and has become he has learned from his culture, from the man-made part of the environment, from other human beings"), Stephen Jay Gould ("[The] brain [is] capable of a full range of behaviors and predisposed to none"), and Jesse Jackson (who blames white racism for the failure of blacks to close the achievement gap between whites and blacks in America). The works on dependency theory in international political economy (with a Marxian influence) and on the Protestant work ethic (by Max Weber) also point to this environmental direction.

- **The Genetic Approach**
  —*Thesis*: It focuses instead, relatively speaking again, on hereditory factors (e.g., genes and evolution) in explaining the achievement gap among individuals and for that matter, countries or regions, when contrasted with the envrionmental factors.
  —*Discourse*: Examples are Hans Eysenck and William Sheldon (in constitutional psychology), Konrad Lorenz (in his work on innate aggressive human nature), Gary Marcus (on the complexities of human thought by a tiny number of genes) and Robert Plomin, together with Michael Owen and Peter McGuffin (on the genetic basis of complex human behaviors).

(continued on next page)

Table 1.24. The Theoretical Debate on Nature vs. Nurture (Part II)

- **The Compromise Approach**
  —*Thesis*: It seeks the middle-of-the-road argument in regard to nature and nurture and regards all differences among individuals and groups as the result of the mixture of both nature and nurture, more or less equally.
  —*Discourse*: Examples include C. Murray and R. Herrnstein ("It seems highly likely to us that both genes and environment have something to do with this issue") and Dan Dennett ("Surely 'everyone knows' that the nature-nurture debate was resolved long ago, and neither side wins since everything – is – a – mixture – of – both – and - it's – all – very -complicated…."

- **The Transcendent Approach**
  —*Thesis*: It goes beyond both nature and nurture (without, however, committing the compromise fallacy) in showing their closely intertwined interactions in producing the behavioral differences as often seen in individual human endeavors on the micro scale, and for that matter, in country (or regional) endeavors on the macro one—in the context of my five theses, namely, (a) the compromise fallacy, (b) no oppression without self-oppression, (c) no success without failure, (d) the factor of randomness, and (e) the post-human vision, to be elaborated in Chapter Six.
  —*Discourse*: Peter Baofu proposed this approach on the basis of his "theory of contrastive advantages" (as an original theoretical contribution to the debate, which was first proposed and analyzed in *The Future of Capitalism and Democracy*). In the end, the human genes will not last, to be eventually superseded by post-human life forms, so the debate between genes and memes has obscured something profoundly important about the future that the world has never known. And the debate is also misleading and faulty in its dichotomy.

Source: From *BNN*. See the book for citations and details.

Table 1.25. Physical Challenges to Hyper-Spatial Consciousness

- **The Understanding of a Higher-Dimensional World of Space-Time**
  —Ex: 4 for traditional aspects of space-time (e.g., length, width, breadth and time) plus 6 more new dimensions in theory of hyper-space, with profound implications for practical applications to new forms of consciousness.

- **The Mastering of Dark Matter and Dark Energy**
  —Ex: "ordinary matter" (e.g., atoms, molecules) as a mere 4.4% of the universe, with 23% made of "cold dark matter" and the rest (about 73%) of mysterious "dark energy," with fundamental significance to questions about the limit of the speed of energy (or info), the availability of energy for use, and the nature of space-time, just to cite some examples.

- **The Exploration of Multiverses**
  —Ex: theoretical speculation of other universes (e.g., "baby universes," "gateways" in black holes, "wave function of the universe," "many worlds," "brane worlds"), with potentially seminary discoveries of different physical laws in relation to matter-energy and space-time, and vital differences to the future of post-human conquest of other universes (for the emergence of new forms of consciousness).

Notes: These examples are solely illustrative (not exhaustive), and some of the items can be reclassified somewhere else. Nor are they always mutually exclusive. Since they are generalities, exceptions are expected. The point here is to give a rough picture of the evolution of consciousness to the hyper-spatial consciousness and others totally unknown to current earthlings. As a note of clarification, it makes no difference to my argument as to whether or not the hyper-spatial consciousness may emerge before, during, and after floating consciousness.
Source: From *Table 4.5* of *FPHC*

Table 1.26. The Theory of Floating Consciousness (Part I)

- **At the Micro-Physical Level**
  —Ex: intelligent life without the human physical-chemical system

- **At the Chemical Level**
  —Ex: space radiation and toxins

- **At the Bio-Psychological Level**
  —Ex: exo-biological evolution in deep space
  —Ex: genetic engineering of new beings

- **At the Institutional Level**
  —Ex: post-capitalism
  —Ex: post-democracy

- **At the Organizational Level**
  —Ex: less legal-formalistic routines

- **At the Structural Level**
  —Ex: alien forms of violence

- **At the Cultural Level**
  —Ex: transcending freedom
  —Ex: transcending equality

(continued on next page)

Table 1.26. The Theory of Floating Consciousness (Part II)

- **At the Cosmological Level**
  —Ex: parallel universes
  —Ex: pocket universes

- **At the Systemic Level**
  —Ex: space habitats (in zero-gravity)

Notes: Each example draws from the works of different scholars in the field. For instance, at the cosmological level, the idea of parallel universes is from the theoretical speculation in quantum cosmology by Stephen Hawking and others, while the one of pocket universes comes from the theoretical work of Allan Guth at MIT. And at the institutional level, I proposed post-capitalism and post-democracy in *FCD* (and later, from *BDPD* and *BCPC*). In addition, the examples are solely illustrative (not exhaustive), and some of the items can be reclassified somewhere else. Nor are they always mutually exclusive. Since they are generalities, exceptions are expected.
Sources: From *FPHC*—and, originally, from *FCD*

Table 1.27. The Potential of Unfolding Unconsciousness

- **Superior Senses**
  - —*Through space*
    - Ex: clair-sentience (in feeling)
    - Ex: clair-voyance (in seeing)
    - Ex: clair-audience (in hearing)
    - Ex: clair-austance (in tasting)
    - Ex: clair-alience (in smelling)
    - Ex: clair-cognizance (in knowing)
  - —*Through time*
    - Ex: pre-cognition (in knowing), pre-sentiment (in feeling)
    - Ex: retro-cognition (in knowing), retro-sentiment (in feeling)

- **Superior Contacts**
  - —*With living minds*
    - Ex: telepathy
  - —*With the dead*
    - Ex: mediumship
  - —*With other-living entities*
    - Ex: telekinesis

Notes: The categories and examples are solely illustrative (not exhaustive), and the comparison is relative (not absolute), nor are they necessarily mutually exclusive. And some can be easily re-classified elsewhere. As generalities, they allow exceptions.
Source: A summary of Ch.5 of *FPHU*

Table 1.28. The Future Exploration of Unfolding Unconsciousness

- **In the Context of Nature**
  —Ex: the higher-dimensional space-time in hyperspace theory
  —Ex: the particle-wave interactions in quantum mechanics
  —Ex: the study of brain waves in electromagnetic theory

- **In the Context of the Mind**
  —Ex: the unconscious fantasies in psychoanalysis
  —Ex: the mind-altering drugs in biochemistry
  —Ex: the manipulation of neural activity in neurobiology

- **In the Context of Culture**
  —Ex: the correlation between anomalous experience and moral/religious/aesthetic interests in culture studies
  —Ex: the role of myths and language in epistemology

- **In the Context of Society**
  —Ex: different organizational agendas in anomalous research
  —Ex: the scholarly divide on anomalous study
  —Ex: interests and propaganda in institutioanl research
  —Ex: the transformative power of technology in research on social systems
  —Ex: the natural and non-natural selection of other worlds in exo-biology
  —Ex: the role of the post-human conscious mind in qualitative demography

Notes: The examples in each category are solely illustrative (not exhaustive), and the comparison is relative (not absolute), nor are they necessarily mutually exclusive. And some can be easily re-classified elsewhere. As generalities, they allow exceptions.
Source: A summary of Chs.2-5 of *FPHU*, in conjunction with the rest of the book

Table 1.29. Creative Techniques and Traits

- **Creative Techniques**
  - —*Comprehensiveness*
    - Ex: Broadness of Scope
    - Ex: In-Depth Analysis
    - Ex: Multifaceted Taxonomy
    - Ex: Numerous Theories
  - —*Arrangement*
    - Ex: Separation (or Subtraction)
    - Ex: Combination (or Addition)
    - Ex: Replacement
    - Ex: Accommodation
    - Ex: Reversal
    - Ex: Stretching
  - —*Serendipity*
    - Ex: Play
    - Ex: Chance

- **Creative Traits**
  - —*Openness / Risk*
    - Ex: Ability to welcome new ideas or to do new things, with risk
  - —*Discipline*
    - Ex: Ability to sacrifice whatever it takes to succeed
  - —*Resilience / Confidence*
    - Ex: Ability to take failures to mind, not to heart
  - —*Trust*
    - Ex: Ability to cooperate with others for team work, if necessary

Notes: The examples in the categories are solely illustrative (not exhaustive), and the comparison is relative (not absolute), nor are they necessarily mutually exclusive. And some can be easily re-classified elsewhere. As generalities, they allow exceptions.
Source: From *Sec.4.2* of *FPHCT*. For more details, also read the rest of the book.

Table 1.30. The Desirability of Creativity, and Its Dark Sides (Part I)

- **In Relation to Instrumental Rationality**
  - —*Desirability*
    - Ex: For the sake of efficiency and effectiveness in this capitalist era of our time.
  - —*Undesirability*
    - Ex: What Max Weber (1930) called the "iron cage" of capitalism, where live the "sensualists without heart, specialists without spirit"—or something which the Frankfurt School has forcefully asked us to be freed from.
- **In Relation to Substantive Rationality**
  - —*Desirability*
    - Ex: For the sake of God, the King, Motherland, or other comparable ideals.
  - —*Undesirability*
    - Ex: Domination and oppression of various forms—something which the moderns had struggled to free themselves from in the first place, since the dawn of modernity.
- **In Relation to Autonomous Rationality**
  - —*Desirability*
    - Ex: For the sake of itself, the autonomy of creative endeavor.
  - —*Undesirability*
    - Ex: The decadence of its own degeneration (e.g., the donwsides of postmodernism in our postmodern times, or what Nietzsche once called the unbearable "unreality" and "falseness" of the autonomous artist's "innermost existence"—and, in other cases, the painful suffering from different mental illnesses for those highly creative individuals).

(continued on next page)

Table 1.30. The Desirability of Creativity, and Its Dark Sides (Part II)

Notes: The examples in the categories are solely illustrative (not exhaustive), and the comparison is relative (not absolute), nor are they necessarily mutually exclusive. And some can be easily re-classified elsewhere. As generalities, they allow exceptions.
Also, I already went to great lenghts to explain the desirability and its dark sides of all these three rationalities (although there may be others too) in the two volumes of *FHC*—and, for that matter, *FCD*.
Source: From *Sec.4.9* of *FPHCT*. For more details, also read the rest of the book.

Table 1.31. Posthuman-Ism, Post-Humanism, and Trans-Humanism

- **Post-Humanism**
  —The neologism "post-human" used in my books should *not* be confused with another term which looks similar but has a totally different meaning in the literature of postmodernism, namely, "post-humanism"—which constitutes a critique of "humanism" as tradionally understood (especially, though not exclusively, in relation to the idea of progress in science and reason in the Enlightenment project). (WK 2008)
  —My works reject the project of "postmodernism" and propose the future world of what I orignally called "after-postmodernity" in *FHC* and *FCD*, for instance.

- **Trans-Humanism**
  —Also, the neologism "post-human" used in my books should *not* be confused with a similar term which is used to champion the ideology of technology for the fturue co-existence between humans and cyborgs in "trans-humanism." (WK 2008a)
  —Instead, my term "post-human" in relation to "posthuman-ism" also rejects "trans-humanism" (especially, though not exclusively, in relation to the promises of technology) and refers to something else altogether, that is, the future extinction of humans and its post-human successors in deep space and beyond unto multiverses.
  —Chapter Two of my book on ethics (*BEPE*) provides a more comprehensive critique of trans-humanism.

- **Posthuman-Ism**
  —With these two clarifications in mind, the "post-humans" (as envisioned in my books) can take different forms, and I proposed, in my different books, some of them, such as "unfolding unconsciousness," "floating consciousness," "hyper-spatial consciousness," "thinking machines," "thinking robots," "genetically altered superior beings," "cyborgs," and others (as already analyzed in my previous works).
  —They will evolve in conjunction with other visions of mine in relation to nature, society, and culture.

Sources: From *Sec.1.6* of *FPHE* (and also *BEPE*). For more details, also read the rest of the books (and other books of mine).

Table 1.32. Three Great Future Transformations of the Martial Body (Part I)

- **Virtual Battle**
  —Ex: virtual fight
  —Ex: virtual memory

- **The Hyper-Martial Body**
  —*In relation to the physical dimension*
  - Ex: striking (e.g., punching, kicking, trapping, acupressure-striking, and so on in an amazing way)
  - Ex: grapping (e.g., throwing, pinning, joint-locking, and so on in an amazing way)
  - Ex: running and walking (e.g., on different surfaces)
  - Ex: jumping (e.g., through walls, trees, etc.)
  - Ex: flying (e.g., through space)
  - Ex: enduring pain (e.g., absorbing punches, kicks, and so on in an amazing way)
  - Ex: using extremely advanced hi-tech weapons
  - Ex: healing (e.g., with special energy, etc.)
  - Ex: entering (e.g., into different dimensions of space)
  - Ex: sensing (e.g., in extraordinary ways through space and time, etc.)
  - Ex: wearing hi-tech suits for defensive and offensive purposes (e.g., like a hi-tech armor)

  —*In relation to the mental dimension*
  - Ex: the ability to relax the martial body in a way that current humans cannot.
  - Ex: the ability to concentrate the martial mind in a way that current humans are not accustomed to.
  - Ex: the ability to breathe and be timely in preparing the martial body for fighting in a way that current humans are not good at.

- **The Post-Martial Floating Mind**
  —Ex: the mind without the human body
  —Ex: the quest for spirituality beyond martial arts

(continued on next page)

Table 1.32. Three Great Future Transformations of the Martial Body (Part II)

Notes: The examples in the categories are solely illustrative (not exhaustive), and the comparison is relative (not absolute), nor are they necessarily mutually exclusive. And some can be easily re-classified elsewhere. As generalities, they allow exceptions.
Source: From *Sec. 2.5.1* of *FPHMA*. See text for citations.

Table 1.33. Three Great Future Transformations of the Sexual Body

- **Virtual Pleasure**
  —Ex: virtual Sex
  —Ex: virtual Recall

- **The Hyper-Sexual Body**
  —*In relation to the physical dimension*
  - Ex: the ability to perform differenet sexual positions without the various physical limitations that humans currently have.
  - Ex: the ability to produce unusual amount of sexual energy to endure in sexual acts in a way that humans currently cannot.
  - Ex: the ability to engage in multiple sexual experiences comparable to (but different from) non-human sexuality (e.g., hermaphrodite, monoecious, sex-switching, and many other types) that current humans cannot.

  —*In relation to the mental dimension*
  - Ex: the ability to relax the sexual body in a way that current humans are not accustomed to.
  - Ex: the ability to concentrate the sexual mind in a way that current humans are not good at.
  - Ex: the ability to breathe and be patient in preparing the sexual body for sexuality in a way that current humans are not able to.

- **The Post-Sexual Floating Mind**
  —Ex: the mind without the human body
  —Ex: the quest for spirituality beyond sexuality

Notes: The examples in the categories are solely illustrative (not exhaustive), and the comparison is relative (not absolute), nor are they necessarily mutually exclusive. And some can be easily re-classified elsewhere. As generalities, they allow exceptions.
Source: From *Sec. 3.4.2* of *FPHS*. See text for more info.

Table 1.34. The Trinity of Pre-Modernity

- **Pre-Free-Spirited Pre-Modernity (Pre-Modernism) and Its Internal Split**
  —Competing worldviews and values both within and between linear centric (e.g., Islamic, Christian, Judaic, Imperial Roman) and cyclical-centric (e.g., Confucian, Taoist, Hindu, and Buddhist) orientations
  —Compare modernism with pre-modernism here in relation to the seven dimensions of human existence like the true and the holy (e.g., different versions of epistemic dogmas and religious superstitions), the everyday and the technological (e.g.,different versions of non-technophilism and non-consumerism), the beautiful/sublime (e.g., different versions of aesthetic non-autonomy), and the good and the just (e.g., different versions of moral particularism).

- **Pre-Capitalist Pre-Modernity (Pre-Modernization) and Its Own Discontents**
  —Competing versions of societal arrangements (e.g., feudalism, monarchism, and the holy order)

- **Hegemonic Pre-Modernity and Its Countervailing Forces**
  —Different power centers and their enemies (e.g., the Roman Empire and the "barbarian hordes," the "Holy Crusades" and the Muslims, the Middle Kingdom and the invading tribes, different social castes in India, and warring Greek city-states)

Notes: The examples in each category are solely illustrative (not exhaustive) nor necessarily mutually exclusive, and the comparison is relative (not absolute). As generalities, they allow exceptions. Also, it does not matter what the "base" era is in the analysis of any trinity. And in the present context, the "base" era is modernity (for instance, with its "free-spirited modernity" and the other two parts). So, for pre-modernity, the trinity takes the form of, say, "pre-free-spirited pre-modernity," together with the other two parts.
Sources: From Ch.2 of *BCIV* and also the 2 volumes of *FHC*

Table 1.35. The Trinity of Modernity (Part I)

- **Free-Spirited Modernity (Modernism) and Its Internal Split**

—*On the True and the Holy*
  - The freedom from the dogmas of the past to the better understanding of, and union with, the world and self (Ch.3 of *FHC*)
  - Alternative discourses: about the true (e.g., anti-science discourses) and the holy (non-mainstream theologies) (Ch.3 of *FHC*)

—*On the Technological and the Everyday*
  - The freedom from life harshness to the higher technophilic, consumeristic lifeform (Ch.2 of *FHC*)
  - Alternative discourses: about the everyday (e.g., transcendental mindsets) and the technological (e.g., Arcadianism) (Ch.2 of *FHC*)

—*On the Good and the Just*
  - The freedom from the theo-aristocratic tyranny to the moral universality for a just society (Ch.5 of *FHC*)
  - Alternative discourses: about the just (e.g., Communism, Anarchism) and the good (e.g., Nazism/Fascism, and Zarathustrianism) (Chs.5-6 of *FHC*)

—*On the Beautiful and the Sublime*
  - The freedom from the external distortion of aesthetic pleasure to the boundless infinity of totality in artistic autonomy (Ch.4 of *FHC*)
  - Alternative discourses: about the beautiful/sublime (e.g., kitsch and historical avant-gardism) (Ch.4 of *FHC*)

- **Capitalist Modernity (Modernization) and Its Own Discontents**

—*During the Industrial Revolution*
  - Ex: Marx on the institution of inequality (Ch.1 of *FHC*)

—*During the Modern Rational-Instrumental Epoch*
  - Ex: Weber on the politics of soft liberal institutions (Ch.5 of *FHC*)

—*During the Great Depression*
  - Ex: Keynes on the myth of the free market (Chs.1-3 of *FHC*)

—*During the Cold War*
  - Ex: Lasch on the narcissistic culture industry (Chs.2-3 of *FHC*)

(continued on next page)

Table 1.35. The Trinity of Modernity (Part II)

- **Hegemonic Modernity and Its Countervailing Forces**
  —*The Legacies of Colonialism and Imperialism*
    - Ex: European colonization of most of the modern world (Ch.1 of *FHC*)

  —*The Struggle for Decolonialization*
    - Ex: The countervailing forces of resentment, rechantment, and regionalism (Chs.1 & 6 of *FHC*)

Notes: The examples in each category are solely illustrative (not exhaustive) nor necessarily mutually exclusive, and the comparison is relative (not absolute). As generalities, they allow exceptions.
Sources: From the 2 volumes of *FHC*—and also from *FCD*

Table 1.36. The Trinity of Post-Modernity

- **Free-Spirited Postmodernity (Postmodernism) and Its Internal Split**

  —*On the True and the Holy*
  - Postmodern performative turn for knowing and its enemies (Ch.3 of *FHC*)
  - Postmodern comparative theology and its opponents (Ch.3 of *FHC*)

  —*On the Technological and the Everyday*
  - Postmodern corporate technological mindset and its adversaries (Ch.2 of *FHC*)
  - Postmodern postmaterialism and its critics (Ch.2 of *FHC*)

  —*On the Good and the Just*
  - Postmodern politics of difference and its foes (Ch.5 of *FHC*)

  —*On the Beautiful and the Sublime*
  - Postmodern deconstruction and its dissenters (Ch.4 of *FHC*)

- **Capitalist Postmodernity (Postmodernization) and Its Own Discontents**

  —*During the Post-Cold War and Beyond*
  - Ex: post-Fordism and its shortcomings (Ch.6 of *FHC*; Chs.6-7 of *FCD*)

- **Hegemonic Postmodernity and Its Countervailing Forces**

  —*The Debate on the Global Village*
  - Ex: uni-civilizationalism vs. multi-civilizationalism (Ch.6 of *FHC*)

  —*The Resistance Movement*
  - Ex: rechantment and the politics of civilizational claims (e.g., Islamic, Confucian and other ethos in relation to the Same) (Ch.6 of *FHC*; Ch.10 of *FCD*)
  - Ex: resentment and the politics of resurgence (e.g., the rising Chinese superpower, the growing EU, and other players in relation to the U.S. and her allies) (Ch.6 of *FHC*; Ch.8 of *FCD*)
  - Ex: regionalism and the politics of inequality (e.g., trans- or inter-national blocs, the North-South divide, NGO's) (Ch.6 of *FHC*; Ch.5 of *FCD*)

Notes: The examples in each category are solely illustrative (not exhaustive) nor necessarily mutually exclusive, and the comparison is relative (not absolute). As generalities, they allow exceptions.
Sources: From *FCD* and the 2 volumes of *FHC*

Table 1.37. The Trinity of After-Postmodernity

- **Free-Spirited After-Postmodernity (After-Postmodernism) and Its Internal Split**
  —The discourse of naked contingency (Ch.10 of *FCD*; Ch.4 of *FPHC*)

- **Post-Capitalist After-Postmodernity (After-Postmodernization) and Its Own Discontents**
  —Different versions of post-capitalism and post-democracy, and their enemies (Ch.10 of *FCD*; Chs.3-4 of *FPHC*)

- **Hegemonic After-Postmodernity and Its Countervailing Forces**
  —The Cyclical Progression of Hegemony in Multiverses (Chs.9-10 of *FCD*; Ch.4 of *FPHC*)

Notes: The examples in each category are solely illustrative (not exhaustive) nor necessarily mutually exclusive, and the comparison is relative (not absolute). As generalities, they allow exceptions.
Sources: From *FCD* and also *FHC*

• PART TWO •

Mind

CHAPTER 2
MENTAL HEALTH AND ITS DUALITY

> [P]erhaps genuine happiness is not something you aim at, but is a by-product of a life well lived, and a life well lived does not settle on the programmed or neatly calibrated [view of positive psychology].
> —K. Schneider (2011)

The Necessity of Mental Health

The study of health care involves both mental health and physical health (in the context of mind and body)—as already indicated in *Sec. 1.3*.

The relationship between mental health and physical health (in the context of mind and body) is dialectic, since there is no mental health without physical health, and vice versa—to be eventually transcended altogether later.

Yet, a scholarly danger here is to reduce the analysis of one to that of the other; thus, this book is to devote a whole chapter on each, with the understanding, of course, that the two are related.

This dialectic interconnection between mental health and physical health (in the context of mind and body) can be revealed by showing how and why the analysis of mental health (in Chapter Two) is inadequate without the inclusion of physical health, just as the examination of physical health (in Chapter Three) is insufficient without the consideration of mental health.

The issues concerning mental health (in the context of the mind) in the study of health care are to be addressed in this chapter (Chapter Two), whereas the issues concerning physical health (in the context of the body) in the study of health care will be analyzed in the next chapter (Chapter Three) instead.

With this dialectic treatment in mind—a good way to examine mental health and its duality (in the context of the mind) in the study of health care is by way of the evaluation of the extent to which it is in fact both possible (or impossible) and desirable (or undesirable).

This can be done by way of a comprehensive analysis of mental health (in the context of the mind) in health care from the four perspectives of the mind, nature, society, and culture (in accordance to my sophisticated methodological holism, as explained in *Sec. 1.9*).

In other words, this chapter is organized in four main sections, namely, in relation to (2.2) mental health and the mind, (2.3) mental health and nature, (2.4) mental health and society, and (2.5) mental health and culture—to be addressed hereafter, in that order (and summarized in *Table 2.1*).

Mental Health and the Mind

Mental health, when examined from the perspective of the mind, can illuminate its possibility (or impossibility) and desirability (or undesirability), and this can be shown by way of two case studies, namely, (2.2.1) mental health, psychotherapy, and medicine, and (2.2.2) mental health, subjective well-being, and genetics—to be addressed in what follows, respectively.

Mental Health, Psychotherapy, and Medicine

A good way to evaluate the possibility (or impossibility) and desirability (or undesirability) of mental health from the perspective of the mind is to explore mental health, psychotherapy, and medicine.

An argument in the literature is that psychotherapy can be used to treat mental health problems, as a form of modern medicine. (WK 2013c)

History of Psychotherapy

Historically, "psychotherapy can be said to have been practiced through the ages, as individuals received psychological counsel and reassurance from others." (WK 2013l)

In antiquity, for Colin Feltham (1997), "the Stoics were one of the main Hellenistic schools of philosophy and therapy, along with the Sceptics and Epicureans. Philosophers and physicians from these schools practised psychotherapy among the Greeks and Romans from about the late 4th century BC to the 4th century AD." (WK 2013l)

But "psychoanalysis was perhaps the first specific school of psychotherapy, developed by Sigmund Freud and others through the early

20th century. Trained as a neurologist, Freud began focusing on problems that appeared to have no discernible organic basis, and theorized that they had psychological causes originating in childhood experiences and the unconscious mind. Techniques such as dream interpretation, free association, transference and analysis of the id, ego and superego were developed. Many theorists, including Anna Freud, Alfred Adler, Carl Jung, Karen Horney, Otto Rank, Erik Erikson, Melanie Klein, and Heinz Kohut, built upon Freud's fundamental ideas and often developed their own systems of psychotherapy. These were all later categorized as psychodynamic, meaning anything that involved the psyche's conscious/unconscious influence on external relationships and the self. Sessions tended to number into the hundreds over several years." (WK 2013l)

Later, "behaviorism developed in the 1920s, and behavior modification as a therapy became popularized in the 1950s and 1960s. Notable contributors were Joseph Wolpe in South Africa, M.B. Shipiro and Hans Eysenck in Britain, and John B. Watson and B.F. Skinner in the United States. Behavioral therapy approaches relied on principles of operant conditioning, classical conditioning and social learning theory to bring about therapeutic change in observable symptoms. The approach became commonly used for phobias, as well as other disorders." (WK 2013l)

Then, there was "the European school of existential philosophy. Concerned mainly with the individual's ability to develop and preserve a sense of meaning and purpose throughout life, major contributors to the field in the U.S. (e.g., Irvin Yalom, Rollo May) and Europe (Viktor Frankl, Ludwig Binswanger, Medard Boss, R. D. Laing, Emmy van Deurzen) and later in the 1960s and 1970s both in the United Kingdom and in Canada, Eugene Heimler attempted to create therapies sensitive to common 'life crises' springing from the essential bleakness of human self-awareness, previously accessible only through the complex writings of existential philosophers (e.g., Søren Kierkegaard, Jean-Paul Sartre, Gabriel Marcel, Martin Heidegger, Friedrich Nietzsche)....A related body of thought in psychotherapy started in the 1950s with Carl Rogers. Based on existentialism and the works of Abraham Maslow and his hierarchy of human needs, Rogers brought person-centered psychotherapy into mainstream focus. The primary requirement of Rogers is that the client should be in receipt of three core 'conditions' from his counsellor or therapist....The aim in using the 'core conditions' is to facilitate therapeutic change within a non-directive relationship conducive to enhancing the client's psychological well being. This type of interaction enables the client to fully experience and express himself. Others developed the approach, like Fritz and Laura Perls in the creation of Gestalt therapy, as well as Marshall Rosenberg, founder of Nonviolent Communication, and Eric Berne, founder of Transactional Analysis. Later these fields of psychotherapy would become what is known as humanistic psychotherapy today. Self-help groups and books became widespread." (WK 2013l; E. Heimler 1975)

By the 1950s, "Albert Ellis originated Rational Emotive Behavior Therapy (REBT). A few years later, psychiatrist Aaron T. Beck developed a form of psychotherapy known as cognitive therapy. Both of these generally included relatively short, structured and present-focused therapy aimed at identifying and changing a person's beliefs, appraisals and reaction-patterns, by contrast with the more long-lasting insight-based approach of psychodynamic or humanistic therapies. Cognitive and behavioral therapy approaches were combined and grouped under the heading and umbrella-term Cognitive behavioral therapy (CBT) in the 1970s....A 'third wave' of cognitive and behavioral therapies developed, including Acceptance and Commitment Therapy and Dialectical behavior therapy, which expanded the concepts to other disorders and/or added novel components and mindfulness exercises. Counseling methods developed, including solution-focused therapy and systemic coaching. During the 1960s and 1970s Eugene Heimler, after training in the new discipline of psychiatric social work, developed Heimler method of Human Social Functioning, a methodology based on the principle that frustration is the potential to human flourishing. Positive psychotherapy (PPT) (since 1968) is the name of the method of the psychotherapeutic modality developed by Nossrat Peseschkian and co-workers." (WK 2013l)

Recently, "postmodern psychotherapies such as Narrative Therapy and Coherence Therapy did not impose definitions of mental health and illness, but rather saw the goal of therapy as something constructed by the client and therapist in a social context. Systems Therapy also developed, which focuses on family and group dynamics—and Transpersonal psychology, which focuses on the spiritual facet of human experience. Other important orientations developed in the last three decades include Feminist therapy, Brief therapy, Somatic Psychology, Expressive therapy, applied Positive psychology and the Human Givens approach...." (WK 2013l; N. Corp 2008)

Forms and Techniques of Psychotherapy

Psychotherapy can come in different forms; for instance, some "use spoken conversation. Some also use various other forms of communication such as the written word, artwork, drama, narrative story or music. Psychotherapy with children and their parents often involves play, dramatization (i.e. role-play), and drawing, with a co-constructed narrative from these non-verbal and displaced modes of interacting." (WK 2013l; D. Schechter 2006)

And psychotherapy also makes good use of different techniques. For instance, "pychotherapists use a range of techniques to influence or persuade the client to adapt or change in the direction the client has chosen. These can be based on clear thinking about their options; experiential relationship building; dialogue, communication and adoption of behavior change strategies. Each is designed to improve the mental health of a client or patient, or to improve group relationships (as in a family)." (WK 2013l)

In general, "because sensitive topics are often discussed during psychotherapy, therapists are expected, and usually legally bound, to respect client or patient confidentiality." (WK 2013l)

Models of Psychotherapy

In addition, psychotherapy have two different models, namely, "medical" and "non-medical."

In a "medical" model, "the client is seen as unwell and the therapist employs their skill to help the client back to health. The extensive use of the DSM-IV, the diagnostic and statistical manual of mental disorders in the United States, is an example of a medically-exclusive model." (WK 2013l)

But in a "non-medical" model, the task is more "humanistic," in striving "to depathologise the human condition. The therapist attempts to create a relational environment conducive to experiential learning and help build the client's confidence in their own natural process resulting in a deeper understanding of themselves. An example would be gestalt therapy." (WK 2013l)

Approaches to Psychotherapy

In practice, however, psychotherapy can draw from different approaches, and some main approaches are shown below.

(a) Psychoanalysis

In psychoanalysis, "Sigmund Freud...explores the dynamic workings of a mind understood to consist of three parts: the hedonistic *id*..., the rational *ego*..., and the moral *superego*....Because the majority of these dynamics are said to occur outside people's awareness, Freudian psychoanalysis seeks to probe the unconscious by way of various techniques, including dream interpretation and free association. Freud maintained that the condition of the unconscious mind is profoundly influenced by childhood experiences. So, in addition to dealing with the defense mechanisms used by an overburdened ego, his therapy addresses fixations and other issues by probing deeply into clients' youth." (WK 2013l)

Later, "other psychodynamic theories and techniques have been developed and used by psychotherapists, psychologists, psychiatrists, personal growth facilitators, occupational therapists and social workers.... This is especially true of the psychodynamic schools of psychotherapy, which today include Jungian therapy and Psychodrama as well as the psychoanalytic schools and object relations theory." (WK 2013l)

(b) Gestalt Therapy

In gestalt therapy, at the beginning, "its founders, Frederick and Laura Perls, called it 'concentration therapy'....Gestalt Therapy stands on top of essentially four load-bearing theoretical walls: phenomenological method, dialogical relationship, field-theoretical strategies, and experimental freedom. Some have considered it an existential phenomenology while others have described it as a phenomenological behaviorism. Gestalt Therapy is a humanistic, holistic, and experiential approach that does not rely on talking alone; instead it facilitates awareness in the various contexts of life by moving from talking about relatively remote situations to action and direct current experience." (WK 2013l)

(c) Positive Psychotherapy

In positive psychotherapy (PPT), as developed by Nossrat Peseschkian and co-workers, the method is based on "humanistic and psychodynamic psychotherapy" and "on a positive image of man, which correlates with a salutogenetic, resource-oriented, humanistic and conflict-centered approach. It is accredited by several institutions (e.g. State Medical Chamber of Hessen, Germany, European Association for Psychotherapy EAP; World Council for Psychotherapy WCP, International Federation of Psychotherapy IFP and other statutory institutions)." (WK 2013l)

(d) Group Psychotherapy

In group psychotherapy, the term was "first used around 1920 by Jacob L. Moreno, whose main contribution was the development of psychodrama, in which groups were used as both cast and audience for the exploration of individual problems by reenactment under the direction of the leader. The more analytic and exploratory use of groups in both hospital and out-patient settings was pioneered by a few European psychoanalysts who emigrated to the USA, such as Paul Schilder, who treated severely neurotic and mildly psychotic out-patients in small groups at Bellevue Hospital, New York." (WK 2013l)

(e) Behavior Therapy

In behavior therapy, the focus is on "modifying overt behavior and helping clients to achieve goals. This approach is built on the principles of learning theory including operant and respondent conditioning, which makes up the area of applied behavior analysis or behavior modification....By nature, behavioral therapies are empirical (data-driven), contextual (focused on the environment and context), functional (interested in the effect or consequence a behavior ultimately has), probabilistic (viewing behavior as statistically predictable), monistic (rejecting mind-body dualism and treating the person as a unit), and relational (analyzing bidirectional interactions)." (WK 2013l; N. Sundberg 2001)

(f) Body-Oriented Psychotherapy

In body-oriented psychotherapy, the focus is "on the link between the mind and the body and try to access deeper levels of the psyche through greater awareness of the physical body and the emotions which gave rise to the various body-oriented based psychotherapeutic approaches, such as Reichian (Wilhelm Reich) Character-Analytic Vegetotherapy and Orgonomy; neo-Reichian Alexander Lowen's Bioenergetic analysis; Peter Levine's Somatic Experiencing; Jack Rosenberg's Integrative body psychotherapy; Ron Kurtz's Hakomi psychotherapy; Pat Ogden's sensorimotor psychotherapy; David Boadella's Biosynthesis psychotherapy; Gerda Boyesen's Biodynamic psychotherapy; etc." (WK 2013l)

(g) Expressive Therapy

In expressive therapy, the task here is to utilize "artistic expression as its core means of treating clients. Expressive therapists use the different disciplines of the creative arts as therapeutic interventions. This includes the modalities dance therapy, drama therapy, art therapy, music therapy, writing therapy, among others. Expressive therapists believe that often the most effective way of treating a client is through the expression of imagination in a creative work and integrating and processing what issues are raised in the act." (WK 2013l)

(h) Interpersonal Psychotherapy

And in interpersonal psychotherapy (IPT), the focus is on "the interpersonal context and on building interpersonal skills. IPT is based on the belief that interpersonal factors may contribute heavily to psychological problems. It is commonly distinguished from other forms of therapy in its emphasis on interpersonal processes rather than intrapsychic processes. IPT aims to change a person's interpersonal behavior by fostering adaptation to current interpersonal roles and situations." (WK 2013l)

Problems with Psychotherapy

However, for the critics, this argument on mental health, psychotherapy, and medicine has some major problems. Consider, for illustration, a few examples below.

Firstly, one main criticism of the argument on mental health, psychotherapy, and medicine is that "there is considerable controversy about which form of psychotherapy is most effective." (WK 2013l)

For instance, for the critics, there exists a "considerable controversy about which form of psychotherapy is most effective, and more specifically, which types of therapy are optimal for treating which sorts of problems. Furthermore, it is controversial whether the form of therapy or the presence of factors common to many psychotherapies best separates effective therapy from ineffective therapy." (WK 2013l; B. Casey 2004)

Secondly, another main criticism of the argument on mental health, psychotherapy, and medicine is that "the dropout rate" of psychotherapeutic patients is "quite high."

For example, for the critics, "the dropout level is quite high; one meta-analysis of 125 studies concluded that the mean dropout rate was 46.86%. The high level of dropout has raised some criticism about the relevance and efficacy of psychotherapy." (WK 2013l; M. Wierzbicki 1993)

Thirdly, still another main criticism of the argument on mental health, psychotherapy, and medicine is that psychotherapy is dispensable.

For instance, "as early as 1952, in one of the earliest studies of psychotherapy treatment, Hans Eysenck reported that two thirds of therapy patients improved significantly or recovered on their own within two years, whether or not they received psychotherapy." (WK 2013l) And "in 1994, the late Frank Pittman, MD questioned "the value of a profession he had practiced for more than three decades" by asking "how perennial psychotherapy customer Woody Allen could have undergone therapy for most of his life and still not have seen anything incestuous in his sexual relationship with his de facto stepdaughter, the sister of his children." (WK 2013l)

Fourthly, an additional main criticism of the argument on mental health, psychotherapy, and medicine is that psychotherapy lacks adequate explanatory power.

For instance, "in 2001, Bruce Wampold of the University of Wisconsin published the book *The Great Psychotherapy Debate*" but concluded that "we do not know why psychotherapy works." (WK 2013l)

And fifthly, another additional main criticism of the argument on mental health, psychotherapy, and medicine is that psychotherapy can be undesirable to the health of the patients.

For instance, "further critiques have emerged from feminist, constructionist and discursive sources. Key to these is the issue of power. In this regard there is a concern that clients are persuaded—both inside and outside the consulting room—to understand themselves and their difficulties in ways that are consistent with therapeutic ideas. This means that alternative ideas (e.g., feminist, economic, spiritual) are sometimes implicitly undermined. Critics suggest that we idealize the situation when we think of therapy only as a helping relation, that it is fundamentally a political practice, in that some cultural ideas and practices are supported while others are undermined or disqualified, and while it is seldom intended, the therapist-client relationship always participates in society's power relations and political dynamics." (WK 2013l; M. Guilfoyle 2005)

Beyond Psychotherapy

These criticisms of psychotherapy should not be misunderstood as a total rejection of its validity but serve to show us the two opposing sides of the debate, such that the possibility (or impossibility) and desirability (or undesirability) of mental health (from the perspective of the mind with mental health, psychotherapy, and medicine as a case study here) are not to the extent that the respective defenders would like us to believe.

Moreover, the analysis of mental health, psychotherapy, and medicine is to shed some light on the ontological principles in existential dialectics, and good examples include the formalness-informalness principle, the absoluteness-relativeness principle, the partiality-totality principle, the predictability-unpredictability principle, the explicability-inexplicability principle, the fiction-reality principle, the cognitiveness-noncognitiveness principle, the finiteness-transfiniteness principle, the preciseness-vagueness principle, the simpleness-complicatedness principle, the openness-hiddenness principle, the denseness-emptiness principle, the prototypicality-variation principle, the change-constancy principle, the order-chaos principle, the slowness-quickness principle, the expansion-contraction principle, the optimality-nonoptimality principle, the theory-praxis principle, the convention-novelty principle, the evolution-transformation principle, the symmetry-asymmetry principle, the softness-hardness principle, the seriousness-playfulness principle, the activeness-inactivess principle, the selfness-otherness principle, the regression-progression principle, the same-difference principle, the stability-reaction principle, the functionality-nonfunctionality principle, and the intentionality-nonintentionality principle.

For instance, in relation to the formalness-informalness principle, if there is formalness (e.g., the formal logical requirement of soundness, completeness, and consistency in a system of ideas, as in the argument for psychotherapy), there is informalness (e.g., the non-formal existence of unsoundness, incompleteness, and inconsistency in the argument for psychotherapy, as shown in the criticisms that "there is considerable controversy about which form of psychotherapy is most effective," that "the dropout rate" of psychotherapeutic patients is quite high, that psychotherapy is dispensable, that psychotherapy lacks adequate explanatory power, and that psychotherapy can be undesirable to the health of the patients, etc.). And the reverse direction also holds true.

In relation to the absoluteness-relativeness principle, if there is absoluteness (e.g., the absolute view on the treatment of mental problems by Freud on the basis of "psychological causes originating in childhood experiences and the unconscious mind"), there is relativeness (e.g., what is right for Freud to treat mental problems on the basis of "psychological causes originating in childhood experiences and the unconscious mind" is not necessarily so for Skinner, who advocated instead "behavioral therapy approaches relied on principles of operant conditioning, classical conditioning and social learning theory to bring about therapeutic change" in patients). (WK 2013l) And the reverse direction also holds true.

In relation to the partiality-totality principle, if there is partiality (e.g., the partial view on health problems by those in Freudian psychoanalysis), there is totality (e.g., the more holistic view on health problems, such that the whole is not the sum of its parts, that is, it cannot be reduced to the sum of opposing views like Freudian psychoanalysis, gestalt therapy, positive psychotherapy, group psychotherapy, behavior therapy, body-oriented psychotherapy, etc., since there will emerge new views in the future not yet known today, just as there are already alternative views nowadays which do not side exclusively with any of them, as is the analysis here). And the reverse direction also holds true.

In relation to the predictability-unpredictability principle, if there is predictability (e.g., the predictable tendency that the dropout rate of psychotherapeutic patients is "quite high"), there is unpredictability (e.g., the more difficult task to predict exactly the extent to which a particular psychotherapeutic patient will stay or drop out on a particular future occasion). And the reverse direction also holds true.

In relation to the explicability-inexplicability principle, if there is explicability (e.g., the explanation, by the practitioners of psychotherapy that psychotherapy can "increase the individual's sense of his/her own well-being" by employing "a range of techniques based on experiential relationship building, dialogue, communication and behavior change"), there is inexplicability (e.g., the lack of sufficient explanation, by the practitioners of psychotherapy of why it is necessarily explainable, since the critic like Bruce Wampold in *The Great Psychotherapy Debate* argued that "we do not know why psychotherapy works"). And the reverse direction also holds true.

In relation to the fiction-reality principle, if there is fiction (e.g., the fictional aspect of psychotherapy, insofar as, "in one of the earliest studies of psychotherapy treatment, Hans Eysenck reported that two thirds of therapy patients improved significantly or recovered on their own within two years, whether or not they received psychotherapy"), there is reality (e.g., the realistic aspect of psychotherapy, insofar as "psychoanalytic psychotherapy has been found to be as effective as Cognitive Behavioral Therapy for immediate relief" of panic disorders). (WK 2013l; B. Milrod 2006; M. Blechner 2007) And the reverse direction also holds true.

In relation to the cognitiveness-noncognitiveness principle, if there is cognitiveness (e.g., a view of things on the basis of reason and evidences, as shown in the empirical research by Wampold that "psychotherapy" can be "effective"), there is noncognitiveness (e.g., a view of things on the basis of non-cognitive factors like envy, jealousy, power, nationality, race, gender, age, class, greed, lust, status, faith, anger, sadness, joy, fear, wish, etc., as shown in the politics of power pointed out by feminist critics, in that "the therapist-client relationship always participates in society's power relations and political dynamics"). (WK 2013l) And the reverse direction also holds true.

In relation to the finiteness-transfiniteness principle, if there is finiteness (e.g., the finite number of the categories of "resources available to a person experiencing emotional distress" like "the friendly support of friends, peers, family members, clergy contacts, personal reading, healthy exercise, research, and independent coping"), there is transfiniteness (e.g., the transfinite number of all the individuals in human history who have ever existed and have used any of the resources available to cope with emotinal distress). And the reverse direction also holds true.

In relation to the preciseness-vagueness principle, if there is preciseness (e.g., the precise identification of 8 main approaches to psychotherapy in the article aforecited), there is vagueness (e.g., the vagueness in the identification of the 8 main approaches to psychotherapy in the article aforecited, since it is not clear why there must be these 8, not 16, 20, 23, 26, 30, and so on). And the reverse direction also holds true.

In relation to the simpleness-complicatedness principle, if there is simpleness (e.g., the relatively simple analysis of the effectiveness of psychotherapy by the advocates), there is complicatedness (e.g., the relatively more complicated analysis of the effectiveness of psychotherapy, by challenging the claims and assumptions, as shown in the problems pointed out by the critics as cited). And the reverse direction also holds true.

In relation to the openness-hiddenness principle, if there is openness (e.g., the open exploration of "uncovering psychotherapy," which "emphasizes facilitating the client's insight into the roots of their difficulties"), there is hiddenness (e.g., the hidden bias in "uncovering psychotherapy," since it neglects the need to "strengthen…the client's defenses and…provid[e]…encouragement and advice," as in "supportive psychotherapy"). (WK 2013l) And the reverse direction also holds true.

In relation to the denseness-emptiness principle, if there is denseness (e.g., the relatively denser concentration of concerns with "childhood experiences and the unconscious mind" by those in "psychoanalysis"), there is emptiness (e.g., the relatively less dense, or more empty, concentration of concerns with "childhood experiences and the unconscious mind" by those in "behavioral therapy"). And the reverse direction also holds true.

In relation to the prototypicality-variation principle, if there is prototypicality (e.g., the prototype, like the example about the original work on psychoanalysis by Freud in the early 20th century), there is variation (e.g., different variants of the protoptye, as shown in many studies of psychoanalysis since then, like the ones built upon Freud's psychoanlaysis by "Anna Freud, Alfred Adler, Carl Jung, Karen Horney, Otto Rank, Erik Erikson, Melanie Klein, and Heinz Kohut," for example, though each with his/er own variation, contribution, and disagreement). And the reverse direction also holds true.

In relation to the change-constancy principle, if there is change (e.g., the ever new ways to treat mental problems, as shown in psychotherapy), there is constancy (e.g., the ever constant existence of different problems with the ever new ways to treat mental problems, as shown in the problems with psychotherapy pointed out by the critics). And the reverse direction also holds true.

In relation to the order-chaos principle, if there is order (e.g., the more or less orderly view on treating health problems, if looked from the sole vantage point of "behavior therapy," with its focus on "modifying overt behavior and helping clients to achieve goals" by way of "operant and respondent conditioning"), there is chaos (e.g., the more or less chaotic view on treating health problems, if looked from the multiple, often conflicting, vantage points of different competing approaches to psychotherapy, each with its own claims and techniques, such that "no comparisons of different psychotherapies with long follow-up times have been done" and they do not really add up to much of anything). (WK 2013; T. Härkänen 2005) And the reverse direction also holds true.

In relation to the slowness-quickness principle, if there is slowness (e.g., the relatively slower speed of a patient to cope with emotional distress if s/he refuses to make good use of "resources available to a person experiencing emotional distress—the friendly support of friends, peers, family members, clergy contacts, personal reading, healthy exercise, research, and independent coping"), there is quickness (e.g., the relatively quicker speed of a patient to cope with emotional distress if s/he makes good use of "resources available to a person experiencing emotional distress—the friendly support of friends, peers, family members, clergy contacts, personal reading, healthy exercise, research, and independent coping"). And the reverse direction also holds true.

In relation to the expansion-contraction principle, if there is expansion (e.g., the relative spread of postmodern psychotherapies in the last 2 decades), there is contraction (e.g., the relative decline of Freudian psychoanalysis in the last 2 decades). And the reverse direction also holds true.

In relation to the optimality-nonoptimality principle, if there is optimality (e.g., the search for highly favorable options, like the quest for optimality in some models of psychotherapy, like the view that "depending on the client's personality, a more supportive or more uncovering approach may be optimal"), there is nonoptimality (e.g., the existence of non-optimal alternatives to optimality, like the argument for more realistic studies by the critics, who pointed out that the search for optimal approaches are unrealistic, because of the different problems aforecited, and some critics even suggested that psychotherapy is dispensable). (WK 2013l) And the reverse direction also holds true.

In relation to the theory-praxis principle, if there is theory (e.g., the theoretical construction of "power relations" in feminism), there is praxis (e.g., the practical application of "power relations" in feminism to the field of psychotherapy, as in feminist therapy). And the reverse direction also holds true.

In relation to the convention-novelty principle, if there is convention (e.g., the conventional wisdom about "uncovering psychotherapy," which "emphasizes facilitating the client's insight into the roots of their difficulties"), there is novelty (e.g., the alternative novel challenge to the conventional wisdom about "uncovering psychotherapy," by the new idea of "feminist, constructionist and discursive sources," which suggest instead that "the therapist-client relationship...participates in society's power relations and political dynamics"). And the reverse direction also holds true.

In relation to the evolution-transformation principle, if there is evolution (e.g., the natural evolution of humans to "deal...with crises, navigat[e]...severe social problems and find...solutions to life problems" in the state of nature), there is transformation (e.g., the technical transformation of human ability to deal...with crises, navigat[e]...severe social problems and find...solutions to life problems" by the invention of different approaches to psychotherapy). And the reverse direction also holds true.

In relation to the symmetry-asymmetry principle, if there is symmetry (e.g., the co-existence of different individuals in psychotherapy, like a therapist and a client), there is asymmetry (e.g., according to "feminist, constructionist and discursive sources," "the therapist-client relationship...participates in society's power relations and political dynamics," with the therapist having power over the client). And the reverse direction also holds true.

In relation to the softness-hardness principle, if there is softness (e.g., the defense of psychotherapy by the advocates aforecited), there is hardness (e.g., the critique of psychotherapy by the critics aforecited). And the reverse direction also holds true.

In relation to the seriousness-playfulness principle, if there is seriousness (e.g., the serious business of those in psychotherapy who try to understand how to treat mental problems), there is playfulness (e.g., the playful part of those in in psychotherapy, when they play around with different models of, and approaches to, psychotherpay over the centuries, as shown in the main examples aforedescribed). And the reverse direction also holds true.

In relation to the activeness-inactivess principle, if there is activeness (e.g., the relative activeness of those who can function well in life after successfully coping with life problems by way of psychotherapy), there is inactiveness (e.g., the relative inactiveness of those who cannot function well in life, because they do not successfully cope with life problems, even after trying psychotherapy and other methods). And the reverse direction also holds true.

In relation to the selfness-otherness principle, if there is selfness (e.g., the tendency to be mostly centered on one's self or group, as shown in those advocates of the effectiveness of psychotherapy, even when the "critics of psychotherapy are skeptical of the healing power of a psychotherapeutic relationship"), there is otherness (e.g., the tendency to be mostly centered on others, as shown in "the American Psychological Association ethics code," in which "confidentiality is an integral part of the therapeutic relationship and psychotherapy in general," as "it includes protecting specific groups of people, like children, while treating private information" in a confidential way). (WK 2013l; J. Masson 1988) And the reverse direction also holds true.

In relation to the regression-progression principle, if there is regression (e.g., the regression made by psychotherapy, as shown in the problems pointed out by the critics), there is progression (e.g., the progress made by psychotherapy, as shown in the contribution to the treatment of mental problems aforecited). And the reverse direction also holds true.

In relation to the same-difference principle, if there is similarity in outcome (e.g., the contribution to the molding and control of beliefs, values, and behaviors, regardless of whether this be done by way of positive psychotherpay, or by way of feminist therapy), there is difference in outcome (e.g., the contribution to the molding and control of beliefs, values, and behaviors by way of positive psychotherpay for a relatively more scientific worldview—but the contribution to the molding and control of beliefs, values, and behaviors by way of feminist therapy for a relatively more social-constructionist worldview). And the reverse direction also holds true.

In relation to the stability-reaction principle, if there is stability (e.g., the relatively more stable condition of the idealized view on the therapist-client relationship in the older days when "we think of therapy only as a helping relation" by a therapist for a client), there is reaction (e.g., the idealized view on the therapist-client relationship in the older days then led to further changes later on, when nowadays, according to "feminist, constructionist and discursive sources,...the therapist-client relationship always participates in society's power relations and political dynamics"). And the reverse direction also holds true.

In relation to the functionality-nonfunctionality principle, if there is functionality (e.g., the presence of action for which something or someone is fitted, as shown in the research by Bruce Wampold who showed that psychotherapy could be effective, which served the function of treating mental prolems in patients), there is nonfunctionality (e.g., the relative lack of action for which something or someone is fitted, as shown in the studies in which, according to "feminist, constructionist and discursive sources,...clients are persuaded—both inside and outside the consulting room—to understand themselves and their difficulties in ways that are consistent with therapeutic ideas," so "alternative ideas...are...implicitly undermined," such that psychotherapy is no longer perceived as functional in treating mental problems nowadays among postmodern therapists, even though it used to be falsely assumed by the advocates in the older days). And the reverse direction also holds true.

In relation to the intentionality-nonintentionality principle, if there is intentionality (e.g., the planning or design of something for a certain outcome, as shown in the original intention of conventional psychotherapists to treat mental problems in patients), there is nonintentionality (e.g., the relative absence of planning or design of something for a certain outcome, such that the outcome can even be counter-intentional in being the opposite of what was originally planned, as shown in the critique by "feminist, constructionist and discursive sources," in that, "while it is seldom intended, the therapist-client relationship always participates in society's power relations and political dynamics"—contrary to the original intention of conventional psychotherapists to treat mental problems in patients). And the reverse direction also holds true.

And in relation to the survivability-nonsurvivability principle, if there is survivability (e.g., the relative survival, nowadays, of "resources available to a person experiencing emotional distress—the friendly support of friends, peers, family members, clergy contacts, personal reading, healthy exercise, research, and independent coping"), there is non-survivability (e.g., the non-survival, nowadays, of the unquestioned, "idealized" view about the "healing power of a psychotherapeutic relationship"). And the reverse direction also holds true.

Mental Health, Subjective Well-Being, and Genetics

Another way to evaluate the possibility (or impossibility) and desirability (or undesirability) of mental health from the perspective of the mind is to explore mental health, subjective well-being, and genetics.

An argument in the literature is that "how people experience the quality of their lives" can be explained on the basis of genetics.

Positive Psychology and Subjective Well-Being

The term "subjective well-being (SWB)" refers to "how people experience the quality of their lives and includes both emotional reactions and cognitive judgments. Psychologists have defined happiness as a combination of life satisfaction and the relative frequency of positive and negative affect. SWB therefore encompasses moods and emotions as well as evaluations of one's satisfaction with general and specific areas of one's life....Positive psychology is particularly concerned with the study of SWB." (WK 2013u; E. Diener 2000, 1999 & 1984)

Positive psychology was proposed by Martin Seligman (2000) and Mihaly Csikszentmihalyi, who "identified that psychology is not just the study of pathology, weakness, and damage; but it is also the study of strength and virtue. Researchers in positive psychology have pointed out that in almost every culture studied the pursuit of happiness is regarded as one of the most valued goals in life. Understanding individual differences in SWB is of key interest in positive psychology, particularly the issue of why some people are happier than others. Some people continue to be happy in the face of adversity whereas others are chronically unhappy at the best of times. Additionally, positive psychology has investigated how people might improve their level of SWB and maintain these improvements over the longer term, rather than returning to baseline." (WK 2013u; S. Lyubomirsky 2001)

Components of Subjective Well-Being

For E. Diener and his colleagues, "the various components of SWB represent distinct constructs that need to be understood separately, even though they are closely related....Definitions of SWB...focus on how a person evaluates their own life, including emotional experiences of pleasure versus pain in response to specific events and cognitive evaluations of what a person considers a good life." (WK 2013u)

Thus, "there are 2 components of SWB. One is Affect Balance and the other is Life Satisfaction. An individual's scores on the 2 measures are summed to produce a total SWB score," as explained below (and summarized in *Table 2.2*). (WK 2013u)

(a) Affect Balance

The first component of SWB is "affect balance," which refers to "the emotions, moods, and feelings a person has. These can be all positive, all negative, or a combination of both positive and negative." (WK 2013u; E. Diener 2008)

In other words, the term "affect" here includes "positive affect (experiencing pleasant emotions and moods) and low negative affect (experiencing unpleasant, distressing emotions and moods), as well as 'overall affect' or 'hedonic balance,' defined as the overall equilibrium between positive and negative affect, and usually measured as the difference between the two. High positive affect and low negative affect are often highly correlated, but not always." (WK 2013u; P. Steel 2008; E. Diener 2008 & 2000)

(b) Life Satisfaction

And the second component of SWB is "life satisfaction," which refers to "global judgments of one's life...and satisfaction with specific life domains (e.g. work satisfaction)," and they "are considered cognitive components of SWB." (WK 2013u)

In this way, the term "happiness" is related to the two components of SWB, because, on the one hand, "happiness" is often "defined variously as 'satisfaction of desires and goals' (therefore related to life satisfaction)" and "as a 'preponderance of positive over negative affect' (therefore related to emotional components of SWB)...." (WK 2013u; E. Diener 1984)

In relation to the two components of SWB, "life satisfaction can also be known as the 'stable' component in one's life. Affective concepts of SWB can be considered in terms of momentary emotional states as well as in terms of longer-term moods and tendencies (i.e. how much positive and/or negative affect a person generally experiences over any given period of time). Life satisfaction and in some research happiness are typically considered over long durations, up to one's lifetime." (WK 2013u; E. Diener 1984 & 1999; P. Steel 2008)

Theories of Subjective Well-Being

There are different theories of the causes of SWB, and hereafter are two main examples (as summarized in *Table 2.2*).

(a) Top-Down Theory

In the top-down theory, "global features of personality influence the way a person perceives events. Individuals may therefore have a global tendency to perceive life in a consistently positive or negative manner, depending on their stable personality traits. Top-down theories of SWB suggest that people have a genetic predisposition to be happy or unhappy and this predisposition determines their SWB 'setpoint.' Set Point theory implies that a person's baseline or equilibrium level of SWB is a consequencc of hereditary characteristics and therefore, almost entirely predetermined at birth. Evidence for this genetic predisposition derives from behavior-genetic studies that have found that positive and negative affectivity each have high heritability (40% and 55% respectively in one study). Numerous twin studies confirm the notion of set point theory, however, they do not rule out the possibility that is it possible for individuals to experience long term changes in SWB." (WK 2013u; K. DeNeve 1999; D. Lykken 1996; M. McGue 1993)

In addition, "further evidence for a genetically influenced predisposition to SWB comes from findings that personality as a large influence on long-term SWB. This has led to the dynamic equilibrium model of SWB. This model proposes that personality provides a baseline for emotional responses. External events may move people away from the baseline, sometimes dramatically, but these movements tend to be of limited duration, with most people returning to their baseline eventually." (WK 2013u; E. Diener 1999)

(b) Bottom-Up Theory

And in the bottom-up theory, "happiness represents an accumulation of happy experiences. Bottom-up influences include external events, and broad situational and demographic factors, including health and marital status. Bottom-up approaches are based on the idea that there are universal basic human needs and that happiness results from their fulfillment. In support of this view, there is evidence that daily pleasurable events are associated with increased positive affect, and daily unpleasant events or hassles are associated with increased negative affect." (WK 2013u)

But "research suggests that external events account for a much smaller proportion of the variance in self-reports of SWB than top-down factors, such as personality. A theory proposed to explain the limited impact of external events on SWB is hedonic adaptation. Based originally on the concept of a 'hedonic treadmill,' this theory proposes that positive or negative external events temporarily increase or decrease feelings of SWB, but as time passes people tend to become habituated to their circumstances and have a tendency to return to a personal SWB 'setpoint' or baseline level." (WK 2013u; E. Diener 1999 & 2000)

Genetics and Subjective Well-Being

This then raises the question concerning the correlation between genetics and SWB.

For instance, "findings from numerous personality studies show that genetics account for 50% of the variance in Five-Factor Model and the variance in subjective well-being is also heritable. Specifically, neuroticism predicts poorer subjective well-being whilst extraversion, agreeableness, conscientiousness and openness to experience tend to predict higher subjective well-being. A meta-analysis found that neuroticism, extraversion, agreeableness, and conscientiousness were significantly related to all facets of SWB examined (positive, negative, and overall affect; happiness; life satisfaction; and quality of life). Neuroticism was the strongest predictor of overall SWB and is the strongest predictor of negative affect." (WK 2013u; T. Bouchard 2001; P. Steel 2008)

DeNeve (1999) and his colleagues argued that "there are three trends in the relationship between personality and SWB. Firstly, SWB is closely tied to traits associated with emotional tendencies (emotional stability, positive affectivity, and tension). Secondly, relationship enhancing traits (e.g. trust, affiliation) are important for subjective well-being. Happy people tend to have strong relationships and be good at fostering them. Thirdly, the way people think about and explain events is important for subjective well-being. Appraising events in an optimistic fashion, having a sense of control, and making active coping efforts facilitates subjective well-being. Trust, a trait substantially related to SWB, as opposed to cynicism involves making positive rather than negative attributions about others. Making positive, optimistic attributions rather than negative pessimistic ones facilitates subjective well-being." (WK 2013u)

In addition, "the related trait of eudaimonia or psychological well-being, is also heritable. Evidence from one study supports 5 independent genetic mechanisms underlying the Ryff facets of psychological well-being, leading to a genetic construct of eudaimonia in terms of general self-control, and four subsidiary biological mechanisms enabling the psychological capabilities of purpose, agency, growth, and positive social relations." (WK 2013u)

Mental Health and Subjective Well-Being

This correlation between genetics and SWB also raises the issue about the relationship between SWB and health.

For instance, "there are substantial positive associations between health and SWB, so that people who rate their general health as 'good' or 'excellent' tend to experience better SWB compared to those who rate their health as 'fair' or 'poor.' A meta-analysis found that self-ratings of general health were more strongly related to SWB than physician ratings of health. The relationship between health and SWB may be bidirectional. There is evidence that good subjective well-being contributes to better health." (WK 2013u; M. Okun 1984; E. Diener 1984)

For illustration, "a review of longitudinal studies found that measures of baseline subjective well-being constructs such as optimism and positive affect predicted longer-term health status and mortality. Conversely, a number of studies found that baseline depression predicted poorer longer-term health status and mortality. Baseline health may well have a causal influence on subjective well-being, so causality is difficult to establish. A number of studies found that positive emotions and optimism had a beneficial impact on cardiovascular health and on immune functioning. Changes in mood are also known to be associated with changes in immune and cardiovascular response. There is evidence that interventions that are successful in improving subjective well-being can have beneficial effects on aspects of health. For example, meditation and relaxation training have been found to increase positive affect and to reduce blood pressure." (WK 2013u; E. Diener 1984 & 2008)

Problems with Genetics and Subjective Well-Being

However, for the critics, this argument on mental health, subjective well-being, and genetics has some major problems. Consider, for illustration, a few examples below (as summarized in *Table 2.2*).

Firstly, one main criticism of the argument on mental health, subjective well-being, and genetics is that it ignores the "objective" conditions of well-being.

For example, as the critics are quick to point out, "due to the specific focus on the subjective aspects of well-being, definitions of SWB typically exclude objective conditions such as material conditions or health." (WK 2013u; E. Diener 1984)

Secondly, another main criticism of the argument on mental health, subjective well-being, and genetics is that the findings are not consistent across studies and across histories.

For instance, the critics like Diener and his colleagues "note that heritability studies are limited in that they describe long-term SWB in a sample of people in a modern western society but may not be applicable to more extreme environments that might influence SWB and do not provide absolute indicators of genetic effects. Additionally, heritability estimates are inconsistent across studies." (WK 2013u)

Thirdly, still another main criticism of the argument on mental health, subjective well-being, and genetics is that much remains uncertain about the nature of SWB.

For instance, for the critics, "the effect of specific types of subjective well-being is not entirely clear. For example, how durable the effects of mood and emotions on health are remains unclear. Whether some types of subjective well-being predict health independently of others is also unclear." (WK 2013u; E. Diener 1984)

Fourthly, an additional main criticism of the argument on mental health, subjective well-being, and genetics is that SWB can be detrimental to health.

For instance, for the critics, in the case of "survival," there is "evidence" which "suggests happiness may actually be sometimes detrimental. It is unclear why exactly research results suggest this is the case, however Diener & Biswas-Diener offer an explanation. It is possible that happy people fail to report symptoms of the illness, which can ultimately lead to no treatment or inadequate treatment. Another possible reason may be that happy people tend to be optimistic, leading them to take their symptoms too lightly, seek treatment too late, and/or follow the doctor's instructions half-heartedly. And lastly, Diener & Biswas-Diener suggest that people with serious illnesses may be more likely to choose to live out the rest of their days without painful or invasive treatments." (WK 2013u; E. Diener 2008)

Fifthly, another additional main criticism of the argument on mental health, subjective well-being, and genetics is that it neglects social factors.

For instance, for the critics, "a person's level of subjective well-being is determined by many different factors and social influences prove to be a strong one. Results from the famous Framingham Heart Study indicate that friends three degrees of separation away (that is, friends of friends of friends) can affect a person's happiness," and it was estimated that "a friend who lives within a mile (about 1.6 km) and who becomes happy increases the probability that a person is happy by 25%." (WK 2013u; J. Fowler 2008)

And sixthly, still another additional main criticism of the argument on mental health, subjective well-being, and genetics is that it does not give sufficient attention to cultural variations.

For instance, for the critics, "although all cultures seem to value happiness, there are variations across cultures in how happiness is defined. There is also evidence that people in more individualistic cultures tend to rate themselves as higher in subjective well-being compared to people in more collectivistic cultures. In Western cultures, predictors of happiness include elements that support personal independence, a sense of personal agency, and self-expression. In Eastern cultures, predictors of happiness focus on an interdependent self that is inseparable from significant others. Compared to people in individualistic cultures, people in collectivistic cultures are more likely to base their judgments of life satisfaction on how significant others appraise their life than on the balance of inner emotions experienced as pleasant versus unpleasant. Pleasant emotional experiences have a stronger social component in East Asian cultures compared to Western ones." (WK 2013u; E. Suh 2008)

Beyond Genetics and Subjective Well-Being

These criticisms of the argument on subjective well-being and genetics do not mean a total rejection of its usefulness but serve to show us the two opposing sides of the debate, such that the possibility (or impossibility) and desirability (or undesirability) of mental health (from the perspective of the mind with mental health, subjective well-being, and genetics as a case study here) are not to the extent that the respective defenders would like us to believe.

In addition, the analysis of mental health, subjective well-being, and genetics can teach us something valuable about the ontological principles in existential dialectics, and good examples include the formalness-informalness principle, the absoluteness-relativeness principle, the partiality-totality principle, the predictability-unpredictability principle, the explicability-inexplicability principle, the fiction-reality principle, the cognitiveness-noncognitiveness principle, the finiteness-transfiniteness principle, the preciseness-vagueness principle, the simpleness-complicatedness principle, the openness-hiddenness principle, the denseness-emptiness principle, the prototypicality-variation principle, the change-constancy principle, the order-chaos principle, the slowness-quickness principle, the expansion-contraction principle, the optimality-nonoptimality principle, the theory-praxis principle, the convention-novelty principle, the evolution-transformation principle, the symmetry-asymmetry principle, the softness-hardness principle, the seriousness-playfulness principle, the activeness-inactivess principle, the selfness-otherness principle, the regression-progression principle, the same-difference principle, the stability-reaction principle, the functionality-nonfunctionality principle, and the intentionality-nonintentionality principle.

For instance, in relation to the formalness-informalness principle, if there is formalness (e.g., the formal logical requirement of soundness, completeness, and consistency in a system of ideas, as in the argument on subjective well-being and genetics), there is informalness (e.g., the non-formal existence of unsoundness, incompleteness, and inconsistency in the argument on subjective well-being and genetics, as shown in the criticisms that it ignores the "objective" conditions of well-being, that the findings are not consistent across studies and across histories, that much remains uncertain about the nature of SWB, that SWB can be detrimental to health, that it neglects social factors, and that it does not give sufficient attention to cultural variations). And the reverse direction also holds true.

In relation to the absoluteness-relativeness principle, if there is absoluteness (e.g., the absolute concern with the "subjective" aspects of well-being by the advocates of SWB), there is relativeness (e.g., what is right for the advocates of SWB to focus on the "subjective" aspects of well-being is not necessarily so for the critics, who call for the need to include "objective conditions such as material conditions or health," and so on). And the reverse direction also holds true.

In relation to the partiality-totality principle, if there is partiality (e.g., the partial view on the nature of well-being by the advocates of SWB), there is totality (e.g., the more holistic view on the nature of well-being, such that the whole is not the sum of its parts, that is, it cannot be reduced to the sum of opposing views like the advocates of SWB, the advocates for the study of the objective conditions of well-being, etc., since there will emerge new views in the future not yet known today, just as there are already alternative views nowadays which do not side exclusively with any of them, as is the analysis here). And the reverse direction also holds true.

In relation to the predictability-unpredictability principle, if there is predictability (e.g., the predictable tendency of some correlation between SWB and health by the advocates of SWB), there is unpredictability (e.g., the more difficult task to predict exactly the extent to which the specific aspects of the correlation between SWB and health are, since the critics pointed out that "how durable the effects of mood and emotions on health are remains unclear," "whether some types of subjective well-being predict health independently of others is also unclear," and so on). And the reverse direction also holds true.

In relation to the explicability-inexplicability principle, if there is explicability (e.g., the explanation by the advocates of SWB that positive SWB can contribute to better health, as shown in the finding that "people who rate their general health as 'good' or 'excellent' tend to experience better SWB compared to those who rate their health as 'fair' or 'poor'"), there is inexplicability (e.g., the lack of convincing explanation, by the advocates of SWB, of why SWB is necessarily desirable for health, since the critics had pointed out that, in the case of "survival," there is "evidence" which "suggests happiness may actually be sometimes detrimental" to health). And the reverse direction also holds true.

In relation to the fiction-reality principle, if there is fiction (e.g., the fictional aspect of "heritability studies," insofar as "they describe long-term SWB in a sample of people in a modern western society but may not be applicable to more extreme environments that might influence SWB and do not provide absolute indicators of genetic effects" and, in addition, "heritability estimates are inconsistent across studies"), there is reality (e.g., the realistic aspect of "heritability studies," insofar as "findings from numerous personality studies show that genetics account for 50% of the variance in Five-Factor Model and the variance in subjective well-being is also heritable"). And the reverse direction also holds true.

In relation to the cognitiveness-noncognitiveness principle, if there is cognitiveness (e.g., a view of things on the basis of reason and evidences, as shown in the research findings that "all cultures seem to value happiness"), there is noncognitiveness (e.g., a view of things on the basis of non-cognitive factors like envy, jealousy, power, nationality, race, gender, age, class, greed, lust, status, faith, anger, sadness, joy, fear, wish, etc., as shown in the "politics" of cultural identity, such that "individualistic versus collectivistic nations reliably differ in a variety of psychological characteristics that are related to SWB," such that this difference cannot be reconciled on the basis of reason and evidences alone, due to the politics in question). And the reverse direction also holds true.

In relation to the finiteness-transfiniteness principle, if there is finiteness (e.g., the finite number of the components of SWB, like the 2 components aforedescribed), there is transfiniteness (e.g., the transfinite number of all the individuals in human history who have ever existed and can be described on the basis of the 2 compnents of SWB). And the reverse direction also holds true.

In relation to the preciseness-vagueness principle, if there is preciseness (e.g., the precise identification of 2 theories of the causes of

SWB in the article aforecited), there is vagueness (e.g., the vagueness in the identification of the 2 theories of the causes of SWB in the article aforecited, since it is not clear why there must be only 2, not 3, 4, 5, 6, and so on). And the reverse direction also holds true.

In relation to the simpleness-complicatedness principle, if there is simpleness (e.g., the relatively simple analysis of SWB by the advocates), there is complicatedness (e.g., the relatively more complicated analysis of SWB, by challenging the claims and assumptions, as shown in the problems pointed out by the critics as cited). And the reverse direction also holds true.

In relation to the openness-hiddenness principle, if there is openness (e.g., the open exploration of the "subjective" aspects of well-being by the advocates of SWB), there is hiddenness (e.g., the hidden bias in the "subjective" aspects of well-being by the advocates of SWB, since they ignore the "objective" aspects). And the reverse direction also holds true.

In relation to the denseness-emptiness principle, if there is denseness (e.g., the relatively denser concentration of concerns with the "genetic predisposition to be happy or unhappy" by those in the Top-down theories of SWB), there is emptiness (e.g., the relatively less dense, or more empty, concentration of concerns with the "genetic predisposition to be happy or unhappy" by those in the bottom-up theories of SWB). And the reverse direction also holds true.

In relation to the prototypicality-variation principle, if there is prototypicality (e.g., the prototype, like the example about the original "hedonic treadmill theory" which "proposed that most people return to a neutral level of SWB [i.e. neither happy nor unhappy] as they habituate to events"), there is variation (e.g., different variants of the protoptye, as shown in many further studies since then, like the "additional refinements to this theory [the original hedonic treadmill theory]" which "have shown that people do not adapt to all life events equally, as people tend to adapt rapidly to some events [e.g. imprisonment], slowly to others [e.g. the death of a loved one], and not at all to others [e.g. noise and sex]"). (WK 2013u; E. Diener 2000) And the reverse direction also holds true.

In relation to the change-constancy principle, if there is change (e.g., the ever new ways to understand the nature of health and well-being, as shown in the research on SWB), there is constancy (e.g., the ever constant existence of different problems with the ever new ways to understand the nature of health and well-being, as shown in the problems with the research on SWB pointed out by the critics). And the reverse direction also holds true.

In relation to the order-chaos principle, if there is order (e.g., the more or less orderly view on health and SWB, if looked from the sole vantage point of the advocates of SWB, in that "SWB constructs are strongly associated with a range of personality traits"), there is chaos (e.g., the more or less chaotic view on health and SWB, if looked from the multiple conflicting vantage points that it ignores the "objective" conditions of well-being, that the findings are not consistent across studies and across histories, that much remains uncertain about the nature of SWB, that SWB can be detrimental to health, that it neglects social factors, that it does not give sufficient attention to cultural variations, and so on). And the reverse direction also holds true.

In relation to the slowness-quickness principle, if there is slowness (e.g., the relatively slower speed of some people who, according to some studies on the hedonic treadmill theory, "tend to adapt…slowly" to some events like "the death of a loved one"), there is quickness (e.g., the relatively quicker speed of some people who, according to some studies on the hedonic treadmill theory, "tend to adapt rapidly to some events [e.g. imprisonment]"). (WK 2013u; E. Diener 2000) And the reverse direction also holds true.

In relation to the expansion-contraction principle, if there is expansion (e.g., the relatively more developed ability of those in Western cultures to express "personal independence, a sense of personal agency, and self-expression"), there is contraction (e.g., the relatively less developed ability of those in Western cultures to express "an interdependent self that is inseparable from significant others" and "to suppress their personal desires when necessary in order to promote collective interests"). (WK 2013u) And the reverse direction also holds true.

In relation to the optimality-nonoptimality principle, if there is optimality (e.g., the search for highly favorable options, like the quest for "a person's baseline or equilibrium level of SWB," which, according to Set Point theory, is "a consequence of hereditary characteristics and therefore, almost entirely predetermined at birth"), there is nonoptimality (e.g., the existence of non-optimal alternatives to optimality, like the argument for more realistic studies by the critics, who pointed out other complicated factors, like "social influence," "cultural variations," "objective" aspects of well-being, Western-centric samples, etc.). And the reverse direction also holds true.

In relation to the theory-praxis principle, if there is theory (e.g., the theoretical construction of "heritability" in genetics), there is praxis (e.g., the practical application of "heritability" in genetics to the field of psychology, like the study on the correlation between genetics and SWB). And the reverse direction also holds true.

In relation to the convention-novelty principle, if there is convention (e.g., the conventional wisdom about the correlation between health and SWB), there is novelty (e.g., the alternative novel challenge to the conventional wisdom about the correlation between health and SWB, by the new idea that, "in the case of "survival," there is "evidence" which "suggests happiness may actually be...detrimental" to health). And the reverse direction also holds true.

In relation to the evolution-transformation principle, if there is evolution (e.g., the natural evolution of humans to experience SWB like "affect balance" and "life satisfaction" in the state of nature in a primitive way), there is transformation (e.g., the technical transformation of human ability to understand SWB like "affect balance" and "life satisfaction" by the invention of "positive psychology" for the systematic study of SWB). And the reverse direction also holds true.

In relation to the symmetry-asymmetry principle, if there is symmetry (e.g., the co-existence of different events that can affect people, like "imprisonment," "the death of a loved one," etc.), there is asymmetry (e.g., according to some studies on the hedonic treadmill theory, "people do not adapt to all life events equally, as people tend to adapt rapidly to some events [e.g. imprisonment], slowly to others [e.g. the death of a loved one], and not at all to others [e.g. noise and sex]"). (WK 2013u) And the reverse direction also holds true.

In relation to the softness-hardness principle, if there is softness (e.g., the defense of SWB by the advocates), there is hardness (e.g., the critique of SWB by the critics). And the reverse direction also holds true.

In relation to the seriousness-playfulness principle, if there is seriousness (e.g., the serious business of those in SWB who try to understand the causes of SWB), there is playfulness (e.g., the playful part of those in SWB who try to understand the causes of SWB, when they play around with different theories over the decades, like the "top-down" and "bottom-up" versions). And the reverse direction also holds true.

In relation to the activeness-inactivess principle, if there is activeness (e.g., the relative activeness of those who can successfully cope with life problems because they often "apprais[e] events in an optimistic fashion" and "hav[e] a sense of control," according to the studies on SWB and genetics), there is inactiveness (e.g., the relative inactiveness of those who cannot successfully cope with life problems because they often show "cynicism" and make "negative attributions about others," so they get stuck with their life problems, according to the studies on SWB and genetics). (WK 2013u) And the reverse direction also holds true.

In relation to the selfness-otherness principle, if there is selfness (e.g., the tendency to be mostly centered on one's self or group, as shown in the studies which showed some "people" who "believe that money does more for happiness than it really does," so they become obsessed with money for themselves), there is otherness (e.g., the tendency to be mostly centered on others, as shown in the studies which showed some "people" who "believe that "spending money on others promotes happiness," so they become more others-oriented). (WK 2013u; M. Norton 2009) And the reverse direction also holds true.

In relation to the regression-progression principle, if there is regression (e.g., the regression made by the study on SWB, as shown in the problems pointed out by the critics), there is progression (e.g., the progress made by the study on SWB, as shown in the contribution to the understanding of the association between genetics and SWB aforecited). And the reverse direction also holds true.

In relation to the same-difference principle, if there is similarity in outcome (e.g., the contribution to the molding and control of beliefs, values, and behaviors, regardless of whether this be done by way of the study on the five factor model and genetics, or by way of the Framingham Heart Study on social influences), there is difference in outcome (e.g., the contribution to the molding and control of beliefs, values, and behaviors by way of the study on the five factor model and genetics for a relatively more biological worldview—but the contribution to the molding and control of beliefs, values, and behaviors by way of the Framingham Heart Study for a relatively more social worldview). And the reverse direction also holds true.

In relation to the stability-reaction principle, if there is stability (e.g., the relatively more stable condition of the popular research on the relationship between genetics and SWB), there is reaction (e.g., the popular research on the relationship between genetics and SWB then led to further changes later on, when nowadays there are new criticisms that it ignores the "objective" conditions of well-being, that the findings are not consistent across studies and across histories, that much remains uncertain about the nature of SWB, that SWB can be detrimental to health, that it neglects social factors, and that it does not give sufficient attention to cultural variations). And the reverse direction also holds true.

In relation to the functionality-nonfunctionality principle, if there is functionality (e.g., the presence of action for which something or someone is fitted, as shown in the popular research on the relationship between genetics and SWB, which serves the function of providing a biological interpretation of human well-being), there is nonfunctionality (e.g., the relative lack of action for which something or someone is fitted, as shown in the criticisms by the critics that the argument on genetics and SWB does not give sufficient attention to social factors and cultural variations, such that the argument is no longer functional nowadays among the critics, who ask for a more balanced approach to take into account of social and cultural factors). And the reverse direction also holds true.

In relation to the intentionality-nonintentionality principle, if there is intentionality (e.g., the planning or design of something for a certain outcome, as shown in the original intention of Seligman and Csikszentmihalyi to study SWB in the context of "personality/genetics," such that "changing one's external circumstances tends to have only a temporary effect on SWB"), there is nonintentionality (e.g., the relative absence of planning or design of something for a certain outcome, such that the outcome can even be counter-intentional in being the opposite of what was originally planned, as shown in the new studies nowadays which show the importance and persistence of "social influences" and "cultural variations" in SWB—contrary to the original intention of Seligman and Csikszentmihalyi to study SWB in the context of "personality/genetics"). And the reverse direction also holds true.

And in relation to the survivability-nonsurvivability principle, if there is survivability (e.g., the relative survival of those patients who "take their symptoms" serioiusly and "seek treatment" early, according to a study by Diener [2008] and his colleagues), there is non-survivability (e.g., the relative non-survival of those patients, who "tend to be optimistic, leading them to take their symptoms too lightly, seek treatment too late, and/or follow the doctor's instructions half-heartedly," according to a study by Diener [2008] and his colleagues). (WK 2013u) And the reverse direction also holds true.

Mental Health and Nature

Mental health, when examined from the perspective of nature, can show us in a controversial way its possibility (or impossibility) and desirability (or undesirability), and this can be shown by way of two case studies, namely, (2.3.1) mental health, evolution, and the environment, and (2.3.2) mental health, zoophilia, and animals —to be addressed in what follows, respectively.

Mental Health, Evolution, and the Environment

A good way to evaluate the possibility (or impossibility) and desirability (or undesirability) of mental health from the perspective of the mind is to explore mental health, evolution, and the environment.

An argument in the literature is that "human psychological traits are evolved adaptations—that is, the functional products of natural selection or sexual selection." (WK 2013m)

Although "adaptationist thinking about physiological mechanisms, such as the heart, lungs, and immune system, is common in evolutionary biology"—"some evolutionary psychologists apply the same thinking to psychology, arguing that the mind has a modular structure similar to that of the body, with different modular adaptations serving different functions. Evolutionary psychologists argue that much of human behavior is the output of psychological adaptations that evolved to solve recurrent problems in human ancestral environments." (WK 2013m; R. Durrant 2003; S. Pinker 2002; J. Tooby 2005).

Scope of Evolutionary Psychology

Evolutionary psychology can be better understood in terms of its "principles" and "premises" (as summarized in *Table 2.3*).

(a) Principles

In regard to principles, "evolutionary psychology is an approach that views human nature as the product of a universal set of evolved psychological adaptations to recurring problems in the ancestral environment. Proponents of EP suggest that it seeks to integrate psychology into the other natural sciences, rooting it in the organizing theory of biology (evolutionary theory), and thus understanding psychology as a branch of biology." (WK 2013m)

Thus, "the purpose of evolutionary psychology is to identify evolved emotional and cognitive adaptations that represent 'human psychological nature'....EP views the human brain as comprising many functional mechanisms, called *psychological adaptations* or evolved cognitive mechanisms or *cognitive modules*, designed by the process of natural selection. Examples include language-acquisition modules, incest-avoidance mechanisms, cheater-detection mechanisms, intelligence and sex-specific mating preferences, foraging mechanisms, alliance-tracking mechanisms, agent-detection mechanisms, and others. Some mechanisms, termed *domain-specific*, deal with recurrent adaptive problems over the course of human evolutionary history. *Domain-general* mechanisms, on the other hand, are proposed to deal with evolutionary novelty." (WK 2013m)

(b) Premises

Evolutionary psychology is based on some main premises, as shown below: (WK 2013m; L. Cosmides 1997)

- "the brain is an information processing device, and it produces behavior in response to external and internal inputs."
- "the brain's adaptive mechanisms were shaped by natural and sexual selection."
- "different neural mechanisms are specialized for solving problems in humanity's evolutionary past."
- "the brain has evolved specialized neural mechanisms that were designed for solving problems that recurred over deep evolutionary time, giving modern humans stone-age minds."
- "most contents and processes of the brain are unconscious; and most mental problems that seem easy to solve are actually extremely difficult problems that are solved unconsciously by complicated neural mechanisms."
- "human psychology consists of many specialized mechanisms, each sensitive to different classes of information or inputs. These mechanisms combine to produce manifest behavior."

These premises of evolutionary psychology are based on "Charles Darwin's work" and other "advances in evolutionary theory in the 20th century," as explained below.

Theoretical Foundations of Evolutionary Psychology

Three major theoretical foundations of evolutionary psychology can be summarized hereafter (and in *Table 2.3*).

(a) C. Darwin's Natural Selection/Sexual Selection

In accordance to evolutionary psychology, "natural selection has provided humans with many psychological adaptations, in much the same way that it generated humans' anatomical and physiological adaptations. As with adaptations in general, psychological adaptations are said to be specialized for the environment in which an organism evolved, the environment of evolutionary adaptedness, or EEA. Sexual selection provides organisms with adaptations related to mating. For male mammals, which have a relatively high maximal potential reproduction rate, sexual selection leads to adaptations that help them compete for females. For female mammals, with a relatively low maximal potential reproduction rate, sexual selection leads to choosiness, which helps females select higher quality mates. Charles Darwin described both natural selection and sexual selection, and he relied on group selection to explain the evolution of altruistic (self-sacrificing) behavior. But group selection was considered a weak explanation, because in any group the less altruistic individuals will be more likely to survive, and the group will become less self-sacrificing as a whole." (WK 2013m; P. Rubin 2003; S. Gaulin 2003)

(b) W. Hamilton's Inclusive Fitness

Later, "in 1964, William D. Hamilton proposed inclusive fitness theory, emphasizing a 'gene's-eye' view of evolution. Hamilton noted that individuals can increase the replication of their genes into the next generation by helping close relatives with whom they share genes survive and reproduce. According to 'Hamilton's rule,' a self-sacrificing behavior can evolve if it helps close relatives so much that it more than compensates for the individual animal's sacrifice. Inclusive fitness theory resolved the issue of how 'altruism' evolved. Other theories also help explain the evolution of altruistic behavior, including evolutionary game theory, tit-for-tat reciprocity, and generalized reciprocity. These theories not only help explain the development of altruistic behavior, but also account for hostility toward cheaters (individuals that take advantage of others' altruism)." (WK 2013m; R. Wright 1995)

(c) Other Advances in Evolutionary Theory

In accordance to "the r/K selection theory,...some species prosper by having many offspring, while others follow the strategy of having fewer offspring but investing much more in each one. Humans follow the second strategy. Parental investment theory explains how parents invest more or less in individual offspring based on how successful those offspring are likely to be, and thus how much they might improve the parents' inclusive fitness. According to the Trivers-Willard hypothesis, parents in good conditions tend to invest more in sons (who are best able to take advantage of good conditions), while parents in poor conditions tend to invest more in daughters (who are best able to have successful offspring even in poor conditions). According to life history theory, animals evolve life histories to match their environments, determining details such as age at first reproduction and number of offspring. Dual inheritance theory posits that genes and human culture have interacted, with genes affecting the development of culture, and culture, in turn, affecting human evolution on a genetic level." (WK 2013m)

Evolved Psychological Mechanisms

With these theoretical foundations in mind, "evolutionary psychology is based on the hypothesis that, just like hearts, lungs, livers, kidneys, and immune systems, cognition has functional structure that has a genetic basis, and therefore has evolved by natural selection. Like other organs and tissues, this functional structure should be universally shared amongst a species, and should solve important problems of survival and reproduction." (WK 2013m)

In other words, "evolutionary psychologists seek to understand psychological mechanisms by understanding the survival and reproductive functions they might have served over the course of evolutionary history. These might include abilities to infer others' emotions, discern kin from non-kin, identify and prefer healthier mates, or cooperate with others. Consistent with the theory of natural selection, evolutionary psychology sees humans as often in conflict with others, including mates and relatives. Even mothers sometimes struggle with their children over weaning, which benefits the mother more than the child. Evolutionary psychology also recognizes the role of kin selection and reciprocity in evolving prosocial traits such as altruism. Like chimps and bonobos, humans have subtle and flexible social instincts, allowing them to form extended families, lifelong friendships, and political alliances. In studies testing theoretical predictions, evolutionary psychologists have made modest findings on topics such as infanticide, intelligence, marriage patterns, promiscuity, perception of beauty, bride price and parental investment." (WK 2013m R. Wright 1995)

Research Methods

The research methods of evolutionary psychology are "heuristic," and "one of the major goals of adaptationist research is to identify which organismic traits are likely to be adaptations." (WK 2013m)

In general, "evolutionary psychologists use several strategies to develop and test hypotheses about whether a psychological trait is likely to be an evolved adaptation," and hereafter are four main ones: (WK 2013m; D. Buss 2011)

- "Cross-Cultural Consistency"—"Characteristics that have been demonstrated to be cross cultural human universals such as smiling, crying, facial expressions are presumed to be evolved psychological adaptations. Several evolutionary psychologists have collected massive datasets from cultures around the world to assess cross-cultural universality."

- "Function to Form (or 'Problem to Solution')"—"The fact that males, but not females, risk potential misidentification of genetic offspring (referred to as 'paternity insecurity') led evolutionary psychologists to hypothesize that, compared to females, male jealousy would be more focused on sexual, rather than emotional, infidelity."
- "Form to Function (Reverse-Engineering or 'Solution to Problem')"—"Morning sickness, and associated aversions to certain types of food, during pregnancy seemed to have the characteristics of an evolved adaptation (complexity and universality). Margie Profet hypothesized that the function was to avoid the ingestion of toxins during early pregnancy that could damage fetus (but which are otherwise likely to be harmless to healthy non-pregnant women)."
- "Corresponding Neurological Modules"—"Evolutionary psychology and cognitive neuropsychology are mutually compatible–evolutionary psychology helps to identify psychological adaptations and their ultimate, evolutionary functions, while neuropsychology helps to identify the proximate manifestations of these adaptations."

Of course, evolutionary psychologists also use other methods like "experiments, archaeological records, data from hunter-gatherer societies, observational studies, self-reports and surveys, public records, and human products." (WK 2013m; D. Buss 2004)

Areas of Research

There are different areas of research in evolutionary psychology, and hereafter are two good examples (as summarized in *Table 2.3*).

(a) Emotion and Motivation

In evolutionary psychology, "motivations direct and energize behavior, while emotions provide the affective component to motivation, positive or negative. In the early 1970s, Paul Ekman and colleagues began a line of research that suggests that many emotions are universal. He found evidence that humans share at least five basic emotions: fear, sadness, happiness, anger, and disgust. Social emotions evidently evolved to motivate social behaviors that were adaptive in the EEA. For example, spite seems to work against the individual but it can establish an individual's reputation as someone to be feared. Shame and pride can motivate behaviors that help one maintain one's standing in a community, and self-esteem is one's estimate of one's status." (WK 2013m; S. Gaulin 2003; R. Wright 1995)

(b) Cognition

In evolutionary psychology, "cognition refers to internal representations of the world and internal information processing. From an EP perspective, cognition is not 'general purpose,' but uses heuristics, or strategies, that generally increase the likelihood of solving problems that the ancestors of present day humans routinely faced. For example, present day humans are far more likely to solve logic problems that involve detecting cheating (a common problem given humans' social nature) than the same logic problem put in purely abstract terms. Since the ancestors of present day humans did not encounter truly random events, present day humans may be cognitively predisposed to incorrectly identify patterns in random sequences. 'Gamblers' Fallacy' is one example of this. Gamblers may falsely believe that they have hit a 'lucky streak' even when each outcome is actually random and independent of previous trials. Most people believe that if a fair coin has been flipped 9 times and Heads appears each time, that on the tenth flip, there is a greater than 50% chance of getting Tails. Humans find it far easier to make diagnoses or predictions using frequency data than when the same information is presented as probabilities or percentages, presumably because the ancestors of present day humans lived in relatively small tribes (usually with fewer than 150 people) where frequency information was more readily available." (WK 2013m; S. Gaulin 2003)

Problems with Evolutionary Adaptedness

However, for the critics, this argument on mental health, evolutionary adaptedness, and the environment has some major problems. Consider, for illustration, a few examples below (as summarized in *Table 2.3*).

Firstly, one main criticism of the argument on mental health, evolutionary adaptedness, and the environment is that there are "non-genetic and non-adaptive explanations" which are not adequately considered.

For instance, for the critics, there are non-adaptive "by-products" (of "an adaptive mechanism with no current or ancestral function," like "white color of bones" or "belly button") and "random noise" (i.e., "random variations in an adaptation or byproduct" like "bumps on the skull, convex or concave belly button shape"), which then led George C Williams (1996) to once suggest that an "adaptation is a special and onerous concept that should only be used where it is really necessary." (WK 2013m)

Secondly, another main criticism of the argument on mental health, evolutionary adaptedness, and the environment is that there is the controversial issues about testability and uncertainty.

For instance, for the critics, "controversies concerning EP involve questions of testability, cognitive and evolutionary assumptions (such as modular functioning of the brain, and large uncertainty about the ancestral environment)." (WK 2013m)

Thirdly, still another main criticism of the argument on mental health, evolutionary adaptedness, and the environment is that it runs the risk of committing "the naturalistic fallacy."

For instance, for the critics, "evolutionary psychology has been entangled in the larger philosophical and social science controversies related to the nature versus nurture debate....For example, eugenics and social darwinism were political philosophies of the early 20th century that were largely based on the naturalistic fallacy—the idea that what is natural is necessarily a moral good. Other critics have expressed concern about EP itself. As an adaptationist, nature-nurture interactionist perspective, it challenged the basic tenets of the predominant paradigms of the social sciences, social learning theory and social constructionism. This view suggested that biology could be pretty much safely ignored when studying human behavior. The result has been sometimes heated discussions between supporters of these two different theoretical paradigms." (WK 2013m; S. Pinker 2002)

Fourthly, an additional main criticism of the argument on mental health, evolutionary adaptedness, and the environment is that it is reductionistic.

For instance, "some critics view evolutionary psychology as a form of genetic reductionism and genetic determinism, a common critique being that evolutionary psychology does not address the complexity of individual development and experience and fails to explain the influence of genes on behavior in individual cases." (WK 2013m; H. Plotkin 2004)

And fifthly, another additional main criticism of the argument on mental health, evolutionary adaptedness, and the environment is that there are disagreements on the "modularity of the mind."

For instance, for the critics, "evolutionary psychology generally presumes that, like the body, the mind is made up of many evolved modular adaptations," but "there is...disagreement within the discipline regarding the degree of general plasticity, or 'generality,' of some modules"—and, in addition, "recent computer simulations of the evolution of neural nets suggests that modularity evolves" or changes over time too. (WK 2013m; R. Kurzban 2011; J. Confer 2010; J. Clune 2012)

Beyond Evolutionary Adaptedness

These criticisms of evolutionary psychology are not to suggest a total rejection of its usefulness but serve to show us the two opposing sides of the debate, such that the possibility (or impossibility) and desirability (or undesirability) of mental health (from the perspective of nature with mental health, evolutionary adaptedness, and the environment as a case study here) are not to the extent that the respective defenders would like us to believe.

In addition, the analysis of mental health, evolutionary adaptedness, and the environment is to shed some light on the ontological principles in existential dialectics, and good examples include the formalness-informalness principle, the absoluteness-relativeness principle, the partiality-totality principle, the predictability-unpredictability principle, the explicability-inexplicability principle, the fiction-reality principle, the cognitiveness-noncognitiveness principle, the finiteness-transfiniteness principle, the preciseness-vagueness principle, the simpleness-complicatedness principle, the openness-hiddenness principle, the denseness-emptiness principle, the prototypicality-variation principle, the change-constancy principle, the order-chaos principle, the slowness-quickness principle, the expansion-contraction principle, the optimality-nonoptimality principle, the theory-praxis principle, the convention-novelty principle, the evolution-transformation principle, the symmetry-asymmetry principle, the softness-hardness principle, the seriousness-playfulness principle, the activeness-inactivess principle, the selfness-otherness principle, the regression-progression principle, the same-difference principle, the stability-reaction principle, the functionality-nonfunctionality principle, and the intentionality-nonintentionality principle.

For instance, in relation to the formalness-informalness principle, if there is formalness (e.g., the formal logical requirement of soundness, completeness, and consistency in a system of ideas, as in the argument on mental health, evolutionary adaptedness, and the environment), there is informalness (e.g., the non-formal existence of unsoundness, incompleteness, and inconsistency in the argument on mental health, evolutionary adaptedness, and the environment, as shown in the criticisms that there are "non-genetic and non-adaptive explanations" which are not adequately considered, that there is the controversial issues about testability and uncertainty, that it runs the risk of committing "the naturalistic fallacy," that it is reductionistic, and that there are disagreements on the "modularity of the mind"). And the reverse direction also holds true.

In relation to the absoluteness-relativeness principle, if there is absoluteness (e.g., the absolute view on psychological adaptations by those in EP), there is relativeness (e.g., what is right for those in EP to focus on psychological adaptations is not necessarily so for the critics, who argued that it suffers from "genetic reductionism"). And the reverse direction also holds truc.

In relation to the partiality-totality principle, if there is partiality (e.g., the partial view on mental health and psychological adaptations by those in EP), there is totality (e.g., the more holistic view on mental health and psychological adaptations, such that the whole is not the sum of its parts, that is, it cannot be reduced to the sum of opposing views by those for EP, those focusing on "the complexity of individual development and experience," those for social learning theory, those for social constructionism, etc., since there will emerge new views in the future not yet known today, just as there are already alternative views nowadays which do not side exclusively with any of them, as is the analysis here). And the reverse direction also holds true.

In relation to the predictability-unpredictability principle, if there is predictability (e.g., the predictable tendency of those in EP to single out the role of psychological adaptation), there is unpredictability (e.g., the more difficult task to predict exactly the extent to which psychological adaptation may apply in a particular individual case, since, for the critics, "evolutionary psychology does not address the complexity of individual development and experience," among other problems aforecited). And the reverse direction also holds true.

In relation to the explicability-inexplicability principle, if there is explicability (e.g., the explanation, by those in EP, of emotion and cognition on the basis of "evolved psychological mechanisms"), there is inexplicability (e.g., the lack of sufficient explanation, by those in EP, of why "evolved psychological mechanisms" is necessarily useful, since, for the critics, "evolutionary psychology…fails to explain the influence of genes on behavior in individual cases," among other problems aforecited). And the reverse direction also holds true.

In relation to the fiction-reality principle, if there is fiction (e.g., the fictional aspect of EP, insofar as there are "non-genetic and non-adaptive explanations" which are not adequately considered), there is reality (e.g., the realistic aspect of EP, insofar as it addresses the role of "evolved psychological mechanisms" in certain relevant cases). And the reverse direction also holds true.

In relation to the cognitiveness-noncognitiveness principle, if there is cognitiveness (e.g., a view of things on the basis of reason and evidences, as shown in research findings about psychological adaptations on "topics such as infanticide, intelligence, marriage patterns, promiscuity," etc.), there is noncognitiveness (e.g., a view of things on the basis of non-cognitive factors like envy, jealousy, power, nationality, race, gender, age, class, greed, lust, status, faith, anger, sadness, joy, fear, wish, etc., as shown in the "politics" of "eugenics and social darwinism" in the early 20th century that were largely based on the naturalistic fallacy," because of the politics in action). And the reverse direction also holds true.

In relation to the finiteness-transfiniteness principle, if there is finiteness (e.g., the finite number of the areas of research in EP, like "cognition" and "emotion/motivation" aforediscussed), there is transfiniteness (e.g., the transfinite number of all the indiviudals in history who have ever existed and whose cognition, emotion, and motivation can be addressed from the standpoint of EP). And the reverse direction also holds true.

In relation to the preciseness-vagueness principle, if there is preciseness (e.g., the precise identification of 4 research methods in the article aforecited), there is vagueness (e.g., the vagueness in the identification of the 4 research methods in the article aforecited, since it is not clear why there must be only 4, not 5, 6, 7, and so on). And the reverse direction also holds true.

In relation to the simpleness-complicatedness principle, if there is simpleness (e.g., the relatively simple analysis of "evolved psychological mechanisms" by the advocates), there is complicatedness (e.g., the relatively more complicated analysis of "evolved psychological mechanisms," by challenging the claims and assumptions, as shown in the problems pointed out by the critics as cited). And the reverse direction also holds true.

In relation to the openness-hiddenness principle, if there is openness (e.g., the open exploration of "evolved psychological mechanisms" in EP), there is hiddenness (e.g., the hidden bias in EP, because, for the critics, it suffers from "genetic reductionism"). And the reverse direction also holds true.

In relation to the denseness-emptiness principle, if there is denseness (e.g., the relatively denser concentration of concerns with "evolved psychological mechanisms" by those in EP), there is emptiness (e.g., the relatively less dense, or more empty, concentration of concerns with "evolved psychological mechanisms" by those in social constructionism). And the reverse direction also holds true.

In relation to the prototypicality-variation principle, if there is prototypicality (e.g., the prototype, like the example about the original evolutionary theory by Charles Darwin), there is variation (e.g., different variants of the protoptye, as shown in many further studies on evolutionary theory since Darwin's original work, like the later theories on "inclusive fitness," "r/K selection," "parental investment," "life history," etc., though each with its own variation, contribution, and disagreement). And the reverse direction also holds true.

In relation to the change-constancy principle, if there is change (e.g., the ever new ways to mental health, as shown in the research on "evolved psychological mechanisms"), there is constancy (e.g., the ever constant existence of different problems with the ever new ways to study mental health, as shown in the problems with the research on "evolved psychological mechanisms" pointed out by the critics). And the reverse direction also holds true.

In relation to the order-chaos principle, if there is order (e.g., the more or less orderly view on health and the environment, if looked from the vantage point of "evolved psychological mechanisms" in EP), there is chaos (e.g., the more or less chaotic view on health and the environment, if looked from the vantage point of "random noise" in evolution, which is not necessarily adaptive at all, together with other conflicting vantage points as pointed out by the critics earlier). And the reverse direction also holds true.

In relation to the slowness-quickness principle, if there is slowness (e.g., the relatively slower speed of someone to "develop close, trusting bonds with others" if s/he did not have "early childhood caregivers" who "could be trusted to provide reliable assistance and attention," according to EP), there is quickness (e.g., the relatively quicker speed of someone to experience "the sweet taste of sugar and the pain of hitting one's knee against concrete," because they are are "the result of fairly obligate psychological adaptations," according to EP). And the reverse direction also holds true.

In relation to the expansion-contraction principle, if there is expansion (e.g., the relative increase of sons to be wanted by parents in good conditions, according to the Trivers-Willard hypothesis, because "parents in good conditions tend to invest more in sons...who are best able to take advantage of good conditions"), there is contraction (e.g., the relative decrease of daughters to be wanted by parents in good conditions, according to the Trivers-Willard hypothesis, because "parents in good conditions tend to invest more in sons...who are best able to take advantage of good conditions"). And the reverse direction also holds true.

In relation to the optimality-nonoptimality principle, if there is optimality (e.g., the search for highly favorable options, like the quest for "inclusive fitness," in that, "according to 'Hamilton's rule,' a self-sacrificing behavior can evolve if it helps close relatives so much that it more than compensates for the individual animal's sacrifice"), there is nonoptimality (e.g., the existence of non-optimal alternatives to optimality, like the argument for more realistic studies by the critics, who pointed out that there are "non-genetic and non-adaptive explanations" which are not adequately considered, that there is the controversial issues about testability and uncertainty, that it runs the risk of committing "the naturalistic fallacy," that it is reductionistic, and that there are disagreements on the "modularity of the mind). And the reverse direction also holds true.

In relation to the theory-praxis principle, if there is theory (e.g., the theoretical construction of "adaptation" in "evolutionary biology"), there is praxis (e.g., the practical application of "adaptation" in "evolutionary biology" to the field of "evolutionary psychology," like the study of "evolved psychological mechanisms"). And the reverse direction also holds true.

In relation to the convention-novelty principle, if there is convention (e.g., the conventional wisdom about "evolved psychological mechanisms" in EP), there is novelty (e.g., the alternative novel challenge to the conventional wisdom about "evolved psychological mechanisms" in EP, by the new idea that EP suffers from "genetic reductionism"). And the reverse direction also holds true.

In relation to the evolution-transformation principle, if there is evolution (e.g., the natural evolution of humans to adapt in the state of nature), there is transformation (e.g., the technical transformation of human ability to understand adaptation by the invention of EP for the systematic study of "evolved psychological mechanisms"). And the reverse direction also holds true.

In relation to the symmetry-asymmetry principle, if there is symmetry (e.g., the co-existence of different traits in humans), there is asymmetry (e.g., not all traits in humans are adaptations, since they "may also be exaptations," "byproducts," "random noise," etc.). (WK 2013m; D. Buss 1998) And the reverse direction also holds true.

In relation to the softness-hardness principle, if there is softness (e.g., the defense of the idea of "evolved psychological mechanisms" by those in EP), there is hardness (e.g., the critique of the idea of "evolved psychological mechanisms" by the critics aforecited). And the reverse direction also holds true.

In relation to the seriousness-playfulness principle, if there is seriousness (e.g., the serious business of those in EP who try to understand "evolved psychological mechanisms"), there is playfulness (e.g., the playful part of those in EP who try to understand "evolved psychological mechanisms," when they play around with different explanations, like "adaptations," "exaptations," "byproducts," "random noise," etc.). And the reverse direction also holds true.

In relation to the activeness-inactivess principle, if there is activeness (e.g., the relative activeness of those who adapt to the environment and successfully cope with life challenges), there is inactiveness (e.g., the relative inactiveness of those who fail to adapt to the environment and become tired, sleepy, sick, injured, etc.).

In relation to the selfness-otherness principle, if there is selfness (e.g., the tendency to be mostly centered on one's self or group, as shown in the study in EP which showed that "mothers sometimes struggle with their children over weaning, which benefits the mother more than the child"), there is otherness (e.g., the tendency to be mostly centered on others, as shown in the study on "inclusive fitness," when "a self-sacrificing behavior can evolve if it helps close relatives so much that it more than compensates for the individual animal's sacrifice"). (WK 2013m) And the reverse direction also holds true.

In relation to the regression-progression principle, if there is regression (e.g., the regression made by evolutionary psychology, as shown in the problems pointed out by the critics), there is progression (e.g., the progress made by evolutionary psychology, as shown in the contribution to the understanding of "evolved psychological mechanisms" aforecited). And the reverse direction also holds true.

In relation to the same-difference principle, if there is similarity in outcome (e.g., the contribution to the molding and control of beliefs, values, and behaviors, regardless of whether this be done by way of evolutionary psychology, or by way of social constructionism), there is difference in outcome (e.g., the contribution to the molding and control of beliefs, values, and behaviors by way of evolutionary psychology for a relatively more genetic-reductionistic worldview—but the contribution to the molding and control of beliefs, values, and behaviors by way of social constructionism for a relatively more social-reductionistic worldview). And the reverse direction also holds true.

In relation to the stability-reaction principle, if there is stability (e.g., the relatively more stable condition of EP in regard to its idea of "evolved psychological mechanisms"), there is reaction (e.g., the established idea of "evolved psychological mechanisms" in EP then led to further changes later on, when nowadays, it receives different criticisms, including the view that it commits "the naturalistic fallacy"). And the reverse direction also holds true.

In relation to the functionality-nonfunctionality principle, if there is functionality (e.g., the presence of action for which something or someone is fitted, as shown in some traits which are "adaptive," as shown by the example of "toddlers' ability to learn to talk with minimal instruction." according to those in EP), there is nonfunctionality (e.g., the relative lack of action for which something or someone is fitted, as shown in some traits which are "non- adaptive," as shown by the example of "within-sex variations in voice pitch," according to those in EP). And the reverse direction also holds true.

In relation to the intentionality-nonintentionality principle, if there is intentionality (e.g., the planning or design of something for a certain outcome, as shown in the original intention of the advocates of EP to use evolutionary theory for the explanation of psychological phenomena like "evolved psychological mechanisms"), there is nonintentionality (e.g., the relative absence of planning or design of something for a certain outcome, such that the outcome can even be counter-intentional in being the opposite of what was originally planned, as shown in the critique by the critics of EP, in that it suffres from "genetic reductionism," among other damaging criticisms aforecited—contrary to the original intention of the advocates of EP to use evolutionary theory for the explanation of psychological phenomena). And the reverse direction also holds true.

And in relation to the survivability-nonsurvivability principle, if there is survivability (e.g., the relative survival, nowadays, of EP), there is non-survivability (e.g., the relative non-survival, nowadays, of "eugenics and social darwinism"). And the reverse direction also holds true.

Mental Health, Zoophilia, and Animals

Another good way to evaluate the possibility (or impossibility) and desirability (or undesirability) of mental health from the perspective of nature is to explore mental health, zoophilia, and animals.

An argument in the literature is that there is a natural attraction of some humans to non-human animals for sexual and other purposes, with implications for mental health.

Concepts on Zoophilia

The word "zoophilia" is a paraphilia involving sexual activity between human and non-human animals or a fixation on such practice," since "the term 'zoophilia' derives from the combination of two nouns in Greek: ζῷον (*zōion*, meaning 'animal') and φιλία (*philia*, meaning 'friendship' or 'love'). (WK 2013v)

However, "zoophilia" should not be confused with some related terms, as shown below (and summarized in *Table 2.4*): (WK 2013v; F. Ascione 2008; SEX 2013; M. Roth 1991; J. MacDonald 1963)

- "Zoophilia"—"was introduced into the field of research on sexuality in *Psychopathia Sexualis* (1886) by Krafft-Ebing, who described a number of cases of 'violation of animals (bestiality),' as well as 'zoophilia erotica,' which he defined as a sexual attraction to animal skin or fur. In general contemporary usage, the term 'zoophilia' may refer to sexual activity between human and non-human animals, the desire to engage in such, or to the specific paraphilia (i.e., the atypical arousal) which indicates a definite preference for non-human animals over humans as sexual partners."
- "Zoosexuality"—"was proposed by Miletski in 2002 as a value-neutral term. Usage of 'zoosexual' as a noun (in reference to a person) is synonymous with zoophile, while the adjectival form of the word – as, for instance, in the phrase 'zoosexual act'—may indicate sexual activity between a human and a non-human animal. The derivative noun 'Zoosexuality' is sometimes used by self-identified zoophiles in both support groups and on internet-based discussion forums to designate sexual orientation manifesting as romantic or emotional involvement with and/or sexual attraction to animals."
- "Bestiality"—was used by "some zoophiles and researchers…to describe the sex acts alone. Confusing the matter yet further, writing in 1962, Masters used the term 'bestialist' specifically in his discussion of zoosadism…, which refers to deriving pleasure (though not necessarily sexual pleasure) from inflicting cruelty to animals. Sephanie LaFarge, an assistant professor of psychiatry at the New Jersey Medical School, and Director of Counseling at the ASPCA, writes that two groups can be distinguished: bestialists, who rape or abuse animals, and zoophiles, who form an emotional and sexual attachment to animals."
- "Zoosadism"—was used by Ernest Bornemann (1990) to refer to "those who derive pleasure—sexual or otherwise—from inflicting

> pain on animals. Zoosadism specifically is one member of the Macdonald triad of precursors to sociopathic behavior."

Of course, there can be other terms, so the ones above are illustrative.

Classifications of Zoophilia

The classification of zoophilia poses another challenge.

For example, "zoophilia is placed in the classification 'paraphilias not otherwise specified' in the DSM-III and IV. The World Health Organization takes the same position, listing a sexual preference for animals in its ICD -10 as 'other disorder of sexual preference.' The DSM-IV (TR) (the Diagnostic and Statistical Manual of the American Psychiatric Association) recommends that the individual does not receive treatment of zoophilia, as with most other paraphilias, unless it is accompanied by distress or interference with normal functioning on the part of the individual." (WK 2013v; APA 2000; J. Milner 2008; J. Money 1988; M. Seto 2000)

In another classification, "the Journal of Forensic and Legal Medicine (Vol. 18, February 2011)...states that there are several kinds of zoophiles," as shown below: (WK 2013v; A. Aggrawal 2013)

1. "Human-animal role-players"
2. "Romantic zoophiles"
3. "Zoophilic fantasizers"
4. "Tactile zoophiles"
5. "Fetishistic zoophiles"
6. "Sadistic bestial"
7. "Opportunistic zoophiles"
8. "Regular zoophiles"
9. "Exclusive zoophiles"

In this classification, "zoophiles in categories 2, 3, and 8 (romantic zoophiles, zoophilic fantisizers, and regular zoophiles) are the most common, while zoophiles found in categories 6 and 7 (sadistic bestials and opportunistic zoophiles) are the least common." (WK 2013v; A. Aggrawal 2013)

More recently, in 2004, Andrea Beetz "described the phenomenon of zoophilia/bestiality as being somewhere between crime, paraphilia and love...." (WK 2013v)

Extent of Occurrence of Zoophilia

This business of conceptual distinctions and classifications aside—a question to ask is, How often does zoophilia occur?

In one study, "the Kinsey reports rated the percentage of people who had sexual interaction with animals at some point in their lives as 8% for men and 3.6% for women, and claimed it was 40–50% in people living near farms." (WK 2013v; D. Laws 2008)

Later, in 1974, "the farm population in the USA had declined by 80 percent compared to 1940, reducing the opportunity to live with animals; Hunt's 1974 study suggests that these demographic changes led to a significant change in reported occurrences of bestiality. The percentage of males who reported sexual interactions with animals in 1974 was 4.9% (1948: 8.3%), and in females in 1974 was 1.9% (1953: 3.6%). Miletski believes this is not due to a reduction in interest but merely a reduction in opportunity." (WK 2013v)

In a different study, this time about zoophilic fantasies (not actual zoophilic acts), "Crépault and Couture (1980) reported that 5.3 percent of the men they surveyed had fantasized about sexual activity with an animal during heterosexual intercourse....Sexual fantasies about zoophilic acts can occur in people who do not have any wish to experience them in real life. Nancy Friday notes that zoophilia as a fantasy may provide an escape from cultural expectations, restrictions, and judgements in regard to sex. A frequent interest in and sexual excitement at watching animals mate is cited as an indicator of latent zoophilia by Massen (1994). Masters (1962) says that some brothel madams used to stage exhibitions of animals mating, as they found it aroused potential clientele...." (WK 2013v; C. Crépault 1980; R. Masters 1962)

In addition, "zoophiles have been described as 'occupying [many] different demographic categories: white, black, Asian, Mormon, Amish, Catholic, atheist, pagan, Jewish, male and female.'" (WK 2013v)

Arguments for Zoophilia

Those who practice zoophilia offer some arguments for their defense (as summarized in *Table 2.4*).

(a) The Issue of Consent

An argument in defense of zoophilia has to do with the issue of "consent," in that "defenders of zoophilia argue that 'consent' is irrelevant because human practices (such as hunting, laboratory testing, artificial insemination, and slaughtering animals for meat) do not involve the consent of the animal." (WK 2013v; L. Wachob 2011)

But some others like Miletski suggested that "'animals are capable of sexual consent—and even initiation—in their own way.' It is not an uncommon practice for dogs to attempt to copulate with ('hump') the legs of people of both genders. Rosenberger (1968) emphasizes that as far as cunnilingus is concerned, dogs require no training, and even Dekkers (1994) and Menninger (1951) admit that sometimes animals take the initiative and do so impulsively." (WK 2013v)

(b) The Issue of Enjoyment

Another argument in defense of zoophilia has to do with the issue of enjoyment, in that "those supporting zoophilia feel animals sometimes even seem to enjoy the sexual attention....Animals such as dogs can be willing participants in sexual activity with humans, and 'seem to enjoy the attention provided by the sexual interaction with a human.' Animal owners normally know what their own pets like or do not like. Most people can tell if an animal does not like how it is being petted, because it will move away. An animal that is liking being petted pushes against the hand, and seems to enjoy it." (WK 2013v)

In this sense, "utilitarian philosopher and animal liberation author Peter Singer argues that zoophilia is not unethical so long as it involves no harm or cruelty to the animal....In the article 'Heavy Petting,' Singer argues that zoosexual activity need not be abusive, and that relationships could form which were mutually enjoyed. Singer and others have argued that people's dislike of bestiality is partly caused by irrational speciesism and anthropocentrism. Because interspecies sex occurs in nature, and because humans are animals, supporters argue that zoosexual activity is not 'unnatural' and is not intrinsically wrong." (WK 2013v)

Zoophilia and Health

The defenders of zoophilia suggested some positive health aspects in the sexual relationships between animals and humans, as Masters (1962) and Beetz (2002) made the following conclusions, as shown below: (WK 2013v; A. Aggrawal 2009)

- "Most zoophiles have (or have also had) long term human relationships as well or at the same time as zoosexual ones, and that zoosexual partners are usually dogs and/or horses."
- "Zoophiles' emotions and care for animals can be real, relational, authentic and (within animals' abilities) reciprocal, and not just a substitute or means of expression. Beetz believes zoophilia is not an inclination which is chosen."

- "Society in general at present is considerably misinformed about zoophilia, its stereotypes, and its meaning. The distinction between zoophilia and zoosadism is a critical one to these researchers, and is highlighted by each of these studies."

In fact, "Masters (1962), Miletski (1999) and Weinberg (2003) each comment significantly on the social harm caused by misunderstandings regarding zoophilia: 'This destroy[s] the lives of many citizens.'" (WK 2013v)

Problems with Zoophilia

However, for the critics, this research on zoophilia has some major problems. Consider, for illustration, a few examples below (as summarized in *Table 2.4*).

Firstly, one main criticism of the research on zoophilia is that there is "self-selection bias" in the research on zoophilia.

For example, in 2004, Andrea Beetz revealed that "as with all volunteer surveys and sexual ones in particular, these studies have a potential for self-selection bias." (WK 2013v; J. Slade 2001) In another study on the Kinsey reports about the occurrence of zoophilia, "some later writers dispute the figures, because the study lacked a random sample in that it included a disproportional amount of prisoners, causing sampling bias." (WK 2013v)

Secondly, another main criticism of the research on zoophilia is that the findings are inconsistent.

For instance, for the critics, on the one hand, "the Kinsey reports rated the percentage of people who had sexual interaction with animals at some point in their lives as 8% for men and 3.6% for women, and claimed it was 40–50% in people living near farms"—but, on the other hand, in a different study, "people who 'grew up in the country around animals were no more likely to become zoophiles than those who grew up in the city without them.'" (WK 2013v; D. Laws 2008)

Thirdly, still another main criticism of the research on zoophilia is that it commits the naturalistic fallacy.

For instance, "because interspecies sex occurs in nature, and because humans are animals, supporters argue that zoosexual activity is not 'unnatural' and is not intrinsically wrong." (WK 2013v) But the problem here is that this is a good example of "the naturalistic fallacy—the idea that what is natural is necessarily a moral good," just as this critique had also been directed against "evolved psychological mechanisms" in evolutionary psychology (as already discussed in the previous section, *Sec. 2.3.1*). (WK 2013m; S. Pinker 2002)

Fourthly, an additional main criticism of research on zoophilia is that there are health and safety concerns in zoophilia.

For instance, for the critics, "zoophilia may reflect...sexual abuse or lack of other avenues of sexual expression....Zoophiles will not usually seek help for their condition, and so do not come to the attention of psychiatrists for zoophilia itself." (WK 2013v; R. Roukema 2003) In addition, "infections that are transmitted from animals to humans are called zoonoses. Some zoonoses may be transferred through casual contact, but others are much more readily transferred by activities that expose humans to the semen, vaginal fluids, urine, saliva, feces and blood of animals. Examples of zoonoses are Brucellosis, Q fever, leptospirosis, and toxocariasis. Therefore sexual activity with animals is, in some instances, a high risk activity. Allergic reactions to animal semen may occur, including anaphylaxis. Bites and other trauma from penetration or trampling may occur." (WK 2013v)

Fifthly, another additional main criticism of research on zoophilia is that there are disagreements about zoophilia across cultures.

For instance, on the affirmative side, "bestiality was accepted in some North American and Middle Eastern indigenous cultures. Sexual intercourse between humans and non-human animals was not uncommon among certain Native American indigenous peoples, including the Hopi. Voget describes the sexual lives of young Native Americans as 'rather inclusive,' including bestiality. In addition, the Copper Inuit people had 'no aversion to intercourse with live animals.'" (WK 2013v; J. Worell 2001; F. Voget 1961; D. Talayesva 1942) But on the negative side, in Europe during "the Middle Ages, zoophilic activity was met with execution, typically burning, and death to the animals involved either the same way or by hanging, as both a violation of Biblical edicts and a degradation of man as a spiritual being rather than one that is purely animal and carnal. Some witches were accused of having congress with the devil in the form of an animal." (WK 2013v; V. Bullough 1994)

Sixthly, still another additional main criticism of research on zoophilia is that the practice can result in violent consequences.

For instance, "in the West, the most explicit records of sex involving humans and animals activity are associated with reports of the murderous sadism, torture and rape of the Roman games and circus, in which some authors estimate that several hundreds of thousands died. Masters believes beasts were specially trained to copulate with women: if the girls or women were unwilling then the animal would attempt rape. A surprising range of creatures was used for such purposes, and taught how to copulate vaginally or anally. Representations of scenes from the sexual lives of the gods, such as Pasiphaë and the Bull, were highly popular, often causing extreme suffering, injury or death. On occasion, the more ferocious beasts were permitted to kill and (if desired) devour their victims afterwards." (WK 2013v)

And seventhly, one last main criticism of the research on zoophilia is that the practice is no longer condoned in our time.

For instance, as the critics are quick to point out, "although sex with animals is not outlawed in some countries, it is not explicitly condoned anywhere. In most countries, bestiality is illegal under animal abuse laws or laws dealing with crimes against nature." (WK 2013v)

Beyond Zoophilia

These criticisms of the research on zoophilia, however, do not imply a total rejection of its usefulness but serve to show us the two opposing sides of the debate, such that the possibility (or impossibility) and desirability (or undesirability) of mental health (from the perspective of nature with mental health, zoophilia, and animals as a case study here) are not to the extent that the respective defenders would like us to believe.

Moreover, the analysis of mental health, zoophilia, and animals is to teach us something important about the ontological principles in existential dialectics, and good examples include the formalness-informalness principle, the absoluteness-relativeness principle, the partiality-totality principle, the predictability-unpredictability principle, the explicability-inexplicability principle, the fiction-reality principle, the cognitiveness-noncognitiveness principle, the finiteness-transfiniteness principle, the preciseness-vagueness principle, the simpleness-complicatedness principle, the openness-hiddenness principle, the denseness-emptiness principle, the prototypicality-variation principle, the change-constancy principle, the order-chaos principle, the slowness-quickness principle, the expansion-contraction principle, the optimality-nonoptimality principle, the theory-praxis principle, the convention-novelty principle, the evolution-transformation principle, the symmetry-asymmetry principle, the softness-hardness principle, the seriousness-playfulness principle, the activeness-inactivess principle, the selfness-otherness principle, the regression-progression principle, the same-difference principle, the stability-reaction principle, the functionality-nonfunctionality principle, and the intentionality-nonintentionality principle.

For instance, in relation to the formalness-informalness principle, if there is formalness (e.g., the formal logical requirement of soundness, completeness, and consistency in a system of ideas, as in the research on zoophilia), there is informalness (e.g., the non-formal existence of unsoundness, incompleteness, and inconsistency in the research on zoophilia, as shown in the criticisms that there is "self-selection bias" in the research on zoophilia, that the findings are inconsistent, that it commits the naturalistic fallacy, that there are health and safety concerns in zoophilia, that there are disagreements about zoophilia across cultures, that the practice can result in violent consequences, and that the practice is no longer condoned in our time"). And the reverse direction also holds true.

In relation to the absoluteness-relativeness principle, if there is absoluteness (e.g., the absolute view on the accpetance of bestiality in some North American and Middle Eastern indigenous cultures in the older days), there is relativeness (e.g., what is right for some North American and Middle Eastern indigenous cultures in the older days to accept bestiality is not necessarily so for Europe during "the Middle Ages, when "zoophilic activity was met with execution, typically burning, and death"). And the reverse direction also holds true.

In relation to the partiality-totality principle, if there is partiality (e.g., the partial view on zoophilia by some North American and Middle Eastern indigenous cultures in the older days for its acceptance), there is totality (e.g., the more holistic view on zoophilia, such that the whole is not the sum of its parts, that is, it cannot be reduced to the sum of opposing views like the acceptance of zoophilia in some North American and Middle Eastern indigenous cultures in the older days, the rejection of zoophilia by those in Europe during "the Middle Ages, and so on, since there will emerge new views in the future not yet known today, just as there are already alternative views nowadays which do not side exclusively with any of them, as is the analysis here). And the reverse direction also holds true.

In relation to the predictability-unpredictability principle, if there is predictability (e.g., the predictable tendency of the political correctness in the foreseeable future that zoophilia "is not explicitly condoned anywhere"), there is unpredictability (e.g., the more difficult task to predict exactly the extent to which form the defense of zoophilia will take in a particular farther future era, in light of the changing history of reacting to zoophilia in the past). And the reverse direction also holds true.

In relation to the explicability-inexplicability principle, if there is explicability (e.g., the explanation, by the defenders of zoophilia, of the extent of its occurrence on the basis of location, in that it was 40–50% in people living near farms," according to "the Kinsey reports"), there is inexplicability (e.g., the lack of sufficient explanation, by the defenders of zoophilia, of why the factor of location necessarily has much explanatory power for the extent of its occurrence, since, for the critics, in a different report, "people who 'grew up in the country around animals were no more likely to become zoophiles than those who grew up in the city without them'"). And the reverse direction also holds true.

In relation to the fiction-reality principle, if there is fiction (e.g., the fictional aspect of the research on zoophilia, insofar as there is "self-selection bias" afore-discussed), there is reality (e.g., the realistic aspect of the research on zoophilia, insofar as "exclusive desire for animals rather than humans is considered a rare paraphilia"). (WK 2013v) And the reverse direction also holds true.

In relation to the cognitiveness-noncognitiveness principle, if there is cognitiveness (e.g., a view of things on the basis of reason and evidences, as shown in the treatment of zoophilia as "a violation of Biblical edicts" during the "Church-oriented" Middle Ages in Europe), there is noncognitiveness (e.g., a view of things on the basis of non-cognitive factors like envy, jealousy, power, nationality, race, gender, age, class, greed, lust, status, faith, anger, sadness, joy, fear, wish, etc., as shown in the "power" of coercion during the "Church-oriented" Middle Ages, when "some witches were accused of having congress with the devil in the form of an animal," and "as with all accusations and confessions extracted under torture in the witch trials in Early Modern Europe, their validity cannot be ascertained"). (WK 2013v; V. Bullough 1994) And the reverse direction also holds true.

In relation to the finiteness-transfiniteness principle, if there is finiteness (e.g., the finite number of the "demographic categories" in the practice of zoophilia, such as "white, black, Asian, Mormon, Amish, Catholic, atheist, pagan, Jewish, male and female"), there is transfiniteness (e.g., the transfinite number of all the individuals in human history who have ever engaged in zoophilia in one form or the other, be it actual, virtual, fantasizing, etc.). And the reverse direction also holds true.

In relation to the preciseness-vagueness principle, if there is preciseness (e.g., the precise identification of 2 main arguments for zoophilia in the article aforecited), there is vagueness (e.g., the vagueness in the identification of the 2 main arguments for zoophilia in the article aforecited, since it is not clear why there must be only 2, not 5, 7, 8, 11, and so on). And the reverse direction also holds true.

In relation to the simpleness-complicatedness principle, if there is simpleness (e.g., the relatively simple analysis of zoophilia by the advocates), there is complicatedness (e.g., the relatively more complicated analysis of zoophilia, by challenging the claims and assumptions, as shown in the problems pointed out by the critics as cited). And the reverse direction also holds true.

In relation to the openness-hiddenness principle, if there is openness (e.g., the open exploration of the extent of occurrence of zoophilia in the research on zoophilia aforecited), there is hiddenness (e.g., the hidden bias in the research on zoophilia aforecited, since there is "self-selection bias" as discovered by Andrea Beetz aforediscussed). And the reverse direction also holds true.

In relation to the denseness-emptiness principle, if there is denseness (e.g., the relatively denser concentration of concerns with the issues of consent and enjoyment by those in the defense of zoophilia aforecited), there is emptiness (e.g., the relatively less dense, or more empty, concentration of concerns with the issues of health and safety by those in the defense of zoophilia aforecited). And the reverse direction also holds true.

In relation to the prototypicality-variation principle, if there is prototypicality (e.g., the prototype, like the example about the term "zoophilia" first introduced by Krafft-Ebing in 1886), there is variation (e.g., different variants of the protoptye, as shown in many ways to define and classify "zoophilia" since the work by Krafft-Ebing, like the ones by the American Psychiatric Association, the World Health Organization, the Journal of Forensic and Legal Medicine, and so on, though each with its own variation, contribution, and disagreement). (WK 2013v) And the reverse direction also holds true.

In relation to the change-constancy principle, if there is change (e.g., the ever new ways to study health, as shown in the research on zoophilia and health), there is constancy (e.g., the ever constant existence of different problems with the ever new ways to study health, as shown in the problems with the research on zoophilia and health pointed out by the critics). And the reverse direction also holds true.

In relation to the order-chaos principle, if there is order (e.g., the more or less orderly view on zoophilia, if looked from the sole vantage point of the defenders, in terms of the issues of consent and enjoyment), there is chaos (e.g., the more or less chaotic view on zoophilia, if looked from the numerous conflictng vantage points as shown in the criticisms from different perspectives aforecited). And the reverse direction also holds true.

In relation to the slowness-quickness principle, if there is slowness (e.g., the relatively slower speed of zoophiles to risk health problems if they are not exposed much or not at all "to the semen, vaginal fluids, urine, saliva, feces and blood of animals"), there is quickness (e.g., the relatively quicker speed of zoophiles to risk health problems if they are exposed "to the semen, vaginal fluids, urine, saliva, feces and blood of animals"). (WK 2013v) And the reverse direction also holds true.

In relation to the expansion-contraction principle, if there is expansion (e.g., the relatively more developed ability of zoophiles to have sex with animals, when they have "exclusive desire for animals rather than humans"), there is contraction (e.g., the relatively less developed ability of zoophiles to have sex with humans, when they have "exclusive desire for animals rather than humans"). And the reverse direction also holds true.

In relation to the optimality-nonoptimality principle, if there is optimality (e.g., the search for highly favorable options, like the quest for the acceptance of zoophilia on maximal utilitarian ground by "utilitarian philosopher and animal liberation author Peter Singer" who "argues that zoophilia is not unethical so long as it involves no harm or cruelty to the animal"), there is nonoptimality (e.g., the existence of non-optimal alternatives to optimality, like the argument for more realistic studies by the critics, who pointed out that "animals might be traumatized even by a non-violent, sexual approach from a human," that it is "profoundly degrading," together with other criticisms aforecited). And the reverse direction also holds true.

In relation to the theory-praxis principle, if there is theory (e.g., the theoretical construction of "consent" in the study of human sexuality on sexual acts between humans), there is praxis (e.g., the practical application of "consent" in the study of human sexuality to the field of zoophilia, as shown in the argument for sexual acts between humans and animals). And the reverse direction also holds true.

In relation to the convention-novelty principle, if there is convention (e.g., the conventional wisdom against zoophilia, as shown in the tendency of "some people [to] express knee-jerk concern or disapproval of sexual interest in non-human animals, sometimes very strongly"), there is novelty (e.g., the alternative novel challenge to the conventional wisdom against zoophilia, by the new idea of defending it on the basis of "consent" and "enjoyment" aforediscussed). And the reverse direction also holds true.

In relation to the evolution-transformation principle, if there is evolution (e.g., the natural evolution of humans to have sex with each other or, in some cases, with animals, in the state of nature), there is transformation (e.g., the technical transformation of human ability to understand sex with each other or, in some cases, with animals by the invention of the field of zoophilia for a systematic study of its practice). And the reverse direction also holds true.

In relation to the symmetry-asymmetry principle, if there is symmetry (e.g., the co-existence of different lifeforms, like animals and humans), there is asymmetry (e.g., "animals don't have the same capacity for thinking as humans," so "they are unable to give full consent," even when humans use them for sex, according to those critics of zoophilia). (WK 2013v) And the reverse direction also holds true.

In relation to the softness-hardness principle, if there is softness (e.g., the defense of zoophilia by the advocates), there is hardness (e.g., the critique of zoophilia by the critics). And the reverse direction also holds true.

In relation to the seriousness-playfulness principle, if there is seriousness (e.g., the serious business of those who try to understand the practice of zoophilia), there is playfulness (e.g., the playful part of those in who try to understand the practice of zoophilia, when they play around with different arguments for and against it over the centuries, like "consent," "enjoyment," "trauma," "degradation," "abuse," etc.). And the reverse direction also holds true.

In relation to the activeness-inactivess principle, if there is activeness (e.g., the relative activeness of those humans who have healthy or safer sex with other humans and do not get sick), there is inactiveness (e.g., the relative inactiveness of those humans who practice risky sex with animals and get very sick because of being exposed to "the semen, vaginal fluids, urine, saliva, feces and blood of animals"). And the reverse direction also holds true.

In relation to the selfness-otherness principle, if there is selfness (e.g., the tendency to be mostly centered on one's self or group, as shown in those zoophiles who practice zoosadism against animals), there is otherness (e.g., the tendency to be mostly centered on others, as shown in those defenders of animal rights against zoosadism). And the reverse direction also holds true.

In relation to the regression-progression principle, if there is regression (e.g., the regression made by zoophilia, as shown in the problems pointed out by the critics), there is progression (e.g., the progress made by zoophilia, as shown in the contribution to the understanding of the history of sexual relationships between humans and animals aforecited). And the reverse direction also holds true.

In relation to the same-difference principle, if there is similarity in outcome (e.g., the contribution to the molding and control of beliefs, values, and behaviors, regardless of whether this be done by way of the medieval sanction against zoophilia in Europe, or by way of the contemporary sanction against zoophilia by the Humane Society of the United States on the ground of the lack of "the same capacity for thinking as humans"), there is difference in outcome (e.g., the contribution to the molding and control of beliefs, values, and behaviors by way of the medieval sanction against zoophilia in Europe for a relatively more religious lifeworld—but the contribution to the molding and control of beliefs, values, and behaviors by way of the medieval sanction against zoophilia in Europe, or by way of the contemporary sanction against zoophilia by the Humane Society of the United States for a relatively more secular lifeworld). And the reverse direction also holds true.

In relation to the stability-reaction principle, if there is stability (e.g., the relatively more stable condition of zoophilia in antiquity, when "bestiality was widespread"), there is reaction (e.g., the stable condition of zoophilia in antiquity then led to further changes later on, when nowadays, "sex with animals…is not explicitly condoned anywhere"). (WK 2013v) And the reverse direction also holds true.

In relation to the functionality-nonfunctionality principle, if there is functionality (e.g., the presence of action for which something or someone is fitted, as shown in the widespread practice of bestiality in antiquity, which served the function of incorporating it "into religious ritual" at that time), there is nonfunctionality (e.g., the relative lack of action for which something or someone is fitted, as shown in the changing condition in our time, when "sex with animals…is not explicitly condoned anywhere," such that the use of bestiality for "religious ritual" is no longer much functional in our itme). (WK 2013v) And the reverse direction also holds true.

In relation to the intentionality-nonintentionality principle, if there is intentionality (e.g., the planning or design of something for a certain outcome, as shown in the original intention of some legal scholars and philosophers to use the idea of "consent" to identify "rape" in human sexual practice), there is nonintentionality (e.g., the relative absence of planning or design of something for a certain outcome, such that the outcome can even be counter-intentional in being the opposite of what was originally planned, as shown in the use of "consent" by the defenders of zoophilia to justify human sexual contacts with animals instead—contrary to the original intention of legal scholars and philosophers to use the idea of "consent" to identify "rape" in human sexual practice). And the reverse direction also holds true.

And in relation to the survivability-nonsurvivability principle, if there is survivability (e.g., the relative survival, nowadays, of the idea that "sex with animals...is not explicitly condoned anywhere"), there is non-survivability (e.g., the relative non-survival, nowadays, of the European medieval practice of punishing zoophiles with "execution, typically burning"). (WK 2013v) And the reverse direction also holds true.

Mental Health and Society

Mental health, when examined from the perspective of society, can reveal to us some powerful features in relation to its possibility (or impossibility) and desirability (or undesirability), and this can be shown by way of two case studies, namely, (2.4.1) mental health, illness, and income inequality, and (2.4.2) mental health, treatment, and technology—to be addressed hereafter.

Mental Health, Illness, and Income Inequality

A good way to evaluate the possibility (or impossibility) and desirability (or undesirability) of mental health from the perspective of society is to explore mental health, illness, and income inequality.

An argument in the literature is the one proposed by Richard G. Wilkinson (2009) and Kate Pickett in *The Spirit Level: Why More Equal Societies Almost Always Do Better* (2009), who argued that there are "pernicious effects that inequality has on societies: eroding trust, increasing anxiety and illness, (and) encouraging excessive consumption," especially in regard to "mental health" (and "physical health," for that matter). (WK 2013o; B. Jarvis 2010)

History of Income Inequality

The term "economic inequality (also known as the gap between rich and poor, income inequality, wealth disparity, or wealth and income differences)" refers to "disparities in the distribution of economic assets (wealth) and income within or between populations or individuals. The term typically refers to inequality among individuals and groups within a society, but can also refer to inequality among countries. The issue of economic inequality is related to the ideas of equity, equality of outcome, and equality of opportunity." (WK 2013w)

Historically, "economic inequality varies between societies and historical periods"; for example, "a study by the World Institute for Development Economics Research at United Nations University reports that the richest 1% of adults alone owned 40% of global assets in the year

2000. The *three* richest people possess more financial assets than the lowest 48 nations combined. The combined wealth of the '10 million dollar millionaires' grew to nearly $41 trillion in 2008. In 2001, 46.4% of people in sub-Saharan Africa were living in extreme poverty. Nearly half of all Indian children are undernourished, however, even among the wealthiest fifth one third of children are malnourished." (WK 2013w; THAI 2008; IND 2007; CAL 2009; ECON 2010)

And in "the two decades prior to the onset of the global financial crisis, real disposable household incomes increased an average of 1.7% a year in its 34 member countries. However, the gap between rich and poor widened in most nations—the OECD journalist resource (2011-05) entitled 'Growing Income Inequality in OECD Countries' states that with the exceptions of only France, Japan and Spain, wages of the 10% best-paid workers have risen relative to those of the 10% least-paid workers and the differential between the top and bottom 10% varies greatly from country to country: 'While this ratio is much lower in the Nordic countries and in many continental European countries, it rises to around 14 to 1 in Israel, Turkey and the United States, to a high of 27 to 1 in Chile and Mexico.'" (WK 2013w; JOUR 2011)

Causes of Income Inequality

Reseachers have pointed out many different causes of income inequality, but "the single most important driver has been greater inequality in wages and salaries." (WK 2013w; A. Gurría 2011)

Consider, for illustration, some main causes of income inequality below (as summarized in *Table 2.5*): (WK 2013w; A. Gurria 2011; L. Bebchuk 2004; J. Bouchaud 2000; I. Meszaros 1995; T. Piketty 2003; TAX 2012; UNRISD 2011; USBLS 2010; B. Charlton 1996)

- "greater inequality in wages and salaries (highly skilled workers earn more than others)"
- "wealth concentration"
- "labor markets (globalization; technological changes; and policy reforms)"
- "more regressive taxation"
- "tax loopholes and shelters such as tax havens"
- "increasing education costs"
- "computerization and increased technology"
- "racial inequality"
- "the gender pay gap"
- "nepotism"

Surely, there can be other causes, so the list above are illustrative.

Effects of Income Inequality (on Health)

Income inequality can produce some important effects on health. For illustration, consider four main examples below (as summarized in *Table 2.5*).

(a) Population Health

The first example of the effects of income inequality on health has to do with "population health."

In fact, "for most of human history higher material living standards—full stomachs, access to clean water and warmth from fuel—led to better health and longer lives. This pattern of higher incomes-longer lives still holds among poorer countries, where life expectancy increases rapidly as per capita income increases, but in recent decades it has slowed down among middle income countries and plateaued among the richest thirty or so countries in the world, where the characteristic most strongly correlated with health is the level of income equality." (WK 2013w; R. Wilkinson 2009)

And "Richard Wilkinson [2011] and Kate Pickett found health and social problems 'more common in countries with bigger income inequalities,' and more common among states in the US with larger income inequalities"—argued that "inequality and social stratification lead to higher levels of psychosocial stress and status anxiety which can lead to depression, chemical dependency, less community life, parenting problems and stress-related diseases." (WK 2013w; R. Booth 2010)

(b) Social Cohesion

The second example of the effects of income inequality on health has to do with "social cohesion."

For instance, "research has shown an inverse link between income inequality and social cohesion. In more equal societies, people are much more likely to trust each other, measures of social capital (the benefits of goodwill, fellowship, mutual sympathy and social connectedness among groups who make up a social units) suggest greater community involvement, and homicide rates are consistently lower." (WK 2013w)

In a study "comparing results from the question 'would others take advantage of you if they got the chance?' in U.S General Social Survey and statistics on income inequality, Eric Uslaner [2002] and Mitchell Brown found there is a high correlation between the amount of trust in society and the amount of income equality. A 2008 article by Andersen and Fetner also found a strong relationship between economic inequality within and across countries and tolerance for 35 democracies." (WK 2013w)

Another researcher "Robert Putnam [1993 & 2000] established links between social capital and economic inequality. His most important studies established these links in both the United States and in Italy." (WK 2013w) And "the economist Joseph Stiglitz has argued that economic inequality has led to distrust of business and government." (WK 2013w)

(c) Crime

The third example of the effects of income inequality on health has to do with "crime."

For instance, "crime rate have...been shown to be correlated with inequality in society. Most studies looking into the relationship have concentrated on homicides—since homicides are almost identically defined across all nations and jurisdictions. There have been over fifty studies showing tendencies for violence to be more common in societies where income differences are larger. Research has been conducted comparing developed countries with undeveloped countries, as well as studying areas within countries. Daly et al. (2001) found that among U.S States and Canadian Provinces, there is a tenfold difference in homicide rates related to inequality. They estimated that about half of all variation in homicide rates can be accounted for by differences in the amount of inequality in each province or state. Fajnzylber et al. (2002) found a similar relationship worldwide." (WK 2013w)

In general, there are two main corrleations between income inequality and crime, as shown below: (WK 2013w; J. Neapolitana 1999; M. Lee 1999)

- "The most consistent finding in cross-national research on homicides has been that of a positive association between income inequality and homicides."
- "Economic inequality is positively and significantly related to rates of homicide despite an extensive list of conceptually relevant controls. The fact that this relationship is found with the most recent data and using a different measure of economic inequality from previous research, suggests that the finding is very robust."

There can be other examples, so the ones above are illustrative.

(d) Social, Cultural, and Civic Participation

And the fourth example of the effects of income inequality on health has to do with "social, cultural, and civic participation."

A good illustration is the correlation that "higher income inequality led to less of all forms of social, cultural, and civic participation among the less wealthy. When inequality is higher, the poor do not shift to less expensive forms of participation." (WK 2013w; B. Lancee 2011)

Problems with the Argument for Less Income Inequality

However, for the critics, this argument on mental health, illness, and income inequality has some major problems. Consider, for illustration, a few examples below (as summarized in *Table 2.5*).

Firstly, one main criticism of the argument on mental health, illness, and income inequality is that it constitutes a very narrow view of social stratification in relation to health care.

For instance, the critic like John Goldthorpe (2009) rebuked by saying that "the book [by Wilkinson and Pickett] elied too heavily on income inequality over other forms of inequality (including broader economic inequality), and demonstrated a one-dimensional understanding of social stratification, with social class being in effect treated as merely a marker for income. He concluded that much more research was needed to support either the Wilkinson and Pickett 'account of the psychosocial generation of the contextual effects of inequality on health or the rival neo-materialist account.'" (WK 2013o)

Secondly, another main criticism of the argument on mental health, illness, and income inequality is that it provides no verification of the claim.

For instance, the critic like "Richard Reeves [2009] in *The Guardian*...said there were problems with the book's approach. 'Drawing a line through a series of data points signals nothing concrete about statistical significance...since they do not provide any statistical analyses, this can't be verified,'" and another critic "John Kay [2009] in *The Financial Times* said that 'the evidence presented in the book is mostly a series of scatter diagrams, with a regression line drawn through them. No data is provided on the estimated equations, or on relevant statistical tests.'" (WK 2013o)

Thirdly, still another main criticism of the argument on mental health, illness, and income inequality is that there is no general agreement on the desirability of income equality (or its reduction).

For instance, "observers differ on both the morality and utility of inequality, whether, and/or how much inequality is necessary in society and how it can be affected. It has been praised as necessary and beneficial, and attacked as a growing social problem." (WK 2013w; T. Garrett 2010) An argument against income equality is the one for "meritocracy," which "favors an eventual society where an individual's success is a direct function of his merit, or contribution. Economic inequality would be a natural consequence of the wide range in individual skill, talent and effort in human population and, being the result of natural variation, individual effort and voluntary exchange, would not be considered ethically problematic in its own right." (WK 2013w)

Fourthly, an additional main criticism of the argument on mental health, illness, and income inequality is that the correlation between health and income level does not always hold.

For instance, for the critics, "Americans live no longer on average (about 77 years in 2004) than Greeks (78 years) or New Zealanders (78), though the USA is almost twice as rich." (WK 2013w)

And fifthly, another additional main criticism of the argument on mental health, illness, and income inequality is that equality can lead to a conformist society.

For instance, in many welfare-oriented (and also communist) countries where the campaign for more income equality is very active, there exists widespread political correctness, to the extent that the society becomes conformist, in the name of higher social capital. The Eastern bloc during the Cold War—and Japan and Nordic countries nowadays—are good examples of higher income equality but also more conformism (higher social capital).

Beyond Less Income Inequality

These criticisms of the argument for the reduction of income inequality, however, should not be misconstrued as a total rejection of its usefulness but serve to show us the two opposing sides of the debate, such that the possibility (or impossibility) and desirability (or undesirability) of mental health (from the perspective of society with mental health, illness, and income inequality as a case study here) are not to the extent that the respective defenders would like us to believe.

Moreover, the analysis of mental health, illness, and income inequality is to shed some light on the ontological principles in existential dialectics, and good examples include the formalness-informalness principle, the absoluteness-relativeness principle, the partiality-totality principle, the predictability-unpredictability principle, the explicability-inexplicability principle, the fiction-reality principle, the cognitiveness-noncognitiveness principle, the finiteness-transfiniteness principle, the preciseness-vagueness principle, the simpleness-complicatedness principle, the openness-hiddenness principle, the denseness-emptiness principle, the prototypicality-variation principle, the change-constancy principle, the order-chaos principle, the slowness-quickness principle, the expansion-contraction principle, the optimality-nonoptimality principle, the theory-praxis principle, the convention-novelty principle, the evolution-transformation principle, the symmetry-asymmetry principle, the softness-hardness principle, the seriousness-playfulness principle, the activeness-inactivess principle, the selfness-otherness principle, the regression-progression principle, the same-difference principle, the stability-reaction principle, the functionality-nonfunctionality principle, and the intentionality-nonintentionality principle.

For instance, in relation to the formalness-informalness principle, if there is formalness (e.g., the formal logical requirement of soundness, completeness, and consistency in a system of ideas, as in the argument for the reduction of income inequality), there is informalness (e.g., the non-formal existence of unsoundness, incompleteness, and inconsistency in the argument for the reduction of income inequality, as shown in the criticisms that the work constitutes a very narrow view of social stratification in relation to health care, that it provides no verification of the claim, that there is no general agreement on the desirability of income equality or its reduction, that the correlation between health and income level does not always hold, and that equality can lead to a conformist society). And the reverse direction also holds true.

In relation to the absoluteness-relativeness principle, if there is absoluteness (e.g., the absolute view on social stratification by Wilkinson and Pickett, because they "relied too heavily on income inequality over other forms of inequality"), there is relativeness (e.g., what is right for Wilkinson and Pickett to focus on "income inequality" is not necessarily so for the critic like John Goldthorpe, who argued for a broader understanding of social stratification by including other forms of inequality too like "broader economic inequality" and others). And the reverse direction also holds true.

In relation to the partiality-totality principle, if there is partiality (e.g., the partial view on social stratification by Wilkinson and Pickett), there is totality (e.g., the more holistic view on social stratification, such that the whole is not the sum of its parts, that is, it cannot be reduced to the sum of opposing views like the one by Wilkinson and Pickett on income inequality, the one by Goldthorpe on "broader economic inequality," etc., since there will emerge new views in the future not yet known today, just as there are already alternative views nowadays which do not side exclusively with any of them, as is the analysis here). And the reverse direction also holds true.

In relation to the predictability-unpredictability principle, if there is predictability (e.g., the predictable tendency of the correlation between health and lesser income inequality, according to Wilkinson and Pickett), there is unpredictability (e.g., the more difficult task to predict exactly the extent to which the correlation between health and lesser income inequality will hold on a particular future occasion, since, for the critics, for example, "Americans live no longer on average [about 77 years in 2004] than Greeks [78 years] or New Zealanders [78], though the USA is almost twice as rich"). And the reverse direction also holds true.

In relation to the explicability-inexplicability principle, if there is explicability (e.g., the explanation, by Wilkinson and Pickett, of the desirability of lesser income inequality on the basis of its positive effects aforecited), there is inexplicability (e.g., the lack of sufficient explanation, by Wilkinson and Pickett, of why lesser income inequality is necessarily desirable, since the critics pointed out that the work constitutes a very narrow view of social stratification in relation to health care, that it provides no verification of the claim, that there is no general agreement on the desirability of income equality or its reduction, that the correlation between health and income level does not always hold, and that equality can lead to a conformist society). And the reverse direction also holds true.

In relation to the fiction-reality principle, if there is fiction (e.g., the fictional aspect of the claim about the correlation between health and lesser income inequality, insofar as there is the counter-example that "Americans live no longer on average [about 77 years in 2004] than Greeks [78 years] or New Zealanders [78], though the USA is almost twice as rich"), there is reality (e.g., the realistic aspect of the claim about some correlation between health and lesser income inequality, insofar as "the most consistent finding in cross-national research on homicides has been that of a positive association between income inequality and homicides"). And the reverse direction also holds true.

In relation to the cognitiveness-noncognitiveness principle, if there is cognitiveness (e.g., a view of things on the basis of reason and evidences, as shown in the research finding that "higher income inequality led to less of all forms of social, cultural, and civic participation among the less wealthy"), there is noncognitiveness (e.g., a view of things on the basis of non-cognitive factors like envy, jealousy, power, nationality, race, gender, age, class, greed, lust, status, faith, anger, sadness, joy, fear, wish, etc., as shown in the ideological politics pointed out by Charles Moore [2010] about the claim by Wilkinson and Pickett, in that their work is "a socialist tract than an objective analysis of poverty"). (WK 2013o) And the reverse direction also holds true.

In relation to the finiteness-transfiniteness principle, if there is finiteness (e.g., the finite number of the causes of income inequality, as shown in the 10 examples aforecited), there is transfiniteness (e.g., the transfinite number of all the individuals in human history who have ever existed and have different income levels with different causes). And the reverse direction also holds true.

In relation to the preciseness-vagueness principle, if there is preciseness (e.g., the precise identification of 4 main effects of income inequality on health in the article aforecited), there is vagueness (e.g., the vagueness in the identification of the 4 main effects of income inequality on health in the article aforecited, since it is not clear why there must be only 4, not 6, 7, 8, 9, 10, 11, and so on). And the reverse direction also holds true.

In relation to the simpleness-complicatedness principle, if there is simpleness (e.g., the relatively simple analysis of the need for lesser income inequality by the advocates), there is complicatedness (e.g., the relatively more complicated analysis of the need for lesser income inequality, by challenging the claims and assumptions, as shown in the problems pointed out by the critics as cited). And the reverse direction also holds true.

In relation to the openness-hiddenness principle, if there is openness (e.g., the open exploration of the correlation between health and lesser income inequality by Wilkinson and Pickett), there is hiddenness (e.g., the hidden bias in the correlation between health and lesser income inequality by Wilkinson and Pickett, since, for the critics, it constitutes a very narrow view of social stratification in relation to health care, it provides no verification of the claim, there is no general agreement on the desirability of income equality or its reduction, the correlation between health and income level does not always hold, and equality can lead to a conformist society). And the reverse direction also holds true.

In relation to the denseness-emptiness principle, if there is denseness (e.g., the relatively denser concentration of concerns with income inequality by Wilkinson and Pickett), there is emptiness (e.g., the relatively less dense, or more empty, concentration of concerns with other forms of inequality like "broader economic inequality" by Wilkinson and Pickett). And the reverse direction also holds true.

In relation to the prototypicality-variation principle, if there is prototypicality (e.g., the prototype, like the example about the original work on income inequality and health by Wilkinson and Pickett in 2009), there is variation (e.g., different variants of the protoptye, as shown in many further views about this work on income inequality by Wilkinson and Pickett since then, like the ones by "the Equality Trust's 'Equality Pledge,'" the article by Ed Miliband, the lecture by David Cameron, etc., though each with its own variation, contribution, and disagreement). And the reverse direction also holds true.

In relation to the change-constancy principle, if there is change (e.g., the ever new ways to understand inequality, as shown in the work by Wilkinson and Pickett), there is constancy (e.g., the ever constant existence of different problems with the ever new ways to understand inequality, as shown in the problems with the work by Wilkinson and Pickett pointed out by the critics). And the reverse direction also holds true.

In relation to the order-chaos principle, if there is order (e.g., the more or less orderly view on the relationship between lesser income inequality and health, if looked from the sole vantage point of Wilkinson and Pickett), there is chaos (e.g., the more or less chaotic view on the relationship between lesser income inequality and health, if looked from the numerous, conflicting vantage points by different advocates and critics alike aforecited). And the reverse direction also holds true.

In relation to the slowness-quickness principle, if there is slowness (e.g., the relatively slower speed of an individual to ever suffer from "psychosocial stress and status anxiety" if he is very rich, according to Wilkinson and Pickett), there is quickness (e.g., the relatively quicker speed of an individual to suffer from "psychosocial stress and status anxiety" if he is very poor, according to Wilkinson and Pickett). And the reverse direction also holds true.

In relation to the expansion-contraction principle, if there is expansion (e.g., the relatively more developed ability of someone to take advantage of others if he suffers from poverty, in accordance to the argument on less income inequality and health), there is contraction (e.g., the relatively less developed ability of someone to trust others if he suffers from poverty, in accordance to the argument on less income inequality and health). And the reverse direction also holds true.

In relation to the optimality-nonoptimality principle, if there is optimality (e.g., the search for highly favorable options, like the quest for reducing income inequality by "Islington's Fairness Commission," following in the footsteps of Wilkinson and Pickett), there is nonoptimality (e.g., the existence of non-optimal alternatives to optimality, like the argument for more realistic studies by the critics, who pointed out that the work by Wilkinson and Pickett is highly problematic, for the reasons aforediscussed). And the reverse direction also holds true.

In relation to the theory-praxis principle, if there is theory (e.g., the theoretical construction of "the spirit level" by Wilkinson and Pickett), there is praxis (e.g., the practical application of "the spirit level" by Wilkinson and Pickett to the field of public politics, as shown in the work of "Islington's Fairness Commission to look at ways of reducing income inequality in the London borough," with Wilkinson being appointed as "the chair"). (WK 2013o; ISL 2011) And the reverse direction also holds true.

In relation to the convention-novelty principle, if there is convention (e.g., the conventional wisdom about laissez-faire capitalism to stress competition between individuals among those on the right wing of the political spectrum), there is novelty (e.g., the alternative novel challenge to the conventional wisdom about laissez-faire capitalism to stress compeition between individuals, by the new idea of Wilkinson and Pickett to reduce income inequality for health and other reasons). And the reverse direction also holds true.

In relation to the evolution-transformation principle, if there is evolution (e.g., the natural evolution of humans to compete and copperate with each other in the state of nature), there is transformation (e.g., the technical transformation of human ability to understand competition and cooperation by the invention of the idea of "the spirit level" for the reduction of income inequality). And the reverse direction also holds true.

In relation to the symmetry-asymmetry principle, if there is symmetry (e.g., the co-existence of different groups in society), there is asymmetry (e.g., income inequality between the rich and the poor in society). And the reverse direction also holds true.

In relation to the softness-hardness principle, if there is softness (e.g., the defense of "the spirit level" by Wilkinson and Pickett), there is hardness (e.g., the critique of "the spirit level" by the critics like Goldthorpe and others). And the reverse direction also holds true.

In relation to the seriousness-playfulness principle, if there is seriousness (e.g., the serious business of those who try to understand income inequality), there is playfulness (e.g., the playful part of those in who try to understand income inequality, when they play around with different views on the causes and effects aforedescribed). And the reverse direction also holds true.

In relation to the activeness-inactivess principle, if there is activeness (e.g., the relative activeness of those who are rich enough to engage fully in life activities without different health problems due to poverty), there is inactiveness (e.g., the relative inactiveness of those who cannot engage fully in life activities because of different health problems due to poverty). (WK 2013w) And the reverse direction also holds true.

In relation to the selfness-otherness principle, if there is selfness (e.g., the tendency to be mostly centered on one's self or group, as shown in those who are rich and want to preserve income inequality vis-a-vis the poor in society), there is otherness (e.g., the tendency to be mostly centered on others, as shown in those who prefer to reduce income inequality between the rich and the poor, like Islington's Fairness Commission). And the reverse direction also holds true.

In relation to the regression-progression principle, if there is regression (e.g., the regression made by the work on "the spirit level," as shown in the problems pointed out by the critics), there is progression (e.g., the progress made by the work on "the spirit level," as shown in the contribution to the debate on the effects of income inequality on health and other problems aforecited). And the reverse direction also holds true.

In relation to the same-difference principle, if there is similarity in outcome (e.g., the contribution to the molding and control of beliefs, values, and behaviors, regardless of whether this be done by way of laissez-faire capitalism, or by way of the "spirit level"), there is difference in outcome (e.g., the contribution to the molding and control of beliefs, values, and behaviors by way of laissez-faire capitalism for a relatively more right-wing worldview—but the contribution to the molding and control of beliefs, values, and behaviors by way of the "spirit level" for a relatively more left-wing worldview). And the reverse direction also holds true.

In relation to the stability-reaction principle, if there is stability (e.g., the relatively more stable condition of laissez-faire capitalism in the older days), there is reaction (e.g., laissez-faire capitalism in the older days then led to further changes later on, when nowadays, there is the socialist tract of "the spirit level" to argue for lesser income inequality). And the reverse direction also holds true.

In relation to the functionality-nonfunctionality principle, if there is functionality (e.g., the presence of action for which something or someone is fitted, as shown in social darwinism in the older days, when it served the function of supporting the ideology of laissez-faire capitalism and other things), there is nonfunctionality (e.g., the relative lack of action for which something or someone is fitted, as shown in the work of "the spirit level" nowadays, which promotes the reduction of income inequality between the rich and the poor, such that the older right-wing ideas like laissez-faire capitalism, social Darwinism, etc. are no longer functional in our time). And the reverse direction also holds true.

In relation to the intentionality-nonintentionality principle, if there is intentionality (e.g., the planning or design of something for a certain outcome, as shown in the original intention of Wilkinson and Pickett to show the close relationship between income inequality and health problems), there is nonintentionality (e.g., the relative absence of planning or design of something for a certain outcome, such that the outcome can even be counter-intentional in being the opposite of what was originally planned, as shown in the criticisms by the critics, who pointed out that the work by Wilkinson and Pickett constitutes a very narrow view of social stratification in relation to health care, that it provides no verification of the claim, that there is no general agreement on the desirability of income equality, that the correlation between health and income level does not really hold, and that equality can lead to a conformist society—contrary to the original intention of Wilkinson and Pickett to show the close relationship between income inequality and health problems). And the reverse direction also holds true.

And in relation to the survivability-nonsurvivability principle, if there is survivability (e.g., the relative survival of the idea of "the spirit level" nowadays), there is non-survivability (e.g., the relative non-survival of social Darwinism nowadays). And the reverse direction also holds true.

Mental Health, Treatment, and Technology

Another good way to evaluate the possibility (or impossibility) and desirability (or undesirability) of mental health from the perspective of society is to explore mental health, treatment, and technology.

An argument in the literature is that "communicative and other new technologies" can be used "as a supplement to mainstream therapies for mental disorders." (WK 2013x)

History of the Use of Technology for Mental Health

In the older days, "traditional methods of helping people with a mental health problem have been to use approaches such as medication, counselling, Cognitive Behavioral Therapy (CBT), exercise and a healthy diet." (WK 2013x)

Nowadays, "the use of communicative and other new technologies as a supplement to mainstream therapies for mental disorders is an emerging mental health treatment field which, it is argued, could improve the accessibility, effectiveness and affordability of mental health care. Mental health technologies used by professionals as an adjunct to mainstream clinical practices include email, SMS, virtual reality, computer programmes, blogs, social networks, the telephone, video conferencing, computer games, instant messaging and podcasts." (WK 2013x; G. Doherty; 2010; K. Anthony 2010)

For instance, "relatively new technology such as mobile phones have…been used to help people with mental health problems by providing timely information. David Haniff produced a computer application that would present media to someone suffering from depression in order to lift their mood; also a computer game has been produced to examine the triggers of depression. For example, pictures of the patient's family or their voice." (WK 2013x; S. Goss 2010; D. Haniff 2007)

In addition, "a key issue in recovery can be sufferers gaining some perspective on their own condition, and self-tracking technology tools appear to enable this. An example is Moodscope, which won the UK government 2011 'Health App' competition, receiving very strong user feedback." (WK 2013x)

Even more so, "as technology improves, it may soon be possible for mobile phones or other devices to sense when sufferers are changing state (e.g. entering a manic or a deeply depressed phase), for instance by noticing a change in voice pattern or usage frequency, or facial tension. It may also become possible to measure physical evidence of levels of distress and suffering, such as changes in hormones or adrenalin in blood, and changes in brain activity. Apps may also be able to predict high stress situations, based on location, time, activity (e.g. purchasing of alcohol) and nearby presence of high risk people. The technology could then send calming messages to sufferers, automatically alert carers and even automatically administer meds." (WK 2013x)

In short, "technology can therefore be used in innovative ways to provide support for those with mental health problems." (WK 2013x) For illustration, consider two main examples in more detail below, namely, (a) virtual reality therapy and (b) telemedicine.

The Case of Virtual Reality Therapy

The first example of the use of technology for mental health to be considered in more detail here concerns "virtual reality therapy" (as summarized in *Table 2.6*). (WK 2013y)

The term "virtual reality therapy (VRT)"—which is "also known as virtual reality immersion therapy (VRIT), Simulation for Therapy(SFT), virtual reality exposure therapy (VRET), and as Computerized CBT (CCBT)"—refers to "a method of psychotherapy that uses virtual reality technology to treat patients with anxiety disorders and phobias where it has proven very effective. It is now one of the primary treatments for PTSD. New technology also allows for the treatment of addictions and other conditions including those caused by lesions." (WK 2013y; H. Hoffman 2004; PSY 1994; K. McAuliffe 2008)

(a) History

Historically, "one of the earliest recorded explorations of VRIT was done by Dr. Ralph Lamson, a USC graduate and now retired clinical psychologist, then at Kaiser Permanente Psychiatry Group, San Rafael, CA in the early 1990s, as a means to solve his own acrophobia or fear of heights. About the same time, Dr. Larry Hodges, then a computer scientist at Georgia Tech active in VR and Dr. Barbara Rothbaum, a psychologist at Emory University, began studying VRT in cooperation with Dr. Max North, who had reported anomalous behavior in flying carpet simulation VR studies and attributed such to phobic response of unknown nature." (WK 2013y; R. Lamson 2005)

In recent years, "Dr. Skip Rizzo of USC's Institute for Creative Technologies, who had, with DOD funding, created a war simulation called Full Spectrum Warrior, with funding from ONR (Office of Naval Research) created an adaptation of that game for the treatment of Posttraumatic Stress Disorder ('PTSD'). Virtual Iraq was subsequently developed under ONR funding and is supported by Virtually Better, Inc. VBI also supports applications of VR-based therapy for fear-of-flying, fear-of-heights, fear-of-public-speaking, and substance abuse. Virtual Iraq proved successful in normalization of over 70% of PTSD sufferers, and that has now become a standard accepted treatment by the Anxiety and Depression Association of America....Military labs have subsequently set up dozens of VRIT labs and treatment centers for treating both PTSD and a variety of other medical conditions." (WK 2013y)

(b) Applications

Virtual reality therapy has been used for different applications. For instance, "there are VRT or Computerised CBT (CCBT) sessions, some immersive and some not, in which the user interacts with computer software (either on a PC, or sometimes via a voice-activated phone service), instead of face to face with a therapist. For people who are embarrassed by their phobias or feeling depressed and withdrawn, the prospect of having to speak to someone about their innermost problems can be unpleasant. In this respect, VIRT/CCBT either in a VR lab or online, is an option. With the huge number of PTSD sufferers and the shortage of available mental health professional, VRIT is expanding. New VR therapy sessions are even being done via the well known VR provider

Second Life. It is becoming well known enough to even be a question on Jeopardy." (WK 2013y; YOUT). 2013 & 2013a)

In 2006, "the UK's National Institute of Health and Clinical Excellence (NICE) recommended that VRIT be made available for use within the NHS across England and Wales, for patients presenting with mild/moderate depression, rather than immediately opting for antidepressant medication. Some areas have developed, or are trialing." (WK 2013y; NHS 2013)

In "at Auckland University [2013] in New Zealand, a team led by Dr. Sally Merry have been developing a computerised CBT fantasy 'serious' game to help tackle depression amongst adolescences. The game is currently undergoing testing…The game has a number of features to help combat depression, where the user takes on a role of a character who travels through a fantasy world, combating 'literal' negative thoughts and learning techniques to manage their depression." (WK 2013y)

In addition, "virtual reality therapy has two promising potential benefits for treatment of hemispatial neglect with lesion patients including: improvement of diagnostic techniques and as a supplement to rehabilitation techniques." (WK 2013y)

(c) Efficacy

Some studies had been done to evaluate the efficacy of virtual reality therapy; for instance, in one study, "of 40 patients treated, 38 showed marked reduction in phobic reaction to heights and self-reported reaching their goals. Research found that VRT allows patients to achieve victory over virtual height situations they could not confront in real life, and that gradually increasing the height and danger in a virtual environment produced increasing victories and greater self-confidence in the patient that they could actually confront the situation in real life." (WK 2013y)

In another study, "virtual therapy interventions empower people. The simulation technology of virtual reality lends itself to mastery oriented treatment...Rather than coping with threats, phobics manage progressively more threatening aspects in a computer generated environment...The range of applications can be extended by enhancing the realness and interactivity so that actions elicit reactions from the environments in which individuals immerse themselves." (WK 2013y)

The Case of Telemedicine

And the second example of the use of technology for mental health to be considered in more detail here concerns "telemedicine" (as summarized in *Table 2.6*).

The term "telemedicine" refers to "the use of telecommunication and information technologies in order to provide clinical health care at a distance. It helps eliminate distance barriers and can improve access to medical services that would often not be consistently available in distant rural communities. It is also used to save lives in critical care and emergency situations." (WK 2013z)

(a) History

In the past, "African villagers used smoke signals to warn people to stay away from the village in case of serious disease. In the early 1900s, people living in remote areas of Australia used two-way radios, powered by a dynamo driven by a set of bicycle pedals, to communicate with the Royal Flying Doctor Service of Australia." (WK 2013z; READ 1990)

However, in spite of these past practices, telemedicine "is essentially a product of 20th century telecommunication and information technologies. These technologies permit communications between patient and medical staff with both convenience and fidelity, as well as the transmission of medical, imaging and health informatics data from one site to another." (WK 2013z)

Over time, "early forms of telemedicine achieved with telephone and radio have been supplemented with videotelephony, advanced diagnostic methods supported by distributed client/server applications, and additionally with telemedical devices to support in-home care." (WK 2013z; I. Sachpazidis 2008)

(b) Types

Telemedicine can be classified in terms of three types, namely, (b1) "store-and-forward," (b2) "remote monitoring," and (b3) "(real-time) interactive services." (WK 2013z)

(b1) "Store-and-forward telemedicine involves acquiring medical data (like medical images, biosignals etc.) and then transmitting this data to a doctor or medical specialist at a convenient time for assessment offline. It does not require the presence of both parties at the same time. Dermatology (cf: teledermatology), radiology, and pathology are common specialties that are conducive to asynchronous telemedicine. A properly structured medical record preferably in electronic form should be a component of this transfer. A key difference between traditional in-person patient meetings and telemedicine encounters is the omission of an actual physical examination and history. The 'store-and-forward' process requires the clinician to rely on a history report and audio/video information in lieu of a physical examination." (WK 2013z; I. Sachpazidis 2008; ATA 2011) (b2) "Remote monitoring, also known as self-monitoring or testing, enables medical professionals to monitor a patient remotely using various technological devices. This method is primarily used for managing chronic diseases or specific conditions, such as heart disease, diabetes mellitus, or asthma. These services can provide comparable health outcomes to traditional in-person patient encounters, supply greater satisfaction to patients, and may be cost-effective." (WK 2013z)

(b3) And "interactive telemedicine services provide real-time interactions between patient and provider, to include phone conversations, online communication and home visits. Many activities such as history review, physical examination, psychiatric evaluations and ophthalmology assessments can be conducted comparably to those done in traditional face-to-face visits. In addition, 'clinician-interactive' telemedicine services may be less costly than in-person clinical visit." (WK 2013z)

(c) Telemedicine and Health Care

Telemedicine has been used in different areas of health care in the past decades.

For instance, in "general health care delivery," telemedicine has been used for "telenursing," "telepharmacy," "telerehabilitation," "teletrauma," etc. (WK 2013z)

And in "specialist care delivery," telemedicine has also been used for "telecardiology," "telepsychiatry," "teleradiology," "telepathology," "teledermatology," "teledentistry," "teleaudiology," "teleophthalmology," etc. (WK 2013z)

Problems with the Use of Technology for Mental Health

However, for the critics, this argument on the use of technology for mental health has some major problems. Consider, for illustration, a few examples below (as summarized in *Table 2.6*).

Firstly, one main criticism of the argument on the use of technology for mental health is that technologies do not necessarily benefit everyone.

For example, for the critics, "one size does not fit all and some technologies may not be suitable for certain people." (WK 2013x)

Secondly, another main criticism of the argument on the use of technology for mental health is that there are "cultural" barriers.

For instance, for the critics, the "adoption of telemedicine in emergency and critical care units" faces "cultural" barriers, which refer to the "barriers occurring from the lack of desire, or unwillingness, of some physicians to adapt clinical paradigms for telemedicine applications." (WK 2013z; PSQH 2013) In fact, "the VA [the U.S. Department of

Veterans Affairs] has continued to emphasize traditional PET (Prolonged exposure therapy) as the treatment of choice, and VR-based therapies have gained only limited adoption, despite active promotion by DOD. This is interesting in view of VRT having much lower cost and apparently higher success rates." (WK 2013y)

Thirdly, still another main criticism of the argument on the use of technology for mental health is that there are "regulatory" barriers.

For instance, for the critics, the "adoption of telemedicine in emergency and critical care units" faces "regulatory challenges related to the difficulty and cost of obtaining licensure across multiple states, malpractice protection and privileges at multiple facilities." (WK 2013z; PSQH 2013) As an example, in the U.S., "if a practitioner serves several states, obtaining this license in each state could be an expensive and time-consuming proposition. Even if the practitioner never practices medicine face-to-face with a patient in another state, he/she still must meet a variety of other individual state requirements, including paying substantial licensure fees, passing additional oral and written examinations, and traveling for interviews." (WK 2013z)

Fourthly, an additional main criticism of the argument on the use of technology for mental health is that there are "financial" barriers.

For instance, for the critics, the "adoption of telemedicine in emergency and critical care units" faces "financial" barriers, which refer to the "lack of acceptance and reimbursement by government payers and some commercial insurance carriers creating a major financial barrier, which places the investment burden squarely upon the hospital or healthcare system." (WK 2013z; PSQH 2013)

Fifthly, another additional main criticism of the argument on the use of technology for mental health is that there are "technical" barriers.

For instance, for the critics, the "adoption of telemedicine in emergency and critical care units" faces "technical" barriers, which refer to "technical training," "poor quality of transmitted records," and "evaluation time"; "for example, it has been estimated that a teledermatology consultation can take up to 30 minutes which contrasts sharply with the 15 minutes allowed for a traditional consultation. Additionally, poor quality of transmitted records, such as images or patient progress reports, and lack of access to relevant clinical information are quality assurance risks that can compromise the quality and continuity of patient care for the reporting doctor." (WK 2013z; RRH 2013; E. Strehle 2006)

And sixthly, still another additional main criticism of the argument on the use of technology for mental health is that virtual reality has its dark side.

For instance, as already discussed in my previous works (e.g., *FHC*, *FCD*, and *BCIV*), "post-civilization will confront psychosis as a primary problem in the culture of virtuality unto the post-human age, just as civilization has neurosis as a primary one of its own (although both neurosis and psychosis are major problems in both)," which is summarized in *Table 4.38*).

Beyond the Use of Technology for Mental Health

These criticisms of the argument on the use of technology for mental health are not to mean a total rejection of its usefulness but serve to show us the two opposing sides of the debate, such that the possibility (or impossibility) and desirability (or undesirability) of mental health (from the perspective of society with mental health, treatment, and technology as a case study here) are not to the extent that the respective defenders would like us to believe.

In fact, the analysis of mental health, treatment, and technology can illuminate the workings of the ontological principles in existential dialectics, and good examples include the formalness-informalness principle, the absoluteness-relativeness principle, the partiality-totality principle, the predictability-unpredictability principle, the explicability-inexplicability principle, the fiction-reality principle, the cognitiveness-noncognitiveness principle, the finiteness-transfiniteness principle, the preciseness-vagueness principle, the simpleness-complicatedness principle, the openness-hiddenness principle, the denseness-emptiness principle, the prototypicality-variation principle, the change-constancy principle, the order-chaos principle, the slowness-quickness principle, the expansion-contraction principle, the optimality-nonoptimality principle, the theory-praxis principle, the convention-novelty principle, the evolution-transformation principle, the symmetry-asymmetry principle, the softness-hardness principle, the seriousness-playfulness principle, the activeness-inactivess principle, the selfness-otherness principle, the regression-progression principle, the same-difference principle, the stability-reaction principle, the functionality-nonfunctionality principle, and the intentionality-nonintentionality principle.

For instance, in relation to the formalness-informalness principle, if there is formalness (e.g., the formal logical requirement of soundness and completeness in a system of ideas, as in the argument on the use of technology for mental health), there is informalness (e.g., the non-formal existence of unsoundness and incompleteness in the argument on the use of technology for mental health, as shown in the criticisms that technologies do not necessarily benefit everyone, that there are "cultural" barriers, that there are "regulatory" barriers, that there are "financial" barriers, that there are "technical" barriers, and that virtual reality has its dark side). And the reverse direction also holds true.

In relation to the absoluteness-relativeness principle, if there is absoluteness (e.g., the absolute view on the use of technology for mental health by the advocates), there is relativeness (e.g., what is right for the advocates to champion the use of technology for mental health is not necessarily so for the critics, who pointed out a lot of different problems afore-described). And the reverse direction also holds true.

In relation to the partiality-totality principle, if there is partiality (e.g., the partial view on the use of technology for mental health by the advocates), there is totality (e.g., the more holistic view on the use of technology for mental health, such that the whole is not the sum of its parts, that is, it cannot be reduced to the sum of opposing views by the advocates, by the critics, etc., since there will emerge new views in the future not yet known today, just as there are already alternative views nowadays which do not side exclusively with any of them, as is the analysis here). And the reverse direction also holds true.

In relation to the predictability-unpredictability principle, if there is predictability (e.g., the predictable tendency of the increasing use of technology for mental health in the foreseeable future), there is unpredictability (e.g., the more difficult task to predict exactly which forms, and to what extent, the use of technology for mental health will take in a particular future era, in light of different barriers and problems in the past afore-described). And the reverse direction also holds true.

In relation to the explicability-inexplicability principle, if there is explicability (e.g., the explanation, by the advocates, of the desirability of the use of technology for mental health on the basis of being "a supplement to mainstream therapies for mental disorders"), there is inexplicability (e.g., the lack of sufficient explanation, by the advocates, of why the use of technology for mental health is necessarily desirable, since, for the critics, there are already different barriers and problems afore-described). And the reverse direction also holds true.

In relation to the fiction-reality principle, if there is fiction (e.g., the fictional aspect of the argument about the use of technology for mental health, insofar as "one size does not fit all and some technologies may not be suitable for certain people," as pointed out by the critics), there is reality (e.g., the realistic aspect of the argument about the use of technology for mental health, insofar as the use of technology for mental health can be used, under certain circumstances, "as a supplement to mainstream therapies for mental disorders"). And the reverse direction also holds true.

In relation to the cognitiveness-noncognitiveness principle, if there is cognitiveness (e.g., a view of things on the basis of reason and evidences, as shown in the empirical problems of "technical training," "poor quality of transmitted records," and "evaluation time" in the "adoption of telemedicine in emergency and critical care units"), there is noncognitiveness (e.g., a view of things on the basis of non-cognitive factors like envy, jealousy, power, nationality, race, gender, age, class, greed, lust, status, faith, anger, sadness, joy, fear, wish, etc., as shown in the politics of "cultural" barriers, which refer to the "barriers occurring from the lack of desire, or unwillingness, of some physicians to adapt clinical paradigms for telemedicine applications," even when the new technologies have "much lower cost and apparently higher success rates"). And the reverse direction also holds true.

In relation to the finiteness-transfiniteness principle, if there is finiteness (e.g., the finite number of the categories of mental health technologies like "email, SMS, virtual reality, computer programmes, blogs, social networks, the telephone, video conferencing, computer games, instant messaging and podcasts"), there is transfiniteness (e.g., the transfinite number of all the individuals, equipments, exchanges, practices, etc. that have ever existed in the history of mental health technologies). And the reverse direction also holds true.

In relation to the preciseness-vagueness principle, if there is preciseness (e.g., the precise identification of 3 types of telemedicine, namely, "store-and-forward," "remote monitoring," and "[real-time] interactive services" in the article aforecited), there is vagueness (e.g., the vagueness in the identification of 3 types of telemedicine in the article aforecited, since it is not clear why there must be only 3, not 4, 5, 6, and so on). And the reverse direction also holds true.

In relation to the simpleness-complicatedness principle, if there is simpleness (e.g., the relatively simple analysis of the use of technology for mental health by the advocates), there is complicatedness (e.g., the relatively more complicated analysis of the use of technology for mental health, by challenging the claims and assumptions, as shown in the problems pointed out by the critics as cited). And the reverse direction also holds true.

In relation to the openness-hiddenness principle, if there is openness (e.g., the open exploration of the use of technology for mental health by the advocates), there is hiddenness (e.g., the hidden bias in the view on the use of technology for mental health by the advocates, because of the different problems aforecited). And the reverse direction also holds true.

In relation to the denseness-emptiness principle, if there is denseness (e.g., the relatively denser concentration of concerns with "email, SMS, virtual reality, computer programmes, blogs, social networks, the telephone, video conferencing, computer games, instant messaging and podcasts" by those advocating "new technologies" aforediscussed), there is emptiness (e.g., the relatively less dense, or more empty, concentration of concerns with "traditional methods" like "medication, counselling, Cognitive Behavioral Therapy, exercise and a healthy diet" by those advocating "new technologies" aforediscussed). And the reverse direction also holds true.

In relation to the prototypicality-variation principle, if there is prototypicality (e.g., the prototype, like the example about the early works on VRT by Ralph Lamson, Larry Hodges, and others), there is variation (e.g., different variants of the protoptye, as shown in many studies on VRT since the early works by by Ralph Lamson, Larry Hodges, and others, like the later ones by Skip Rizzo for DOD, Sally Merry at Auckland University, and so on, though each with his own variation, contribution, and disagreement). And the reverse direction also holds true.

In relation to the change-constancy principle, if there is change (e.g., the ever new ways to treat mental health, as shown in the use of new technologies aforediscussed), there is constancy (e.g., the ever constant existence of different problems with the ever new ways to treat mental health, as shown in the problems with the use of new technologies pointed out by the critics). And the reverse direction also holds true.

In relation to the order-chaos principle, if there is order (e.g., the more or less orderly view on the use of new technologies for mental health, if looked from the sole vantage point of the advocates), there is chaos (e.g., the more or less chaotic view on the use of new technologies for mental health, if looked from the multiple, conflicting vantage points of different advocates and critics alike, as discussed earlier). And the reverse direction also holds true.

In relation to the slowness-quickness principle, if there is slowness (e.g., the relatively slower speed of patients suffering from acrophobia to be cured without any VRT, as shown in the "randomized, tightly controlled, acrophobia treatment trials at Kaiser Permanente…conducted in 1993-4"), there is quickness (e.g., the relatively quicker speed of patients suffering from acrophobia to be cured if put in the "randomized, tightly controlled, acrophobia treatment trials at Kaiser Permanente," which "provided >90% effectiveness, conducted in 1993-4"). (WK 2013y) And the reverse direction also holds true.

In relation to the expansion-contraction principle, if there is expansion (e.g., the relatively more developed ability to deal with new technologies among those practitioning the use of technology to treat mental disorders), there is contraction (e.g., the relatively less developed ability to deal with traditional methods among those practitioning the use of technology to treat mental disorders). And the reverse direction also holds true.

In relation to the optimality-nonoptimality principle, if there is optimality (e.g., the search for highly favorable options, like the quest for ">90% effectiveness" in the "randomized, tightly controlled, acrophobia treatment trials at Kaiser Permanente...in 1993-4"), there is nonoptimality (e.g., the existence of non-optimal alternatives to optimality, like the argument for more realistic studies by the critics, who pointed out different barriers and problems confronting the use of new technologies to treat mental health aforedescribed). And the reverse direction also holds true.

In relation to the theory-praxis principle, if there is theory (e.g., the theoretical construction of "virtual reality" in computer science), there is praxis (e.g., the practical application of"virtual reality" in computer science to the field of medicine, like the use of emails to treat mental disorders). And the reverse direction also holds true.

In relation to the convention-novelty principle, if there is convention (e.g., the conventional wisdom about using "medication, counselling, Cognitive Behavioral Therapy, exercise and a healthy diet" to treat mental problems), there is novelty (e.g., the alternative novel challenge to the conventional wisdom about using "medication, counselling, Cognitive Behavioral Therapy, exercise and a healthy diet" to treat mental problems, by the new idea of new technologies for mental health aforecited). And the reverse direction also holds true.

In relation to the evolution-transformation principle, if there is evolution (e.g., the natural evolution of humans to sometimes suffer from mental problems in the state of nature), there is transformation (e.g., the technical transformation of human ability to treat mental problems by the invention of VRT and telemedicine). And the reverse direction also holds true.

In relation to the symmetry-asymmetry principle, if there is symmetry (e.g., the co-existence of different agents in the world of using new technologies for mental health, like practitioners and regulatory agencies), there is asymmetry (e.g., practitioners have to comply with the requirements as imposed by regulatory agencies, like "paying substantial licensure fees, passing additional oral and written examinations, and traveling for interviews"). And the reverse direction also holds true.

In relation to the softness-hardness principle, if there is softness (e.g., the defense of the use of new technologies for mental health by the advocates), there is hardness (e.g., the critique of the use of new technologies for mental health, as shown in the problems pointed out by the critics as cited). And the reverse direction also holds true.

In relation to the seriousness-playfulness principle, if there is seriousness (e.g., the serious business of those who try to understand and treat mental problems), there is playfulness (e.g., the playful part of those who try to understand and treat mental problems, when they play around with different methods over the decades, like the use of "medication, counselling, Cognitive Behavioral Therapy, exercise and a healthy diet" as well as "email, SMS, virtual reality, computer programmes, blogs, social networks, the telephone, video conferencing, computer games, instant messaging and podcasts"). And the reverse direction also holds true.

In relation to the activeness-inactivess principle, if there is activeness (e.g., the relative activeness of those who get cured of acrophobia, so they can now go to high places), there is inactiveness (e.g., the relative inactiveness of those who suffer from acrophobia and never receive any VRT and other methods, so they cannot now go to high places).

In relation to the selfness-otherness principle, if there is selfness (e.g., the tendency to be mostly centered on one's self or group, as shown in DOD, which funded the project to use VRT "for the treatment of Posttraumatic Stress Disorder" suffered by American soldiers), there is otherness (e.g., the tendency to be mostly centered on others, as shown in the work at Auckland University to "develop…a computerised CBT fantasy 'serious' game to help tackle depression amongst adolescences," as an advance in the field of medicine). And the reverse direction also holds true.

In relation to the regression-progression principle, if there is regression (e.g., the regression made by the use of new technologies for mental health, as shown in the problems pointed out by the critics), there is progression (e.g., the progress made by the use of new technologies for mental health, as shown in the contribution to the treatment of acrophobia and other mental problems aforecited). And the reverse direction also holds true.

In relation to the same-difference principle, if there is similarity in outcome (e.g., the contribution to the molding and control of beliefs, values, and behaviors, regardless of whether this be done by way of medication, counselling, exercise and a healthy diet to treat mental health problems, or by way of virtual reality therapy), there is difference in outcome (e.g., the contribution to the molding and control of beliefs, values, and behaviors by way of medication, counselling, exercise and a healthy diet to treat mental health problems for a relatively more traditional lifeworld—but the contribution to the molding and control of beliefs, values, and behaviors by way of virtual reality therapy for a relatively more imaginative lifeworld). And the reverse direction also holds true.

In relation to the stability-reaction principle, if there is stability (e.g., the relatively more stable condition of traditional methods in the older days, when "medication, counselling, Cognitive Behavioral Therapy, exercise and a healthy diet" were used to treat mental problems), there is reaction (e.g., traditional methods in the older days then led to further changes later on, when nowadays new technologies are used instead, like "email, SMS, virtual reality, computer programmes, blogs, social networks, the telephone, video conferencing, computer games, instant messaging and podcasts"). And the reverse direction also holds true.

In relation to the functionality-nonfunctionality principle, if there is functionality (e.g., the presence of action for which something or someone is fitted, as shown in the use of"medication, counselling, Cognitive Behavioral Therapy, exercise and a healthy diet" to treat mental problems in the older days, which served the function of supporting traditional methods for a relatively less advanced technological society), there is nonfunctionality (e.g., the relative lack of action for which something or someone is fitted, as shown in the use of new technologies to treat mental problems nowadays, such that the traditional methods in the older days are no longer much functional in our time, with its relatively more advanced technological environment). And the reverse direction also holds true.

In relation to the intentionality-nonintentionality principle, if there is intentionality (e.g., the planning or design of something for a certain outcome, as shown in the original intention of the early pioneers like Ralph Lamson, Larry Hodges, and others to use VRT for the treatment of mental disorders), there is nonintentionality (e.g., the relative absence of planning or design of something for a certain outcome, such that the outcome can even be counter-intentional in being the opposite of what was originally planned, as shown in the current decision of "the VA [the U.S. Department of Veterans Affairs]" to "continue...to emphasize traditional PET [prolonged exposure therapy] as the treatment of choice, and VR-based therapies have gained only limited adoption, despite active promotion by DOD [even though]...VRT having much lower cost and apparently higher success rates"—contrary to the original intention of the early pioneers to use VRT for the treatment of mental disorders). And the reverse direction also holds true.

And in relation to the survivability-nonsurvivability principle, if there is survivability (e.g., the relative survival, nowadays, of using high technologies like "telenursing," "telepharmacy," "telepsychiatry," etc. to treat health problems), there is non-survivability (e.g., the relative non-survival, nowadays, of using "smoke signals to warn people to stay away...in case of serious disease"). And the reverse direction also holds true.

Mental Health and Culture

Mental health, when examined from the perspective of culture, can cast an illuminating light on its possibility (or impossibility) and desirability (or undesirability), and this can be shown by way of two case studies, namely, (2.5.1) mental health, alternative medicine, and culture, and (2.5.2) mental health, mindfulness, and religion—to be addressed hereafter, in that order.

Mental Health, Alternative Medicine, and Culture

An excellent case study here to understand mental health from the perspective of culture has to do with mental health, alternative medicine, and culture.

An argument in the literature is that "alternative medicine" like "homeopathy, Ayurveda, chiropractic, and acupuncture" in different cultures (or subcultures) can be used to yield "the healing effects of medicine" but is "usually based on religion, tradition, superstition, belief in supernatural energies," and other "treatments...that are not part of the conventional, science-based healthcare system." (WK 2013q; NSF 2002; W. Sampson 1995; B. Beyerstein 2001; NCCAM 2005; USIM 2005)

History of Alternative Medicines

Historically, "according to Robert Jutte, labels used to describe health belief systems other than modern, scientific, Western medicine, are either misleading or carry semantic load, as for example 'alternative,' 'marginal,' 'fringe,' 'unorthodox,' or 'irregular,' and historians have had some difficulty simply to name and describe without connotative judgement. Jutte found that in the period from the mid-nineteenth century to the first two decades of the twentieth, the opposition of the developing medical establishment in

Germany, based on modern scientific medicine, had resulted in the threat from homoepaths, naturopaths, mesmerists and others being stemmed by legal and organizational measures." (WK 2013q)

By the 1970s, "in North America, Great Britain and elsewhere, there has been a tendency for the terms 'alternative' and 'complementary' to be used interchangeably to describe a wide diversity of therapies that attempt to use the self-healing powers of the body by amplifying natural recuperative processes to restore health. By 1990, approximately 60 million Americans had used one or more complementary or alternative therapies to address health issues, according to a nationwide survey in the United States published in 1993 by David Eisenberg. A study published in the November 11, 1998 issue of the Journal of the American Medical Association reported that 42% of Americans had used complementary and alternative therapies, up from 34% in 1990." (WK 2013q; D. Eisenberg 1993 & 1998)

In general, "alternative medicine practices and beliefs are diverse in their foundations and methodologies. Methods may incorporate or base themselves on traditional medicine, folk knowledge, spiritual beliefs, ignorance or misunderstanding of scientific principles, errors in reasoning, or newly conceived approaches claiming to heal. African, Caribbean, Pacific Island, Native American, and other regional cultures have traditional medical systems as diverse as their diversity of cultures." (WK 2013q; W. Sampson 1995; B. Beyerstein 2001; D. Acharya 2008; NCCAM 2005)

An illustrative list of alternative medicines is shown below: (WK 2013q)

- "Prayer to Heal"—"is the most common alternative medicine in many western countries, and faith healing is a part of many religions."
- "Meditation"—is believed by some to "affect…health."
- "Yoga"—is "a healing practice involves stretching, exercise and meditation related to the Hindu religion, and makes claims to healing in the spiritual realm."
- "Traditional Chinese Medicine/Ayurvedic Medicine of India"—"are complex systems developed over thousands of years, both based on regional supernatural belief systems and traditional use of herbs and other substances."
- "Acupuncture"—"is a part of Traditional Chinese medicine in which needles are inserted in the body to alter the flow of supernatural energy believed to propel the blood and influence health."

- "Chiropractic Manipulation of the Spine"—"was developed in the United States, and involves manipulating the spine to influence supernatural energies believed to cause disease."
- "Homeopathy"—"was developed in Europe before the existence of science of chemistry."
- "Magnets and Light"—"are used in therapies based on a misunderstanding of electricity and magnetism."
- "Dietary Supplements"—"that are unproven by science are considered alternative medicines."

Of course, there can be other examples, so the ones above are illustrative.

Types of Alternative Medicines

This list of alternative medicines then raises the question about the classification of its different types. Over the years, some researchers have come up with five different types, as shown below (and summarized in *Table 2.7*).

(a) Alternative Medical Systems

The first type of alternative medicines to be introduced here concerns "alternative medical systems," which refer to "complete health systems with their own approaches to diagnosis and treatment that differ from the conventional biomedical approach to health. Some are cultural systems such as Ayurveda and Traditional Chinese Medicine, while others, such as Homeopathy and Naturopathy are relatively recent and were developed in the West." (WK 2013q; M. Goldrosen 2004)

There are four sub-types of alternative medical systems, as described below.

(a1) "Ayurvedic medicine" is "a traditional medicine of India and has strong links with Buddhism and Hinduism. It is based on the belief that health is controlled by 3 'humours' with disease caused by an imbalance of these 'humours.' The basis of treatment has some similarities with 'Western medicine.' Rememdies are mainly plant based with some use of animal materials. Safety concerns have been raised about Ayurveda, with two U.S. studies finding about 20 percent of Ayurvedic Indian-manufactured patent medicines contained toxic levels of heavy metals such as lead, mercury and arsenic. Other concerns include the use of herbs containing toxic compounds and the lack of quality control in Ayurvedic facilities." (WK 2013q; R. Saper 2008; M. Valiathan 2006)

(a2) "Traditional Chinese medicine" is "based on a concept of 'spirit' called qi, considerations of Chinese Astrology as in acupuncture, traditional use of herbs and other substances found in China, and a belief that a map of the body is contained on the tongue, which reflects changes in the body." (WK 2013q; P. Ho 2000; J. Needham 2002; G. Cia 1995)

(a3) "Homeopathy" is "based on the belief that a disease can be cured by a very low dose of substance that creates similar symptoms in a healthy person. These ideas are known as 'like cures like' and the 'law of the minimum dose' This conflicts with fundamental concepts of physics and chemistry and there is no good evidence from reviews of research to support its use." (WK 2013q; S. Hahnemann 1833; E. Ernst 2002)

(a4) "Naturopathy" is "based on a belief in vitalism, which posits that a special energy called vital energy or vital force guides bodily processes such as metabolism, reproduction, growth, and adaptation. Naturopathy favors a holistic approach with non-invasive treatment and, similar to conventional medicine, encourages minimal use of surgery and drugs." (WK 2013q; J. Sarris 2010)

(b) Energy Therapies

The second type of alternative medicines to be introduced here concerns "energy therapies," which "are designed to influence energy fields (biofields) that practitioners believe surround and enter the body. Some energy therapies involve the use of crystals, while others use magnets and electric fields." (WK 2013q)

For instance, "biofield therapies are intended to influence energy fields that, it is purported, surround and penetrate the body," and "chiropractic was developed in the belief that manipulating the spine affects the flow of a supernatural vital energy and thereby affects health and disease." (WK 2013q; NCCAM 2005)

And "bioelectromagnetic-based therapies use…electromagnetic fields, such as pulsed fields, alternating-current, or direct-current fields in an unconventional manner. Magnetic healing does not claim existence of supernatural energies, but asserts that magnets can be used to defy the laws of physics to influence health and disease." (WK 2013q; NCCAM 2005)

(c) Mind Body Therapies

The third type of alternative medicines to be introduced here concerns "mind body therapies," which refers to the attempt "to use the mind to affect bodily symptoms and functions; examples include yoga, spirituality and relaxation." (WK 2013q)

In other words, "mind-body medicine takes a holistic approach to health that explores the interconnection between the mind, body, and spirit. It works under the premise that the mind can affect 'bodily functions and symptoms.' Mind body medicines includes healing claims made in yoga, meditation, deep-breathing exercises, guided imagery, hypnotherapy, progressive relaxation, qi gong, and tai chi." (WK 2013q; NCCAM 2005)

And "yoga, a method of traditional stretches, excercises, and meditations in Hinduism, may also be classified as an energy medicine insofar as its healing effects are believed by to be due to a healing 'life energy' that is absorbed into the body through the breath, and is thereby believed to treat a wide variety of illnesses and complaints." (WK 2013q; J. Raub 2002)

(d) Herbs, Diet and Vitamins

The fourth type of alternative medicines to be introduced here concerns "herbs, diet, and vitamins," which refer to "the use of herbal medicines, special diets or very high doses of vitamins." (WK 2013q)

This type of alternative medicine makes good use of "substances found in nature such as herbs, foods, non-vitamin supplments and megavitmins, and minerals, and includes traditional herbal remedies with herbs specific to regions in which the cultural practices arose. 'Herbal' remedies in this case, may include use of nonherbal toxic chemicals from a nonbiological sources, such as use of the poison lead in Traditional Chinese Medicine. Nonvitamin supplements include fish oil, Omega-3 fatty acid, glucosamine, echinacea, flaxseed oil or pills, and ginseng, when used under a claim to have healing effects." (WK 2013q; NCCAM 2005)

(e) Body manipulation

And the fifth type of alternative medicines to be introduced here concerns "body manipulation," which refers to "body-based therapies such as massage, chiropractic and osteopathy use movement and physical manipulation of joints and muscles." (WK 2013q)

In this way, "manipulative and body-based practices feature manipulation or movement of body parts, such as is done in chiropractic manipulation." (WK 2013q)

Use of Alternative Medicines

The use of alternative medicines can be widespread.

For instance, "about 50% of people in developed countries use some kind of complementry and alternative medicine other than prayer for health. About 40% of cancer patients use some form of Complementary and Alternative Medicine. The use of alternative medicine in developed countries is increasing, with a 50 percent increase in expenditures and a 25 percent increase in the use of alternative therapies between 1990 and 1997 in America. Americans spend many billions on the therapies annually. Most Americans used CAM to treat and/or prevent musculoskeletal conditions or other conditions associated with chronic or recurring pain. In America, women were more likely than men to use CAM., with the biggest difference in use of mind-body therapies including prayer specifically for health reasons. In 2008, more than 37% of American hospitals offered alternative therapies, up from 26.5 percent in 2005, and 25% in 2004. More than 70% of the hospitals offering CAM were in urban areas." (WK 2013q; P. Barnes 2004; J. Astin 1998; D. Eisenberg 1998; CBS 2006)

Regulation of Alternative Medicines

Alternative medicines are regulated, of course, but the regulations vary from country to country and from type to type.

For instance, "some fields of alternative practice are regulated in a manner similar to that governing science-based medicine, and some have no regulation at all. Regulation and licensing of alternative medicine ranges widely from country to country, and state to state." (WK 2013q)

In the U.S., for instance, "government bodies...have published information or guidance about alternative medicine. One of those is the U.S. Food and Drug Administration (FDA), which mentions specifically homeopathic products, traditional Chinese medicine and Ayurvedic products." (WK 2013q)

Problems with Alternative Medicine

However, for the critics, the argument on mental health, alternative medicine, and culture has some major problems. Consider, for illustration, a few examples below (as summarized in *Table 2.7*).

Firstly, one main criticism of the argument on mental health, alternative medicine, and culture is that altnerative medicine is not scientific.

For instance, "the United States' National Science Foundation [2002] has defined alternative medicine as 'all treatments that have not been proven effective using scientific methods,'" (WK 2013q)

Secondly, another main criticism of the argument on mental health, alternative medicine, and culture is that its practice is unethical.

For instance, "in November 2011 Edzard Ernst [2011] stated that the 'level of misinformation about alternative medicine has now reached the point where it has become dangerous and unethical. So far, alternative medicine has remained an ethics-free zone. It is time to change this.'" (WK 2013q)

Thirdly, still another main criticism of the argument on mental health, alternative medicine, and culture is that alternative medicine often uses "ambiguous" words to mislead.

For instance, the critic Wallace Sampson (1995) pointed out that "proponents of alternative medicine often use terminology which is loose or ambiguous to create the appearance that a choice between 'alternative' effective treatments exists when it does not, that there is effectiveness or scientific validity when it does not exist, to suggest that a dichotomy exists when it does not, or to suggest that consistency with science exists when it may not." (WK 2013q)

Fourthly, an additional main criticism of the argument on mental health, alternative medicine, and culture is that alternative medicine is not effective as claimed.

For instance, "Edzard Ernst, a professor of complementary medicine, characterizes the evidence for many alternative techniques as weak, nonexistent, or negative. Ernst has concluded that 95% of the alternative treatments he and his team have studied, including acupuncture, herbal medicine, homeopathy, and reflexology, are, according to The Economist, 'statistically indistinguishable from placebo treatments.'" (WK 2013q; E. Ernst 2013; ECON 2011)

Fifthly, another additional main criticism of the argument on mental health, alternative medicine, and culture is that its practice is manipulative, in "using plausibility of one practice to support implausible other practices." (WK 203q)

For instance, for the critics, "a group of prominent scientists argued before the federal government that plausibility of interventions such as diet, relaxation, yoga and botanical remedies, should not be used to support research on implausible interventions based on superstition and belief in the supernatural, and that the plausible methods can be studied just as well in other parts of NIH, where they should be made to compete on an equal footing with other research projects." (WK 2013q; D. Brown 2009)

And sixthly, still another additional main criticism of the argument on mental health, alternative medicine, and culture is that its practitioners play trick on patients.

For instance, for the critics, "academic proponents of integrative medicine [combining alternative medicine with evidence based medicine] sometimes recommend misleading patients by using known placebo treatments in order to achieve a placebo effect," and "integrative medicine has been criticized in that its practitioners, trained in science based medicine, deliberately mislead patients by pretending placebos are not." (WK 2013q; B. Berman 2010)

Beyond Alternative Medicine

These criticisms of alternative medicine, however, do not imply a total rejection of its usefulness but serve to show us the two opposing sides of the debate, such that the possibility (or impossibility) and desirability (or undesirability) of mental health (from the perspective of culture with mental health, alternative medicine, and culture as a case study here) are not to the extent that the respective defenders would like us to believe.

Moreover, the analysis of mental health, alternative medicine, and culture can teach us something valuable about the ontological principles in existential dialectics, and good examples include the formalness-informalness principle, the absoluteness-relativeness principle, the partiality-totality principle, the predictability-unpredictability principle, the explicability-inexplicability principle, the fiction-reality principle, the cognitiveness-noncognitiveness principle, the finiteness-transfiniteness principle, the preciseness-vagueness principle, the simpleness-complicatedness principle, the openness-hiddenness principle, the denseness-emptiness principle, the prototypicality-variation principle, the change-constancy principle, the order-chaos principle, the slowness-quickness principle, the expansion-contraction principle, the optimality-nonoptimality principle, the theory-praxis principle, the convention-novelty principle, the evolution-transformation principle, the symmetry-asymmetry principle, the softness-hardness principle, the seriousness-playfulness principle, the activeness-inactivess principle, the selfness-otherness principle, the regression-progression principle, the same-difference principle, the stability-reaction principle, the functionality-nonfunctionality principle, and the intentionality-nonintentionality principle.

For instance, in relation to the formalness-informalness principle, if there is formalness (e.g., the formal logical requirement of soundness, completeness, and consistency in a system of ideas, as in the argument for alternative medicine), there is informalness (e.g., the non-formal existence of unsoundness, incompleteness, and inconsistency in the argument for alternative medicine, as shown in the criticisms that altnerative medicine is not scientific, that its practice is unethical, that alternative medicine often uses "ambiguous" words to mislead, that alternative medicine is not effective as claimed, and that its practice is manipulative, that its practitioners play trick on patients). And the reverse direction also holds true.

In relation to the absoluteness-relativeness principle, if there is absoluteness (e.g., the absolute view on "like cures like" and the "law of the minimum dose" by the advocates of "homeopathy"), there is relativeness (e.g., what is right for the advocates of "homeopathy" to claim "like cures like" and the "law of the minimum dose" is not necessarily so for the critcs, who consider "homeopathy...to be quackery"). And the reverse direction also holds true.

In relation to the partiality-totality principle, if there is partiality (e.g., the partial view on alternative medicines by the advocates), there is totality (e.g., the more holistic view on alternative medicines, such that the whole is not the sum of its parts, that is, it cannot be reduced to the sum of opposing views by the advocates, the critics, etc., since there will emerge new views in the future not yet known today, just as there are already alternative views nowadays which do not side exclusively with any of them, as is the analysis here). And the reverse direction also holds true.

In relation to the predictability-unpredictability principle, if there is predictability (e.g., the predictable tendency of more or less "50% of people in developed countries" to "use some kind of complementry and alternative medicine other than prayer for health" in the foreseeable future), there is unpredictability (e.g., the more difficult task to predict exactly which particular types, and to what extent, alternative medicines will take in a particular future era, in light of its controversical past history with different problems aforediscussed). And the reverse direction also holds true.

In relation to the explicability-inexplicability principle, if there is explicability (e.g., the explanation, by the critics of alternative medicines, that they are undesirable because of the criticisms that altnerative medicine is not scientific, that its practice is unethical, that alternative medicine often uses "ambiguous" words to mislead, that alternative medicine is not effective as claimed, and that its practice is manipulative, that its practitioners play trick on patients, etc.), there is inexplicability (e.g., the lack of sufficient explanation, by the critics of of alternative medicines, of why "alternative medicine can be on the rise 'in countries where Western science and scientific method generally are accepted as the major foundations for healthcare" and this anomaly "has been described as an 'enigma' in the Medical Journal of Australia"). (WK 2013q; I. Coulter 2004) And the reverse direction also holds true.

In relation to the fiction-reality principle, if there is fiction (e.g., the fictional aspect of alternative medicine, insofar as "academic proponents...sometimes recommend misleading patients by using known placebo treatments in order to achieve a placebo effect"), there is reality (e.g., the realistic aspect of alternative medicine, insofar as a small percentage of alternative treatments were found effective, although the rest, 95%, were not, according to the study by Ernst). And the reverse direction also holds true.

In relation to the cognitiveness-noncognitiveness principle, if there is cognitiveness (e.g., a view of things on the basis of reason and evidences, as shown in empirical finding that "about 50% of people in developed countries use some kind of complementry and alternative medicine other than prayer for health"), there is noncognitiveness (e.g., a view of things on the basis of non-cognitive factors like envy, jealousy, power, nationality, race, gender, age, class, greed, lust, status, faith, anger, sadness, joy, fear, wish, etc., as shown in the politics of "faith" by "alternative medicine users," who "appear to be doing so largely because 'they find these healthcare alternatives to be more congruent with their own values, beliefs, and philosophical orientations toward health and life,'" even though "95%" of alternative treatments were not effective, according to the study by Ernst). (WK 2013q) And the reverse direction also holds true.

In relation to the finiteness-transfiniteness principle, if there is finiteness (e.g., the finite number of the categories of substances used in alternative medicines, like "herbs, foods, non-vitamin supplments and megavitmins, and minerals," as well as "seed oil or pills, and ginseng," for example), there is transfiniteness (e.g., the transfinite number of all the individual pieces of "herbs, foods, non-vitamin supplments and megavitmins, and minerals," as well as "seed oil or pills, and ginseng," that have ever existed in history and used for alternative medicines). (WK 2013q) And the reverse direction also holds true.

In relation to the preciseness-vagueness principle, if there is preciseness (e.g., the precise identification of 5 types of alternative medecines in the article aforecited), there is vagueness (e.g., the vagueness in the identification of the 5 types of alternative medecines in the article aforecited, since it is not clear why there must be only 5, not 6, 7, 8, and so on). And the reverse direction also holds true.

In relation to the simpleness-complicatedness principle, if there is simpleness (e.g., the relatively simple analysis of alternative medicines by the advocates), there is complicatedness (e.g., the relatively more complicated analysis of alternative medicines, by challenging the claims and assumptions, as shown in the problems pointed out by the critics as cited). And the reverse direction also holds true.

In relation to the openness-hiddenness principle, if there is openness (e.g., the open exploration of the use of "a very low dose of substance that creates similar symptoms in a healthy person" to cure disease, according to those in homeopathy), there is hiddenness (e.g., the hidden bias in homeopathy, since "this conflicts with fundamental concepts of physics and chemistry and there is no good evidence from reviews of research to support its use" and "within the medical community homeopathy is now considered to be quackery"). (WK 2013q) And the reverse direction also holds true.

In relation to the denseness-emptiness principle, if there is denseness (e.g., the relatively denser concentration of concerns with "religion, tradition, superstition, belief in supernatural energies," etc. by those in alternative medicines), there is emptiness (e.g., the relatively less dense, or more empty, concentration of concerns with "modern scientific reasoning" by those in alternative medicines). And the reverse direction also holds true.

In relation to the prototypicality-variation principle, if there is prototypicality (e.g., the prototype, like the example about the original "traditional Chinese medicine" based "on a tradition of more than 2,000 years" ago), there is variation (e.g., different variants of the protoptye, as shown in many further developments of "traditional Chinese medicine" since then, like the ones "modernized in the People's Republic of China so as to integrate many anatomical and pathological notions with scientific medicine," though each with its own variation, contribution, and disagreement). (WK 2013aa) And the reverse direction also holds true.

In relation to the change-constancy principle, if there is change (e.g., the ever new ways to treat health problems, as shown in the use of alternative medicines), there is constancy (e.g., the ever constant existence of different problems with the ever new ways to treat health problems, as shown in the problems with the use of alternative medicines pointed out by the critics). And the reverse direction also holds true.

In relation to the order-chaos principle, if there is order (e.g., the more or less orderly view on the treatment of disease, if looked from the sole vantage point of "like cures like" and the "law of the minimum dose" in homeopathy), there is chaos (e.g., the more or less chaotic view on the treatment of disease, if looked from all the multiple, conflicting vantage points of numerous types of alternative medicines and different versions of "evidence-based medicine"). And the reverse direction also holds true.

In relation to the slowness-quickness principle, if there is slowness (e.g., the relatively slower speed of a patient to recover if he does not receive a "placebo" and also does not receive any treatment from any other sources), there is quickness (e.g., the relatively quicker speed of a patient to recover if he receives a "placebo," especially for those who believe that "placebos can have both psychological and physical benefits"). (WK 2013q) And the reverse direction also holds true.

In relation to the expansion-contraction principle, if there is expansion (e.g., the relatively more developed ability of those in "evidence-based medicine" to deal with scientific methods in treating patients), there is contraction (e.g., the relatively less developed ability of those in "evidence-based medicine" to deal with "religion, tradition, superstition,...supernatural energies," etc. in treating patients). And the reverse direction also holds true.

In relation to the optimality-nonoptimality principle, if there is optimality (e.g., the search for highly favorable options, like the quest for effective scientific treatments by the National Science Foundation when it advocated only "evidence-based medicine" and dismissed "alternative medicine" as "all treatments that had not been proven effective using scientific methods"), there is nonoptimality (e.g., the existence of non-optimal alternatives to optimality, like the argument for more realistic studies by the critics, who pointed out that the focus on "evidence-based medicine" is questionable, since "alternative medicine can be on the rise 'in countries where Western science and scientific method generally are accepted as the major foundations for healthcare" and this anomaly "has been described as an 'enigma' in the Medical Journal of Australia"). (WK 2013q) And the reverse direction also holds true.

In relation to the theory-praxis principle, if there is theory (e.g., the theoretical construction of "Chinese astrology" in ancient times), there is praxis (e.g., the practical application of "Chinese astrology" in ancient times to the field of medicine, as in "traditional Chinese medicine"). And the reverse direction also holds true.

In relation to the convention-novelty principle, if there is convention (e.g., the conventional wisdom about "traditional Chinese medicine" in ancient times), there is novelty (e.g., the alternative novel challenge to the conventional wisdom about traditional Chinese medicine" in ancient times, by the new idea nowadays that "many of its assumptions, including the model of the body, or concept of disease, are not supported by modern evidence-based medicine"). (WK 2013aa) And the reverse direction also holds true.

In relation to the evolution-transformation principle, if there is evolution (e.g., the natural evolution of humans to sometimes get sick in the state of nature), there is transformation (e.g., the technical transformation of human ability to cure sickness by the invention of "alternative medicines"). And the reverse direction also holds true.

In relation to the symmetry-asymmetry principle, if there is symmetry (e.g., the co-existence of different types of medicines, be they "evidence-based" or "alternative"), there is asymmetry (e.g., "evidence-based medicine" is more domiannt than "alternative medicine" in developed countries nowadays). And the reverse direction also holds true.

In relation to the softness-hardness principle, if there is softness (e.g., the use of yoga and meditation to fight disease), there is hardness (e.g., the use of painful, invasive surgery to fight disease). And the reverse direction also holds true.

In relation to the seriousness-playfulness principle, if there is seriousness (e.g., the serious business of those who try to understand the role of herbs to treat diseases), there is playfulness (e.g., the playful part of those who try to understand the role of herbs to treat diseases, when they play around with different options over the centuries, like "herbs, foods, non-vitamin supplments and megavitmins, and minerals," as well as "seed oil or pills, and ginseng," for example). And the reverse direction also holds true.

In relation to the activeness-inactivess principle, if there is activeness (e.g., the relative activeness of those who recover from illness, with the help of alternative medicines, and can now engage in full life activities), there is inactiveness (e.g., the relative inactiveness of those who do not recover from illness, even with the help of alternative medicines and other sources, so they cannot now engage in full life activities).

In relation to the selfness-otherness principle, if there is selfness (e.g., the tendency to be mostly centered on one's self or group, as shown in those practitioners who have misled about "alternative medicine," to "the piont where it has become dangerous and unethical," as pointed out by Ernst [2011]"), there is otherness (e.g., the tendency to be mostly centered on others, as shown in the call by "a group of prominent scientists," who "argued before the federal government that plausibility of interventions such as diet, relaxation, yoga and botanical remedies, should not be used to support research on implausible interventions based on superstition" and other questionable practices, for the advancement of medical knowledge). And the reverse direction also holds true.

In relation to the regression-progression principle, if there is regression (e.g., the regression made by alternative medicines, as shown in the problems pointed out by the critics), there is progression (e.g., the progress made by alternative medicines, as shown in the contribution to the use of "diet, relaxation, yoga and botanical remedies" to treat health problems aforecited). And the reverse direction also holds true.

In relation to the same-difference principle, if there is similarity in outcome (e.g., the contribution to the molding and control of beliefs, values, and behaviors, regardless of whether this be done by way of "evidence-based medicine," or by way of "alternative medicine"), there is difference in outcome (e.g., the contribution to the molding and control of beliefs, values, and behaviors by way of "evidence-based medicine" for a relatively more scientific lifeworld—but the contribution to the molding and control of beliefs, values, and behaviors by way of "alternative medicine" for a relatively more traditional lifeworld). And the reverse direction also holds true.

In relation to the stability-reaction principle, if there is stability (e.g., the relatively more stable condition of alternative medicines in the older days), there is reaction (e.g., alternative medicines in the older days then led to further changes later on, when nowadays, they are challenged by "evidence-based medicine"). And the reverse direction also holds true.

In relation to the functionality-nonfunctionality principle, if there is functionality (e.g., the presence of action for which something or someone is fitted, as shown in the widespread use of alternative medicines in the older days, which served the function of maintaining the world of "religion, tradition, and superstition" at that time), there is nonfunctionality (e.g., the relative lack of action for which something or someone is fitted, as shown in the rise of "evidence-based medicine" nowadays, such that the world of "religion, tradition, and superstition" in the older days is no longer functional in our time, with its relatively more scientific expectations). And the reverse direction also holds true.

In relation to the intentionality-nonintentionality principle, if there is intentionality (e.g., the planning or design of something for a certain outcome, as shown in the original intention of the advocates of traditional Chinese Medicine in ancient times to use "Chinese astrology as in acupuncture" to treat health problems), there is nonintentionality (e.g., the relative absence of planning or design of something for a certain outcome, such that the outcome can even be counter-intentional in being the opposite of what was originally planned, as shown in the rejection of "many of its assumptions, including the model of the body, or concept of disease" which "are not supported by modern evidence-based medicine"—contrary to the original intention of the advocates of traditional Chinese Medicine in ancient times to use "Chinese astrology as in acupuncture" to treat health problems). (WK 2013q & 2013aa) And the reverse direction also holds true.

And in relation to the survivability-nonsurvivability principle, if there is survivability (e.g., the relative survival, nowadays, of "evidence-based medicine" in developed countries), there is non-survivability (e.g., the relative non-survival, nowadays, of homeopathy in developed countries, because "within the medical community homeopathy is now considered to be quackery"). And the reverse direction also holds true.

Mental Health, Mindfulness, and Religion

Another way to evaluate the possibility (or impossibility) and desirability (or undesirability) of mental health from the perspective of culture concerns mental health, mindfulness, and religion.

An argument in the literature is that "the concept of mindfulness" in Buddhist meditation can be used for "clinical psychology and psychiatry" to treat health problems. (WK 2013bb)

Definitions of Mindfulness

The term "mindfulness" in Buddhism can be defined in different ways; for instance, in one definition, "mindfulness" can refer to the following: (WK 2013bb; R. Baer 2013)

- "bringing one's complete attention to the present experience on a moment-to-moment basis"
- "paying attention in a particular way: on purpose, in the present moment, and nonjudgmentally"

Others provided a different definition, and a good example is the one by S. Bishop (2004) and his colleagues, which "offered a two-component model of mindfulness," as shown below (and summarized in *Table 2.8*): (WK 2013bb)

- "The First Component"—"involves the self-regulation of attention so that it is maintained on immediate experience, thereby allowing for increased recognition of mental events in the present moment."
- "The Second Component"—"involves adopting a particular orientation toward one's experiences in the present moment, an orientation that is characterized by curiosity, openness, and acceptance."

Thus, "in this two-component model, self-regulated attention (the first component) involves conscious awareness of one's current thoughts, feelings, and surroundings, which can result in metacognitive skills for controlling concentration. Orientation to experience (the second component) involves accepting one's mindstream, maintaining open and curious attitudes, and thinking in alternative categories (developing upon Ellen Langer's research on decision-making). Training in mindfulness and mindfulness-based practices, oftentimes as part of a quiet meditation session, results in the development of a Beginner's mind, or, looking at experiences as if for the first time." (WK 2013bb; J. Teasdale 1999)

In this way, "practicing mindfulness can help people to begin to recognise their habitual patterns of mind, which have developed out of awareness over time and this allows practitioners to respond in new rather than habitual ways to their life." (WK 2013bb; MIND 2013)

History of Mindfulness Practices

The history of mindfulness practices (from Buddhism) in the West is more recent.

For instance, "Thich Nhat Hanh [1975] has brought mindfulness to the attention of Westerners. It was on a retreat he led in the United States that an American doctor, Jon Kabat-Zinn, first realised the appropriateness of mindfulness in the treatment of chronic medical conditions. Kabat-Zinn later adapted Hanh's teachings on mindfulness into the structured eight-week Mindfulness Based Stress Reduction course, which has since spread throughout the western World." (WK 2013bb)

With this influence from the teachings of Thich Nhat Hanh—"in 1979, Dr. Jon Kabat-Zinn [1982] founded the Mindfulness-Based Stress Reduction program at the University of Massachusetts to treat the chronically ill, which sparked a growing interest and application of mindfulness ideas and practices in the medical world for the treatment of a variety of conditions in people both healthy and unhealthy." (WK 2013bb)

The program "was inspired by teachings from the East, and particularly from the Buddhist traditions, where mindfulness is one of the eight constituents of the Noble Eightfold Path taught by Siddhartha Gautama, the Buddha, who founded Buddhism almost 2,500 years ago. Although originally articulated as a part of what is known in the West as Buddhism, there is nothing inherently religious about mindfulness, and it is often taught independent of religious or cultural connotation." (WK 2013bb; J. Kabat-Zinn 1982)

Later, "mindfulness and other Buddhist meditation techniques receive support in the West" from other figures like "the teacher Jack Kornfield, the teacher Joseph Goldstein, the psychologist Tara Brach, the writer Alan Clements, and the teacher Sharon Salzberg, who have been widely attributed with playing a significant role in integrating the healing aspects of Buddhist meditation practices with the concept of psychological awareness and healing. Psychotherapists have adapted and developed mindfulness techniques into promising cognitive behavioral therapies" like "Acceptance and Commitment Therapy (ACT, pronounced act). ACT was recently reviewed by SAMHSA's National Registry of Evidence-Based Programs and Practices." (WK 2013bb; S. Hayes 2004; R. Harris 2008)

Scientific Research on Mindfulness

In the past three decades, "there has been an increase in the number of published studies on mindfulness." (WK 2013bb) For illustration, consider the following examples (as summarized in *Table 2.8*).

(a) Mindfulness Scales

In the research on "mindfulness scales"—"researchers attempt to define and measure the results of mindfulness primarily through controlled, randomised studies of mindfulness intervention on various dependent variables. The participants in mindfulness interventions measure many of the outcomes of such interventions subjectively. For this reason, several mindfulness inventories or scales (a set of questions posed to a subject…) have arisen. Twelve such methods are detailed at Mindfulness Research Guide. The most prominent include": (WK 2013bb)

- "the Mindful Attention Awareness Scale (MAAS)"
- "the Freiburg Mindfulness Inventory"
- "the Kentucky Inventory of Mindfulness Skills"
- "the Cognitive and Affective Mindfulness Scale"

With "these scales—which can illuminate self-reported changes in levels of mindfulness, the measurement of other correlated inventories in fields such as subjective well-being, and the measurement of other correlated variables such as health and performance—researchers have produced studies that investigate the nature and effects of mindfulness." (WK 2013bb)

(b) Stress Reduction

In the research on "stress reduction"—the concern is with "human response to stressors in the environment," which "produces emotional and physiological changes in individual human bodies in order to cope with that stress. This process most likely evolved to help us attend to immediate concerns in our environment to better our chances of survival, but in modern society, much of the stress felt is not beneficial in this way. Stress has been shown to have several negative effects on health, happiness, and overall wellbeing." (WK 2013bb)

Several important findings are shown below: (WK 2013bb)

- "Jain and Shapiro (2007) conducted a study to show that mindfulness meditation may be specific in its ability to 'reduce distractive and ruminative thoughts and behaviours,' which may provide a 'unique mechanism by which mindfulness meditation reduces distress.'"
- "Arch (2006) found emotional regulation following focused breathing. A breathing group provided moderately positive responses to emotionally neutral visual slides, while 'unfocused attention and worry' groups both responded significantly more negatively to neutral slides."
- "Brown (2003) found declines in mood disturbance and stress following mindfulness interventions."
- "Jha (2010) found that a sufficient meditation training practice may protect against functional impairments associated with high-stress contexts."
- "Garland (2009) found declines in stress after mindfulness interventions, which are potentially due to the positive re-appraisals of what were at first appraised as stressors."

Of course, there can be other examples, so the ones above are illustrative.

(c) Elevation of Positive Emotions and Outcomes

In the research on the "elevation of positive emotions and outcomes"—"evidence indicates that mindfulness meditation leads to well-being through increases in awareness. Shapiro, Oman, Thoresen, Plante, and Flinders (2008) found that the Mindfulness Based Stress Reduction (MBSR) and the Eight Point Program (EPP) interventions increased levels of well-being in participants." (WK 2013bb)

For instance, "Schoormans and Nyklicek (2011) compared well-being measures for two groups that had each practiced a different meditation—mindfulness meditation (MM) or transcendental meditation (TM). MM explicitly seeks to enhance mindfulness, while TM uses the repetition of a mantra. Authors believed that MM would increase mindfulness and psychological well-being more than would the TM. In fact, MM and TM practitioners had very similar mindfulness and well-being outcomes. The only predictor of higher mindfulness and reduced stress was the number of days meditated per week, with more days associated with higher mindfulness and reduced stress. These studies demonstrate that MM and TM are both associated with heightened well-being. Meditation may increase well-being due to increases in personal resources." (WK 2013bb)

And "Frederickson (2008) assessed a loving-kindness meditation and found an increase in positive emotions and life satisfaction when controlling for personal resources. These results indicated that daily activities, such as specific forms of meditation, may only increase life satisfaction if they also develop personal resources. Personal resources, which may be increased by meditation, prepare people to deal with threatening situations, which may lead to increased well-being." (WK 2013bb)

(d) Mindfulness Meditation as Cross-Modal Adaptation

In the research on "mindfulness meditation as cross-modal adaptation"—"Bedford (2012) proposed a novel psychological theory of how mindfulness meditation leads to healing based in the field of perception. According to the theory, mindful meditation along with guided imagery creates a conflict between a visual image and the immune system, the latter of which is argued to be a sensory modality. This cross-modal visual-immune system conflict now acts like any cross-modal conflict in perception: one of the modalities must change to realign the two modalities. When the immune system is the modality that changes, healing can occur. In this view, there is no 'mind' over 'matter'; what appears as the mind influencing the body is actually just low level interaction of multiple perceptual modalities/senses, which they evolved to do to maintain perceptual accuracy." (WK 2013bb)

Specific Mindfulness-Based Therapy Programs

Over the decades, mindfulness research has yielded interesting therapy programs to fight health problems; for example, "since 2006 research supports promising mindfulness-based therapies for a number of medical and psychiatric conditions, notably chronic pain (McCracken et al. 2007), stress (Grossman et al. 2004), anxiety and depression (Hofmann et al. 2010), substance abuse (Melemis 2008…), and recurrent suicidal behavior (Williams et al. 2006)." (WK 2013bb)

Hereafter are a few specific mindfulenss-based therapy programs to fight health problems: (WK 2013bb)

- "Morita Therapy"—was proposed by "the Japanese psychiatrist Shoma Morita, who trained in Zen meditation" and "developed Morita therapy upon principles of mindfulness and non-attachment." (WK 2013bb)
- "Gestalt Therapy"—focuses on "awareness," which "has been an essential part of its theory and practice," especially "since the beginnings...in the early 1940s." (WK 2013bb)
- "Adaptation Practice"—was proposed by the "British doctor, Clive Sherlock," who "developed Adaptation practice in 1977" for "a structured programme of self-discipline." (WK 2013bb; A. Garvey 2004)
- "Mindfulness-Based Stress Reduction"—was proposed by "Jon Kabat-Zinn...over a ten-year period at the University of Massachusetts Medical School," for "all the regular, disciplined practice of moment-to-moment awareness or mindfulness, the complete 'owning' of each moment of your experience, good, bad, or ugly." (WK 2013bb)
- "Mindfulness-Based Cognitive Therapy"—"combines cognitive therapy with mindfulness techniques as a treatment for major depressive disorder and many other disorders." (WK 2013bb; S. Hofmann 2011)
- "Acceptance and Commitment Therapy"—was proposed by "Steven C. Hayes and others" who "have developed acceptance and commitment therapy (ACT), originally called 'comprehensive distancing,' which uses strategies of mindfulness, acceptance, and behavior change." (WK 2013bb)
- "Dialectical Behavior Therapy"—was proposed by Marsha M. Linehan to focuse on "mindfulness" as a "core" exercise for "treating people with borderline personality disorder," and the treatment is "dialectic,...in the sense of 'the reconciliation of opposites in a continual process of synthesis.'" (WK 2013bb)
- "Hakomi"—was proposed by "Ron Kurtz and others," for "a somatic psychology based upon Asian philosophical precepts of mindfulness and nonviolence." (WK 2013bb)

Again, there can be other examples, so the ones above are illustrative.

Problems with Mindfulness-Based Therapy

However, for the critics, the argument for mindfulness-based therapy has some major problems. Consider, for illustration, a few examples below (as summarized in *Table 2.8*).

Firstly, one main criticism of the argument for mindfulness-based therapy is that the research works are often incomplete.

For example, for the critics, in the research on the "elevation of positive emotions and outcomes"—"the study did not address specific differences between the interventions, and how these differences may relate to well-being." (WK 2013bb)

Secondly, another main criticism of the argument for mindfulness-based therapy is that the practices are not so effective.

For instance, for the critics, "the effects of these meditations may become nonexistent once practice ceases," and "Diener, Lucas, and Scollon (2006) claimed that emotional techniques used successfully in the lab may not translate to life outside of the lab...." (WK 2013bb)

Thirdly, still another main criticism of the argument for mindfulness-based therapy is that its terms are often not clearly defined and can mean different things.

For instance, for the critics, "much of the terminology used in such research has no cohesive definition. For example, there is a lack of differentiation between 'attention' and 'awareness' and an interchangeable use of the two in modern descriptions. Buddhist contemplative psychology however, differentiates more clearly, as 'attention' in that context signifies an ever-changing factor of consciousness, while 'awareness' refers to a stable and specific state of consciousness." (WK 2013bb)

Fourthly, an additional main criticism of the argument for mindfulness-based therapy is that the idea of "mindfulness" in mindfulness-based therapy programs deviates significantly from the original Buddhist version.

For instance, for the critics, "B. Alan Wallace [2006] has stated that an influential definition of mindfulness in the psychology literature (by Bishop et al.) differs in significant ways from how mindfulness was defined by the Buddha himself, and by much of Buddhist tradition. Wallace concludes that 'The modern description and practice of mindfulness are certainly valuable, as thousands of people have discovered for themselves through their own practice. But this doesn't take away from the fact that the modern understanding departs significantly from the Buddha's own account of sati, and from those of the most authoritative commentators in the Theravada and Indian Mahayana traditions.'" (WK 2013bb) And "Eleanor Rosch [2007] has stated that contemporary 'therapeutic systems that include mindfulnes...could as much be called wisdom-based as mindfulness-based," because "mindfulness would seem to play two roles: as a part of the therapy itself and as an umbrella justification ('empirical') for the inclusion of other aspects of wisdom that may be beyond our present cultural assumptions. Where in this is mindfulness in its original sense of the mind adhering to an object of consciousness with a clear mental focus?" (WK 2013bb)

And fifthly, another additional main criticism of the argument for mindfulness-based therapy is that, because of its connection with alternative medicine, mindfulness-based therapy programs have been criticized as not being scientific.

For instance, for the critics, "Ayurvedic medicine is a traditional medicine of India and has strong links with Buddhism and Hinduism," just as mindfulness-based therapy programs are linked to Buddhism, but alternative medicines (including those linked to Buddhism) have been criticized for "the lack of critical thinking and scientific rigor." (WK 2013q; B. Cassileth 1999)

Beyond Mindfulness-Based Therapy

These criticisms of mindfulness-based therapy, however, should not be misunderstood as a total rejection of its usefulness but serve to show us the two opposing sides of the debate, such that the possibility (or impossibility) and desirability (or undesirability) of mental health (from the perspective of culture with mental health, mindfulness, and religion as a case study here) are not to the extent that the respective defenders would like us to believe.

Furthermore, the analysis of mental health, mindfulness, and religion is to shed some light on the ontological principles in existential dialectics, and good examples include the formalness-informalness principle, the absoluteness-relativeness principle, the partiality-totality principle, the predictability-unpredictability principle, the explicability-inexplicability principle, the fiction-reality principle, the cognitiveness-noncognitiveness principle, the finiteness-transfiniteness principle, the preciseness-vagueness principle, the simpleness-complicatedness principle, the openness-hiddenness principle, the denseness-emptiness principle, the prototypicality-variation principle, the change-constancy principle, the order-chaos principle, the slowness-quickness principle, the expansion-contraction principle, the optimality-nonoptimality principle, the theory-praxis principle, the convention-novelty principle, the evolution-transformation principle, the symmetry-asymmetry principle, the softness-hardness principle, the seriousness-playfulness principle, the activeness-inactivess principle, the selfness-otherness principle, the regression-progression principle, the same-difference principle, the stability-reaction principle, the functionality-nonfunctionality principle, and the intentionality-nonintentionality principle.

For instance, in relation to the formalness-informalness principle, if there is formalness (e.g., the formal logical requirement of soundness, completeness, and consistency in a system of ideas, as in the argument for mindfulness-based therapy), there is informalness (e.g., the non-formal existence of unsoundness, incompleteness, and inconsistency in the argument for mindfulness-based therapy, as shown in the criticisms that the research works are often incomplete, that the practices are not so effective, that its terms are often not clearly defined and can mean different things, that the idea of "mindfulness" in mindfulness-based therapy programs deviates significantly from the original Buddhist version, and that because of its connection with alternative medicine, mindfulness-based therapy programs have been criticized as not being scientific). And the reverse direction also holds true.

In relation to the absoluteness-relativeness principle, if there is absoluteness (e.g., the absolute view on Mindfulness-Based Stress Reduction program by Jon Kabat-Zinn "for the treatment of a variety of conditions in people both healthy and unhealthy"), there is relativeness (e.g., what is right for Jon Kabat-Zinn in regard to his Mindfulness-Based Stress Reduction program is not necessarily so for the critics, who pointed out different problems associated with mindfulness-based therapy aforediscussed). And the reverse direction also holds true.

In relation to the partiality-totality principle, if there is partiality (e.g., the partial view on mindfulness-based therapy by the advocates), there is totality (e.g., the more holistic view on mindfulness-based therapy, such that the whole is not the sum of its parts, that is, it cannot be reduced to the sum of opposing views by the advocates, by the critics, etc., since there will emerge new views in the future not yet known today, just as there are already alternative views nowadays which do not side exclusively with any of them, as is the analysis here). And the reverse direction also holds true.

In relation to the predictability-unpredictability principle, if there is predictability (e.g., the predictable tendency by the advocates, of the working of the mindfulness-based therapy for the "elevation of positive emotions and outcomes"), there is unpredictability (e.g., the more difficult task to predict exactly the extent to which the mindfulness-based therapy on the "elevation of positive emotions and outcomes" will necessarily work on a particular future occasion, since, for the critics, "the study did not address specific differences between the interventions, and how these differences may relate to well-being," and, in addition, "the effects of these meditations may become nonexistent once practice ceases"). And the reverse direction also holds true.

In relation to the explicability-inexplicability principle, if there is explicability (e.g., the explanation, by the advocates, of the desirability of the scientific research on mindfulness on the basis of its practical use for therapy), there is inexplicability (e.g., the lack of sufficient explanation, by the advocates, of why the scientific research on mindfulness is necessarily desirable, since, for the critics, it suffers from the problems that the research works are often incomplete, that the practices are not so effective, that its terms are often not clearly defined and can mean different things, and that because of its connection with alternative medicine, mindfulness-based therapy programs have been criticized as not being scientific). And the reverse direction also holds true.

In relation to the fiction-reality principle, if there is fiction (e.g., the fictional aspect of mindfulness-based therapy, insofar as, for the critics, "the effects of these meditations may become nonexistent once practice ceases," and "Diener, Lucas, and Scollon claimed that emotional techniques used successfully in the lab may not translate to life outside of the lab…."), there is reality (e.g., the realistic aspect of mindfulness-based therapy, insofar as the study by "Brown [2003] found declines in mood disturbance and stress following mindfulness interventions," under certain conditions). And the reverse direction also holds true.

In relation to the cognitiveness-noncognitiveness principle, if there is cognitiveness (e.g., a view of things on the basis of reason and evidences, as shown in the empirical work by Wallace, who pointed out that "the modern description and practice of mindfulness are certainly valuable, as thousands of people have discovered for themselves through their own practice"), there is noncognitiveness (e.g., a view of things on the basis of non-cognitive factors like envy, jealousy, power, nationality, race, gender, age, class, greed, lust, status, faith, anger, sadness, joy, fear, wish, etc., as shown in the politics of historical revisionism in regard to how "mindfulness has been defined or represented in recent western psychology publications," which "differs in significant ways from how mindfulness was defined by the Buddha himself, and by much of Buddhist tradition," as pointed out by Wallace). (WK 2013bb) And the reverse direction also holds true.

In relation to the finiteness-transfiniteness principle, if there is finiteness (e.g., the finite number of the components in mindfullness, like "attention," "openness," etc.), there is transfiniteness (e.g., the transfinite number of all the individuals in history who have ever existed and shared the traits of "attention, "openness," etc.). And the reverse direction also holds true.

In relation to the preciseness-vagueness principle, if there is preciseness (e.g., the precise identification of 8 mindfulness-based therapy programs in the article aforecited), there is vagueness (e.g., the vagueness in the identification of the 8 mindfulness-based therapy programs in the article aforecited, since it is not clear why there must be only 8, not 10, 13, 14, 16, and so on). And the reverse direction also holds true.

In relation to the simpleness-complicatedness principle, if there is simpleness (e.g., the relatively simple analysis of mindfulness-based therapy programs by the advocates), there is complicatedness (e.g., the relatively more complicated analysis of mindfulness-based therapy programs, by challenging the claims and assumptions, as shown in the problems pointed out by the critics as cited). And the reverse direction also holds true.

In relation to the openness-hiddenness principle, if there is openness (e.g., the open exploration of using mindfulness to cure health problems), there is hiddenness (e.g., the hidden bias in the mindfulness-based therapy programs, since, for the critics, the research works are often incomplete, the practices are not so effective, and because of its connection with alternative medicine, mindfulness-based therapy programs have been criticized as not being scientific). And the reverse direction also holds true.

In relation to the denseness-emptiness principle, if there is denseness (e.g., the relatively denser concentration of concerns with "attention" and "openness" by those in mindfulness-based therapy programs), there is emptiness (e.g., the relatively less dense, or more empty, concentration of concerns with "pre-judgement" and "past-centered awareness" by those in mindfulness-based therapy programs). And the reverse direction also holds true.

In relation to the prototypicality-variation principle, if there is prototypicality (e.g., the prototype, like the example about the original work on "mindfulness" in "the Noble Eightfold Path taught by Siddhartha Gautama," that is, "the Buddha, who founded Buddhism almost 2,500 years ago"), there is variation (e.g., different variants of the protoptye, as shown in many studies about the Buddhist tradition since then, like the ones by Jon Kabat-Zinn, Thich Nhat Hanh, Jack Kornfield, Joseph Goldstein, Tara Brach, Alan Clements, and Sharon Salzberg,, etc., though each with his own variation, contribution, and disagreement). And the reverse direction also holds true.

In relation to the change-constancy principle, if there is change (e.g., the ever new ways to understand therapy, as shown in the mindfulness-based therapy programs), there is constancy (e.g., the ever constant existence of different problems with the ever new ways to understand therapy, as shown in the problems with mindfulness-based therapy programs pointed out by the critics). And the reverse direction also holds true.

In relation to the order-chaos principle, if there is order (e.g., the more or less orderly view on therapy, if looked from the sole vantage point of "attention" and "openness" by those in mindfulness-based therapy), there is chaos (e.g., the more or less chaotic view on therapy, if looked from the multiple, conflicting vantage points of the advocates, the critics, and so on, as shown in the debates on the different problems afore-discussed). And the reverse direction also holds true.

In relation to the slowness-quickness principle, if there is slowness (e.g., the relatively slower speed of those patients to recover from their health problems if they have never used "mindfulness-based therapy" or any other programs, as studied by Wallace), there is quickness (e.g., the relatively quicker speed of "thousands of people" to "discover…for themselves through the…practice" of mindfulness-based therapy, as studied by Wallace). And the reverse direction also holds true.

In relation to the expansion-contraction principle, if there is expansion (e.g., the relatively more developed ability of those in mindfulness-based therapy to deal with "attention" and "a clear mental focus"), there is contraction (e.g., the relatively less developed ability of those in mindfulness-based therapy to deal with wealth acquisition, colonial conquest, etc.). (WK 2013bb; E. Rosch 2007) And the reverse direction also holds true.

In relation to the optimality-nonoptimality principle, if there is optimality (e.g., the search for highly favorable options, like the quest by Jon Kabat-Zinn for "the Mindfulness-Based Stress Reduction program," which can treat "a variety of conditions in people both healthy and unhealthy"), there is nonoptimality (e.g., the existence of non-optimal alternatives to optimality, like the argument for more realistic studies by the critics, who pointed out that the research works are often incomplete, that the practices are not so effective, that its terms are often not clearly defined and can mean different things, that the idea of "mindfulness" in mindfulness-based therapy programs deviates significantly from the original Buddhist version, and that because of its connection with alternative medicine, mindfulness-based therapy programs have been criticized as not being scientific). (WK 2013bb) And the reverse direction also holds true.

In relation to the theory-praxis principle, if there is theory (e.g., the theoretical construction of "mindfulness" in Buddhism), there is praxis (e.g., the practical application of "mindfulness" in Buddhism to the field of therapy, as shown in mindfulness-based therapy programs). And the reverse direction also holds true.

In relation to the convention-novelty principle, if there is convention (e.g., the conventional wisdom about "mindfulness" in Buddhism), there is novelty (e.g., the alternative novel challenge to the conventional wisdom about "mindfulness" in Buddhism, by the new idea of using it for therapy, as proposed by Jon Kabat-Zinn and others). And the reverse direction also holds true.

In relation to the evolution-transformation principle, if there is evolution (e.g., the natural evolution of humans to suffer from health problems at times in the state of nature), there is transformation (e.g., the technical transformation of human ability to deal with health problems by the invention of mindfulness-based therapy). And the reverse direction also holds true.

In relation to the symmetry-asymmetry principle, if there is symmetry (e.g., the co-existence of different agents in a mindfulness-based therapy relationship, like a Buddhist teacher and his patient), there is asymmetry (e.g., the Buddhist teacher has authority over his patient in a mindfulness-based therapy relationship). And the reverse direction also holds true.

In relation to the softness-hardness principle, if there is softness (e.g., the defense of mindfulness-based therapy by the advocates), there is hardness (e.g., the critique of mindfulness-based therapy, as shown in the problems pointed out by the critics as cited). And the reverse direction also holds true.

In relation to the seriousness-playfulness principle, if there is seriousness (e.g., the serious business of those who try to use mindfulness in Buddhism for mindfulness-based therapy), there is playfulness (e.g., the playful part of those who try to use mindfulness in Buddhism for mindfulness-based therapy, when they play around with different options over the decades, like the the 8 therapy programs afore-described). And the reverse direction also holds true.

In relation to the activeness-inactivess principle, if there is activeness (e.g., the relative activeness of those who learn how to bring "a complete attention" with the help of "mindfulness-based therapy," so he can now engage in life activities better), there is inactiveness (e.g., the relative inactiveness of those who suffer from "attention-deficit disorder" and has not received any help from "mindfulness-based therapy" or any other source, so he cannot concentrate well on life activities).

In relation to the selfness-otherness principle, if there is selfness (e.g., the tendency to be mostly centered on one's self or group, as shown in those captialists who have no problem in pursuing "greed" and other materialistic desires for themselves), there is otherness (e.g., the tendency to be mostly centered on others, as shown in those who pursue a more spiritual lifestyle with the help of "mindfulness-based therapy" for "a clear mental focus" with "wisdom," away from "greed, hatred, and delusion"). (WK 2013cc) And the reverse direction also holds true.

In relation to the regression-progression principle, if there is regression (e.g., the regression made by "mindfulness-based therapy," as shown in the problems pointed out by the critics), there is progression (e.g., the progress made by "mindfulness-based therapy," as shown in the contribution to the therapy for "attention" and "openness" afore-described). And the reverse direction also holds true.

In relation to the same-difference principle, if there is similarity in outcome (e.g., the contribution to the molding and control of beliefs, values, and behaviors, regardless of whether this be done by way of the Mindfulness-Based Stress Reduction program, or by way of the Noble Eightfold Path taught by the Buddha), there is difference in outcome (e.g., the contribution to the molding and control of beliefs, values, and behaviors by way of the Mindfulness-Based Stress Reduction program for a relatively more secular-therapeutic lifeworld—but the contribution to the molding and control of beliefs, values, and behaviors by way of the Noble Eightfold Path taught by the Buddha for a relatively more spiritual lifeworld). And the reverse direction also holds true.

In relation to the stability-reaction principle, if there is stability (e.g., the relatively more stable condition of the Buddhist tradition as shown in the Noble Eightfold Path taught by the Buddha in the older days), there is reaction (e.g., the Buddhist tradition in the older day then led to further changes later on, when nowadays, it is revised for "mindfulness-based therapy" instead). And the reverse direction also holds true.

In relation to the functionality-nonfunctionality principle, if there is functionality (e.g., the presence of action for which something or someone is fitted, as shown in the Noble Eightfold Path taught by the Buddha in the older days, which served the function of advocating the spiritual life away from "greed, hatred, and delusion" at that time), there is nonfunctionality (e.g., the relative lack of action for which something or someone is fitted, as shown in the use of the Buddhist tradition for "mindfulness-based therapy," such that the Noble Eightfold Path taught by the Buddha in the older days is no longer functional in the contemporary Western psychotherapeutic community, whose "modern understanding departs significantly from the Buddha's own account of sati"). (WK 2013bb) And the reverse direction also holds true.

In relation to the intentionality-nonintentionality principle, if there is intentionality (e.g., the planning or design of something for a certain outcome, as shown in the original intention of the Buddha to teach the Noble Eightfold Path so as to strive for the spiritual life away from "greed, hatred, and delusion"), there is nonintentionality (e.g., the relative absence of planning or design of something for a certain outcome, such that the outcome can even be counter-intentional in being the opposite of what was originally planned, as shown in the use of the Buddhist tradition for "mindfulness-based therapy" nowadays to enhance "attention" and "openness"—contrary to the original intention of the Buddha to teach the Noble Eightfold Path so as to strive for the spiritual life away from "greed, hatred, and delusion" instead). And the reverse direction also holds true.

And in relation to the survivability-nonsurvivability principle, if there is survivability (e.g., the relative survival, nowadays, of using the Buddhist tradition for "mindfulness-based therapy" to cope with health problems like "chronic pain," "stress," "anxiety and depression," "substance abuse," and "recurrent suicidal behavior" in the contemporary Western psychotherapeutic community), there is non-survivability (e.g., the relative non-survival, nowadays, of using the Buddhist tradition for a spiritual life to cope with health problems like "greed," "pleasures of the flesh," etc. in the contemporary Western psychotherapeutic community). And the reverse direction also holds true.

The Contingency of Mental Health

This comprehensive analysis of the possibility (or impossibility) and desirability (or undesirability) of mental health in the context of health care, from the perspectives of the mind, nature, society, and culture, is important to show us the different ways in which mental health is both possible and desirable, but not to the extent that the spokespersons from each side would like us to believe.

Mental health thus has its necessity, just as it has its contingency too, as the other side of the same coin.

But this is only one part of a larger story, since there is also physical health, the other concern of health care. Since this chapter already deals with mental health, the next chapter will therefore address physical health.

These dual analyses should not be underestimated, because those on the side of mental health often downgrade physical health merely as the other concern of health care without really appreciating it from the vantage point of physical health too—and vice versa.

With this in mind, let's now turn to Chapter Three for the study of physical health and its ambivalence—for which we now turn to chapter three.

Table 2.1. Mental Health and its Duality

- **Mental Health and the Mind**
  - —Ex: mental health, psychotherapy, and medicine
  - —Ex: mental health, subjective well-being, and genetics

- **Mental Health and Nature**
  - —Ex: mental health, evolution, and the environment
  - —Ex: mental health, zoophilia, and animals

- **Mental Health and Society**
  - —Ex: mental health, illness, and income inequality
  - —Ex: mental health, treatment, and technology

- **Mental Health and Culture**
  - —Ex: mental health, alternative medicine, and culture
  - —Ex: mental health, mindfulness, and religion

Notes: The examples in the categories are solely illustrative (not exhaustive), and the comparison is relative (not absolute), nor are they necessarily mutually exclusive. And some can be easily re-classified elsewhere. As generalities, they allow exceptions.
Source: A summary of Ch.2 of *FPHHC*

Table 2.2. Mental Health, Subjective Well-Being, and Genetics

- **Components of Subjective Well-Being**
  —Ex: affect balance
  —Ex: life satisfaction

- **Genetic Theories of Subjective Well-Being**
  —Ex: top-down theory
  —Ex: bottom-up theory

- **Problems with Genetics and Subjective Well-Being**
  —Firstly, one main criticism of the argument on mental health, subjective well-being, and genetics is that it ignores the "objective" conditions of well-being.
  —Secondly, another main criticism of the argument on mental health, subjective well-being, and genetics is that the findings are not consistent across studies and across histories.
  —Thirdly, still another main criticism of the argument on mental health, subjective well-being, and genetics is that much remains uncertain about the nature of SWB.
  —Fourthly, an additional main criticism of the argument on mental health, subjective well-being, and genetics is that SWB can be detrimental to health.
  —Fifthly, another additional main criticism of the argument on mental health, subjective well-being, and genetics is that it neglects social factors.
  —And sixthly, still another additional main criticism of the argument on mental health, subjective well-being, and genetics is that it does not give sufficient attention to cultural variations.

Notes: The examples in the categories are solely illustrative (not exhaustive), and the comparison is relative (not absolute), nor are they necessarily mutually exclusive. And some can be easily re-classified elsewhere. As generalities, they allow exceptions.
Source: From *Sec. 2.2.2* of *FPHHC*. See book for citations.

Table 2.3. Mental Health, Evolution, and the Environment

- **Scope of Evolutionary Psychology**
  —Ex: principles
  —Ex: premises

- **Theoretical Foundations of Evolutionary Psychology**
  —Ex: C. Darwin's natural selection/sexual selection
  —Ex: W. Hamilton's inclusive fitness
  —Ex: other advances in evolutionary theory

- **Areas of Research**
  —Ex: emotion and motivation
  —Ex: cognition

- **Problems with Evolutionary Adaptedness**
  —Firstly, one main criticism of the argument on mental health, evolutionary adaptedness, and the environment is that there are "non-genetic and non-adaptive explanations" which are not adequately considered.
  —Secondly, another main criticism of the argument on mental health, evolutionary adaptedness, and the environment is that there is the controversial issues about testability and uncertainty.
  —Thirdly, still another main criticism of the argument on mental health, evolutionary adaptedness, and the environment is that it runs the risk of committing "the naturalistic fallacy."
  —Fourthly, an additional main criticism of the argument on mental health, evolutionary adaptedness, and the environment is that it is reductionistic.
  —And fifthly, another additional main criticism of the argument on mental health, evolutionary adaptedness, and the environment is that there are disagreements on the "modularity of the mind."

Notes: The examples in the categories are solely illustrative (not exhaustive), and the comparison is relative (not absolute), nor are they necessarily mutually exclusive. And some can be easily re-classified elsewhere. As generalities, they allow exceptions.
Source: From *Sec. 2.3.1* of *FPHHC*. See book for citations.

Table 2.4. Mental Health, Zoophilia, and Animals

- **Concepts on Zoophilia**
  —Ex: zoophilia
  —Ex: zoosexuality
  —Ex: bestiality
  —Ex: zoosadism

- **Arguments for Zoophilia**
  —Ex: the issue of consent
  —Ex: the issue of enjoyment

- **Problems with Zoophilia**
  —Firstly, one main criticism of the research on zoophilia is that there is "self-selection bias" in the research on zoophilia.
  —Secondly, another main criticism of the research on zoophilia is that the findings are inconsistent.
  —Thirdly, still another main criticism of the research on zoophilia is that it commits the naturalistic fallacy.
  —Fourthly, an additional main criticism of research on zoophilia is that there are health and safety concerns in zoophilia.
  —Fifthly, another additional main criticism of research on zoophilia is that there are disagreements about zoophilia across cultures.
  —Sixthly, still another additional main criticism of research on zoophilia is that the practice can result in violent consequences.
  —And seventhly, one last main criticism of the research on zoophilia is that the practice is no longer condoned in our time.

Notes: The examples in the categories are solely illustrative (not exhaustive), and the comparison is relative (not absolute), nor are they necessarily mutually exclusive. And some can be easily re-classified elsewhere. As generalities, they allow exceptions.
Source: From *Sec. 2.3.2* of *FPHHC*. See book for citations.

Table 2.5. Mental Health, Illness, and Income Inequality

- **Causes of Income Inequality**
  —Ex: "greater inequality in wages and salaries"
  —Ex: "wealth concentration"
  —Ex: "labor markets"
  —Ex: "more regressive taxation"
  —Ex: "increasing education costs"
  —Ex: "racial inequality"
  —Ex: "nepotism"

- **Effects of Income Inequality (on Health)**
  —Ex: "population health"
  —Ex: "social cohesion"
  —Ex: "crime"
  —Ex: "social, cultural, and civic participation"

- **Problems with the Argument for Less Income Inequality**
  —Firstly, one main criticism of the argument on mental health, illness, and income inequality is that it constitutes a very narrow view of social stratification in relation to health care.
  —Secondly, another main criticism of the argument on mental health, illness, and income inequality is that it provides no verification of the claim.
  —Thirdly, still another main criticism of the argument on mental health, illness, and income inequality is that there is no general agreement on the desirability of income equality (or its reduction).
  —Fourthly, an additional main criticism of the argument on mental health, illness, and income inequality is that the correlation between health and income level does not always hold.
  —And fifthly, another additional main criticism of the argument on mental health, illness, and income inequality is that equality can lead to a conformist society.

Notes: The examples in the categories are solely illustrative (not exhaustive), and the comparison is relative (not absolute), nor are they necessarily mutually exclusive. And some can be easily re-classified elsewhere. As generalities, they allow exceptions.
Source: From *Sec. 2.4.1* of *FPHHC*. See book for citations.

Table 2.6. Mental Health, Treatment, and Technology

- **The Case of Virtual Reality Therapy**
  —History
  —Applications
  —Efficacy

- **The Case of Telemedicine**
  —History
  —Types
  —Telemedicine and health care

- **Problems with the Use of Technology for Mental Health**
  —Firstly, one main criticism of the argument on the use of technology for mental health is that technologies do not necessarily benefit everyone.
  —Secondly, another main criticism of the argument on the use of technology for mental health is that there are "cultural" barriers.
  —Thirdly, still another main criticism of the argument on the use of technology for mental health is that there are "regulatory" barriers.
  —Fourthly, an additional main criticism of the argument on the use of technology for mental health is that there are "financial" barriers.
  —Fifthly, another additional main criticism of the argument on the use of technology for mental health is that there are "technical" barriers.
  —And sixthly, still another additional main criticism of the argument on the use of technology for mental health is that virtual reality has its dark side.

Notes: The examples in the categories are solely illustrative (not exhaustive), and the comparison is relative (not absolute), nor are they necessarily mutually exclusive. And some can be easily re-classified elsewhere. As generalities, they allow exceptions.
Source: From *Sec. 2.4.2* of *FPHHC*. See book for citations.

Table 2.7. Mental Health, Alternative Medicine, and Culture

- **Types of Alternative Medicines**
  —Ex: "alternative medical systems"
  —Ex: "energy therapies"
  —Ex: "mind body therapies"
  —Ex: "herbs, diet and vitamins"
  —Ex: "body manipulation"

- **Problems with Alternative Medicine**
  —Firstly, one main criticism of the argument on mental health, alternative medicine, and culture is that altnerative medicine is not scientific.
  —Secondly, another main criticism of the argument on mental health, alternative medicine, and culture is that its practice is unethical.
  —Thirdly, still another main criticism of the argument on mental health, alternative medicine, and culture is that alternative medicine often uses "ambiguous" words to mislead.
  —Fourthly, an additional main criticism of the argument on mental health, alternative medicine, and culture is that alternative medicine is not effective as claimed.
  —Fifthly, another additional main criticism of the argument on mental health, alternative medicine, and culture is that its practice is manipulative, in "using plausibility of one practice to support implausible other practices." (WK 203q)
  —And sixthly, still another additional main criticism of the argument on mental health, alternative medicine, and culture is that its practitioners play trick on patients.

Notes: The examples in the categories are solely illustrative (not exhaustive), and the comparison is relative (not absolute), nor are they necessarily mutually exclusive. And some can be easily re-classified elsewhere. As generalities, they allow exceptions.
Source: From *Sec. 2.5.1* of *FPHHC*. See book for citations.

Table 2.8. Mental Health, Mindfulness, and Religion

- **Definitions of Mindfulness**
  —"The first component involves the self-regulation of attention so that it is maintained on immediate experience, thereby allowing for increased recognition of mental events in the present moment."
  —The second component involves adopting a particular orientation toward one's experiences in the present moment, an orientation that is characterized by curiosity, openness, and acceptance."

- **Scientific Research on Mindfulness**
  —Ex: "mindfulness scales"
  —Ex: "stress reduction"
  —Ex: "elevation of positive emotions and outcomes"
  —Ex: "mindfulness meditation as cross-modal adaptation"

- **Problems with Mindfulness-Based Therapy**
  —Firstly, one main criticism of the argument for mindfulness-based therapy is that the research works are often incomplete.
  —Secondly, another main criticism of the argument for mindfulness-based therapy is that the practices are not so effective.
  —Thirdly, still another main criticism of the argument for mindfulness-based therapy is that its terms are often not clearly defined and can mean different things.
  —Fourthly, an additional main criticism of the argument for mindfulness-based therapy is that the idea of "mindfulness" in mindfulness-based therapy programs deviates significantly from the original Buddhist version.
  —And fifthly, another additional main criticism of the argument for mindfulness-based therapy is that, because of its connection with alternative medicine, mindfulness-based therapy programs have been criticized as not being scientific.

Notes: The examples in the categories are solely illustrative (not exhaustive), and the comparison is relative (not absolute), nor are they necessarily mutually exclusive. And some can be easily re-classified elsewhere. As generalities, they allow exceptions.
Source: From *Sec. 2.5.2* of *FPHHC*. See book for citations.

• PART THREE •

Body

CHAPTER 3
PHYSICAL HEALTH AND ITS AMBIVALENCE

> Too much exercise can be harmful....Inappropriate exercise can do more harm than good....Stopping excessive exercise suddenly can also create a change in mood."
> —Wikipedia (WK 2013a)

The Use of Physical Health

The study of health care involves both mental health and physical health (in the context of mind and body)—as already indicated in *Sec. 1.3*.

The relationship between mental health and physical health (in the context of mind and body) is dialectic, since there is no mental health without physical health, and vice versa—to be eventually transcended altogether later.

As already stressed in *Sec. 2.1*, a scholarly danger here is to reduce the analysis of one to that of the other; thus, this book is to devote a whole chapter on each, with the understanding, of course, that the two are related.

This dialectic interconnection between mental health and physical health (in the context of mind and body) can be revealed by showing how and why the analysis of mental health (in Chapter Two) is inadequate without the inclusion of physical health, just as the examination of physical health (in Chapter Three) is insufficient without the consideration of mental health.

The issues concerning mental health (in the context of the mind) in the study of health care were already addressed in Chapter Two—whereas the issues concerning physical health (in the context of the body) in the study of health care will be analyzed in this chapter (Chapter Three).

With this dialectic treatment in mind—a good way to examine physical health and its ambivalence (in the context of the body) in the study of health care is by way of the evaluation of the extent to which it is in fact both possible (or impossible) and desirable (or undesirable).

This can be done by way of a comprehensive analysis of physical health (in the context of the body) in health care from the four perspectives of the mind, nature, society, and culture (in accordance to my sophisticated methodological holism, as explained in *Sec. 1.9*).

In other words, this chapter is organized in four main sections, namely, in relation to (3.2) physical health and the mind, (3.3) physical health and nature, (3.4) physical health and society, and (3.5) physical health and culture—to be addressed hereafter, in that order (and summarized in *Table 3.1*).

Physical Health and the Mind

Physical health, when examined from the perspective of the mind, can illuminate its possibility (or impossibility) and desirability (or undesirability), and this can be shown by way of two case studies, namely, (3.2.1) physical health, exercise, and effects, and (3.2.2) physical health, abuse, and children—to be addressed in what follows, respectively.

Physical Health, Exercise, and Effects

A good way to evaluate the possibility (or impossibility) and desirability (or undesirability) of physical health from the perspective of the mind is to explore physical health, exercise, and effects.

An argument in the literature is that "physical exercise is important for maintaining physical fitness and can contribute positively to maintaining a healthy weight, building and maintaining healthy bone density, muscle strength, and joint mobility, promoting physiological well-being, reducing surgical risks, and strengthening the immune system." (WK 2013a)

History of Physical Exercise

Historically, "the benefits of exercise have been known since antiquity. Marcus Cicero, around 65 BC, stated: 'It is exercise alone that supports the spirits, and keeps the mind in vigor.' However, the link between physical health and exercise (or lack of it) was only discovered in 1949 and reported in 1953 by a team led by Jerry Morris. Dr. Morris noted that men of similar social class and occupation (bus conductors versus bus drivers) had markedly different rates of heart attacks, depending on the level of exercise they got: bus drivers had a sedentary occupation and a higher incidence of heart disease, while bus conductors were forced to move continually and had a lower incidence of heart disease. This link had not previously been noted and was later confirmed by other researchers." (WK 2013a; S. Kuper 2009; J. Morris 1953)

In general, "physical exercise…enhances or maintains physical fitness and overall health and wellness. It is performed for various reasons including strengthening muscles and the cardiovascular system, honing athletic skills, weight loss or maintenance, as well as for the purpose of enjoyment. Frequent and regular physical exercise boosts the immune system, and helps prevent the 'diseases of affluence' such as heart disease, cardiovascular disease, Type 2 diabetes and obesity. It also improves mental health, helps prevent depression, helps to promote or maintain positive self-esteem, and can even augment an individual's sex appeal or body image, which is also found to be linked with higher levels of self-esteem. Childhood obesity is a growing global concern and physical exercise may help decrease some of the effects of childhood and adult obesity. Health care providers often call exercise the 'miracle' or 'wonder' drug—alluding to the wide variety of proven benefits that it provides." (WK 2013a; M. Stampfer 2000; F. Hu 2001; NCBI 2010)

Types of Physical Exercise

With this introductory history in mind, "physical exercises are generally grouped into three types, depending on the overall effect they have on the human body," as shown below (and summarized in *Table 3.2*): (WK 2013a; D. O'Connor 2005; J. Wilmore 2003.; N. de Vos 2005)

- "Flexibility Exercises"—"such as stretching, improve the range of motion of muscles and joints."
- "Aerobic Exercises"—"such as cycling, swimming, walking, skipping rope, rowing, running, hiking or playing tennis, focus on increasing cardiovascular endurance."
- "Anaerobic Exercises"—"such as weight training, functional training, eccentric training or sprinting and high-intensity interval training, increase short-term muscle strength."

Besides types, physical exercise can also be classified in terms of categories (to be described in the next sub-section).

Categories of Physical Exercise

In general, "physical exercise is used to improve physical skills," which "fall into the following general categories" (as summarized in *Table 3.2*): (WK 2013a; CRO 2002)

- "Cardiovascular/respiratory endurance"
- "Stamina"
- "Power"
- "Strength"
- "Coordination"
- "Balance"
- "Agility"
- "Speed"
- "Flexibility"
- "Accuracy"

Other categories like "dynamic" and "static" are sometimes used, in that "'dynamic' exercises such as steady running, tend to produce a lowering of the diastolic blood pressure during exercise, due to the improved blood flow. Conversely, 'static' exercise (such as weight-lifting) can cause the systolic pressure to rise significantly (during the exercise)." (WK 2013a)

Health Effects of Physical Exercise

"Physical exercise" can produce good health effects, since it "is important for maintaining physical fitness and can contribute positively to maintaining a healthy weight, building and maintaining healthy bone density, muscle strength, and joint mobility, promoting physiological well-being, reducing surgical risks, and strengthening the immune system." (WK 2013a)

For illustration, consider five main health effects below (as summarized in *Table 3.2*).

(a) Cardiovascular System

The first health effect of physical exercise to be illustrated here concerns "cardiovascular system."

For instance, "there is a direct relation between physical inactivity and cardiovascular mortality, and physical inactivity is an independent risk factor for the development of coronary artery disease. There is a dose-response relation between the amount of exercise performed from approximately 700 to 2000 kcal of energy expenditure per week and all-cause mortality and cardiovascular disease mortality in middle-aged and elderly populations. The greatest potential for reduced mortality is in the sedentary who become moderately active. Most beneficial effects of physical activity on cardiovascular disease mortality can be attained through moderate-intensity activity (40% to 60% of maximal oxygen uptake, depending on age)," and "persons who modify their behavior after myocardial infarction to include regular exercise have improved rates of survival....Persons who remain sedentary have the highest risk for all-cause and cardiovascular disease mortality." (WK 2013a)

(b) Immune System

The second health effect of physical exercise to be illustrated here concerns "immune system."

For instance, "epidemiological evidence suggests that moderate exercise has a beneficial effect on the human immune system; an effect which is modeled in a J curve. Moderate exercise has been associated with a 29% decreased incidence of upper respiratory tract infections (URTI).... Biomarkers of inflammation such as C-reactive protein, which are associated with chronic diseases, are reduced in active individuals relative to sedentary individuals, and the positive effects of exercise may be due to its anti-inflammatory effects. The depression in the immune system following acute bouts of exercise may be one of the mechanisms for this anti-inflammatory effect." (WK 2013a; M. Gleeson 2007)

(c) Brain Function

The third health effect of physical exercise to be illustrated here concerns "brain function."

For instance, "a 2008 review of cognitive enrichment therapies (strategies to slow or reverse cognitive decline) concluded that 'physical activity, and aerobic exercise in particular, enhances older adults' cognitive function.'" (WK 2013a; C. Hertzog 2008)

Even "in mice, exercise improves cognitive functioning via improvement of hippocampus-dependent spatial learning, and enhancement of synaptic plasticity and neurogenesis. In addition, physical activity has been shown to be neuroprotective in many neurodegenerative and neuromuscular diseases. For instance, it reduces the risk of developing dementia. Furthermore, anecdotal evidence suggests that frequent exercise may reverse alcohol-induced brain damage." (WK 2013a; H. van Praag 1999; C. Grondard 2005)

In fact, "there are several possibilities for why exercise is beneficial for the brain. Examples are as follows": (WK 2013a; J. Hunsberger 2007; T. Parker-Pope 2001; H. van Praag 1999)

- "increasing the blood and oxygen flow to the brain"
- "increasing growth factors that help create new nerve cells and promote synaptic plasticity"
- "increasing chemicals in the brain that help cognition, such as dopamine, glutamate, norepinephrine, and serotonin"

And "physical activity is thought to have other beneficial effects related to cognition as it increases levels of nerve growth factors, which support the survival and growth of a number of neuronal cells." (WK 2013a; E. McAuley 2004)

(d) Depression

The fourth health effect of physical exercise to be illustrated here concerns "depression."

For instance, "a number of factors may contribute to depression including being overweight, low self-esteem, stress, and anxiety. Endorphins act as a natural pain reliever and antidepressant in the body. Endorphins have long been regarded as responsible for what is known as 'runner's high,' a euphoric feeling a person receives from intense physical exertion. However, recent research indicates that anandamide may possibly play a greater role than endorphins in 'runner's high.' When a person exercises, levels of both circulating serotonin and endorphins are increased. These levels are known to stay elevated even several days after exercise is discontinued, possibly contributing to improvement in mood, increased self-esteem, and weight management. Exercise alone is a potential prevention method and/or treatment for mild forms of depression. Research has also shown that when exercise is done in the presence of other people (familiar or not), it can be more effective in reducing stress than simply exercising alone." (WK 2013a; K. Johnsgard 2004; M. Thase 2007; A. Byrd 1999; T. Plante 2001; P. Sparling 2003; A. Burfoot 2004)

(e) Sleep

And the fifth health effect of physical exercise to be illustrated here concerns "sleep."

For instance, "a 2010 review of published scientific research suggested that exercise generally improves sleep for most people, and helps sleep disorders such as insomnia. The optimum time to exercise may be 4 to 8 hours before bedtime, though exercise at any time of day is beneficial, with the possible exception of heavy exercise taken shortly before bedtime, which may disturb sleep." (WK 2013a)

And "according to a 2005 study, exercise is the most recommended alternative to sleeping pills for resolving insomnia. Sleeping pills are more costly than to make time for a daily routine of staying fit, and may have dangerous side effects in the long run. Exercise can be a healthy, safe and inexpensive way to achieve more and better sleep." (WK 2013a; S. Youngstedt 2005)

Problems with Physical Exercise

However, for the critics, the argument on physical health, exercise, and effects has some major problems. Consider, for illustration, a few examples below (as summarized in *Table 3.2*).

Firstly, one main criticism of the argument on physical health, exercise, and effects is that vigorous exercise can have its downside.

For instance, for the critics, "some studies have shown that vigorous exercise...for long periods of time, or without proper warmup beforehand and cooldown afterwards, can lead to an increased risk of injury and overtraining." (WK 2013a; P. Sparling 2003; A. Burfoot 2004)

Secondly, another main criticism of the argument on physical health, exercise, and effects is that some individuals can be exercise-resistant.

For instance, for the critics, "not everyone benefits equally from exercise. There is tremendous variation in individual response to training; where most people will see a moderate increase in endurance from aerobic exercise, some individuals will as much as double their oxygen uptake, while others can never augment endurance." (WK 2013a; C. Bouchard 1999; G. Kolata 2002) In fact, "a number of studies of both rodents and humans have demonstrated that individual differences in both ability and propensity for exercise (i.e., voluntary exercise) have some genetic basis." (WK 2013a; T. Garland 2011)

Thirdly, still another main criticism of the argument on physical health, exercise, and effects is that the findings are inconsistent.

For instance, for the critic, on the relationship between physical exercise and "immune system"— "another study did not find the effect. Immune cell functions are impaired following acute sessions of prolonged, high-intensity exercise, and some studies have found that athletes are at a higher risk for infections....Athletes may have slightly elevated natural killer cell count and cytolytic action, but these are unlikely to be clinically significant." (WK 2013a; M. Gleeson 2007)

Fourthly, an additional main criticism of the argument on physical health, exercise, and effects is that there is often "insufficient evidence" for any firm conclusion.

For instance, for the critics, on the relationship between physical exercise and "sleep"—"there is, in any case, insufficient evidence to draw detailed conclusions about the relationship between exercise and sleep." (WK 2013a)

Fifthly, another additional main criticism of the argument on physical health, exercise, and effects is that there are alternative categories of physical exercise.

For instance, for the critics, there are other ways to classify physical exercise, and an alternative list of categories include "eccentric training," "interval training," "continuous training," etc. (WK 2013a)

And sixthly, still another additional main criticism of the argument on physical health, exercise, and effects is that some effects of physical exercise remain unknown.

For instance, for the critics, "as of 2011 the effects of community wide interventions to increase exercise levels at the population level is unknown." (WK 2013a; P. Baker 2011)

Beyond Physical Exercise

These criticisms of physical exercise, however, should not be misunderstood as a total rejection of its validity but serve to show us the two opposing sides of the debate, such that the possibility (or impossibility) and desirability (or undesirability) of physical health (from the perspective of the mind with physical health, exercise, and effects as a case study here) are not to the extent that the respective defenders would like us to believe.

Moreover, the analysis of physical health, exercise, and effects is to shed some light on the ontological principles in existential dialectics, and good examples include the formalness-informalness principle, the absoluteness-relativeness principle, the partiality-totality principle, the predictability-unpredictability principle, the explicability-inexplicability principle, the fiction-reality principle, the cognitiveness-noncognitiveness principle, the finiteness-transfiniteness principle, the preciseness-vagueness principle, the simpleness-complicatedness principle, the openness-hiddenness principle, the denseness-emptiness principle, the prototypicality-variation principle, the change-constancy principle, the order-chaos principle, the slowness-quickness principle, the expansion-contraction principle, the optimality-nonoptimality principle, the theory-praxis principle, the convention-novelty principle, the evolution-transformation principle, the symmetry-asymmetry principle, the softness-hardness principle, the seriousness-playfulness principle, the activeness-inactivess principle, the selfness-otherness principle, the regression-progression principle, the same-difference principle, the stability-reaction principle, the functionality-nonfunctionality principle, and the intentionality-nonintentionality principle.

For instance, in relation to the formalness-informalness principle, if there is formalness (e.g., the formal logical requirement of soundness, completeness, and consistency in a system of ideas, as in the argument on physical health, exercise, and effects), there is informalness (e.g., the non-formal existence of unsoundness, incompleteness, and inconsistency in the argument on physical health, exercise, and effects, as shown in the criticisms that vigorous exercise can have its downside, that some individuals can be exercise-resistant, that the findings are inconsistent, that there is often "insufficient evidence" for any firm conclusion, that there are alternative categories of physical exercise, and that some effects of physical exercise remain unknown). And the reverse direction also holds true.

In relation to the absoluteness-relativeness principle, if there is absoluteness (e.g., the absolute view on physical exercise and health effects by the advocates), there is relativeness (e.g., what is right for the advocates in regard to physical exercise and health effects is not necessarily so for the critics, who pointed out the different problems aforedescribed). And the reverse direction also holds true.

In relation to the partiality-totality principle, if there is partiality (e.g., the partial view on physical exercise and health effects by the advocates), there is totality (e.g., the more holistic view on physical exercise and health effects, such that the whole is not the sum of its parts, that is, it cannot be reduced to the sum of opposing views by the advocates, the critics, and so on, since there will emerge new views in the future not yet known today, just as there are already alternative views nowadays which do not side exclusively with any of them, as is the analysis here). And the reverse direction also holds true.

In relation to the predictability-unpredictability principle, if there is predictability (e.g., the predictable tendency of the relationship between physical exercise and improved "immune system," as pointed out by the advocates aforecited), there is unpredictability (e.g., the more difficult task to predict exactly the extent to which physical exercise will improve "immune system" on a particular future occasion, since, for the critics, "another study did not find the effect," in that "immune cell functions are impaired following acute sessions of prolonged, high-intensity exercise, and some studies have found that athletes are at a higher risk for infections....Athletes may have slightly elevated natural killer cell count and cytolytic action, but these are unlikely to be clinically significant"). And the reverse direction also holds true.

In relation to the explicability-inexplicability principle, if there is explicability (e.g., the explanation, by the advocates, of the desirability of physical exercise on the basis of its positive effects on physical health), there is inexplicability (e.g., the lack of sufficient explanation, by the advocates, of why physical exercise is necessarily desirable, since, for the critics, vigorous exercise can have its downside, besides other problems aforecited). And the reverse direction also holds true.

In relation to the fiction-reality principle, if there is fiction (e.g., the fictional aspect of physical exercise on health, insofar as vigorous exercise can have its downside, some individuals can be exercise-resistant, etc.), there is reality (e.g., the realistic aspect of physical exercise on health, insofar as "epidemiological evidence suggests that moderate exercise has a beneficial effect on the human immune system"). And the reverse direction also holds true.

In relation to the cognitiveness-noncognitiveness principle, if there is cognitiveness (e.g., a view of things on the basis of reason and evidences, as shown in the research finding that "when a person exercises, levels of both circulating serotonin and endorphins are increased"), there is noncognitiveness (e.g., a view of things on the basis of non-cognitive factors like envy, jealousy, power, nationality, race, gender, age, class, greed, lust, status, faith, anger, sadness, joy, fear, wish, etc., as shown in the "euphoric feeling" when someone "exercises" and his "levels of both circulating serotonin and endorphins are increased," but his improvement in mood, that is, the "euphoric feeling," does not automatically reflect an improvement of his social conditions). (WK 2013a) And the reverse direction also holds true.

In relation to the finiteness-transfiniteness principle, if there is finiteness (e.g., the finite number of the categories of cells in immune systems, like "natural killer cells," "cytotoxic T cells," etc.), there is transfiniteness (e.g., the transfinite number of all the individual cells in immune systems that have ever existed in history, be they "natural killer cells," "cytotoxic T cells," etc.). (WK 2013a & 2013dd) And the reverse direction also holds true.

In relation to the preciseness-vagueness principle, if there is preciseness (e.g., the precise identification of 5 main health effects of physical exercise in the article aforecited), there is vagueness (e.g., the vagueness in the identification of the 5 main health effects of physical exercise in the article aforecited, since it is not clear why there must be only 5, not 6, 10, 13, 17, and so on). And the reverse direction also holds true.

In relation to the simpleness-complicatedness principle, if there is simpleness (e.g., the relatively simple analysis of the health effects of physical exercise by the advocates), there is complicatedness (e.g., the relatively more complicated analysis of the health effects of physical exercise, by challenging the claims and assumptions, as shown in the problems pointed out by the critics as cited). And the reverse direction also holds true.

In relation to the openness-hiddenness principle, if there is openness (e.g., the open exploration of the health effects of physical exercise by the advocates), there is hiddenness (e.g., the hidden bias in the claim on the health effects of physical exercise by the advocates, since, for the critics, vigorous exercise can have its downside, some individuals can be exercise-resistant, the findings are inconsistent, there is often "insufficient evidence" for any firm conclusion, some effects of physical exercise remain unknown, etc.). And the reverse direction also holds true.

In relation to the denseness-emptiness principle, if there is denseness (e.g., the relatively denser concentration of concerns with flexibility, aerobics, and anaerobics by the advocates of physical exercise), there is emptiness (e.g., the relatively less dense, or more empty, concentration of concerns with mental exercise by the advocates of physical exercise). And the reverse direction also holds true.

In relation to the prototypicality-variation principle, if there is prototypicality (e.g., the prototype, like the example about the original work on the link "between physical health and exercise…in 1953 by a team led by Jerry Morris"), there is variation (e.g., different variants of the protoptye, as shown in many studies since the original work on the link "between physical health and exercise…in 1953 by a team led by Jerry Morris," like other subsequent studies aforecited, though each with its own variation, contribution, and disagreement). And the reverse direction also holds true.

In relation to the change-constancy principle, if there is change (e.g., the ever new ways to study exercise, as shown in the work on the link "between physical health and exercise"), there is constancy (e.g., the ever constant existence of different problems with the ever new ways to study exercise, as shown in the problems with the work on the link "between physical health and exercise" pointed out by the critics). And the reverse direction also holds true.

In relation to the order-chaos principle, if there is order (e.g., the more or less orderly view on physical exercise, if looked from the sole vantage point of the advocates on the link "between physical health and exercise"), there is chaos (e.g., the more or less chaotic view on physical exercise, if looked from the multiple, conflicting vantage points of both the different advocates and the critics aforecited). And the reverse direction also holds true.

In relation to the slowness-quickness principle, if there is slowness (e.g., the relatively slower speed to sleep by someone, if he has "heavy exercise…shortly before bedtime, which may disturb sleep"), there is quickness (e.g., the relatively quicker speed to sleep by someone, if he exercises "4 to 8 hours before bedtime"). And the reverse direction also holds true.

In relation to the expansion-contraction principle, if there is expansion (e.g., the relatively more developed ability of a bus conductor to lead a physically active workstyle), there is contraction (e.g., the relatively less developed ability of a bus conductor to lead a sedentary workstyle). And the reverse direction also holds true.

In relation to the optimality-nonoptimality principle, if there is optimality (e.g., the search for highly favorable options, like the quest for "the optimum time to exercise," by those who studied physical exercise, as they claimed that it "may be 4 to 8 hours before bedtime, though exercise at any time of day is beneficial"), there is nonoptimality (e.g., the existence of non-optimal alternatives to optimality, like the argument for more realistic studies by the critics, who pointed out the different problems with physical exercise aforedescribed). And the reverse direction also holds true.

In relation to the theory-praxis principle, if there is theory (e.g., the theoretical construction of "synaptic plasticity" in neurobiology), there is praxis (e.g., the practical application of "synaptic plasticity" in neurobiology to the field of physical exercise, in that exercise increases "growth factors that help create new nerve cells and promote synaptic plasticity"). And the reverse direction also holds true.

In relation to the convention-novelty principle, if there is convention (e.g., the conventional wisdom about the link "between physical health and exercise"), there is novelty (e.g., the alternative novel challenge to the conventional wisdom about the link "between physical health and exercise," by the new idea that vigorous exercise can have its downside, or that some individuals can be exercise-resistant). And the reverse direction also holds true.

In relation to the evolution-transformation principle, if there is evolution (e.g., the natural evolution of humans to walk, run, jump, etc. in the state of nature), there is transformation (e.g., the technical transformation of human ability to walk, run, jump, etc. by the invention of physical exercise for the systematic study of its types, categories, effects, etc.). And the reverse direction also holds true.

In relation to the symmetry-asymmetry principle, if there is symmetry (e.g., the co-existence of different individuals in society who try to exercise), there is asymmetry (e.g., some individuals like athletes are good in physical exercise—but some other individuals are "exercise-resistant" and "can never augment endurance" in exercise). And the reverse direction also holds true.

In relation to the softness-hardness principle, if there is softness (e.g., the defense of physical exercise by the advocates), there is hardness (e.g., the critique of physical exercise by the critics as cited). And the reverse direction also holds true.

In relation to the seriousness-playfulness principle, if there is seriousness (e.g., the serious business of those who try to understand the nature of exercise), there is playfulness (e.g., the playful part of those who try to understand the nature of exercise, when they play around with different types and categories aforeindicated over the decades). And the reverse direction also holds true.

In relation to the activeness-inactivess principle, if there is activeness (e.g., the relative activeness of those who do a lot of different exercises), there is inactiveness (e.g., the relative inactiveness of those who are "exercise-resistant" and cannot engage in much of any exercise at all).

In relation to the selfness-otherness principle, if there is selfness (e.g., the tendency to be mostly centered on one's self or group, as shown in those who are obsessed with physical exercise to improve health, such that they engage in "too much exercise," which "can be harmful," because "without proper rest, the chance of stroke or other circulation problems increases," for example), there is otherness (e.g., the tendency to be mostly centered on others, as shown in those researchers who warn others from engaging in "excessive exercise" which has its own downside, as an advancement in the knowledge of physical health). And the reverse direction also holds true.

In relation to the regression-progression principle, if there is regression (e.g., the regression made by physical exercise, as shown in the problems pointed out by the critics), there is progression (e.g., the progress made by physical exercise, as shown in the contribution to health aforecited). And the reverse direction also holds true.

In relation to the same-difference principle, if there is similarity in outcome (e.g., the contribution to the molding and control of beliefs, values, and behaviors, regardless of whether this be done by way of bus driving, or by way of bus conducting), there is difference in outcome (e.g., the contribution to the molding and control of beliefs, values, and behaviors by way of bus driving for a relatively more sedentary work life—but the contribution to the molding and control of beliefs, values, and behaviors by way of bus conducting for a relatively more active work life). And the reverse direction also holds true.

In relation to the stability-reaction principle, if there is stability (e.g., the relatively more stable condition of the belief about the link between physical health and exercise in the older days), there is reaction (e.g., the belief about the link between physical health and exercise in the older days then led to further changes later on, when nowadays "a number of studies of both rodents and humans have demonstrated that individual differences in both ability and propensity for exercise [i.e., voluntary exercise] have some genetic basis," and vigorous exercise can have its downside). And the reverse direction also holds true.

In relation to the functionality-nonfunctionality principle, if there is functionality (e.g., the presence of action for which something or someone is fitted, as shown in the link between physical health and exercise, which serves the function of "increasing the blood and oxygen flow to the brain," "increasing growth factors that help create new nerve cells," etc.), there is nonfunctionality (e.g., the relative lack of action for which something or someone is fitted, as shown in the critique of physical exercise, in that it can become non-functional too, since "a number of studies of both rodents and humans have demonstrated that individual differences in both ability and propensity for exercise [i.e., voluntary exercise] have some genetic basis," such that some individuals are in fact exercise-resistant). And the reverse direction also holds true.

In relation to the intentionality-nonintentionality principle, if there is intentionality (e.g., the planning or design of something for a certain outcome, as shown in the original intention in 1953 of a team led by Jerry Morris, who showed "the link between physical health and exercise," so as to encourage people to exercise more for health benefits), there is nonintentionality (e.g., the relative absence of planning or design of something for a certain outcome, such that the outcome can even be counter-intentional in being the opposite of what was originally planned, as shown in more recent findings that vigorous exercise can have its downside, that some individuals can be exercise-resistant, that the findings are inconsistent, that there is often "insufficient evidence" for any firm conclusion, and that some effects of physical exercise remain unknown—contrary to the original intention of Jerry Morris and his team, who encouraged people to exercise more for health benefits). And the reverse direction also holds true.

And in relation to the survivability-nonsurvivability principle, if there is survivability (e.g., the relative survival, nowadays, of the belief in the link between physical health and exercise), there is non-survivability (e.g., the relative non-survival, nowadays, of "physically demanding work" which requries a lot of people to be physically active, since "worldwide there has been a large shift towards less physically demanding work" in our time). (WK 2013a; WHO 2008a) And the reverse direction also holds true.

Physical Health, Abuse, and Children

Another way to evaluate the possibility (or impossibility) and desirability (or undesirability) of physical health from the perspective of the mind is to explore physical health, abuse, and children.

An argument in the literature is that "child abuse can occur in a child's home, or in the organizations, schools or communities the child interacts with" and can be prevented and treated. (WK 2013ee)

Types of Child Abuse

The term "child abuse" refers to "the physical, sexual or emotional mistreatment or neglect of a child or children. In the United States, the Centers for Disease Control and Prevention (CDC) and the Department for Children And Families (DCF) define child maltreatment as any act or series of acts of commission or omission by a parent or other caregiver that results in harm, potential for harm, or threat of harm to a child. Child abuse can occur in a child's home, or in the organizations, schools or communities the child interacts with." (WK 2013ee; R. Leeb 2008)

In general, child abuse can take four major forms, as described below (and summarized in *Table 3.3*).

(a) Physical Abuse

The first form of child abuse to be described here concerns "physical abuse."

By definition, "physical abuse involves physical aggression directed at a child by an adult. Most nations with child-abuse laws consider the deliberate infliction of serious injuries, or actions that place the child at obvious risk of serious injury or death, to be illegal. Physical abuse is the intentional or non-accidental production of a physical injury. Bruises, scratches, burns, broken bones, lacerations, as well as repeated 'mishaps,' and rough treatment that could cause physical injury, are the results of physical abuse." (WK 2013ee; D. Theoklitou 2011)

Some professionals claim that cultural norms that sanction physical punishment are one of the causes of child abuse, and have undertaken campaigns to redefine such norms." (WK 2013ee; R. Barth 1994; J. Durrant 1996)

(b) Sexual Abuse

The second form of child abuse to be described here concerns "sexual abuse."

By definition, "child sexual abuse (CSA) is a form of child abuse in which an adult or older adolescent abuses a child for sexual stimulation. Sexual abuse refers to the participation of a child in a sexual act aimed toward the physical gratification or the financial profit of the person committing the act. Forms of CSA include asking or pressuring a child to engage in sexual activities (regardless of the outcome), indecent exposure of the genitals to a child, displaying pornography to a child, actual sexual contact with a child, physical contact with the child's genitals, viewing of the child's genitalia without physical contact, or using a child to produce child pornography. Selling the sexual services of children may be viewed and treated as child abuse with services offered to the child rather than simple incarceration." (WK 2013ee; D. Theoklitou 2011; J. Martin 1993; P. Brown 2011)

Child sexual abuse can provide negative effects like "guilt and self-blame, flashbacks, nightmares, insomnia, fear of things associated with the abuse (including objects, smells, places, doctor's visits, etc.), self-esteem issues, sexual dysfunction, chronic pain, addiction, self-injury, suicidal ideation, somatic complaints, depression, post-traumatic stress disorder, anxiety, other mental illnesses including borderline personality disorder and dissociative identity disorder, propensity to re-victimization in adulthood, bulimia nervosa, physical injury to the child, among other problems." (WK 2013ee; M. Roosa 1999; C. Widom 1999; R. Levitan 2003; T. Messman-Moore 2000; S. Dinwiddie 2000)

(c) Psychological/Emotional Abuse

The third form of child abuse to be described here concerns "psychological/emotional abuse."

By definition, "emotional abuse" refers to "the production of psychological and social deficits in the growth of a child as a result of behavior such as loud yelling, coarse and rude attitude, inattention, harsh criticism, and denigration of the child's personality. Other examples include name-calling, ridicule, degradation, destruction of personal belongings, torture or killing of a pet, excessive criticism, inappropriate or excessive demands, withholding communication, and routine labeling or humiliation." (WK 2013ee; D. Theoklitou 2011)

In response, "victims of emotional abuse may react by distancing themselves from the abuser, internalizing the abusive words, or fighting back by insulting the abuser. Emotional abuse can result in abnormal or disrupted attachment development, a tendency for victims to blame themselves (self-blame) for the abuse, learned helplessness, and overly passive behavior." (WK 2013ee; D. Theoklitou 2011)

(d) Neglect

And the fourth form of child abuse to be described here concerns "neglect."

By definition, "child neglect is the failure of a parent or other person with responsibility for the child to provide needed food, clothing, shelter, medical care, or supervision to the degree that the child's health, safety, and well-being are threatened with harm. Neglect is also a lack of attention from the people surrounding a child, and the non-provision of the relevant and adequate necessities for the child's survival, which would be a lacking in attention, love, and nurture. Some of the observable signs in a neglected child include: the child is frequently absent from school, begs or steals food or money, lacks needed medical and dental care, is consistently dirty, lacks sufficient clothing for the weather." (WK 2013ee; D. Theoklitou 2011)

As a consequence, "neglected children may experience delays in physical and psychosocial development, possibly resulting in psychopathology and impaired neuropsychological functions including executive function, attention, processing speed, language, memory and social skills. Researchers investigating maltreated children have repeatedly found that neglected children in foster and adoptive populations manifest different emotional and behavioral reactions to regain lost or secure relationships and are frequently reported to have disorganized attachments and a need to control their environment. Such children are not likely to view caregivers as being a source of safety, and instead typically show an increase in aggressive and hyperactive behaviors which may disrupt healthy or secure attachment with their adopted parents. These children have apparently learned to adapt to an abusive and inconsistent caregiver by becoming cautiously self-reliant, and are often described as glib, manipulative and disingenuous in their interactions with others as they move through childhood. Children who are victims of neglect have a more difficult time forming and maintaining relationships, such as romantic or friendship, later in life due to the lack of attachment they had in their earlier stages of life." (WK 2013ee; J. Golden 2009)

Prevalence of Child Abuse

In an estimate by the (American) National Committee to Prevent Child Abuse, "in 1997 neglect represented 54% of confirmed cases of child abuse, physical abuse 22%, sexual abuse 8%, emotional maltreatment 4%, and other forms of maltreatment 12%." (WK 2013ee; NCPCA 1998)

In a UNICEF report on child wellbeing in the United States and the United Kingdom, "child neglect and child abuse were far more common in single-parent families than in families where both parents are present." (WK 2013ee)

In another study, this time by the U.S. Department of Health and Human Services, "for each year between 2000 and 2005, 'female parents acting alone' were most likely to be perpetrators of child abuse." (WK 2013ee)

In 2011, "United States reported 676,569 victims of child abuse and neglect. Race and ethnicity of victims in 2011: 43.9% of all victims were White, 21.5% were African American, and 22.1% were Hispanic." (WK 2013ee; USDHHS 2011)

And "according to Manas Akmatov [2011], 'a median of 83, 64 and 43% of children in the African region experienced psychological, and moderate and severe physical abuse, respectively. A considerably lower percentage of children in transitional countries experienced these forms of abuse (56, 46 and 9%, respectively).'" (WK 2013ee)

Causes of Child Abuse

Child abuse have different causes, and hereafter are a few of them for illustration (as summarized in *Table 3.3*):

- "Parents who physically abuse their spouses are more likely than others to physically abuse their children." (WK 2013ee; S. Ross 1996)
- "Children resulting from unintended pregnancies are more likely to be abused or neglected....In addition, unintended pregnancies are more likely than intended pregnancies to be associated with abusive relationships, and there is an increased risk of physical violence during pregnancy. They also result in poorer maternal mental health,

and lower mother-child relationship quality." (WK 2013ee; L. Bethea 1999; L. Eisenberg 1995; J. Hathaway 2000: HEAL 2011)

- "A study on child abuse sought to determine: the forms of child abuse perpetrated on children with disabilities; the extent of child abuse; and the causes of child abuse of children with disabilities...in Botswana. The study found that the majority of participants were involved in doing domestic chores. They were also sexually, physically and emotionally abused by their teachers. This study showed that children with disabilities were vulnerable to child abuse in their schools." (WK 2013ee; A. Shumba 2011)
- "Substance abuse can be a major contributing factor to child abuse. One U.S. study found that parents with documented substance abuse, most commonly alcohol, cocaine, and heroin, were much more likely to mistreat their children, and were also much more likely to reject court-ordered services and treatments." (WK 2013ee; J. Murphy 1991)
- "A 2010 article in the BBC reports that thousands of African children have been abandoned, tortured and murdered because they are believed to be witches." (WK 2013ee; BBC 2010)
- "Unemployment and financial difficulties are associated with increased rates of child abuse. In 2009 CBS News reported that child abuse in the United States had increased during the economic recession." (WK 2013ee)
- "A 1988 study of child murders in the US found that children are 100 times more often killed by a 'non-biological parent (e.g. step-parent, co-habitee or boyfriend/girlfriend of a biological parent)' than by a biological parent. An evolutionary psychology explanation for this is that using resources in order to take care of another person's biological child is likely not a good strategy for increasing reproductive success. More generally, stepchildren have a much higher risk of being abused which is sometimes referred to as the Cinderella effect. The Cinderella Effect is often regarded as one of the great successes of Evo Psych research. It attempts to explain the observation that parents are more likely to kill their stepchildren than their biological children using evolutionary logic—as described by Daly and Wilson: 'research concerning animal social behaviour provide a rationale for expecting parents to be discriminative in their care and affection, and more specifically, to discriminate in favour of their own young.'" (WK 2013ee; M. Samsa 2010)

- "Psychologists conducted a study in the United States in 2010 which examined over 200 regular church attendees from eleven different denominations of Christianity, most of whom were educated, upper-middle class White Americans, found that extrinsic religious orientation was associated with a greater risk of physical child abuse. Those with a more extrinsic religious orientation who also adhered to greater social conformity were particularly more likely to share characteristics with physically abusive subjects. Subjects who adhered to Biblical literalism exhibited a higher potential of physical child abuse. Those who had a more intrinsic religious orientation were not found to be at a greater risk of child abuse, although they sometimes exhibited greater social conformity or a greater propensity for holding literal interpretations of the Bible. Approximately 85% of the study's subjects were parents." WK 2013ee; C. Rodriguez 2010)

Surely, there can be other studies, so the ones above are illustrative.

Effects of Child Abuse

Child abuse can have serious effects, and hereafter are two main examples (as summarized in *Table 3.3*).

(a) Psychological Effects

Psychologically, "children who have a history of neglect or physical abuse are at risk of developing psychiatric problems, or a disorganized attachment style. Disorganized attachment is associated with a number of developmental problems, including dissociative symptoms, as well as anxiety, depressive, and acting out symptoms. A study by Dante Cicchetti found that 80% of abused and maltreated infants exhibited symptoms of disorganized attachment. When some of these children become parents, especially if they suffer from posttraumatic stress disorder (PTSD), dissociative symptoms, and other sequelae of child abuse, they may encounter difficulty when faced with their infant and young children's needs and normative distress, which may in turn lead to adverse consequences for their child's social-emotional development." (WK 2013ee; L. Gauthier 1996; R. Malinosky-Rummell 1993; K. Lyons-Ruth 1999; M. Main 1990; D. Schechter 2008)

In addition, "victims of childhood abuse…suffer from different types of physical health problems later in life. Some reportedly suffer from some type of chronic head, abdominal, pelvic, or muscular pain with no identifiable reason. Even though the majority of childhood abuse victims know or believe that their abuse is, or can be, the cause of different health problems in their adult life, for the great majority their abuse was not directly associated with those problems, indicating that sufferers were most likely diagnosed with other possible causes for their health problems, instead of their childhood abuse. One long-term study found that up to 80% of abused people had at least one psychiatric disorder at age 21, with problems including depression, anxiety, eating disorders, and suicide attempts. One Canadian hospital found that between 36% and 76% of women mental health outpatients had been abused, as had 58% of women and 23% of men schizophrenic inpatients." (WK 2013ee)

(b) Physical Effects

Physically, "children who are...abused are likely to receive bone fractures, particularly rib fractures, and may have a higher risk of developing cancer. Children who experience child abuse and neglect are 59% more likely to be arrested as juveniles, 28% more likely to be arrested as adults, and 30% more likely to commit violent crime." (WK 2013ee; A. Kemp 2008; E. Fuller-Thomson 2009)

Of course, "the immediate physical effects of abuse or neglect can be relatively minor (bruises or cuts) or severe (broken bones, hemorrhage, or even death). In some cases the physical effects are temporary; however, the pain and suffering they cause a child should not be discounted." (WK 2013ee)

Some possible long-term effects of child abuse are shown below: (WK 2013ee)

- "Shaken Baby Syndrome"—"Shaking a baby is a common form of child abuse that often results in permanent neurological damage (80% of cases) or death (30% of cases). Damage results from intracranial hypertension (increased pressure in the skull) after bleeding in the brain, damage to the spinal cord and neck, and rib or bone fractures." (WK 2013ee; Y. Morad 2010)
- "Impaired Brain Development"—"Child abuse and neglect have been shown, in some cases, to cause important regions of the brain to fail to form or grow properly, resulting in impaired development....These alterations in brain maturation have long-term consequences for cognitive, language, and academic abilities....NSCAW found more than three-quarters of foster children between 1 and 2 years of age to be at medium to high risk for problems with brain development, as opposed to less than half of children in a control sample." (WK 2013ee)

- "Poor Physical Health"—"Several studies have shown a relationship between various forms of household dysfunction (including childhood abuse) and poor health. Adults who experienced abuse or neglect during childhood are more likely to suffer from physical ailments such as allergies, arthritis, asthma, bronchitis, high blood pressure, and ulcers." (WK 2013ee)

Again, there can be other effects, so the examples above are illustrative.

Prevention/Treatment of Child Abuse

For many health-care providers, child abuse can be prevented.

For instance, "a support-group structure is needed to reinforce parenting skills and closely monitor the child's well-being. Visiting home nurse or social-worker visits are also required to observe and evaluate the progress of the child and his/her caretaking situation. The support-group structure and visiting home nurse or social-worker visits are not mutually exclusive. Many studies have demonstrated that the two measures must be coupled together for the best possible outcome." (WK 2013ee; MEDI 2012)

And "children's school programs regarding 'good touch...bad touch' can provide children with a forum in which to role-play and learn to avoid potentially harmful scenarios. Unintended conception increases the risk of subsequent child abuse, and large family size increases the risk of child neglect. Thus a comprehensive study for the National Academy of Sciences concluded that affordable contraceptive services should form the basis for child abuse prevention. 'The starting point for effective child abuse programming is pregnancy planning,' according to an analysis for US Surgeon General C. Everett Koop." (WK 2013ee; L. Eisenberg 1995; T. Cron 1986)

Child abuse can also be treated, and good examples include "group therapy, play therapy, and art therapy. Each of these types of treatment can be used to better assist the client, depending on the form of abuse they have experienced. Play therapy and art therapy are ways to get children more comfortable with therapy by working on something that they enjoy (coloring, drawing, painting, etc.). The design of a child's artwork can be a symbolic representation of what they are feeling, relationships with friends or family, and more. Being able to discuss and analyze a child's artwork can allow a professional to get a better insight of the child." (WK 2013ee)

Problems with the Study of Child Abuse

However, for the critics, this study of child abuse has some major problems. Consider, for illustration, a few examples below (as summarized in *Table 3.3*).

Firstly, one main criticism of the study of child abuse is that scholars disagree over what constitutes child abuse.

For example, for the critcs, "the distinction between child discipline and abuse is often poorly defined," and "among professionals as well as the wider public, people do not agree on what behaviors constitute abuse." (WK 2013ee; H. Noh Anh 1994)

Secondly, another main criticism of the study of child abuse is that the alleged causes of child abuse can be questionable.

For instance, for the critics, "it is impossible to know whether marital strife is a cause of child abuse, or if both the marital strife and the abuse are caused by tendencies in the abuser." (WK 2013ee; S. Ross 1996)

Thirdly, still another main criticism of the study of child abuse is that the long-term effects of child abuse remains unknown.

For instance, as the critics were quick to point out, "the long-term impact of child abuse and neglect on physical health is just beginning to be explored" and remains inconclusive. (WK 2013ee)

Fourthly, an additional main criticism of the study of child abuse is that the alleged causes do not determine the often cited consequences.

For instance, for the critics, "there are some children who are raised in child abuse, but who manage to do unexpectedly well later in life regarding the preconditions. Such children have been termed dandelion children, as inspired from the way that dandelions seem to prosper irrespective of soil, sun, drought, or rain. Such children (or currently grown-ups) are of high interest in finding factors that mitigate the effects of child abuse." (WK 2013ee; B. Ellis 2008)

Fifthly, another additional main criticism of the study of child abuse is that the prevention of child abuse can be limited.

For instance, for the critics, "resources for child-protection services are...limited. According to Hosin (2007), 'a considerable number of traumatized abused children do not gain access to protective child-protection strategies.' Briere (1992) argues that only when 'lower-level violence' of children ceases to be culturally tolerated will there be changes in the victimization and police protection of children." (WK 2013ee)

And sixthly, still another additional main criticism of the study of child abuse is that there is cultural bias in the studies.

For instance, for the critics, "Asian parenting perspectives, specifically, hold different ideals from American culture....Balancing disciplinary responsibilities within parenting is common in many Asian cultures, including China, Japan, Singapore, Vietnam and Korea. To some cultures, forceful parenting may be seen as abuse, but in other societies such as these, the use of force is looked at as a reflection of parental devotion." (WK 2013ee; A. Lau 2006)

Beyond Child Abuse

These criticisms of child abuse, however, do not imply a total rejection of its usefulness but serve to show us the two opposing sides of the debate, such that the possibility (or impossibility) and desirability (or undesirability) of physical health (from the perspective of the mind with physical health, abuse, and children as a case study here) are not to the extent that the respective defenders would like us to believe.

In addition, the analysis of physical health, abuse, and children can teach us something valuable about the ontological principles in existential dialectics, and good examples include the formalness-informalness principle, the absoluteness-relativeness principle, the partiality-totality principle, the predictability-unpredictability principle, the explicability-inexplicability principle, the fiction-reality principle, the cognitiveness-noncognitiveness principle, the finiteness-transfiniteness principle, the preciseness-vagueness principle, the simpleness-complicatedness principle, the openness-hiddenness principle, the denseness-emptiness principle, the prototypicality-variation principle, the change-constancy principle, the order-chaos principle, the slowness-quickness principle, the expansion-contraction principle, the optimality-nonoptimality principle, the theory-praxis principle, the convention-novelty principle, the evolution-transformation principle, the symmetry-asymmetry principle, the softness-hardness principle, the seriousness-playfulness principle, the activeness-inactivess principle, the selfness-otherness principle, the regression-progression principle, the same-difference principle, the stability-reaction principle, the functionality-nonfunctionality principle, and the intentionality-nonintentionality principle.

For instance, in relation to the formalness-informalness principle, if there is formalness (e.g., the formal logical requirement of soundness, completeness, and consistency in a system of ideas, as in the argument on child abuse), there is informalness (e.g., the non-formal existence of unsoundness, incompleteness, and inconsistency in the argument on child abuse, as shown in the criticisms that scholars disagree over what constitutes child abuse, that the alleged causes of child abuse can be questionable, that the long-term effects of child abuse remains unknown, and that the alleged causes do not determine the often cited consequences, that the prevention of child abuse can be limited, and that there is cultural bias in the studies). And the reverse direction also holds true.

In relation to the absoluteness-relativeness principle, if there is absoluteness (e.g., the absolute view on child abuse by the abusers), there is relativeness (e.g., what is right for the abusers in regard to child abuse is not necessarily so for the child victims, with subsequent health problems aforecited). And the reverse direction also holds true.

In relation to the partiality-totality principle, if there is partiality (e.g., the partial view on child abuse by the abusers), there is totality (e.g., the more holistic view on child abuse, such that the whole is not the sum of its parts, that is, it cannot be reduced to the sum of opposing views by the child abusers, the child victims, the child abuse researchers, etc., since there will emerge new views in the future not yet known today, just as there are already alternative views nowadays which do not side exclusively with any of them, as is the analysis here). And the reverse direction also holds true.

In relation to the predictability-unpredictability principle, if there is predictability (e.g., the predictable tendency of child abuse to have certain causes in accordance to the studies aforecited), there is unpredictability (e.g., the more difficult task to predict exactly the extent to which that the causal relationship in regard to child abuse will hold on a particular future occasion, since, for the critics, the alleged causes of child abuse can be questionable, the long-term effects of child abuse remains unknown, and the alleged causes do not determine the often cited consequences). And the reverse direction also holds true.

In relation to the explicability-inexplicability principle, if there is explicability (e.g., the explanation, by a child abuser, of the desirability of child abuse on the basis of "sexual stimulation" and so on), there is inexplicability (e.g., the lack of sufficient explanation, by a child abuser, of why child abuse is necessarily desirable, since, for the victims, there are negative health effects aforedescribed). And the reverse direction also holds true.

In relation to the fiction-reality principle, if there is fiction (e.g., the fictional aspect of the studies on child abuse, insofar as scholars disagree over what constitutes child abuse, the alleged causes of child abuse can be questionable, and the alleged causes do not determine the often cited consequences), there is reality (e.g., the realistic aspect of the studies on child abuse, insofar as, in an estimate by the [American] National Committee to Prevent Child Abuse, "in 1997 neglect represented 54% of confirmed cases of child abuse, physical abuse 22%, sexual abuse 8%, emotional maltreatment 4%, and other forms of maltreatment 12%"). And the reverse direction also holds true.

In relation to the cognitiveness-noncognitiveness principle, if there is cognitiveness (e.g., a view of things on the basis of reason and evidences, as shown in the existence of a debate in the U.S. during the 2000s on "the parental rights of abusive parents or caretakers with regard to their children, particularly in medical settings"), there is noncognitiveness (e.g., a view of things on the basis of non-cognitive factors like envy, jealousy, power, nationality, race, gender, age, class, greed, lust, status, faith, anger, sadness, joy, fear, wish, etc., as shown in the politics of "parental rights" advocated by "abusive parents or caretakers with regard to their children, particularly in medical settings"). (WK 2013ee) And the reverse direction also holds true.

In relation to the finiteness-transfiniteness principle, if there is finiteness (e.g., the finite number of the categories of child abuse effects, like "physical effects" and "psychological effects" in the article aforecited), there is transfiniteness (e.g., the transfinite number of all the individuals, young or old, who have ever existed in history and have been abused, in one way or the other, regardless of whether the incident of an abuse is minor or serious). And the reverse direction also holds true.

In relation to the preciseness-vagueness principle, if there is preciseness (e.g., the precise identification of 2 child abuse effects, that is, "physical effects" and "psychological effects," in the article aforecited), there is vagueness (e.g., the vagueness in the identification of the 2 child abuse effects in the article aforecited, since it is not clear why there must be only 2, not 3, 4, 5, 6, and so on). And the reverse direction also holds true.

In relation to the simpleness-complicatedness principle, if there is simpleness (e.g., the relatively simple analysis of the nature of child abuse by the advocates of child protection), there is complicatedness (e.g., the relatively more complicated analysis of the nature of child abuse, by challenging the claims and assumptions, as shown in the problems pointed out by the critics as cited). And the reverse direction also holds true.

In relation to the openness-hiddenness principle, if there is openness (e.g., the open exploration of the types, causes, and effects of child abuse in the studies aforecited), there is hiddenness (e.g., the hidden bias in the studies on child abuse, since the critics pointed out that scholars disagree over what constitutes child abuse, that the alleged causes of child abuse can be questionable, that the long-term effects of child abuse remains unknown, and that the alleged causes do not determine the often cited consequences, and that the prevention of child abuse can be limited). And the reverse direction also holds true.

In relation to the denseness-emptiness principle, if there is denseness (e.g., the relatively denser concentration of concerns with "forceful parenting...in many Asian cultures, including China, Japan, Singapore, Vietnam and Korea"), there is emptiness (e.g., the relatively less dense, or more empty, concentration of concerns with Western tolerant parenting "in many Asian cultures, including China, Japan, Singapore, Vietnam and Korea"). And the reverse direction also holds true.

In relation to the prototypicality-variation principle, if there is prototypicality (e.g., the prototype, like the example about the original 1973 work by psychiatrist P. D. Scott on the link "between stepparents and child maltreatment," now known as "the Cinderella effect"), there is variation (e.g., different variants of the protoptye, as shown in many studies since the work on "the Cinderella effect" by Scott in 1973, like the subsequent ones by Martin Daly, Margo Wilson, Greg Tooley, and so on, though each with his own variation, contribution, and disagreement). (WK 2013ff) And the reverse direction also holds true.

In relation to the change-constancy principle, if there is change (e.g., the ever new ways to study abuse, as shown in the research on child abuse), there is constancy (e.g., the ever constant existence of different problems with the ever new ways to study abuse, as shown in the problems with the research on child abuse pointed out by the critics earlier). And the reverse direction also holds true.

In relation to the order-chaos principle, if there is order (e.g., the more or less orderly view on child abuse, if looked from the sole vantage point of its opponents, who simplistically pointed out its causes, effects, and prevention methods aforecited), there is chaos (e.g., the more or less chaotic view on child abuse, if looked from the multiple, conflicting vantage points of both the opponents and their critics alike, as shown in their disagrements aforecited). And the reverse direction also holds true.

In relation to the slowness-quickness principle, if there is slowness (e.g., the relatively slower speed for a child to suffer abuse, if he has not experienced any of the causes aforecited), there is quickness (e.g., the relatively quicker speed for a child to suffer abuse, if he is unlucky enough to experience many of the causes aforecited). And the reverse direction also holds true.

In relation to the expansion-contraction principle, if there is expansion (e.g., the relatively more developed ability of "a medical professional" against the "confidentiality" of a child in child abuse cases to be able "to testify in court as to otherwise privileged evidence about suspected child abuse despite the wishes of the child and his/her family"), there is contraction (e.g., the relatively less developed ability of "a medical professional" against the "confidentiality" of a child in child abuse cases to insist the "standard requirements for confidentiality and legal privileges in instances of child abuse"). (WK 2013ee) And the reverse direction also holds true.

In relation to the optimality-nonoptimality principle, if there is optimality (e.g., the search for highly favorable options, like the quest for "optimal caregiving" to prevent "child abuse" by researchers like Baumrind and others), there is nonoptimality (e.g., the existence of non-optimal alternatives to optimality, like the argument for more realistic studies by the critics, who pointed out that scholars disagree over what constitutes child abuse, that the alleged causes of child abuse can be questionable, that the long-term effects of child abuse remains unknown, and that the alleged causes do not determine the often cited consequences, that the prevention of child abuse can be limited, and that there is cultural bias in the studies). (WK 2013ee) And the reverse direction also holds true.

In relation to the theory-praxis principle, if there is theory (e.g., the theoretical construction of "rights" in ethics), there is praxis (e.g., the practical application of "rights" in ethics to the field of health care and the law, as shown in "the 2008 New Hampshire case of Andrew Bedner" about "the parental rights of abusive parents or caretakers with regard to their children, particularly in medical settings"). (WK 2013ee) And the reverse direction also holds true.

In relation to the convention-novelty principle, if there is convention (e.g., the conventional wisdom about protecting child victims from abuse), there is novelty (e.g., the alternative novel challenge to the conventional wisdom about protecting child victims from abuse, by the new idea of "the 2008 New Hampshire case of Andrew Bedner" about "the parental rights of abusive parents or caretakers with regard to their children, particularly in medical settings"). And the reverse direction also holds true.

In relation to the evolution-transformation principle, if there is evolution (e.g., the natural evolution of humans to treat each other, which can "result…in harm, potential for harm, or threat of harm to a child," in the state of nature), there is transformation (e.g., the technical transformation of human ability to treat each other by the invention of ethics and jurisprudence, like "the 2008 New Hampshire case of Andrew Bedner" about "the parental rights of abusive parents or caretakers with regard to their children, particularly in medical settings"). And the reverse direction also holds true.

In relation to the symmetry-asymmetry principle, if there is symmetry (e.g., the co-existence of different entities in a social relationship, like a child and an adult), there is asymmetry (e.g., an adult, on average, can abuse a child in a way that a child cannot do the same to an adult, especially when the child is dependent on the adult for caretaking). And the reverse direction also holds true.

In relation to the softness-hardness principle, if there is softness (e.g., the defense of the prevention of child abuse by the advocates), there is hardness (e.g., the critique of the studies on child abuse by the critics afore-cited). And the reverse direction also holds true.

In relation to the seriousness-playfulness principle, if there is seriousness (e.g., the serious business of those researchers who try to understand the nature of child abuse), there is playfulness (e.g., the playful part of those researchers who try to understand the nature of child abuse, when they play around with diffferent ideas in regards to its types, causes, effects, and prevention programs over the decades). And the reverse direction also holds true.

In relation to the activeness-inactivess principle, if there is activeness (e.g., the relative activeness of those children who are lucky enough to not suffer from any child abuse and can engage both physically and psychologically in life activities in a healthy way), there is inactiveness (e.g., the relative inactiveness of those children who are not lucky and have sufferred from different forms of child abuse, so that they cannot engage both physically and psychologically in life activities in a healthy way, because of the negative health effects aforecited).

In relation to the selfness-otherness principle, if there is selfness (e.g., the tendency to be mostly centered on one's self or group, as shown in the abusive act of an abuser to abuse a child for his own pleasure), there is otherness (e.g., the tendency to be mostly centered on others, as shown in the work by The National Alliance of Children's Trust Funds and Prevent Child Abuse America to protect children from abuse). And the reverse direction also holds true.

In relation to the regression-progression principle, if there is regression (e.g., the regression made by the studies on child abuse, as shown in the problems pointed out by the critics), there is progression (e.g., the progress made by the studies on child abuse, as shown in the contribution to the understanding of its types, causes, and effects aforecited). And the reverse direction also holds true.

In relation to the same-difference principle, if there is similarity in outcome (e.g., the contribution to the molding and control of beliefs, values, and behaviors, regardless of whether this be done by way of child abuse, or by way of child protection), there is difference in outcome (e.g., the contribution to the molding and control of beliefs, values, and behaviors by way of child abuse for a relatively more amoral lifeworld—but the contribution to the molding and control of beliefs, values, and behaviors by way of child protection for a relatively more moral lifeworld). And the reverse direction also holds true.

In relation to the stability-reaction principle, if there is stability (e.g., the relatively more stable condition of "the Soviet period," when there was "the emphasis on equality within the sexes" in regard to child care), there is reaction (e.g., "the Soviet period" then led to further changes later on, when, nowadays in the post-Soviet period, "controlling parenting may be less of a concern," but "financial difficulty, unemployment, and substance abuse" are the "dominating factors in child abuse throughout Eastern Europe"). (WK 2013ee) And the reverse direction also holds true.

In relation to the functionality-nonfunctionality principle, if there is functionality (e.g., the presence of action for which something or someone is fitted, as shown in "the emphasis on equality within the sexes" during the Soviet period, which served the ideological function of championing Communist ideals at that time), there is nonfunctionality (e.g., the relative lack of action for which something or someone is fitted, as shown in the post-Soviet period, when "financial difficulty, unemployment, and substance abuse" are the "dominating factors in child abuse throughout Eastern Europe," which reflect the transitional period to a more market-oriented open society nowadays, such that the older Communist ideals are no longer functional). And the reverse direction also holds true.

In relation to the intentionality-nonintentionality principle, if there is intentionality (e.g., the planning or design of something for a certain outcome, as shown in the original intention of the Eastern European leaders in the Soviet era to uphold "equality within the sexes" in regard to child care, as part of their Communist propaganda at the time), there is nonintentionality (e.g., the relative absence of planning or design of something for a certain outcome, such that the outcome can even be counter-intentional in being the opposite of what was originally planned, as shown in the changes in Eastern Europe nowadays, when "there is a new openness and acceptance regarding parenting styles and close relationships with children," and, although "controlling parenting may be less of a concern, financial difficulty, unemployment, and substance abuse still remain to be dominating factors in child abuse throughout Eastern Europe"—contrary to the original intention of the Eastern European leaders in the Soviet era to uphold "equality within the sexes" as part of their Communist propaganda at the time). And the reverse direction also holds true.

And in relation to the survivability-nonsurvivability principle, if there is survivability (e.g., the relative survival of the post-Soviet period nowadays, in regard to the fact that "financial difficulty, unemployment, and substance abuse" are the "dominating factors in child abuse throughout Eastern Europe"), there is non-survivability (e.g., the relative non-survival of "the emphasis on equality within the sexes" in Eastern Europe nowadays, though it was the case in the Soviet period). And the reverse direction also holds true.

Physical Health and Nature

Physical health, when examined from the perspective of nature, can show us in a controversial way its possibility (or impossibility) and desirability (or undesirability), and this can be shown by way of two case studies, namely, (3.3.1) physical health, astral travel, and higher dimensions, and (3.3.2) physical health, infectious disease, and animals—to be addressed in what follows, respectively.

Physical Health, Astral Travel, and Higher Dimensions,

A good way to evaluate the possibility (or impossibility) and desirability (or undesirability) of physical health from the perspective of nature is to explore physical health, astral travel, and higher dimensions.

An argument in the literature is that a person can leave his "physical body" and travel to his "subtle body (or dreambody or astral body) into 'higher' realms," especially when he suffers from "illness" and "surgical operations," or simply does so for some "spiritual" or other reasons. (WK 2013gg)

A Brief History

The term "astral projection (or astral travel)" refers to "an interpretation of out-of-body experience (OBE) that assumes the existence of an 'astral body' separate from the physical body and capable of traveling outside it. Astral projection or travel denotes the astral body leaving the physical body to travel in the astral plane" (in higher realms). (WK 2013gg)

Historically, "the idea of astral travel is rooted in common worldwide religious accounts of the afterlife in which the consciousness' or soul's journey or 'ascent' is described in such terms as 'an... out-of body experience, wherein the spiritual traveller leaves the physical body and travels in his/her subtle body (or dreambody or astral body) into 'higher' realms," so "it is…associated with near death experiences and is also frequently reported as spontaneously experienced in association with sleep and dreams, illness, surgical operations, drug experiences, sleep paralysis and forms of meditation." (WK 2013gg; R. Woolger 2008)

Sometimes, "it is…attempted out of curiosity, or may be believed to be necessary to, or the result of, some forms of spiritual practice. It may involve 'travel to higher realms' called astral planes but is commonly used to describe any sensation of being 'out of the body' in the everyday world, even seeing one's body from outside or above. It may be reported in the form of an apparitional experience, a supposed encounter with a doppelgänger, some living person also seen somewhere else at the same time." (WK 2013gg; R. Wilhelm 1930; J. Melton 1996; P. Yogananda 1946)

By the 1960s and 1970s, "surveys reported percentages ranging from 8 percent to as many as 50 percent (in certain groups) of respondents who state they had such an experience." (WK 2013gg; S. Blackmore 1991)

"Astral" vs. "Etheric"

In the history of the study about "astral travel" (or "astral projection'), there is a distinction between "astral" and "etheric" meanings.

(a) The "Astral" Meaning

In regard to the "astral" meaning—especially "for the Golden Dawn and some Theosophists, it retained the classical and medieval philosophers' meaning of journeying to other worlds, heavens, hells, the astrological spheres and other imaginal landscapes, but outside these circles the term was increasingly applied to non-physical travel around the physical world." (WK 2013gg; A. Powell 2008; H. Corbin 1969; W. Judge 1893)

In fact, "the astral environment may also be divided into levels or sub-planes by theorists, but there are many different views in various traditions concerning the overall structure of the astral planes: they may include heavens and hells and other after-death spheres, transcendent environments or other less-easily characterized states." (WK 2013gg; R. Monroe 1977; R. Bruce 1999)

(b) The "Etheric" Meaning

And in regard to the "etheric" meaning—especially "used by some later Theosophists," it "offers a useful distinction. Some experients say they visit different times and/or places: 'etheric,' then, is used to represent the sense of being 'out of the body' in the physical world, whereas 'astral' may connote some alteration in time-perception. Robert Monroe describes the former type of projection as 'Locale I' or the 'Here-Now,' involving people and places that actually exist: Robert Bruce calls it the 'Real Time Zone' (RTZ) and describes it as the non-physical dimension-level closest to the physical. This etheric body is usually, though not always, invisible but is often perceived by the experient as connected to the physical body during separation by a 'silver cord.' Some link 'falling' dreams with projection." (WK 2013gg)

For some researchers like Max Heindel (1911), "the etheric 'double' serves as a medium between the astral and physical realms. In his system the ether, also called prana, is the 'vital force' that empowers the physical forms to change. From his descriptions it can be inferred that, to him, when one views the physical during an out-of-body experience, one is not technically 'in' the astral realm at all." (WK 2013gg)

Western Sources

This distinction between "astral" and "etheric" meanings aside—in the Western tradition, there are different sources to understand "astral travel."

For example, "according to classical, medieval and renaissance Hermeticism, Neoplatonism, and later Theosophist and Rosicrucian thought, the astral body is an intermediate body of light linking the rational soul to the physical body while the astral plane is an intermediate world of light between Heaven and Earth, composed of the spheres of the planets and stars. These astral spheres were held to be populated by angels, demons and spirits." (WK 2013gg; W. Pagel 1967)

In this way, "the subtle bodies, and their associated planes of existence, form an essential part of the esoteric systems that deal with astral phenomena. In the neo-platonism of Plotinus, for example, the individual is a microcosm ('small world') of the universe (the macrocosm or 'great world'). 'The rational soul...is akin to the great Soul of the World' while 'the material universe, like the body, is made as a faded image of the Intelligible.' Each succeeding plane of manifestation is causal to the next, a world-view called emanationism; 'from the One proceeds Intellect, from Intellect Soul, and from Soul—in its lower phase, or Nature—the material universe.'" (WK 2013gg)

Often enough, "these bodies and their planes of existence are depicted as a series of concentric circles or nested spheres, with a separate body traversing each realm. The idea of the astral figured prominently in the work of the nineteenth-century French occultist Eliphas Levi, whence it was adopted and developed further by Theosophy, and used afterwards by other esoteric movements." (WK 2013gg; A. Besant 1897)

Even in the Bible, "some have claimed that the Bible contains mentions of astral projection. Carrington, Muldoon, Peterson, and Williams claim that the subtle body is attached to the physical body by means of a psychic silver cord. The final chapter of the Biblical Book of Ecclesiastes is often cited in this respect: 'Before the silver cord be loosed, or the golden bowl be broken, or the pitcher be shattered at the fountain, or the wheel be broken at the cistern.' Scherman, however, contends that the context points to this being merely a metaphor, comparing the body to a machine, with the silver cord referring to the spine." (WK 2013gg; S. Muldoon 1961; N. Scherman 2011)

And "Paul's Second Epistle to the Corinthians is more generally agreed to refer to the astral planes; 'I know a man in Christ, fourteen years ago, (whether in the body I know not, or out of the body I know not, God knows) such a one caught up to the third heaven….' This statement gave rise to the *Visio Pauli*, a tract that offers a vision of heaven and hell, a forerunner of visions attributed to Adomnan and Tnugdalus as well as of Dante's *Divine Comedy*." (WK 2013gg)

Islamic Sources

In the Islamic tradition, "many sects and offshoots belonging to Islamic mysticism interpret Muhammad's night ascent—the Isra and Mi'raj—to be an out of body experience through nonphysical environments, unlike the Sunni Muslims or mainstream Islam. In view of the references from the Qur'an and Hadith, the Sunni Muslims reject this saying the Isra and Mi'raj, the night journey—mentioned in the Qur'an and Hadith was physical yet spiritual. He was taken to the Masjid Al Aqsa, where he performed prayer leading all previous prophets and then taken to the heavens in a journey. The mystics claim Muhammad was transported to Jerusalem and onward to seven heavens, even though 'the apostle's body remained where it was.'" (WK 2013gg; B. McNeely 2013; D. Brown 2003)

In fact, "Islamic spiritual system called Sufism also have some similar practices. There are stories about the sufis that they were seen on multiple places at the same time. There are hundreds of such stories. It is believed that the sufis make their soul pure and light by surrendering themselves to Allah (God). And Allah in return gives them some special powers including this." (WK 2013gg)

Eastern Sources

In the Eastern tradition, there is no lack of works on astral travel.

For example, in China, “Taoist alchemical practice involves creation of an energy body by breathing meditations, drawing energy into a 'pearl' that is then 'circulated.' 'Xiangzi ... with a drum as his pillow fell fast asleep, snoring and motionless. His primordial spirit, however, went straight into the banquet room,” so he said: “My lords, here I am again.” (WK2013gg; M. Chia 1989) And “when Tuizhi walked…with the officials to take a look, there really was a Daoist sleeping on the ground and snoring like thunder. Yet inside, in the side room, there was another Daoist beating a fisher drum and singing Daoist songs. The officials all said, 'Although there are two different people, their faces and clothes are exactly alike. Clearly he is a divine immortal who can divide his body and appear in several places at once'….At that moment, the Daoist in the side room came walking out, and the Daoist sleeping on the ground woke up. The two merged into one.” (WK 2013gg; E. Yang 2007)

In India, “similar ideas such as the Lin'ga S'ari-ra are found in ancient Hindu scriptures such as the YogaVashishta-Maharamayana of Valmiki. Modern Indians who have vouched for astral projection include Paramahansa Yogananda who witnessed Swami Pranabananda doing a miracle through a possible astral projection and Osho (Bhagwan Shree Rajneesh) who practiced it himself.” (WK 2013gg; E. Yang 2007)

And in Japan, “an ikiryō (生霊?) (also read *shōryō*, *seirei*, or *ikisudama*) is a manifestation of the soul of a living person separately from their body. Traditionally, if someone holds a sufficient grudge against another person, it is believed that a part or the whole of their soul can temporarily leave their body and appear before the target of their hate in order to curse or otherwise harm them, similar to an evil eye. Souls are also believed to leave a living body when the body is extremely sick or comatose; such ikiryō are not malevolent.” (WK 2013gg; P. Clarke 2000)

Problems with the Views on Astral Travel

However, for the critics, these views on astral travel have some major problems. Consider, for illustration, a few examples below.

Firstly, one main criticism of the views on astral travel is that the experience is subjective.

For example, for the critics, “the subjective nature of the experience permits explanations that do not rely on the existence of an 'astral' body and plane.” (WK 2013gg) In fact, “Robert Todd Carroll [2003] writes that the main evidence to support claims of astral travel is anecdotal and comes 'in the form of testimonials of those who claim to have experienced being out of their bodies when they may have been out of their minds.'" (WK 2013gg)

Secondly, another main criticism of the views on astral travel is that there are competing interpretations of astral travel.

For instance, for the critics, there are different competing interpretations of astral travel over the centuries, as shown in the different traditions (Western, Islamic, Eastern, etc.) aforediscussed.

Thirdly, still another main criticism of the views on astral travel is that the claims are "contrary to the limits of science."

For instance, the critic Bob Bruce argued that "astral projection is 'just imagining,' or 'a dream state.' Although there is rigorous mathematical support for parallel universes, Bruce writes that the existence of an astral plane is contrary to the limits of science. 'We know how many possibilities there are for dimensions and we know what the dimensions do. None of it correlates with things like astral projection.' Bruce attributes astral experiences such as 'meetings' alleged by practitioners to confirmation bias and coincidences." (WK 2013gg; P. Frazer 2010)

And fourthly, an additional main criticism of the views on astral travel is that the claims are not accurate.

For instance, the critic "Arthur W. Wiggins, writing in *Quantum Leaps in the Wrong Direction: Where Real Science Ends...and Pseudoscience Begins* [2001], said that purported evidence of the ability to astral travel great distances and give descriptions of places visited" is not accurate; in response to this critique, "in 1978, Ingo Swann provided a test of his alleged ability to astral travel to Jupiter and observe details of the planet. Actual findings and information were later compared to Swann's claimed observations. According to an evaluation by James Randi, Swann's accuracy was 'unconvincing and unimpressive' with an overall score of 37 percent. Wiggins considers astral travel an illusion, and looks to neuroanatomy, human belief, imagination and prior knowledge to provide prosaic explanations for those claiming to experience it." (WK 2013gg)

Beyond Astral Travel

These criticisms of the claims on astral travel, however, should not be misconstrued as a total rejection of their usefulness but serve to show us the two opposing sides of the debate, such that the possibility (or impossibility) and desirability (or undesirability) of physical health (from the perspective of nature with physical health, astral travel, and higher dimensions as a case study here) are not to the extent that the respective defenders would like us to believe.

In fact, the analysis of physical health, astral travel, and higher dimensions can shed some light on the ontological principles in existential dialectics, and good examples include the formalness-informalness principle, the absoluteness-relativeness principle, the partiality-totality principle, the predictability-unpredictability principle, the explicability-inexplicability principle, the fiction-reality principle, the cognitiveness-noncognitiveness principle, the finiteness-transfiniteness principle, the preciseness-vagueness principle, the simpleness-complicatedness principle, the openness-hiddenness principle, the denseness-emptiness principle, the prototypicality-variation principle, the change-constancy principle, the order-chaos principle, the slowness-quickness principle, the expansion-contraction principle, the optimality-nonoptimality principle, the theory-praxis principle, the convention-novelty principle, the evolution-transformation principle, the symmetry-asymmetry principle, the softness-hardness principle, the seriousness-playfulness principle, the activeness-inactivess principle, the selfness-otherness principle, the regression-progression principle, the same-difference principle, the stability-reaction principle, the functionality-nonfunctionality principle, and the intentionality-nonintentionality principle.

For instance, in relation to the formalness-informalness principle, if there is formalness (e.g., the formal logical requirement of soundness, completeness, and consistency in a system of ideas, as in the claims on astral travel), there is informalness (e.g., the non-formal existence of unsoundness, incompleteness, and inconsistency in the claims on astral travel, as shown in the criticisms that the experience is subjective, that there are competing interpretations of astral travel, that the claims are "contrary to the limits of science," and that the claims are not accurate). And the reverse direction also holds true.

In relation to the absoluteness-relativeness principle, if there is absoluteness (e.g., the absolute view on astral travel by the advocates like Ingo Swann), there is relativeness (e.g., what is right for the advocates like Ingo Swann in regard to the alleged ability to astral travel is not necessarily so for the critics, who pointed out that the experience is subjective, that there are competing interpretations of astral travel, that the claims are "contrary to the limits of science," and that the claims are not accurate). And the reverse direction also holds true.

In relation to the partiality-totality principle, if there is partiality (e.g., the partial view on astral travel by the advocates), there is totality (e.g., the more holistic view on astral travel, such that the whole is not the sum of its parts, that is, it cannot be reduced to the sum of opposing views by the advocates, the critics, the in-between researchers, etc., since there will emerge new views in the future not yet known today, just as there are already alternative views nowadays which do not side exclusively with any of them, as is the analysis here). And the reverse direction also holds true.

In relation to the predictability-unpredictability principle, if there is predictability (e.g., the predictable tendency of the advocates like Ingo Swann to claim the alleged ability to astral travel), there is unpredictability (e.g., the more difficult task to predict exactly the extent to which a claim about astral travel will be like in a particular distant future era, since some critics already pointed out that there are competing interpretations of astral travel over time, depending on different historical traditions, etc.). And the reverse direction also holds true.

In relation to the explicability-inexplicability principle, if there is explicability (e.g., the explanation, by those advocates like Ingo Swann to claim the alleged ability to astral travel travel on the basis of his account of "Jupiter and observe details of the planet"), there is inexplicability (e.g., the lack of sufficient explanation, by those advocates like Ingo Swann to claim the alleged ability to astral travel on the basis of his account of "Jupiter and observe details of the planet," of why the claims are necessarily true, since the critics were quick to reveal that the claims are not accurate, as they are merely "neuroanatomy, human belief, imagination and prior knowledge to provide prosaic explanations"). And the reverse direction also holds true.

In relation to the fiction-reality principle, if there is fiction (e.g., the fictional aspect of astral travel, insofar as the claims by the advocates like Ingo Swann are not accurate, based on "neuroanatomy, human belief, imagination and prior knowledge" pointed out by the critics), there is reality (e.g., the realistic aspect of astral travel, insofar as there are different historical sources to offer details about astral travel aforecited, although this does not imply that the claims must be true). And the reverse direction also holds true.

In relation to the cognitiveness-noncognitiveness principle, if there is cognitiveness (e.g., a view of things on the basis of reason and evidences, as shown in different historical sources, be they Western, Islamic, or Eastern, to offer details about astral travel aforecited), there is noncognitiveness (e.g., a view of things on the basis of non-cognitive factors like envy, jealousy, power, nationality, race, gender, age, class, greed, lust, status, faith, anger, sadness, joy, fear, wish, etc., as shown in the wishful imagination by those advocates of astral travel, whose "subjective nature of the experience permits explanations that do not rely on the existence of an 'astral' body and plane," which can be true or false but is irrelevat in this context). And the reverse direction also holds true.

In relation to the finiteness-transfiniteness principle, if there is finiteness (e.g., the finite number of the categories of historical sources about astral travel, namely, Western, Islamic, and Eastern), there is transfiniteness (e.g., the transfinite number of all the individual stories, individuals, incidents, etc. that have ever existed in history and are related to astral travel). And the reverse direction also holds true.

In relation to the preciseness-vagueness principle, if there is preciseness (e.g., the precise identification of 3 main historical sources about astral travel, namely, Western, Islamic, and Eastern, in the article aforecited), there is vagueness (e.g., the vagueness in the identification of the 3 main historical sources about astral travel, namely, Western, Islamic, and Eastern, in the article aforecited, since it is not clear why there must be only 3, not 5, 7, 10, 11, 13, and so on). And the reverse direction also holds true.

In relation to the simpleness-complicatedness principle, if there is simpleness (e.g., the relatively simple analysis of astral travel by the advocates), there is complicatedness (e.g., the relatively more complicated analysis of astral travel, by challenging the claims and assumptions, as shown in the problems pointed out by the critics as cited). And the reverse direction also holds true.

In relation to the openness-hiddenness principle, if there is openness (e.g., the open exploration of "out-of-body experience" like "astral travel"), there is hiddenness (e.g., the hidden bias in the claims on "out-of-body experience" like "astral travel," because of the different problems pointed out by the critics aforecited). And the reverse direction also holds true.

In relation to the denseness-emptiness principle, if there is denseness (e.g., the relatively denser concentration of concerns with "out-of-body experience" by the advocates of "astral travel"), there is emptiness (e.g., the relatively less dense, or more empty, concentration of concerns with ordinary travel as a tourist by the advocates of "astral travel"). And the reverse direction also holds true.

In relation to the prototypicality-variation principle, if there is prototypicality (e.g., the prototype, like the example about the original historical sources on astral travel, be they Western, Islamic, or Eastern), there is variation (e.g., different variants of the protoptye, as shown in many studies since the original historical sources on astral travel, like the contemporary ones by Robert Monroe, Oliver Fox, Sylvan Muldoon,

Hereward Carrington, etc., though each with his own variation, contribution, and disagreement). (WK 2013gg) And the reverse direction also holds true.

In relation to the change-constancy principle, if there is change (e.g., the ever new ways to travel, as shown in the claims about astral travel), there is constancy (e.g., the ever constant existence of different problems with the ever new ways to travel, as shown in the problems with the claims about astral travel pointed out by the critics). And the reverse direction also holds true.

In relation to the order-chaos principle, if there is order (e.g., the more or less orderly view on astral travel, if looked from the sole vantage point of someone like Ingo Swann about his travel "to Jupiter and observe details of the planet"), there is chaos (e.g., the more or less chaotic view on astral travel, if looked from the multiple, conflicting vantage points of different advocates and their critics alike, as shown in the different interpretations and disagreements aforecited). And the reverse direction also holds true.

In relation to the slowness-quickness principle, if there is slowness (e.g., the relatively slower speed for someone to travel to Jupiter by an ordinary spacecraft, not through "astral travel," if this were to become possible), there is quickness (e.g., the relatively quicker speed for someone to travel to Jupiter through "astral travel," if this were to become real). And the reverse direction also holds true.

In relation to the expansion-contraction principle, if there is expansion (e.g., the relative expansion of the belief in astral travel in the pre-modern era, when science was not as well developed), there is contraction (e.g., the relative decline of the belief in astral travel in our time, when the scientific way of thinking is more dominant. especially in the scientific community). And the reverse direction also holds true.

In relation to the optimality-nonoptimality principle, if there is optimality (e.g., the search for highly favorable options, like the quest for some preferred "levels or sub-planes" in astral travel, like "heavens" over "hells"), there is nonoptimality (e.g., the existence of non-optimal alternatives to optimality, like the argument for more realistic studies by the critics, who pointed out that the experience is subjective, that there are competing interpretations of astral travel, that the claims are "contrary to the limits of science," and that the claims are not accurate). (WK 2013gg) And the reverse direction also holds true.

In relation to the theory-praxis principle, if there is theory (e.g., the theoretical construction of "heavens and hells" in different religions), there is praxis (e.g., the practical application of "heavens and hells" in different religions to the field of "out-of-body experience" like "astral travel"). And the reverse direction also holds true.

In relation to the convention-novelty principle, if there is convention (e.g., the conventional wisdom about astral travel "in classical philosophy and in various myths and religious scriptures"), there is novelty (e.g., the alternative novel challenge to the conventional wisdom about astral travel "in classical philosophy and in various myths and religious scriptures," by the new idea of science nowadays that the claims are "contrary to the limits of science" and that the claims are not accurate). (WK 2013gg) And the reverse direction also holds true.

In relation to the evolution-transformation principle, if there is evolution (e.g., the natural evolution of humans to wander to different places in the state of nature in a primitive way), there is transformation (e.g., the technical transformation of human ability to wander to different places by the invention of the idea of astral travel "in classical philosophy and in various myths and religious scriptures"). And the reverse direction also holds true.

In relation to the symmetry-asymmetry principle, if there is symmetry (e.g., the co-existence of different ways to understand astral travel), there is asymmetry (e.g., the scientific interpretaton of astral travel is more dominant or persuasive in the academic community nowadays than the sacred interpretation based on "various myths and religious scriptures"). (WK 2013gg) And the reverse direction also holds true.

In relation to the softness-hardness principle, if there is softness (e.g., the defense of the idea of astral travel by the advocates), there is hardness (e.g., the critique of the idea of astral travel, as shown in the problems pointed out by the critics as cited). And the reverse direction also holds true.

In relation to the seriousness-playfulness principle, if there is seriousness (e.g., the serious business of the advocates who try to understand the nature of astral travel), there is playfulness (e.g., the playful part of the advocates who try to understand the nature of astral travel, when they play around with different versions and interpretations over the centuries, as shown in different historical sources aforecited). And the reverse direction also holds true.

In relation to the activeness-inactivess principle, if there is activeness (e.g., the relative activeness of those in dreams when they encounter "the out-of-body experience" like "flying or ascending" in different "higher realms"), there is inactiveness (e.g., the relative inactiveness of those in dreams when they do not encounter "the out-of-body experience" like "flying or ascending" in different "higher realms" nor have any other dream related to intense activities). (WK 2013gg) And the reverse direction also holds true.

In relation to the selfness-otherness principle, if there is selfness (e.g., the tendency to be mostly centered on one's self or group, as shown in the exaggered claim by Ingo Swann about his alleged ability to astral travel travel on the basis of his account of "Jupiter and observe details of the planet," which were rejected by scientists as not accurate), there is otherness (e.g., the tendency to be mostly centered on others, as shown in the skepticism by scientists like Bob Bruce of the Queensland Skeptics Association, when he showed that "the existence of an astral plane is contrary to the limits of science," as an advancement in the knowledge of different possible worlds). And the reverse direction also holds true.

In relation to the regression-progression principle, if there is regression (e.g., the regression made by the claims on astral travel, as shown in the problems pointed out by the critics), there is progression (e.g., the progress made by the claims on astral travel, as shown in the contribution to the imagination of traveling to "higher realms" aforecited). And the reverse direction also holds true.

In relation to the same-difference principle, if there is similarity in outcome (e.g., the contribution to the molding and control of beliefs, values, and behaviors, regardless of whether this be done by way of the defense of "astral travel," or by way of the critique of "astral travel"), there is difference in outcome (e.g., the contribution to the molding and control of beliefs, values, and behaviors by way of the defense of "astral travel" for a relatively more mystical or religious worldview—but the contribution to the molding and control of beliefs, values, and behaviors by way of the critique of "astral travel" for a relatively more scientific worldview). And the reverse direction also holds true.

In relation to the stability-reaction principle, if there is stability (e.g., the relatively more stable condition of some "twentieth century publications on astral projection," which are "widely cited," like the works by Robert Monroe, Oliver Fox, Sylvan Muldoon and Hereward Carrington," for example), there is reaction (e.g., some "twentieth century publications on astral projection" then led to further changes later on, when, nowadays, the critics are quick to point out that the experience is subjective, that there are competing interpretations of astral travel, that the claims are "contrary to the limits of science," and that the claims are not accurate). And the reverse direction also holds true.

In relation to the functionality-nonfunctionality principle, if there is functionality (e.g., the presence of action for which something or someone is fitted, as shown in the widespread belief in astral travel in the older days, like the different historical sources aforedescribed, which served the function of maintaining the old-fashioned worldview of "witchcraft and shamanism" as well as "classical philosophy and...various myths and religious scriptures" at that time), there is nonfunctionality (e.g., the relative lack of action for which something or someone is fitted, as shown in the relatively more skeptical reception of the claims on astral travel nowadays, such that the old-fashioned worldview of "witchcraft and shamanism" as well as "classical philosophy and...various myths and religious scriptures" is no longer much functional in our relatively more advanced scientific age, especially in the scientific community). And the reverse direction also holds true.

In relation to the intentionality-nonintentionality principle, if there is intentionality (e.g., the planning or design of something for a certain outcome, as shown in the original intention of the historical sources of astral travel to propound the possibility of "out-of-body experience"), there is nonintentionality (e.g., the relative absence of planning or design of something for a certain outcome, such that the outcome can even be counter-intentional in being the opposite of what was originally planned, as shown in the relatively more skeptical reception of the claims on astral travel in the scientific community nowadays—contrary to the original intention of the historical sources of astral travel to propound the possibility of "out-of-body experience"). And the reverse direction also holds true.

And in relation to the survivability-nonsurvivability principle, if there is survivability (e.g., the relative survival, nowadays, of the skeptical reception of the claims on astral travel in the scientific community), there is non-survivability (e.g., the relative non-survival of the claim by Ingo Swann about the alleged ability to astral travel on the basis of his account of "Jupiter and observe details of the planet," which is now discredited as being not quite accurate by the critics aforedescribed). And the reverse direction also holds true.

Physical Health, Infectious Disease, and Animals

Another good way to evaluate the possibility (or impossibility) and desirability (or undesirability) of physical health from the perspective of nature is to explore physical health, infectious disease, and animals.

An argument in the literature is that there are certain "infectious diseases," like "zoonotic diseases," which can be "transmitted...from animals other than humans to humans.'" (WK 2013n; L. Taylor 2001)

History of Zoonotic Diseases

Historically, "most human prehistory was spent as groups of hunter-gatherers usually with fewer than 150 individuals that were not often in contact with other bands. Because of this, epidemic or pandemic diseases, which depend on a constant influx of humans who have not developed an immune response, tended to burn out after their first run through a population. To survive, a biological pathogen had to be a chronic infection, stay alive in the host for long periods, or have a non-human reservoir in which to live while waiting for new hosts to pass by. In fact, for many 'human' diseases, the human is actually an accidental victim and a dead-end host....This is the case with rabies, anthrax, tularemia, West Nile virus, and many others....Thus, much of human development has been in relation to zoonotic, not epidemic, diseases." (WK 2013n)

Therefore, "many modern diseases, even epidemic diseases, started out as zoonotic diseases. It is hard to be certain which diseases jumped from other animals to humans, but there is good evidence that measles, smallpox, influenza, HIV, and diphtheria came to us this way. The common cold, and tuberculosis may also have started in other species." (WK 2013n)

What makes zoonoses important is that "they are often previously unrecognized diseases or have increased virulence in populations lacking immunity. The West Nile virus appeared in the United States in 1999 in the New York City area, and moved through the country in the summer of 2002, causing much distress. Bubonic plague is a zoonotic disease, as are salmonella, Rocky Mountain spotted fever, and Lyme disease." (WK 2013n; B. Meerburg 2009)

In this way, "the major factor contributing to the appearance of new zoonotic pathogens in human populations is increased contact between humans and wildlife. This can be caused either by encroachment of human activity into wilderness areas or by movement of wild animals into areas of human activity. An example of this is the outbreak of Nipah virus in peninsular Malaysia in 1999, when intensive pig farming began on the habitat of infected fruit bats. Unidentified infection of the pigs amplified the force of infection, eventually transmitting the virus to farmers and causing 105 human deaths." (WK 2013n; H. Field 2001; P. Daszak 2001)

More recently, "avian influenza and West Nile virus have spilled over into human populations probably due to interactions between the carrier host and domestic animals. Highly mobile animals such as bats and birds may present a greater risk of zoonotic transmission than other animals due to the ease with which they can move into areas of human habitation." (WK 2013n)

However, "diseases like malaria, African schistosomiasis, river blindness, and elephantiasis are *not* zoonotic, even though they may be transmitted by insects or use intermediate hosts vectors, because they depend on the human host for part of their life-cycle." (WK 2013n)

In any event, nowadays, "the emerging interdisciplinary field of conservation medicine, which integrates human and veterinary medicine, and environmental sciences, is largely concerned with zoonoses." (WK 2013n)

Examples of Carriers

With this history in mind—there are different examples of carriers of zoonotic diseases, that is, those animals which "can carry zoonotic infectious organisms" to humans, as shown below (and summarized in *Table 3.4*): (WK 2013n)

- Ex: "apes"
- Ex: "bats"
- Ex: "birds"
- Ex: "cats"
- Ex: "cattle"
- Ex: "dogs"
- Ex: "fish"
- Ex: "fleas"
- Ex: "foxes"
- Ex: "geese"
- Ex: "hamsters"
- Ex: "horses"
- Ex: "mice"
- Ex: "monkeys"
- Ex: "pigs"
- Ex: "rabbits and hares"
- Ex: "rodents"
- Ex: "sheep"
- Ex: "snails"
- Ex: "wolves"

Of couse, there can be other examples, so the ones above are illustrative.

Types of Agents

Besides examples—zoonoses can also be classified "by infectious agent type," as shown below (and summarized in *Table 3.4*): (WK 2013n)

- "parasites"
- "fungi"
- "bacteria"
- "viruses"
- "pria"

Each of these types can be further sub-classified, of course; for example, parasites can include "protozoa," "nematodes," "cestodes," and "trematodes." (WK 2013n)

Cases of Zoonoses

In additon, zoonoses can also be classified in terms of different specific cases, as shown below (and summarized in *Table 3.4*): (WK 2013n)

- Ex: "anthrax"
- Ex: "Bolivian hemorrhagic fever"
- Ex: "Borna virus infection"
- Ex: "bovine tuberculosis"
- Ex: "cat scratch disease"
- Ex: "cholera"
- Ex: "ebola"
- Ex: "Eastern equine encephalitis virus"
- Ex: "henipavirus"
- Ex: "human immunodeficiency virus (HIV)"
- Ex: "Kyasanur forest disease"
- Ex: "Marburg fever"
- Ex: "Mediterranean spotted fever"
- Ex: "monkey B"
- Ex: "plague"
- Ex: "rabies"
- Ex: "Salmonellosis"
- Ex: "West Nile virus"
- Ex: "Yellow fever"

Surely, there can be other cases, so the ones here are illustrative.

Outbreaks of Zoonotic Diseases

In general, "outbreaks of zoonoses have been traced to human interaction with and exposure to animals at fairs, petting zoos, and other settings. In 2005, the Centers for Disease Control and Prevention (CDC) issued an updated list of recommendations for preventing zoonosis transmission in public settings." (WK 2013n; CDCP 2005)

For example, "in 1988, a person became ill with swine influenza virus (swine flu) and died after visiting the display area of the pig barn at a Wisconsin county fair. Three healthcare personnel treating the case patient also developed flu-like illness with laboratory evidence of swine influenza virus infection. Investigators from the CDC indicated in their final report that the swine flu had been transmitted directly from pig to human host." (WK 2013n; D. Hopfensperger 1991; CDCP 1998)

In another outbreak, this time in 1994, "seven cases of *E. coli* O157:H7 infection were traced to a farm in Leicestershire, United Kingdom. An epidemiological investigation into the outbreak revealed that the strain of *E. coli* O157:H7 isolated from nine animals on the farm was indistinguishable from the strain isolated from human samples. Investigators concluded that the most likely cause of this outbreak was direct human contact with animals." (WK 2013n; R. Shukla 1995)

In the following year, "in 1995, 43 children who had visited a rural farm in Wales became ill with Cryptosporidiosis. Cryptosporidium was isolated from seven of the ill children. An epidemiological investigation indicated that the source of the children's illness was contact with calves at the farm." (WK 2013n; M. Evans 1996)

Worse, "in 1999, what is believed to be the largest outbreak of waterborne *E. coli* O157:H7 illness in United States history occurred at the Washington County, New York fair. The New York State Department of Health identified 781 individuals who were suspected of being infected with either *E. coli* O157:H7 or Campylobacter jejuni. An investigation into the outbreak revealed that consumption of beverages purchased from vendors supplied with water drawn from an unchlorinated fairgrounds well was associated with illness. In all, 127 outbreak victims were confirmed ill with *E. coli* O157:H7 infections; 71 were hospitalized, 14 developed HUS, and two died." (WK 2013n)

A year later, "in 2000, 51 people became ill with confirmed or suspected *E. coli* O157:H7 infections after visiting a dairy farm in Pennsylvania. Eight children developed HUS. A case-control study among visitors to the dairy was conducted jointly by the CDC, Pennsylvania Department of Health, and the Montgomery County Health Department. The study's authors concluded that *E. coli* was transmitted to visitors as a result of contamination on animal hides and in the environment." (WK 2013n; CDCP 2001)

Then in 2002, "what is believed to be the largest *E. coli* O157:H7 outbreak in Oregon history occurred among attendees at the Lane County fair in 2002. An Oregon Department of Human Services-Health Services investigation led to the belief that the *E. coli* outbreak originated from exposure in the sheep and goat barn. In all, 79 people were confirmed ill with *E. coli* infections as part of the outbreak; 22 were hospitalized, and 12 suffered HUS." (WK 2013n; ODHS 2002)

And "in 2005, a petting zoo that exhibited at two Florida fairs and a festival was traced as the source of an *E. coli* O157:H7 outbreak. Sixty-three people who had visited either the Florida State Fair, the Central Florida Fair, or the Florida Strawberry Festival reported illness to investigators for the Florida Department of Health, including 20 who were culture-confirmed and 7 with HUS. A case-control study revealed that illness was associated with exposure to a petting zoo exhibit present at all three events." (WK 2013n; CDCP 2005a)

Problems with the Research on Zoonotic Diseases

However, for the critics, this argument on physical health, infectious disease, and animals has some major problems. Consider, for illustration, a few examples below (as summarized in *Table 3.4*).

Firstly, one main criticism of the argument on physical health, infectious disease, and animals is that zoonotic diseases can be historically contingent.

For instance, for the critics, "most human prehistory was spent as groups of hunter-gatherers usually with fewer than 150 individuals that were not often in contact with other bands. Because of this, epidemic or pandemic diseases, which depend on a constant influx of humans who have not developed an immune response, tended to burn out after their first run through a population. To survive, a biological pathogen had to be a chronic infection, stay alive in the host for long periods, or have a non-human reservoir in which to live while waiting for new hosts to pass by. In fact, for many 'human' diseases, the human is actually an accidental victim and a dead-end host." (WK 2013n)

Secondly, another main criticism of the argument on physical health, infectious disease, and animals is that there are infectious diseases which can go in the opposite direction.

For instance, for the critics, "in a systematic review of 1,415 pathogens known to infect humans," 39% were not zoonotic at all and occurred in the opposite direction, that is, "from humans to other animals" instead, in what is now known as "reverse zoonosis or anthroponosis." (WK 2013n; L. Taylor 2001)

Thirdly, still another main criticism of the argument on physical health, infectious disease, and animals is that the causes of zoonotic diseases can be more complicated than previously thought.

For instance, the critics are quick to point out that "the environmental causes of health problems are complex, global, and poorly understood," such that "conservation medicine," which is "largely concerned with zoonoses," has to take into account of "diverse disciplines, including microbiologists, pathologists, landscape analysts, marine biologists, toxicologists, epidemiologists, climate biologists, anthropologists, economists, and political scientists." (WK 2013n &2013hh)

And fourthly, an additional main criticism of the argument on physical health, infectious disease, and animals is that the acceptance of the findings in zoonotic research can be based on the politics of social impact.

For instance, for the critics, "the broad topic of suburban sprawl is made more relevant when seen in terms of the immediate imbalance it brings to rural ecosystems, which increases population densities and forces humans into closer contact with, certain animals (like rodents), increasing the risk of new cross-species diseases. When tied to actual cases (like SARS or HIV/AIDS), this holistic outlook seems likely to resonate more powerfully with the public than the more abstract explanations of environmental and health issues that are currently common." (WK 2013hh)

Beyond Zoonotic Diseases

These criticisms of the studies on zoonotic diseases, however, do not suggest a total rejection of their usefulness but serve to show us the two opposing sides of the debate, such that the possibility (or impossibility) and desirability (or undesirability) of physical health (from the perspective of nature with physical health, infectious disease, and animals as a case study here) are not to the extent that the respective defenders would like us to believe.

Moreover, the analysis of physical health, infectious disease, and animals can further illuminate the ontological principles in existential dialectics, and good examples include the formalness-informalness principle, the absoluteness-relativeness principle, the partiality-totality principle, the predictability-unpredictability principle, the explicability-inexplicability principle, the fiction-reality principle, the cognitiveness-noncognitiveness principle, the finiteness-transfiniteness principle, the preciseness-vagueness principle, the simpleness-complicatedness principle, the openness-hiddenness principle, the denseness-emptiness principle, the prototypicality-variation principle, the change-constancy principle, the order-chaos principle, the slowness-quickness principle, the expansion-contraction principle, the optimality-nonoptimality principle, the theory-praxis principle, the convention-novelty principle, the evolution-transformation principle, the symmetry-asymmetry principle, the softness-hardness principle, the seriousness-playfulness principle, the activeness-inactivess principle, the selfness-otherness principle, the regression-progression principle, the same-difference principle, the stability-reaction principle, the functionality-nonfunctionality principle, and the intentionality-nonintentionality principle.

For instance, in relation to the formalness-informalness principle, if there is formalness (e.g., the formal logical requirement of soundness and completeness in a system of ideas, as in the argument on zoonotic diseases), there is informalness (e.g., the non-formal existence of unsoundness and incompleteness in the argument on zoonotic diseases, as shown in the criticisms that zoonotic diseases can be historically contingent, that there are infectious diseases which can go in the opposite direction, that the causes of zoonotic diseases can be more complicated than previously thought, and that the acceptance of the findings in zoonotic research can be based on the politics of social impact). And the reverse direction also holds true.

In relation to the absoluteness-relativeness principle, if there is absoluteness (e.g., the absolute view on zoonotic diseases by those in the public, based on the politics of social impact), there is relativeness (e.g., what is right for those in the public, based on the politics of social impact, is not necessarily so for the critics, who pointed out that "actual cases [like SARS or HIV/AIDS]...resonate more powerfully with the public than the more abstract explanations of environmental and health issues," but then this public perception of the cases is distorted). And the reverse direction also holds true.

In relation to the partiality-totality principle, if there is partiality (e.g., the partial view on zoonotic diseases by the practitioners), there is totality (e.g., the more holistic view on zoonotic diseases, such that the whole is not the sum of its parts, that is, it cannot be reduced to the sum of opposing views by the practitioners, the critcs, the public, etc., since there will emerge new views in the future not yet known today, just as there are already alternative views nowadays which do not side exclusively with any of them, as is the analysis here). And the reverse direction also holds true.

In relation to the predictability-unpredictability principle, if there is predictability (e.g., the predictable tendency of those working on zoonotic diseases to link human health with infectious diseases from animals), there is unpredictability (e.g., the more difficult task to predict exactly the extent to which the causes of zoonotic diseases and their effects are on a particular future occasion, since the critics are quick to point out that "the environmental causes of health problems are complex, global, and poorly understood," such that the causes and effects of zoonotic diseases can be more complicated than previously thought). And the reverse direction also holds true.

In relation to the explicability-inexplicability principle, if there is explicability (e.g., the explanation, by the advocates, of the occurrence of zoonotic diseases on the basis of "infectious diseases...transmitted...from animals"), there is inexplicability (e.g., the lack of sufficient explanation, by the advocates, of the more complicated nature of the causes and effects of zoonotic diseases, since, for the critics, "the environmental causes of health problems are complex, global, and poorly understood"). And the reverse direction also holds true.

In relation to the fiction-reality principle, if there is fiction (e.g., the fictional aspect of the perception of zoonotic diseases, insofar as there is the politics of social impact aforedescribed), there is reality (e.g., the realistic aspect of the perception of zoonotic diseases, insofar as there were in fact "actual cases" like "SARS or HIV/AIDS"). And the reverse direction also holds true.

In relation to the cognitiveness-noncognitiveness principle, if there is cognitiveness (e.g., a view of things on the basis of reason and evidences, as shown in the empirical findings on outbreaks of zoonotic diseases aforecited), there is noncognitiveness (e.g., a view of things on the basis of non-cognitive factors like envy, jealousy, power, nationality, race, gender, age, class, greed, lust, status, faith, anger, sadness, joy, fear, wish, etc., as shown in the politics of social impact, such that "actual cases [like SARS or HIV/AIDS]...resonate more powerfully with the public than the more abstract explanations of environmental and health issues," regardless of whether the perception is accurate or not). And the reverse direction also holds true.

In relation to the finiteness-transfiniteness principle, if there is finiteness (e.g., the finite number of "infectious agent types," like "parasites," "fungi," "bacteria," "viruses," and "pria"), there is transfiniteness (e.g., the transfinite number of all the individual "parasites," "fungi," "bacteria," "viruses," and "pria" that have ever existed in history). And the reverse direction also holds true.

In relation to the preciseness-vagueness principle, if there is preciseness (e.g., the precise identification of 20 examples of carriers of zoonotic diseases in the article aforecited), there is vagueness (e.g., the vagueness in the identification of the 20 examples of carriers of zoonotic diseases in the article aforecited, since it is not clear why there must be only these 20 or so examples, not 40, 54, 64, 100, 143, and so on). And the reverse direction also holds true.

In relation to the simpleness-complicatedness principle, if there is simpleness (e.g., the relatively simple analysis of the causes of zoonotic diseases by the practitioners), there is complicatedness (e.g., the relatively more complicated analysis of the causes of zoonotic diseases, by challenging the claims and assumptions, as shown in the problems pointed out by the critics as cited). And the reverse direction also holds true.

In relation to the openness-hiddenness principle, if there is openness (e.g., the open exploration of the link between human health and infectious diseases from animals), there is hiddenness (e.g., the hidden bias in the studies on the link between human health and infectious diseases from animals, since, for the critics, zoonotic diseases can be historically contingent, there are infectious diseases which can go in the opposite direction, the causes of zoonotic diseases can be more complicated than previously thought, and the acceptance of the findings in zoonotic research can be based on the politics of social impact). And the reverse direction also holds true.

In relation to the denseness-emptiness principle, if there is denseness (e.g., the relatively denser concentration of "zoonotic diseases" in much of human history), there is emptiness (e.g., the relatively less dense, or more empty, concentration of "epidemic diseases" in much of human history). (WK 2013n) And the reverse direction also holds true.

In relation to the prototypicality-variation principle, if there is prototypicality (e.g., the prototype, like the example about the first cases of "HIV-1 and HIV-2," which "originated in non-human primates in West-central Africa and...transferred to humans...in the early 20th century"), there is variation (e.g., different variants of the protoptye, as shown in many studies since the first cases of "HIV-1 and HIV-2" in West-central Africa—like the later findings on the cases of "AIDS" spread to the United States in the 1980s, though each with its own variation, because "HIV differs from many viruses in that it has very high genetic variability"). (WK 2013ii) And the reverse direction also holds true.

In relation to the change-constancy principle, if there is change (e.g., the ever new ways to understand diseases, as shown in the work on zoonotic diseases), there is constancy (e.g., the ever constant existence of different problems with the ever new ways to understand diseases, as shown in the problems with the work on zoonotic diseases pointed out by the critics). And the reverse direction also holds true.

In relation to the order-chaos principle, if there is order (e.g., the more or less orderly view on zoonotic diseases, if looked from the vantage point of "HIV" which predictably "infects vital cells in the human immune system such as helper T cells [specifically CD4+ T cells], macrophages, and dendritic cells"), there is chaos (e.g., the more or less chaotic view on zoonotic diseases, if looked from the vantage point of "HIV," which "differs from many viruses in that it has very high genetic variability," in that it has "a high mutation rate of approximately 3 x 10−5 per nucleotide base per cycle of replication and recombinogenic properties of reverse transcriptase," so "this...leads to the generation of many variants of HIV in a single infected patient in the course of one day"). (WK 2013ii) And the reverse direction also holds true.

In relation to the slowness-quickness principle, if there is slowness (e.g., the relatively slower speed for modern cities of many million individuals to ever get wiped out by infectious diseases), there is quickness (e.g., the relatively quicker speed for "hunter-gatherers usually with fewer than 150 individuals" to "burn out after the...first run through a population" by "epidemic or pandemic diseases"). (WK 2013n) And the reverse direction also holds true.

In relation to the expansion-contraction principle, if there is expansion (e.g., the relative spread of "the West Nile virus...in 1999 in the New York City area"), there is contraction (e.g., the relative decline of "the West Nile virus...in the New York City area" nowadays). And the reverse direction also holds true.

In relation to the optimality-nonoptimality principle, if there is optimality (e.g., the search for highly favorable options, like the understanding of the optimal conditions of infectious agents to survive and cause damage to human populations, in that "a biological pathogen had to be a chronic infection, stay alive in the host for long periods, or have a non-human reservoir in which to live while waiting for new hosts to pass by"), there is nonoptimality (e.g., the existence of non-optimal alternatives to optimality, like the argument for more realistic studies by the critics, who pointed out that zoonotic diseases can be historically contingent, that there are infectious diseases which can go in the opposite direction, that the causes of zoonotic diseases can be more complicated than previously thought, and that the acceptance of the findings in zoonotic research can be based on the politics of social impact). (WK 2013n) And the reverse direction also holds true.

In relation to the theory-praxis principle, if there is theory (e.g., the theoretical construction of "zoonotic diseases" in conservation medicine), there is praxis (e.g., the practical application of the understanding of "zoonotic diseases" in conservation medicine to the field of public health, as shown in 2006, when "a conference held in Berlin was focusing on the issue of zoonotic pathogen effects on food safety, urging governments to intervene, and the public to be vigilant towards the risks of catching food-borne diseases from farm-to-dining table"). (WK 2013n) And the reverse direction also holds true.

In relation to the convention-novelty principle, if there is convention (e.g., the conventional wisdom about the link between human health and infectious diseases from animals), there is novelty (e.g., the alternative novel challenge to the conventional wisdom about the link between human health and infectious diseases from animals, by the new idea that zoonotic diseases can be historically contingent, that there are infectious diseases which can go in the opposite direction, that the causes of zoonotic diseases can be more complicated than previously thought, and that the acceptance of the findings in zoonotic research can be based on the politics of social impact). And the reverse direction also holds true.

In relation to the evolution-transformation principle, if there is evolution (e.g., the natural evolution of humans to suffer from infectious diseases at times in the state of nature in a primitive way), there is transformation (e.g., the technical transformation of human ability to deal with infectious diseases by the invention of "conservation medicine" to deal largely with "zoonoses"). And the reverse direction also holds true.

In relation to the symmetry-asymmetry principle, if there is symmetry (e.g., the co-existence of different directions for infectoius diseases to spread, that is, from humans to animals and from animals to humans), there is asymmetry (e.g., "in a systematic review of 1,415 pathogens known to infect humans," 61% were zoonotic [from animals to humans] but 39% were reverse-zoonotic [from humans to animals]). (WK 2013n) And the reverse direction also holds true.

In relation to the softness-hardness principle, if there is softness (e.g., the defense of the studies on zoonotic diseases by the advocates aforecited), there is hardness (e.g., the critique of the studies on zoonotic diseases, as shown in the problems pointed out by the critics as cited). And the reverse direction also holds true.

In relation to the seriousness-playfulness principle, if there is seriousness (e.g., the serious business of those researchers who try to understand the nature of zoonotic diseases), there is playfulness (e.g., the playful part of those researchers who try to understand the nature of zoonotic diseases, when they play around with different lists, examples, and interpretations over the decades aforecited). And the reverse direction also holds true.

In relation to the activeness-inactivess principle, if there is activeness (e.g., the relative activeness of those who are not infected with any zoonotic or non-zoonotic diseases and can engage fully in life activities), there is inactiveness (e.g., the relative inactiveness of those who are not lucky to have infected with zoonotic and/or non-zoonotic diseases, so they cannot engage fully in life activities).

In relation to the selfness-otherness principle, if there is selfness (e.g., the tendency to be mostly centered on one's self or group, as shown in those infectious agents like "parasites", who survive at the expense of the hosts), there is otherness (e.g., the tendency to be mostly centered on others, as shown in those working in conservation medicine to counter the threat of zoonotic diseases, for the advancement in human health). And the reverse direction also holds true.

In relation to the regression-progression principle, if there is regression (e.g., the regression made by the studies on zoonotic diseases, as shown in the problems pointed out by the critics), there is progression (e.g., the progress made by the studies on zoonotic diseases, as shown in the contribution to the understanding of the carriers and agents of zoonotic diseases aforecited). And the reverse direction also holds true.

In relation to the same-difference principle, if there is similarity in outcome (e.g., the contribution to the molding and control of beliefs, values, and behaviors, regardless of whether this be done by way of zoonosis, or by way of reverse-zoonosis), there is difference in outcome (e.g., the contribution to the molding and control of beliefs, values, and behaviors by way of zoonosis for a relatively more animal-centric lifeworld—but the contribution to the molding and control of beliefs, values, and behaviors by way of reverse-zoonosis for a relatively more human-centric lifeworld). And the reverse direction also holds true.

In relation to the stability-reaction principle, if there is stability (e.g., the relatively more stable condition of "zoonotic pathogens causing foodborne diseases" like "*Escherichia coli* O157:H7, *Campylobacter*, *Caliciviridae*, and *Salmonella*"), there is reaction (e.g., "zoonotic pathogens causing foodborne diseases" then led to further changes later on, when "in 2006, a conference held in Berlin was focusing on the issue of zoonotic pathogen effects on food safety, urging governments to intervene, and the public to be vigilant towards the risks of catching food-borne diseases from farm-to-dining table"). (WK 2013n) And the reverse direction also holds true.

In relation to the functionality-nonfunctionality principle, if there is functionality (e.g., the presence of action for which something or someone is fitted, as shown in the infection, by HIV, of "vital cells in the human immune system such as helper T cells [specifically CD4+ T cells], macrophages, and dendritic cells," which serves the function of spreading zoonotic diseases), there is nonfunctionality (e.g., the relative lack of action for which something or someone is fitted, as shown in the adoption of different "prevention strategies" nowadays, such that HIV is no longer functional in causing zoonotic diseases to the extent as seen in the older days). (WK 2013ii & 2013jj) And the reverse direction also holds true.

In relation to the intentionality-nonintentionality principle, if there is intentionality (e.g., the planning or design of something for a certain outcome, as shown in the original intention of those working in conservation medicine to successfully cope with the threat of zoonotic diseases), there is nonintentionality (e.g., the relative absence of planning or design of something for a certain outcome, such that the outcome can even be counter-intentional in being the opposite of what was originally planned, as shown in the realization nowadays by the critics of conservation medicine that "the environmental causes of health problems are complex, global, and poorly understood," such that the causes and effects of zoonotic diseases can be more complicated than previously thought—contrary to the original intention of those working in conservation medicine to successfully cope with the threat of zoonotic diseases). (WK 2013hh) And the reverse direction also holds true.

And in relation to the survivability-nonsurvivability principle, if there is survivability (e.g., the relative survival of those individuals who suffer from infectious diseases but are benefited from different "prevention strategies" to fight them), there is non-survivability (e.g., the relative non-survival of those unlucky individuals who suffer from infectious diseases, when "the human is actually an accidental victim and a dead-end host"). (WK 2013n & 2013jj) And the reverse direction also holds true.

Physical Health and Society

Physical health, when examined from the perspective of society, can reveal to us some powerful features in relation to its possibility (or impossibility) and desirability (or undesirability), and this can be shown by way of two case studies, namely, (3.4.1) physical health, drug use, and the law, and (3.4.2) physical health, domestic violence, and society—to be addressed hereafter.

Physical Health, Drug Use, and the Law

A good way to evaluate the possibility (or impossibility) and desirability (or undesirability) of physical health from the perspective of society is to explore physical health, drug use, and the law.

An argument in the literature is that, as suggested by "advocates of drug prohibition,...particular drugs should be illegal because they are harmful. Drug Free Australia, for example, argues 'that illicit drugs are inherently harmful substances....' The U.S. government has argued that illegal drugs are 'far more deadly than alcohol' saying 'although alcohol is used by seven times as many people as drugs, the number of deaths induced by those substances is not far apart.'" (WK 2013p; DRA 2010)

In general, the debate on drug use and physical health can touch on different contentious issues. For illustration, consider a few main examples below.

1st Contentious Issue: Efficacy

The first contentious issue in the debate on drug use and physical health concerns "efficacy." As is true in any debate, there are two sides, as shown below.

(a) The Affirmative Side

On the affirmative side (for the idea of efficacy)—"supporters of prohibition claim that prohibitive drug laws have a successful track record suppressing illicit drug use since they were introduced 100 years ago. The licit drug alcohol has current (last 12 months) user rates as high as 80-90% in populations over 14 years of age, and tobacco has historically had current use rates up to 60% of adult populations, yet the percentages currently using illicit drugs in OECD countries are generally below 1% of the population excepting cannabis where most are between 3% and 10%, with six countries between 11% and 17%." (WK 2013p; DRA 2010; D. Gerstein 1998)

(b) The Negative Side

On the negative side (against the idea of efficacy)—the critic like "August Vollmer, founder of the School of Criminology at University of California, Irvine and former president of the International Association of Chiefs of Police" argued in his 1936 book *The Police and Modern Society* that "stringent laws, spectacular police drives, vigorous prosecution, and imprisonment of addicts and peddlers have proved not only useless and enormously expensive as means of correcting this evil, but they are also unjustifiably and unbelievably cruel in their application to the unfortunate drug victims. Repression has driven this vice underground and produced the narcotic smugglers and supply agents, who have grown wealthy out of this evil practice and who, by devious methods, have stimulated traffic in drugs. Finally, and not the least of the evils associated with repression, the helpless addict has been forced to resort to crime in order to get money for the drug which is absolutely indispensable for his comfortable existence." (WK 2013p)

2nd Contentious Issue: Deterrence

The second contentious issue in the debate on drug use and physical health concerns "deterrence." As is true in any debate, there are two sides, as shown below.

(a) The Affirmative Side

On the affirmative side (for the idea of deterrence)—"a 2001 Australian study of 18-29 year olds by the NSW Bureau of Crime Statistics and Research suggests that prohibition deters illicit drug use. 29% of those who had never used cannabis cited the illegality of the substance as their reason for never using the drug, while 19% of those who had ceased use of cannabis cited its illegality as their reason." (WK 2013p; NSW 2010)

And Gil Kerlikowske, Director of the US ONDCP, argued that "controls and prohibitions help to keep prices higher, and higher prices help keep use rates relatively low, since drug use, especially among young people, is known to be sensitive to price. The relationship between pricing and rates of youth substance use is well-established with respect to alcohol and cigarette taxes. There is literature showing that increases in the price of cigarettes triggers declines in use." (WK 2013p; G. Kerlikowske 2010)

(b) The Negative Side

On the negative side (against the idea of deterrence)—"according to a 2009 annual report by the European Monitoring Centre for Drugs and Drug Addiction, the Dutch are among the lowest users of marijuana or cannabis in Europe, despite the Netherlands' policy on soft drugs being one of the most liberal in Europe, allowing for the sale of marijuana at 'coffee shops,' which the Dutch have allowed to operate for decades, and possession of less than 5 grams (0.18 oz)." (WK 2013p; R. Stevenson 2009)

And "the use of drugs by minors is much more difficult to control with drugs prohibited. To effectively regulate the sellers of drugs so as to ensure that they only sell drugs to adults, drugs must be legalized, and the sellers licensed. With drugs prohibited, sellers are 'underground' and therefore nearly impossible to control. Licensed sellers in a community sometimes attempt to increase their income by selling to minors, but when the community suspects such activity, it is a trivial task to discover which of the licensed sellers is breaking the law, and then put them out of business. Underground sellers may adhere to a 'code or honor' and not sell to minors, but, when they do sell to minors, it is very difficult to expose. The difficulty results from the somewhat sophisticated culture of underground drug sales and use that has evolved, with one of the most fundamental adaption mechanisms of this culture that the sellers and consumers act such in such a manner so as to make it as difficult as possible for outsiders to discover information about their activities, including, of course, who is selling to whom." (WK 2013p)

3rd Contentious Issue: Gateway

The third contentious issue in the debate on drug use and physical health concerns "gateway." As is true in any debate, there are two sides, as shown below.

(a) The Affirmative Side

On the affirmative side (for the idea of gateway)—"the US Drug Enforcement Agency's '2008 Marijuana Sourcebook' argues that recent research supports the gateway hypothesis that certain drugs (such as cannabis) act as gateways to use of 'harder' drugs such as heroin, either because of social contact or because of an increasing search for a better high. Proponents cite studies such as that of 311 same sex twins, where only one twin smoked cannabis before age 17, and where such early cannabis smokers were five times more likely than their twin to move on to harder drugs." (WK 2013p; M. Lynskey 2003)

(b) The Negative Side

On the negative side (against the idea of gateway)—"several research studies have addressed the question whether cannabis leads to the use of harder drugs such as cocaine and heroin, and concluded that it does not act as a gateway drug. A study of drug users in Amsterdam over a 10-year period conducted by Jan van Ours of Tilburg University in the Netherlands concluded that cannabis is not a stepping stone to using cocaine or heroin. The study found that there was little difference in the probability of an individual taking up cocaine as to whether or not he or she had used cannabis." (WK 2013p)

In addition, "the US Institute of Medicine found no conclusive evidence that the drug effects of marijuana are causally linked to the subsequent abuse of other illicit drugs. In the American Journal of Public

Health, Andrew Golub and Bruce Johnson of the National Development and Research Institute in New York wrote that young people who smoked marijuana in the generations before and after the baby boomers did not appear to be likely to move on to harder drugs." (WK 2013p; DRUG 2006)

4th Contentious Issue: Medical Use

The fourth contentious issue in the debate on drug use and physical health concerns "medical use." As is true in any debate, there are two sides, as shown below.

(a) The Affirmative Side

On the affirmative side (for the idea of medical use)—"most of the psychoactive drugs now prohibited in modern societies have had medical uses in history. In natural plant drugs like opium, coca, cannabis, mescaline, and psilocybin, the medical history usually dates back thousands of years and through a variety of cultures." (WK 2013p; L. Grinspoon 2013)

And "psychedelics such as LSD and psilocybin (the main ingredient in most hallucinogenic mushrooms) are the subject of renewed research interest because of their therapeutic potential. They could ease a variety of difficult-to-treat mental illnesses, such as chronic depression, post-traumatic stress disorder, and alcohol dependency. MDMA (Ecstasy) has been used for cognitive enhancement in people with Parkinson's Disease, and has shown potential in treating Posttraumatic Stress Disorder." (WK 2013p; D. Brown 2007; S. Pekkanen 1992; NEWS 2006; T. Shroder 2007)

(b) The Negative Side

On the negative side (against the idea of medical use)—"according to Janet D. Lapey, M.D., of Concerned Citizens For Drug Prevention, 'due to a placebo effect, a patient may erroneously believe a drug is helpful when it is not. This is especially true of addictive, mind-altering drugs like marijuana. A marijuana withdrawal syndrome occurs, consisting of anxiety, depression, sleep and appetite disturbances, irritability, tremors, diaphoresis, nausea, muscle convulsions, and restlessness. Often, persons using marijuana erroneously believe that the drug is helping them combat these symptoms without realizing that actually marijuana is the cause of these effects. Therefore, when a patient anecdotally reports a drug to have medicinal value, this must be followed by objective scientific studies.'" (WK 2013p)

And "the US Drug Enforcement Administration also says: 'There is a growing misconception that some illegal drugs can be taken safely. For example, savvy drug dealers have learned how to market drugs like Ecstasy to youth. Some in the Legalization Lobby even claim such drugs have medical value, despite the lack of conclusive scientific evidence.'" (WK 2013p)

5th Contentious Issue: Cost

The fifth contentious issue in the debate on drug use and physical health concerns "cost." As is true in any debate, there are two sides, as shown below.

(a) The Affirmative Side

On the affirmative side (for cost)—"the DEA argues that 'compared to the social costs of drug abuse and addiction—whether in taxpayer dollars or in pain and suffering—government spending on drug control is minimal.'" (WK 2013p)

Antonio Maria Costa, executive director of the United Nations Office on Drugs and Crime, added further that "the economic argument is also based on poor fiscal logic: any reduction in the cost of drug control (due to lower law enforcement expenditure) will be offset by much higher expenditure on public health (due to the surge of drug consumption)." (WK 2013p)

(b) The Negative Side

On the negative side (against cost)—"the United States efforts at drug prohibition started out with a US$ 350 million budget in 1971, and was in 2006 a US$ 30 billion campaign. These numbers only include direct prohibition enforcement expenditures, and as such only represent part of the total cost of prohibition. This $ 30 billion figure rises dramatically once other issues, such as the economic impact of holding 400,000 prisoners on prohibition violations, are factored in." (WK 2013p; CSDP 2007 & 2007a)

Moreover, "the war on drugs is extremely costly to such societies that outlaw drugs in terms of taxpayer money, lives, productivity, the inability of law enforcement to pursue mala in se crimes, and social inequality. Some proponents of decriminalization say that the financial and social costs of drug law enforcement far exceed the damages that the drugs themselves cause. For instance, in 1999 close to 60,000 prisoners (3.3% of the total incarcerated population) convicted of violating marijuana laws were behind bars at a cost to taxpayers of some $ 1.2 billion per year. In 1980, the total jail and prison population was 540,000, about one-quarter the size it is today. Drug offenders accounted for 6% of all prisoners.

According to the Federal Bureau of Prisons, drug offenders now account for nearly 51%." (WK 2013p; M. Friedman 2013)

6th Contentious Issue: Social Order

The sixth contentious issue in the debate on drug use and physical health concerns "social order." As is true in any debate, there are two sides, as shown below.

(a) The Affirmative Side

On the affirmative side (for the idea of social order)—"while concerns are sometimes expressed that the 'war on drugs' can never be won, there is a failure to recognize that other justifiably costly policing wars such as 'blitzes' on speeding can likewise never be won. Such blitzes reduce and contain speeding, as with policing of illicit drug use. Failure to police speeding drivers simply allows inordinate harm to be inflicted on other individuals. Speeding is not legalized simply because it can never be eradicated. There is an argument that much crime and terrorism is drug related or drug funded and that prohibition should reduce this." (WK 2013p; DRA 2010)

And the US Drug Enforcement Administration argued that "crime, violence and drug use go hand in hand. Six times as many homicides are committed by people under the influence of drugs, as by those who are looking for money to buy drugs. Most drug crimes aren't committed by people trying to pay for drugs; they're committed by people on drugs." (WK 2013p)

(b) The Negative Side

On the negative side (against the idea of social order)—"prohibition protects the drug cartel insofar as it keeps the distribution in the black market and creates the risk that makes smuggling profitable." (WK 2013p; A. Trebach 1992)

And "Michael Levine states in relation to his undercover work with Colombian cocaine cartels,from Lamar: 'I learned that not only did they not fear our war on drugs, they *counted on it* to increase the market price and to weed out the smaller, inefficient drug dealers. They found U.S. interdiction efforts laughable. The only U.S. action they feared was an effective demand reduction program. On one undercover tape-recorded conversation, a top cartel chief, Jorge Roman, expressed his gratitude for the drug war, calling it 'a sham put on for the American taxpayer' that was actually 'good for business.'" (WK 2013p; T. Lynch 2000)

7th Contentious Issue: Political Calculation

And the seventh contentious issue in the debate on drug use and physical health concerns "political calculation." As is true in any debate, there are two sides, as shown below.

(a) The Affirmative Side

On the affirmative side (for political calculation)—"John Donnelly, writing for the *Boston Globe* on the presidential race of 2000, suggested that the candidates' silence on drug policy may stem from a widely shared belief that any position even hinting at reducing penalties for drug use would be political suicide. Charles R. Schuster, director of the National Institute on Drug Abuse under Presidents Reagan and Bush (Snr.), was reported as saying in 1997, 'Talking sense about drug policy in today's climate of opinion can be political suicide.'" (WK 2013p)

And "Scott Morgan [2008] reports how he once attended a discussion of Peter Reuter and David Boyum's book 'An Analytic Assessment of U.S. Drug Policy,' in which the authors admitted ignoring the legalization option in their analysis. Boyum claimed that there was no legitimate political support for ending the drug war and that he and Reuter had therefore confined themselves to recommendations that they thought were politically viable." (WK 2013p)

(b) The Negative Side

On the negative side (against political calculation)—"two teenagers deaths in March 2010 triggered nationwide concern about the drug mephedrone in the UK. The Advisory Council on the Misuse of Drugs (ACMD) recommended a ban on 29 March, which was quickly passed into law, but the decision was criticised for being politically rather than scientifically driven and led to the resignation of the ACMD's Eric Carlin, the eighth member of the council to leave in five months in protest at what was seen as political interference. Toxicology reports released later in May 2010 revealed that the boys had never taken the drug." (WK 2013p)

Thus, this led Professor David Nutt, the former chairman of the ACMD, to say that "the previous government's rush to ban mephedrone never had any serious scientific credibility—it looks much more like a decision based on a short-term electoral calculation. This news demonstrates why it's so important to base drug classification on the evidence, not fear, and why the police, media and politicians should only make public pronouncements once the facts are clear." (WK 2013p; J. Laurance 2010)

Beyond Drug Prohibition

These criticisms of both sides in the debate on drug prohibition, however, do not mean a total rejection of its usefulness but serve to show us the two opposing sides of the debate, such that the possibility (or impossibility) and desirability (or undesirability) of physical health (from the perspective of society with physical health, drug use, and the law as a case study here) are not to the extent that the respective defenders would like us to believe.

Furthermore, the analysis of physical health, drug use, and the law is to reveal the refreshing insights of the ontological principles in existential dialectics, and good examples include the formalness-informalness principle, the absoluteness-relativeness principle, the partiality-totality principle, the predictability-unpredictability principle, the explicability-inexplicability principle, the fiction-reality principle, the cognitiveness-noncognitiveness principle, the finiteness-transfiniteness principle, the preciseness-vagueness principle, the simpleness-complicatedness principle, the openness-hiddenness principle, the denseness-emptiness principle, the prototypicality-variation principle, the change-constancy principle, the order-chaos principle, the slowness-quickness principle, the expansion-contraction principle, the optimality-nonoptimality principle, the theory-praxis principle, the convention-novelty principle, the evolution-transformation principle, the symmetry-asymmetry principle, the softness-hardness principle, the seriousness-playfulness principle, the activeness-inactivess principle, the selfness-otherness principle, the regression-progression principle, the same-difference principle, the stability-reaction principle, the functionality-nonfunctionality principle, and the intentionality-nonintentionality principle.

For instance, in relation to the formalness-informalness principle, if there is formalness (e.g., the formal logical requirement of soundness, completeness, and consistency in a system of ideas, as in the debate on drug prohibition), there is informalness (e.g., the non-formal existence of unsoundness, incompleteness, and inconsistency in the debate on drug prohibition, as shown in the different disagreements by both sides on 7 contentious issues aforedescribed). And the reverse direction also holds true.

In relation to the absoluteness-relativeness principle, if there is absoluteness (e.g., the absolute view on the idea of social order by the affirmative side in the debate on drug prohibition), there is relativeness (e.g., what is right for the affirmative side in regard to the idea of social order is not necessarily so for the negative side in the debate on drug prohibition). And the reverse direction also holds true.

In relation to the partiality-totality principle, if there is partiality (e.g., the partial view on deterrence by the affirmative side), there is totality (e.g., the more holistic view on deterrence, such that the whole is not the sum of its parts, that is, it cannot be reduced to the sum of opposing views by the affirmative side, the negative side, etc., since there will emerge new views in the future not yet known today, just as there are already alternative views nowadays which do not side exclusively with any of them, as is the analysis here). And the reverse direction also holds true.

In relation to the predictability-unpredictability principle, if there is predictability (e.g., the predictable tendency of "The United States Drug Enforcement Administration [DEA]...to suggest that illegal drugs are 'far more deadly than alcohol'" for drug prohibition), there is unpredictability (e.g., the more difficult task to predict exactly the extent to which the health statistics by DEA will be accurate on a particular future occasion, because of the tendency of DEA to engage in "misleading health statistics," in that "the DEA's use of such figures is questionable," for example). (WK 2013p) And the reverse direction also holds true.

In relation to the explicability-inexplicability principle, if there is explicability (e.g., the explanation, by those in the DEA, of the desirability of drug prohibition, on the ground that "compared to the social costs of drug abuse and addiction—whether in taxpayer dollars or in pain and suffering—government spending on drug control is minimal"), there is inexplicability (e.g., the lack of sufficient explanation, by those in the DEA, of why their calculation of "cost" in the enforcement of drug prohibition is accurate, since, for the critics, "these numbers only include direct prohibition enforcement expenditures, and as such only represent part of the total cost of prohibition," but "rise...dramatically once other issues, such as the economic impact of holding 400,000 prisoners on prohibition violations, are factored in" and "the war on drugs is extremely costly to such societies that outlaw drugs in terms of taxpayer money, lives, productivity, the inability of law enforcement to pursue mala in se crimes, and social inequality"). And the reverse direction also holds true.

In relation to the fiction-reality principle, if there is fiction (e.g., the fictional aspect of the figures on "drug-induced deaths" in 2000 povided by the Centers for Disease Control and Prevention, insofar as the actual "number deaths caused by alcohol in year 2000" was "85,000—over four and a half times greater than the DEA's preferred figure," according to "the Journal of the American Medical Association"), there is reality (e.g., the realistic aspect of the figures on "drug-induced deaths" in 2000 provided by the Centers for Disease Control and Prevention, insofar as in

2000, there were quite a few thousand drug-induced deaths). (WK 2013p) And the reverse direction also holds true.

In relation to the cognitiveness-noncognitiveness principle, if there is cognitiveness (e.g., a view of things on the basis of reason and evidences, as shown in the empirical finding by Scott Morgan that "there was no legitimate political support for ending the drug war" in the U.S. in 2008), there is noncognitiveness (e.g., a view of things on the basis of non-cognitive factors like envy, jealousy, power, nationality, race, gender, age, class, greed, lust, status, faith, anger, sadness, joy, fear, wish, etc., as shown in the "political calculation" by Peter Reuter and David Boyum, who in their book *An Analytic Assessment of U.S. Drug Policy* "admitted ignoring the legalization option in their analysis," because "there was no legitimate political support for ending the drug war" at the time, regardless of whether or not they personally believed in the legalization option). And the reverse direction also holds true.

In relation to the finiteness-transfiniteness principle, if there is finiteness (e.g., the finite number of the categories of "natural plant drugs," namely, "opium, coca, cannabis, mescaline, and psilocybin," for example), there is transfiniteness (e.g., the transfinite number of all the individual pieces of "opium, coca, cannabis, mescaline, and psilocybin" that have ever existed in history). And the reverse direction also holds true.

In relation to the preciseness-vagueness principle, if there is preciseness (e.g., the precise identification of 7 contentious issues in the debate on drug prohibition in the article aforecited), there is vagueness (e.g., the vagueness in the identification of the 7 contentious issues in the debate on drug prohibition in the article aforecited, since it is not clear why there must be only these 7, not 13, 16, 19, 21, 24, 27, and so on). And the reverse direction also holds true.

In relation to the simpleness-complicatedness principle, if there is simpleness (e.g., the relatively simple analysis of drug prohibition by the affirmative side), there is complicatedness (e.g., the relatively more complicated analysis of drug prohibition, by challenging the claims and assumptions, as shown in the problems pointed out by the negative side as cited). And the reverse direction also holds true.

In relation to the openness-hiddenness principle, if there is openness (e.g., the open exploration of the relationship between drug use and death by "The United States Drug Enforcement Administration [DEA]"), there is hiddenness (e.g., the hidden bias in the figures on drug-induced deaths by the DEA, since the critics revealed the tendency of DEA to engage in "misleading health statistics," in that "the DEA's use of such figures is questionable," for example). And the reverse direction also holds true.

In relation to the denseness-emptiness principle, if there is denseness (e.g., the relatively denser concentration of concerns with supporting "the gateway hypothesis that certain drugs [such as cannabis] act as gateways to use of 'harder' drugs such as heroin" by "the US Drug Enforcement Agency's '2008 Marijuana Sourcebook'"), there is emptiness (e.g., the relatively less dense, or more empty, concentration of concerns with supporting "the gateway hypothesis" by the "study of drug users in Amsterdam over a 10-year period conducted by Jan van Ours of Tilburg University in the Netherlands," which "concluded that cannabis is not a stepping stone to using cocaine or heroin"). And the reverse direction also holds true.

In relation to the prototypicality-variation principle, if there is prototypicality (e.g., the prototype, like the example about the original medical uses of "natural plant drugs like opium, coca, cannabis, mescaline, and psilocybin," which can be dated "back thousands of years and through a variety of cultures" in antiquity), there is variation (e.g., different variants of the protoptye, as shown in many studies and uses of natural plant drugs since the orignal medical uses thousands of years ago, like the modern use of these drugs in American and European countries nowadays, though each country with its own variations, purposes, and regulations). And the reverse direction also holds true.

In relation to the change-constancy principle, if there is change (e.g., the ever new ways to understand drug use, as shown in the debate on physical health and drug use afore-discussed), there is constancy (e.g., the ever constant existence of different problems with the ever new ways to understand drug use, as shown in the contentious disagreements between both sides in the debate on physical health and drug use afore-discussed). And the reverse direction also holds true.

In relation to the order-chaos principle, if there is order (e.g., the more or less orderly view on physical health and drug use, if looked from the sole vantage point of the contribution to "social order" aforedescribed), there is chaos (e.g., the more or less chaotic view on physical health and drug use, if looked from the multiple, conflicting vantage points of both sides in the debate on social order and other contentious issues aforediscussed). And the reverse direction also holds true.

In relation to the slowness-quickness principle, if there is slowness (e.g., the relatively slower speed for an individual to ever get "addictive" if he consumes an extremely small dose of "opium, coca, cannabis, mescaline, and psilocybin" or none at all), there is quickness (e.g., the relatively quicker speed for an individual to get "addictive" if he consumes a lot of "opium, coca, cannabis, mescaline, and psilocybin"). (WK 2013p) And the reverse direction also holds true.

In relation to the expansion-contraction principle, if there is expansion (e.g., the relative expansion of "the 'Just Say No' campaign, initiated under the patronage of Nancy Reagan" in the 1980s), there is contraction (e.g., the relative decline of "illicit drug use…from 14.1% in 1979 to 5.8% in 1992, a drop of 60%" after "the 'Just Say No' campaign"). (WK 2013p) And the reverse direction also holds true.

In relation to the optimality-nonoptimality principle, if there is optimality (e.g., the search for highly favorable options, like the quest for the most effective deterrence against drug use, in that, as explained by Gil Kerlikowske, Director of the US ONDCP, "controls and prohibitions help to keep prices higher, and higher prices help keep use rates relatively low, since drug use, especially among young people, is known to be sensitive to price"), there is nonoptimality (e.g., the existence of non-optimal alternatives to optimality, like the argument for more realistic studies by the critics, who pointed out the negative side of the debate, against the idea of deterrence aforecited). And the reverse direction also holds true.

In relation to the theory-praxis principle, if there is theory (e.g., the theoretical construction of "cost," "price," "demand," etc. in economics), there is praxis (e.g., the practical application of "cost," "price," "demand," etc. in economics to the field of drug prohibition, as shown in the debate on "cost"). And the reverse direction also holds true.

In relation to the convention-novelty principle, if there is convention (e.g., the conventional wisdom about drug prohibition for "social order"), there is novelty (e.g., the alternative novel challenge to the conventional wisdom about drug prohibition for "social order," by the new idea that "prohibition protects the drug cartel insofar as it keeps the distribution in the black market and creates the risk that makes smuggling profitable"). And the reverse direction also holds true.

In relation to the evolution-transformation principle, if there is evolution (e.g., the natural evolution of humans to consume plants, including "natural plant drugs," in the state of nature), there is transformation (e.g., the technical transformation of human ability to deal with plants, including "natural plant drugs," by the invention of the knowledge discourse on different contentious issues about drug prohibition). And the reverse direction also holds true.

In relation to the symmetry-asymmetry principle, if there is symmetry (e.g., the co-existence of different agents in regard to drug prohibition, like drug users and law enforcement authorities), there is asymmetry (e.g., law enforcement authorities can arrest and detain drug users under certain legal conditions). And the reverse direction also holds true.

In relation to the softness-hardness principle, if there is softness (e.g., the defense of drug prohibition for social order by the affirmative side), there is hardness (e.g., the critique of drug prohibition for social order, as shown in the problems pointed out by the negative side as cited). And the reverse direction also holds true.

In relation to the seriousness-playfulness principle, if there is seriousness (e.g., the serious business of those who try to cope with the problem of drug use), there is playfulness (e.g., the playful part of those in who try to cope with the problem of drug use, when they play around with different arguments over the centuires, as shown in the debate on 7 contentious issues by both sides afore-discussed). And the reverse direction also holds true.

In relation to the activeness-inactivess principle, if there is activeness (e.g., the relative activeness of those who do not suffer from any drug-induced problems and can fully engage in life activities), there is inactiveness (e.g., the relative inactiveness of those who suffer from drug-induced problems to the point of death, so they cannot engage fully in life activities).

In relation to the selfness-otherness principle, if there is selfness (e.g., the tendency to be mostly centered on one's self or group, as shown in those illicit drug users, who in the process negatively affect others close or related to them like "children, parents, grandparents, friends, colleagues, work, victims of drugged drivers, crime victims, elder abuse, sexual victims etc.," so that "illicit drug use is no less victimless than alcoholism"), there is otherness (e.g., the tendency to be mostly centered on others, as shown in the argument by Aldous Huxley, and Terence McKenna, who argued that "persons should be able to do whatever they want with their bodies, including the recreational use of drugs, as long as they do not harm others," as an advancement in civil rights for all). (WK 2013p) And the reverse direction also holds true.

In relation to the regression-progression principle, if there is regression (e.g., the regression made by drug prohibition, as shown in the problems pointed out by the negative side), there is progression (e.g., the progress made by drug prohibition, as shown in the positive effects pointed out by the affirmative side). And the reverse direction also holds true.

In relation to the same-difference principle, if there is similarity in outcome (e.g., the contribution to the molding and control of beliefs, values, and behaviors, regardless of whether this be done by way of appealing to the argument on cost, or by way of appealing to the argument on social order), there is difference in outcome (e.g., the contribution to the molding and control of beliefs, values, and behaviors by way of appealing to the argument on cost for a relatively more economic worldview—but the contribution to the molding and control of beliefs, values, and behaviors by way of appealing to the argument on social order for a relatively more political worldview). And the reverse direction also holds true.

In relation to the stability-reaction principle, if there is stability (e.g., the relatively more stable condition of using "natural plant drugs like opium, coca, cannabis, mescaline, and psilocybin" for medical uses in antiquity), there is reaction (e.g., using "natural plant drugs like opium, coca, cannabis, mescaline, and psilocybin" for medical uses in antiquity then led to further changes later on, when nowadays in the U.S., there are regulations concerning drug use). And the reverse direction also holds true.

In relation to the functionality-nonfunctionality principle, if there is functionality (e.g., the presence of action for which something or someone is fitted, as shown in the use of "natural plant drugs like opium, coca, cannabis, mescaline, and psilocybin" in antiquity, which served the function of medical and other uses at that time), there is nonfunctionality (e.g., the relative lack of action for which something or someone is fitted, as shown in the "political calculation" by Peter Reuter and David Boyum, who in their book *An Analytic Assessment of U.S. Drug Policy* "admitted ignoring the legalization option in their analysis," because "there was no legitimate political support for ending the drug war," such that the old-fashioned use of "natural plant drugs like opium, coca, cannabis, mescaline, and psilocybin" in antiquity is no longer functional in contemporary American society). And the reverse direction also holds true.

In relation to the intentionality-nonintentionality principle, if there is intentionality (e.g., the planning or design of something for a certain outcome, as shown in the original intention of those pushing for laws to prohibit drug use, so as to get rid of organized crime associated with it, since the US Drug Enforcement Administration argued that "crime, violence and drug use go hand in hand"), there is nonintentionality (e.g., the relative absence of planning or design of something for a certain outcome, such that the outcome can even be counter-intentional in being the opposite of what was originally planned, as shown in the unintended consequence of "drug prohibition," which ends up protecting "the drug cartel insofar as it keeps the distribution in the black market and creates the risk that makes smuggling profitable"—contrary to the original intention of those pushing for laws to prohibit drug use, so as to get rid of organized crime associated with it). And the reverse direction also holds true.

And in relation to the survivability-nonsurvivability principle, if there is survivability (e.g., the relative survival of those minimal drug users who do not suffer much from drug-induced problems, let alone death), there is non-survivability (e.g., the relative non-survival of those heavy drug users who died due to drug-induced deaths). And the reverse direction also holds true.

Physical Health, Domestic Violence, and Society

Another good way to evaluate the possibility (or impossibility) and desirability (or undesirability) of physical health from the perspective of society is to explore physical health, domestic violence, and society.

An argument in the literature is that "domestic violence" (which "involves the abuse by one partner against another in an intimate relationship such as marriage, cohabitation, dating or within the family") is to be prevented in society. (WK 2013kk)

Definitions of Domestic Violence

There are different definitions of "domestic violence." For illustration, consider four main examples below (as summarized in *Table 3.5*).

(a) Government Definitions

In regard to "government definitions"—"the US Office on Violence Against Women (OVW) defines domestic violence as a 'pattern of abusive behavior in any relationship that is used by one partner to gain or maintain power and control over another intimate partner.' The definition adds that domestic violence 'can happen to anyone regardless of race, age, sexual orientation, religion, or gender,' and can take many forms, including physical abuse, sexual abuse, emotional, economic, and psychological abuse." (WK 2013kk; OVW 2007)

And "the Children and Family Court Advisory and Support Service in the United Kingdom in its 'Domestic Violence Policy' uses domestic violence to refer to a range of violent and abusive behaviours, defining it as: 'Patterns of behaviour characterised by the misuse of power and control by one person over another who are or have been in an intimate relationship. It can occur in mixed gender relationships and same gender relationships and has profound consequences for the lives of children, individuals, families and communities. It may be physical, sexual, emotional and/or psychological. The latter may include intimidation, harassment, damage to property, threats and financial abuse.'" (WK 2013kk; CFCASS 2007)

(b) Dynamics Classification

In regard to "dynamics classification"—"violence by a person against their intimate partner is often done as a way for controlling their partner, even if this kind of violence is not the most frequent. Many types of intimate partner violence occur, including violence between gay and lesbian couples, and by women against their male partners." (WK 2013kk; D. Laroche 2004; C. Renzetti 1996; M. Johnson 2000)

(c) Intimate Partner Violence Types

In regard to "intimate partner violence types"—"Michael P. Johnson [1995 & 2006] argues for four major types of intimate partner violence, which is supported by subsequent research and evaluation as well as independent researchers," as shown below: (WK 2013kk)

- "Common Couple Violence (CCV)"—"is not connected to general control behavior, but arises in a single argument where one or both partners physically lash out at the other."
- "Intimate Terrorism (IT)"—"may also involve emotional and psychological abuse. Intimate terrorism is one element in a general pattern of control by one partner over the other. Intimate terrorism is less common than common couple violence, more likely to escalate over time, not as likely to be mutual, and more likely to involve serious injury. IT batterers include two types: 'Generally-violent-antisocial' and 'dysphoric-borderline.' The first type includes people with general psychopathic and violent tendencies. The second type are people who are emotionally dependent on the relationship. Support for this typology has been found in subsequent evaluations."
- "Violent Resistance (VR)"—is "sometimes thought of as 'self-defense'" and "is violence perpetrated by victims against their abusive partners."
- "Mutual Violent Control (MVC)"—"is rare type of intimate partner violence occurring when both partners act in a violent manner, battling for control."

Of course, there can be other types, so the ones above are illustrative.

(d) Other Definitions

For example, "the US Centers for Disease Control...divide[s] domestic violence into two types: reciprocal, in which both partners are violent, and non-reciprocal violence, in which one partner is violent; it is possible that the former is more common." (WK 2013kk; D. Whitaker 2007; M. Straus 2006)

Forms of Domestic Violence

These definitions aside—domestic violence can come in different shapes and sizes. Hereafter are some illustrative examples (as summarized in *Table 3.5*).

(a) Physical

In relation to the "physical" form of domestic violence—"physical abuse is abuse involving contact intended to cause feelings of intimidation, pain, injury, or other physical suffering or bodily harm. Physical abuse includes hitting, slapping, punching, choking, pushing, burning and other types of contact that result in physical injury to the victim. Physical abuse can also include behaviors such as denying the victim of medical care when needed, depriving the victim of sleep or other functions necessary to live, or forcing the victim to engage in drug/alcohol use against his/her will. If a person is suffering from any physical harm then they are experiencing physical abuse. This pain can be experienced on any level. It can also include inflicting physical injury onto other targets, such as children or pets, in order to cause psychological harm to the victim." (WK 2013kk)

(b) Sexual

In relation to the "sexual" form of domestic violence—"sexual abuse is any situation in which force or threat is used to obtain participation in unwanted sexual activity. Coercing a person to engage in sexual activity against their will, even if that person is a spouse or intimate partner with whom consensual sex has occurred, is an act of aggression and violence." (WK 2013kk)

In addition, "marital rape, also known as spousal rape, is non-consensual sex in which the perpetrator is the victim's spouse. As such, it is a form of partner rape, of domestic violence, and of sexual abuse. In the US spousal rape is illegal in all 50 states. In Canada, spousal rape was outlawed in 1983, when several legal changes were made, including changing the rape statute to sexual assault, and making the laws gender neutral." (WK 2013kk; J. Barden 1987)

(c) Emotional

In relation to the "emotional" form of domestic violence—"emotional abuse (also called psychological abuse or mental abuse) can include humiliating the victim privately or publicly, controlling what the victim can and cannot do, withholding information from the victim, deliberately doing something to make the victim feel diminished or embarrassed, isolating the victim from friends and family, implicitly blackmailing the victim by harming others when the victim expresses independence or happiness, or denying the victim access to money or other basic resources and necessities. Degradation in any form can be considered psychological abuse." (WK 2013kk)

Also, "emotional abuse can include verbal abuse and is defined as any behavior that threatens, intimidates, undermines the victim's self-worth or self-esteem, or controls the victim's freedom. This can include threatening the victim with injury or harm, telling the victim that they will be killed if they ever leave the relationship, and public humiliation. Constant criticism, name-calling, and making statements that damage the victim's self-esteem are also common verbal forms of emotional abuse....Emotional abuse includes conflicting actions or statements which are designed to confuse and create insecurity in the victim. These behaviors also lead the victims to question themselves, causing them to believe that they are making up the abuse or that the abuse is their fault." (WK 2013kk; D. Follingstad 2000)

(d) Verbal

In relation to the "verbal" form of domestic violence— "verbal abuse is a form of emotionally abusive behavior involving the use of language. Verbal abuse can also be referred to as the act of threatening. Through threatening a person can blatantly say they will harm you in any way and will also be considered as abuse. It may include profanity but can occur with or without the use of expletives." (WK 2013kk)

For instance, "verbal abuse may include aggressive actions such as name-calling, blaming, ridicule, disrespect, and criticism, but there are also less obviously aggressive forms of verbal abuse. Statements that may seem benign on the surface can be thinly veiled attempts to humiliate; falsely accuse; or manipulate others to submit to undesirable behavior, make others feel unwanted and unloved, threaten others economically, or isolate victims from support systems." (WK 2013kk)

(e) Economic

In relation to the "economic" form of domestic violence—"economic abuse is a form of abuse when one intimate partner has control over the other partner's access to economic resources. Economic abuse may involve preventing a spouse from resource acquisition, limiting the amount of resources to use by the victim, or by exploiting economic resources of the victim. The motive behind preventing a spouse from acquiring resources is to diminish victim's capacity to support his/herself, thus forcing him/her to depend on the perpetrator financially, which includes preventing the victim from obtaining education, finding employment, maintaining or advancing their careers, and acquiring assets." (WK 2013kk; A. Adams 2008; M. Brewster 2003)

Moreover, "the abuser may also put the victim on an allowance, closely monitor how the victim spends money, spend victim's money without his/her consent and creating debt, or completely spend victim's savings to limit available resources." (WK 2013kk)

Causes of Domestic Violence

There are various causes of domestic violence. Consider, for example, the following ones (as summarized in *Table 3.5*).

(a) Biological

In relation to the "biological" cause of domestic violence—"these factors include genetics and brain dysfunction and are studied by neuroscience," and the work by C. Patrick (2008) on "psychophysiological correlates of aggression and violence" is a good case in point.

(b) Psychological

In relation to the "psychological" cause of domestic violence—"psychological theories focus on personality traits and mental characteristics of the offender. Personality traits include sudden bursts of anger, poor impulse control, and poor self-esteem. Various theories suggest that psychopathology and other personality disorders are factors, and that abuse experienced as a child leads some people to be more violent as adults. Correlation has been found between juvenile delinquency and domestic violence in adulthood. Studies have found high incidence of psychopathy among abusers." (WK 2013kk)

Two good case studies are about "mental illness" and "marital conflict disorder," as shown below: (WK 2013kk; R. Siemieniuk 2010)

- "Mental Illness"—refers to "any psychiatric disorders" which "are risk factors for domestic violence, including several personality disorders: all Cluster B PDs, (especially antisocial), paranoid and passive-aggressive. Bipolar disorder, schizophrenia, drug abuse, alcoholism and poor impulse control are also risk factors. It is estimated that at least one-third of all abusers have some type of mental illness."

- "Marital Conflict Disorder"—refers to "marital disorders" which "sometimes come to clinical attention because the couple recognize long-standing dissatisfaction with their marriage and come to the clinician on their own initiative or are referred by an astute health care professional. Secondly, there is serious violence in the marriage which is—'usually the husband battering the wife.'"

Surely, there can be other case studies too, like the one about "jealousy," in which "one partner is either suspected of being unfaithful or is planning to leave the relationship," so domestic violence occurs subsequently. (WK 2013kk; J. Roach 2011; A. Goetz 2010)

(c) Behavioral

In relation to the "behavioral" cause of domestic violence—"behavioral theories draw on the work of behavior analysts. Applied behavior analysis uses the basic principles of learning theory to change behavior. Behavioral theories of domestic violence focus on the use of functional assessment with the goal of reducing episodes of violence to zero rates. This program leads to behavior therapy. Often by identifying the antecedents and consequences of violent action, the abusers can be taught self control. Recently more focus has been placed on prevention and a behavioral prevention theory." (WK 2013kk; R. Shorey 2008)

(d) Social

And in relation to the "social" cause of domestic violence—there are different focuses on social factors. Consider, for illustration, the following examples:

- "Resource"—refers to the focus "suggested by William Goode [1971]. Women who are most dependent on the spouse for economic well being (e.g. homemakers/housewives, women with handicaps, the unemployed), and are the primary caregiver to their children, fear the increased financial burden if they leave their marriage. Dependency means that they have fewer options and few resources to help them cope with or change their spouse's behavior." (WK 2013kk)
- "Social Stress"—refers to stress which "may be increased when a person is living in a family situation, with increased pressures. Social stresses, due to inadequate finances or other such problems in a family may further increase tensions. Violence is not always caused

by stress, but may be one way that some people respond to stress. Families and couples in poverty may be more likely to experience domestic violence, due to increased stress and conflicts about finances and other aspects." (WK 2013kk; J. Seltzer 1988; C. Aneshensel 1992; R. Jewkes 2002)

- "Social Learning"—refers to the learning that people have "from observing and modeling after others' behavior. With positive reinforcement, the behavior continues. If one observes violent behavior, one is more likely to imitate it. If there are no negative consequences (e. g. victim accepts the violence, with submission), then the behavior will likely continue. Often, violence is transmitted from generation to generation in a cyclical manner." (WK 2013kk; D. Doumas 1994)
- "Power and control"—refers to an "abusive relationship," in which "violence is posited to arise out of a need for power and control of one partner over the other. An abuser will use various tactics of abuse (e.g., physical, verbal, emotional, sexual or financial) in order to establish and maintain control over the partner. Abusers' efforts to dominate their partners have been attributed to low self-esteem or feelings of inadequacy, unresolved childhood conflicts, the stress of poverty, hostility and resentment toward women (misogyny), hostility and resentment toward men (misandry), personality disorders, genetic tendencies and sociocultural influences, among other possible causative factors." (WK 2013kk)

Of course, there can be other causes, so the ones above are illustrative.

Effects of Domestic Violence

Regardless of the causes, domestic violence can produce some effects. Consider, for illustration, some main ones below (as summarized in *Table 3.5*).

(a) Physical

In relation to the "physical" effect of domestic violence—"bruises, broken bones, head injuries, lacerations, and internal bleeding are some of the acute effects of a domestic violence incident that require medical attention and hospitalization. Some chronic health conditions that have been linked to victims of domestic violence are arthritis, irritable bowel syndrome, chronic pain, pelvic pain, ulcers, and migraines. Victims who are pregnant during a domestic violence relationship experience greater risk of miscarriage, pre-term labor, and injury to or death of the fetus." (WK 2013kk; R. Jones 1997; D. Berrios 1991)

(b) Psychological

In relation to the "psychological" effect of domestic violence—"among victims who are still living with their perpetrators high amounts of stress, fear, and anxiety are commonly reported. Depression is also common, as victims are made to feel guilty for 'provoking' the abuse and are frequently subjected to intense criticism. It is reported that 60% of victims meet the diagnostic criteria for depression, either during or after termination of the relationship, and have a greatly increased risk of suicidality." (WK 2013kk; O. Barnett 2001)

In addition, "victims of domestic violence also commonly experience long-term anxiety and panic, and are likely to meet the diagnostic criteria for Generalized Anxiety Disorder and Panic Disorder. The most commonly referenced psychological effect of domestic violence is Post-Traumatic Stress Disorder (PTSD). PTSD (as experienced by victims) is characterized by flashbacks, intrusive images, exaggerated startle response, nightmares, and avoidance of triggers that are associated with the abuse. These symptoms are generally experienced for a long span of time after the victim has left the dangerous situation. Many researchers state that PTSD is possibly the best diagnosis for those suffering from psychological effects of domestic violence, as it accounts for the variety of symptoms commonly experienced by victims of trauma." (WK 2013kk; S. Vitanza 1995)

(c) Financial

In relation to the "financial" effect of domestic violence—"due to economic abuse and isolation, the victim usually has very little money of their own and few people on whom they can rely when seeking help. This has been shown to be one of the greatest obstacles facing victims of DV, and the strongest factor that can discourage them from leaving their perpetrators." (WK 2013kk)

Also, "victims of DV often lack specialized skills, education, and training that are necessary to find gainful employment, and also may have several children to support. In 2003,...one out of every three homeless women are homeless due to having left a DV relationship. If a victim is able to secure rental housing, it is likely that her apartment complex will have 'zero tolerance' policies for crime; these policies can cause them to face eviction even if they are the victim (not the perpetrator) of violence. While the number of shelters and community resources available to DV victims has grown tremendously, these agencies often have few employees and hundreds of victims seeking assistance which causes many victims to remain without the assistance they need." (WK 2013kk)

(d) Long-Term

And in relation to the "long-term" effect of domestic violence—"domestic violence can trigger many different responses in victims, all of which are very relevant for any professional working with a victim." (WK 2013kk)

A good case study concerns the effects on "children," because "there has been an increase in acknowledgment that a child who is exposed to domestic abuse during their upbringing will suffer in their developmental and psychological welfare. Because of the awareness of domestic violence that some children have to face, it also generally impacts how the child develops emotionally, socially, behaviorally as well as cognitively." (WK 2013kk; L. Dodd 2009; A. Lazenbatt 2009)

In fact, "some emotional and behavioral problems that can result due to domestic violence include increased aggressiveness, anxiety, and changes in how a child socializes with friends, family, and authorities. Depression, as well as self-esteem issues, can follow due to traumatic experiences. Problems with attitude and cognition in schools can start developing, along with a lack of skills such as problem-solving. Correlation has been found between the experience of abuse and neglect in childhood and perpertrating domestic violence and sexual abuse in adulthood." (WK 2013kk; L. Dodd 2009)

Prevention of Domestic Violence

With these effects of domestic violence in mind—"there are many community organizations which work to prevent domestic violence by offering safe shelter, crisis intervention, advocacy, and education and prevention programs. Community screening for domestic violence can be more systematic in cases of animal abuse, healthcare settings, emergency departments, behavioral health settings and court systems. Tools are being developed to facilitate domestic violence screening such as mobile apps." (WK 2013kk)

In addition, major programs for prevention also include "medical response," "law enforcement," "counseling for person affected," and "counseling for offenders." (WK 2013kk)

Problems with the Study on Domestic Violence

However, for the critics, this study of physical health, domestic violence, and society has some major problems. Consider, for illustration, a few examples below (as summarized in *Table 3.5*).

Firstly, one main criticism of the study of physical health, domestic violence, and society is that there are competing defintions of "domestic violence."

For example, for the critics, the different definitions (as discussed earlier) reveals different views of what constitutes domestic violence.

Secondly, another main criticism of the study of physical health, domestic violence, and society is that there is too much attention to domestic violence by men against women, but not by women against men.

For instance, for the critics, in the case about "marital conflict"—"there is current considerable controversy over whether male-to-female marital violence is best regarded as a reflection of male psychopathology and control or whether there is an empirical base and clinical utility for conceptualizing these patterns as relational." (WK 2013kk) In fact, "modern research into predictors of injury from domestic violence finds that the strongest predictor of injury by domestic violence is participation in reciprocal domestic violence, and that this pattern of domestic violence is more often initiated by the female in the relationship." (WK 2013kk; D. Whitaker 2007) And "there has been controversy as the Duluth framework depends on a strict 'patriarchal violence' model and presumes that all violence in the home and elsewhere has a male perpetrator and female victim. Also evidence of success of the model is limited, with scholarly analysis and critique." (WK 2013kk)

Thirdly, still another main criticism of the study of physical health, domestic violence, and society is that the theories are "disputed."

For instance, for the critics, "the...psychological theories [about the causes of domestic violence] are disputed: Gelles suggests that psychological theories are limited, and points out that other researchers have found that only 10% (or less) fit this psychological profile." (WK 2013kk)

Fourthly, an additional main criticism of the study of physical health, domestic violence, and society is that each approach is limited to itself.

For instance, "critics of the...model [of power and control] argue that it ignores research linking domestic violence to substance abuse and psychological problems. Some modern research into the patterns in DV has found that women are more likely to be physically abusive towards their partner in relationships in which only one partner is violent, which draws the effectiveness of using concepts like male privilege to treat domestic violence into question." (WK 2013kk; M. Straus 2006; D. Whitaker 2007; M. Twohey 2009)

Fifthly, another additional main criticism of the study of physical health, domestic violence, and society is that the prevention of domestic violence is not as successful as claimed.

For instance, for the critics, "The health care professional has not always met this role, with uneven quality of care, and in some cases misunderstandings about domestic violence." (WK 2013kk; P. Abbott 1999) And "Washaw (1993) suggests that many doctors prefer not to get involved in people's 'private' lives. Clifton, Jacobs, and Tulloch (1996) found that training for general practitioners in the United States about domestic violence was very limited or they had no training. Abbott and Williamson found that knowledge and understanding of domestic violence was very limited among health care professionals in a Midlands, United Kingdom county, and that they do not see themselves as being able to play a major role in helping women in regards to domestic violence. Furthermore, in the biomedical model of health care, injuries are often just treated and diagnosed…." (WK 2013kk)

Sixthly, still another additional main criticism of the study of physical health, domestic violence, and society is that the prevention of domestic violence may only be temporary.

For instance, for the critics, "in the replication studies which were far more broad and methodologically sound in both size and scope, arrest seemed to help in the short run in certain cases, but those arrested experienced double the rate of violence over the course of one year." (WK 2013kk; J. Schmidt 1993) Even "criminologists do not fully understand the reasons why deterrent effects do not last over time." (WK 2013kk)

Seventhly, still another additional main criticism of the study of physical health, domestic violence, and society is that the call for the prevention of domestic violence is culturally relative.

For instance, "in 2010, the United Arab Emirates's Supreme Court ruled that a man has the right to physically discipline his wife and children as long as he doesn't leave physical marks." (WK 2013kk; CNN 2010) And "according to a UNICEF survey, the percentage of *women* aged 15–49 who think that a husband is justified in hitting or beating his wife under certain circumstances is, for example: 90% in Jordan, 85.6% in Guinea, 85.4% in Zambia, 85% in Sierra Leone, 81.2% in Laos, 81% in Ethiopia." (WK 2013kk)

And eighthly, one last main criticism of the study of physical health, domestic violence, and society is that the victims are not so completely innocent as conventionally assumed.

For instance, for the critics, "domestic abuse crosses all racial, ethnic and economic boundaries….Why do these women stay and endure so much violence from their men? When they finally complain to law enforcement authorities, they often recant, refusing to cooperate with the criminal justice system and actually protect their abusers…." (R. Klieman 2013)

Beyond Domestic Violence

These criticisms of the studies on domestic violence, however, should not be misunderstood as a total rejection of their usefulness but serve to show us the two opposing sides of the debate, such that the possibility (or impossibility) and desirability (or undesirability) of physical health (from the perspective of society with physical health, domestic violence, and society as a case study here) are not to the extent that the respective defenders would like us to believe.

In addition, the analysis of physical health, domestic violence, and society can cast a bright light on the ontological principles in existential dialectics, and good examples include the formalness-informalness principle, the absoluteness-relativeness principle, the partiality-totality principle, the predictability-unpredictability principle, the explicability-inexplicability principle, the fiction-reality principle, the cognitiveness-noncognitiveness principle, the finiteness-transfiniteness principle, the preciseness-vagueness principle, the simpleness-complicatedness principle, the openness-hiddenness principle, the denseness-emptiness principle, the prototypicality-variation principle, the change-constancy principle, the order-chaos principle, the slowness-quickness principle, the expansion-contraction principle, the optimality-nonoptimality principle, the theory-praxis principle, the convention-novelty principle, the evolution-transformation principle, the symmetry-asymmetry principle, the softness-hardness principle, the seriousness-playfulness principle, the activeness-inactivess principle, the selfness-otherness principle, the regression-progression principle, the same-difference principle, the stability-reaction principle, the functionality-nonfunctionality principle, and the intentionality-nonintentionality principle.

For instance, in relation to the formalness-informalness principle, if there is formalness (e.g., the formal logical requirement of soundness, completeness, and consistency in a system of ideas, as in the studies on domestic violence), there is informalness (e.g., the non-formal existence of unsoundness, incompleteness, and inconsistency in the studies on domestic violence, as shown in the criticisms that there are competing defintions of "domestic violence," that there is too much attention to domestic violence by men against women [but not by women against men too], that the theories are "disputed," that each approach is limited to itself, that the prevention of domestic violence is not as successful as claimed, that the prevention of domestic violence may only be temporary, the call for the prevention of domestic violence is culturally relative, and the victims are not so completely innocent as conventionally assumed). And the reverse direction also holds true.

In relation to the absoluteness-relativeness principle, if there is absoluteness (e.g., the absolute view on domestic violence by men against women by the feminists), there is relativeness (e.g., what is right for the feminists in regard to their obsession with domestic violence by men against women is not necessarily so for the critcs, who pointed out that "modern research into predictors of injury from domestic violence finds that the strongest predictor of injury by domestic violence is participation in reciprocal domestic violence, and that this pattern of domestic violence is more often initiated by the female in the relationship"). (WK 2013kk) And the reverse direction also holds true.

In relation to the partiality-totality principle, if there is partiality (e.g., the partial view on domestic violence by men against women by the feminists), there is totality (e.g., the more holistic view on domestic violence, such that the whole is not the sum of its parts, that is, it cannot be reduced to the sum of opposing views by the feminists, the masculinists, the critics, etc., since there will emerge new views in the future not yet known today, just as there are already alternative views nowadays which do not side exclusively with any of them, as is the analysis here). And the reverse direction also holds true.

In relation to the predictability-unpredictability principle, if there is predictability (e.g., the predictable tendency of the advocates of "the…psychological theories [about the causes of domestic violence]" to focus on such issues like "mental illness" and "marital conflict disorder"), there is unpredictability (e.g., the more difficult task to predict exactly the extent to which "the…psychological theories" are appropriate on a particular future occasion, since the critic like Gelles showed that "psychological theories are limited" and that "only 10% [or less] fit this psychological profile"). And the reverse direction also holds true.

In relation to the explicability-inexplicability principle, if there is explicability (e.g., the explanation, by the advocates of the "strict 'patriarchal violence' model," that "all violence in the home and elsewhere has a male perpetrator and female victim"), there is inexplicability (e.g., the lack of sufficient explanation, by the advocates of the "strict 'patriarchal violence' model," of why this model is necessarily valid, since, for the critics, "modern research into predictors of injury from domestic violence finds that the strongest predictor of injury by domestic violence is participation in reciprocal domestic violence, and that this pattern of domestic violence is more often initiated by the female in the relationship"). And the reverse direction also holds true.

In relation to the fiction-reality principle, if there is fiction (e.g., the fictional aspect of the "model" of power and control, insofar as "it ignores research linking domestic violence to substance abuse and psychological problems"), there is reality (e.g., the realistic aspect of the "model" of power and control, insofar as some cases in which "violence is posited to arise out of a need for power and control of one partner over the other" did occur). And the reverse direction also holds true.

In relation to the cognitiveness-noncognitiveness principle, if there is cognitiveness (e.g., a view of things on the basis of reason and evidences, as shown in the report that "in 2003,...one out of every three homeless women are homeless due to having left a DV relationship"), there is noncognitiveness (e.g., a view of things on the basis of non-cognitive factors like envy, jealousy, power, nationality, race, gender, age, class, greed, lust, status, faith, anger, sadness, joy, fear, wish, etc., as shown in the politics of feminism by some advocates of the "strict 'patriarchal violence' model," in that "all violence in the home and elsewhere has a male perpetrator and female victim," regardless of whether it is true or false). And the reverse direction also holds true.

In relation to the finiteness-transfiniteness principle, if there is finiteness (e.g., the finite number of the forms of domestic violence like "hitting, kicking, biting, shoving, restraining, slapping, throwing objects, battery..., sexual abuse, emotional abuse, controlling or domineering, intimidation, stalking, passive/covert abuse," etc.), there is transfiniteness (e.g., the transfinite number of all the individual instances of "hitting, kicking, biting, shoving, restraining, slapping, throwing objects, battery..., sexual abuse, emotional abuse, controlling or domineering, intimidation, stalking, passive/covert abuse," etc. that have ever existed in history). And the reverse direction also holds true.

In relation to the preciseness-vagueness principle, if there is preciseness (e.g., the precise identification of 4 causes of domestic violence in the article aforecited), there is vagueness (e.g., the vagueness in the identification of the 4 causes of domestic violence in the article aforecited, since it is not clear why there must be only these 4, not 7, 10, 14, 21, and so on). And the reverse direction also holds true.

In relation to the simpleness-complicatedness principle, if there is simpleness (e.g., the relatively simple analysis of domestic violence by the feminists), there is complicatedness (e.g., the relatively more complicated analysis of domestic violence , by challenging the claims and assumptions, as shown in the problems pointed out by the critics as cited). And the reverse direction also holds true.

In relation to the openness-hiddenness principle, if there is openness (e.g., the open exploration of domestic violence by men against women by the advocates of the "strict 'patriarchal violence' model"), there is hiddenness (e.g., the hidden bias in the "strict 'patriarchal violence' model," since, for the critics, "modern research into predictors of injury from domestic violence finds that the strongest predictor of injury by domestic violence is participation in reciprocal domestic violence, and that this pattern of domestic violence is more often initiated by the female in the relationship"). And the reverse direction also holds true.

In relation to the denseness-emptiness principle, if there is denseness (e.g., the relatively denser concentration of concerns with domestic violence by men against women by the advocates of the "strict 'patriarchal violence' model"), there is emptiness (e.g., the relatively less dense, or more empty, concentration of concerns with domestic violence by women against men by the advocates of the "strict 'patriarchal violence' model"). And the reverse direction also holds true.

In relation to the prototypicality-variation principle, if there is prototypicality (e.g., the prototype, like the example about the original work on "power and control" in the "Duluth Domestic Abuse Intervention Project"), there is variation (e.g., different variants of the protoptye, as shown in many studies since the original work on "power and control" in the "Duluth Domestic Abuse Intervention Project," like the later ones by M. Twohey, M. Straus, etc., though each with his own variation, contribution, and disagreement). (WK 2013kk; NAT 2011) And the reverse direction also holds true.

In relation to the change-constancy principle, if there is change (e.g., the ever new ways to study violence, as shown in the research on domestic violence aforedescribed), there is constancy (e.g., the ever constant existence of different problems with the ever new ways to study violence, as shown in the problems with the research on domestic violence pointed out by the critics). And the reverse direction also holds true.

In relation to the order-chaos principle, if there is order (e.g., the more or less orderly view on domestic violence, if looked from the vantage point of "a strict 'patriarchal violence' model," which presumes that "all violence in the home and elsewhere has a male perpetrator and female victim"), there is chaos (e.g., the more or less chaotic view on domestic violence, if looked from the vantage point of "borderline personalities" with their "unusual variability and depth of moods," which are often unpredictable and correlate with the "psychological profile of men who abuse their wives"). (WK 2013kk & 2013ll) And the reverse direction also holds true.

In relation to the slowness-quickness principle, if there is slowness (e.g., the relatively slower speed for a woman to encounter domestic violence during her honeymoon, since "the period immediately following a marital separation is the period of greatest risk for the women," according to a study), there is quickness (e.g., the relatively quicker speed for a woman to encounter domestic violence in "the period immediately following a marital separation," which is "the period of greatest risk for the women," according to a study). (WK 2013kk) And the reverse direction also holds true.

In relation to the expansion-contraction principle, if there is expansion (e.g., the relative spread of prevention and intervention programs against domestic violence against women in the Western world nowadays), there is contraction (e.g., the relative decline of men who believe that "a husband is justified in hitting or beating his wife under certain circumstances" in the Western world nowadays). (WK 2013kk) And the reverse direction also holds true.

In relation to the optimality-nonoptimality principle, if there is optimality (e.g., the search for highly favorable options, like the research on "the period immediately following a marital separation," which was found to be "the period of greatest risk for the women," according to a study), there is nonoptimality (e.g., the existence of non-optimal alternatives to optimality, like the argument for more realistic studies by the critics, who pointed out that there is too much attention to domestic violence by men against women [but not by women against men too], that the theories are "disputed," that each approach is limited to itself, that the prevention of domestic violence is not as successful as claimed, that the prevention of domestic violence may only be temporary, and the call for the prevention of domestic violence is culturally relative). And the reverse direction also holds true.

In relation to the theory-praxis principle, if there is theory (e.g., the theoretical construction of "borderline personalities" in psychology), there is praxis (e.g., the practical application of "borderline personalities" in psychology to the field of "domestic violence" for causal explanations). And the reverse direction also holds true.

In relation to the convention-novelty principle, if there is convention (e.g., the conventional wisdom about domestic violence by men against women by the feminists), there is novelty (e.g., the alternative novel challenge to the conventional wisdom about domestic violence by men against women, by the new idea of "modern research into predictors of injury from domestic violence," which "finds that the strongest predictor of injury by domestic violence is participation in reciprocal domestic violence, and that this pattern of domestic violence is more often initiated by the female in the relationship"). And the reverse direction also holds true.

In relation to the evolution-transformation principle, if there is evolution (e.g., the natural evolution of humans to be violent towards each other at times in the state of nature), there is transformation (e.g., the technical transformation of human ability to to be violent towards each other by the invention of different "prevention and intervention" programs against domestic violence). And the reverse direction also holds true.

In relation to the symmetry-asymmetry principle, if there is symmetry (e.g., the co-existence of different views about domestic violence in the world), there is asymmetry (e.g., "in most developed countries domestic violence is considered unacceptable by most people" nowadays—but "in many regions of the world the views are different: according to a UNICEF survey, the percentage of *women* aged 15–49 who think that a husband is justified in hitting or beating his wife under certain circumstances is, for example: 90% in Jordan, 85.6% in Guinea, 85.4% in Zambia, 85% in Sierra Leone, 81.2% in Laos, 81% in Ethiopia"). (WK 2013kk) And the reverse direction also holds true.

In relation to the softness-hardness principle, if there is softness (e.g., the defense of the "prevention and intervention" programs against domestic violence by the advocates), there is hardness (e.g., the critique of the "prevention and intervention" programs against domestic violence by the critics, as shown in the problems pointed out earlier). And the reverse direction also holds true.

In relation to the seriousness-playfulness principle, if there is seriousness (e.g., the serious business of the researchers who work hard to understand the causes and effects of domestic violence), there is playfulness (e.g., the playful part of the researchers who work hard to understand the causes and effects of domestic violence, when they play around with different views and interpretations about the causes and effects over the decades aforediscussed). And the reverse direction also holds true.

In relation to the activeness-inactivess principle, if there is activeness (e.g., the relative activeness, in relation to their husbands, of those women who are not dependent at all on their spouse, so that they can leave their marriage if they want to and are therefore able to "cope with or change their spouse's behavior," according to the "power and control" model), there is inactiveness (e.g., the relative inactiveness, in relation to their husbands, of those women who "are most dependent on the spouse for economic well being" and "fear the increased financial burden if they leave their marriage," so that "they have fewer options and few resources to help them cope with or change their spouse's behavior," according to the "power and control" model). (WK 2013kk) And the reverse direction also holds true.

In relation to the selfness-otherness principle, if there is selfness (e.g., the tendency to be mostly centered on one's self or group, as shown in "an abuser," who "use[s] various tactics of abuse [e.g., physical, verbal, emotional, sexual or financial] in order to establish and maintain control over the partner," according to the "power and control" model), there is otherness (e.g., the tendency to be mostly centered on others, as shown in recemt "criminal and civil justice systems" which "have created policies to hold offenders accountable and keep the victims safe," as an advancement in the prevention of domestic violence). (WK 2013kk) And the reverse direction also holds true.

In relation to the regression-progression principle, if there is regression (e.g., the regression made by the works on domestic violence, as shown in the problems pointed out by the critics), there is progression (e.g., the progress made by the works on domestic violence, as shown in the contribution to its prevention aforecited). And the reverse direction also holds true.

In relation to the same-difference principle, if there is similarity in outcome (e.g., the contribution to the molding and control of beliefs, values, and behaviors, regardless of whether this be done by way of feminism, or by way of patriarchalism, in regard to domestic violence), there is difference in outcome (e.g., the contribution to the molding and control of beliefs, values, and behaviors by way of feminism, in regard to domestic violence, for a relatively more egalitarian lifeworld—but the contribution to the molding and control of beliefs, values, and behaviors by way of patriarchalism, in regard to domestic violence, for a relatively more inegalitarian lifeworld). And the reverse direction also holds true.

In relation to the stability-reaction principle, if there is stability (e.g., the relatively more stable condition of the pre-1800 era, when "most legal systems accepted wife beating as a valid exercise of a husband's authority over his wife"), there is reaction (e.g., the pre-1800 era, when "most legal systems accepted wife beating as a valid exercise of a husband's authority over his wife," then led to further changes later on, when "modern attention to domestic violence began in the women's movement of the

1970s, particularly within the contexts of feminism and women's rights, as concern about wives being beaten by their husbands gained attention" in the Western world). (WL 2013kk) And the reverse direction also holds true.

In relation to the functionality-nonfunctionality principle, if there is functionality (e.g., the presence of action for which something or someone is fitted, as shown in domestic violence by men against women due to jealousy, which, according to "an evolutionary psychology explanation," serves the "male attempts to control female reproduction and ensure sexual exclusivity through violence or the threat of violence"), there is nonfunctionality (e.g., the relative lack of action for which something or someone is fitted, as shown in "the women's movement of the 1970s, particularly within the contexts of feminism and women's rights, as concern about wives being beaten by their husbands gained attention," such that the old-fashioned domestic violence by men against women due to jealousy in the older days is no longer functional in the Western world nowadays). (WK 2013kk) And the reverse direction also holds true.

In relation to the intentionality-nonintentionality principle, if there is intentionality (e.g., the planning or design of something for a certain outcome, as shown in the original intention of the advocates to campaign for "law enforcement" against domestic violence), there is nonintentionality (e.g., the relative absence of planning or design of something for a certain outcome, such that the outcome can even be counter-intentional in being the opposite of what was originally planned, as shown in some recent findings about "law enforcement," in that "arrest seemed to help in the short run in certain cases, but those arrested experienced double the rate of violence over the course of one year," and "criminologists do not fully understand the reasons why deterrent effects do not last over time"—contrary to the original intention of the advocates to campaign for "law enforcement" against domestic violence). (WK 2013kk) And the reverse direction also holds true.

And in relation to the survivability-nonsurvivability principle, if there is survivability (e.g., the relative survival of "the women's movement" against domestic violence in the Western world nowadays), there is non-survivability (e.g., the relative non-survival, nowadays in the Western world, of the practice often found in the pre-1800 era, when "most legal systems accepted wife beating as a valid exercise of a husband's authority over his wife"). And the reverse direction also holds true.

Physical Health and Culture

Physical health, when examined from the perspective of culture, can cast an illuminating light on its possibility (or impossibility) and desirability (or undesirability), and this can be shown by way of two case studies, namely, (3.5.1) physical health, torture, and culture, and (3.5.2) physical health, medical practice, and ethics—to be addressed hereafter, in that order.

Physical Health, Torture, and Culture

An excellent case study here to understand physical health from the perspective of culture has to do with physical health, torture, and culture.

An argument in the literature is that, as shown in many "national and international legal prohibitions on torture" in our time, as part of the global culture against torture, there is "a consensus that torture and similar ill-treatment are immoral, as well as impractical," since those who are physically violated are very unlikely to offer valuable information to the torturers. (WK 2013r; AMN 2005)

Definitions of Torture

The word "torture" has different definitions. Consider, for illustration, the following four examples (as summarized in *Table 3.6*):

- "The 1984 United Nations Convention Against Torture"—defines torture as "any act by which severe pain or suffering, whether physical or mental, is intentionally inflicted on a person for such purposes as obtaining from him, or a third person, information or a confession, punishing him for an act he or a third person has committed or is suspected of having committed, or intimidating or coercing him or a third person, or for any reason based on discrimination of any kind, when such pain or suffering is inflicted by or at the instigation of or with the consent or acquiescence of a public official or other person acting in an official capacity." (WK 2013r; UNCT 1984)
- "The World Health Organization" (1986)—defined torture as part of "the concept of organized violence," which refers to "the inter-human infliction of significant, avoidable pain and suffering by an organized group according to a declared or implied strategy and/or system of ideas and attitudes. It comprises any violent action that is

unacceptable by general human standards, and relates to the victims' feelings." (WK 2013r; WHO 1986)

- "The 1975 Declaration of Tokyo"—defined torture as "the deliberate, systematic or wanton infliction of physical or mental suffering by one or more persons acting alone or on the orders of any authority, to force another person to yield information, to make a confession, or for any other reason." (WK 2013r; WMA 1975)
- "Amnesty International"—"has adopted," since 1973, "the simplest, broadest definition of torture," in that "torture is the systematic and deliberate infliction of acute pain by one person on another, or on a third person, in order to accomplish the purpose of the former against the will of the latter." (WK 2013r; AMN 2005)

Of course, there can be other definitions, so the ones above are illustrative.

History of Torture in the West

With these different definitions in mind—the history of torture in the West is also long.

(a) Antiquity

In the history of the West, "the ancient Greeks and Romans used torture for interrogation. Until the 2nd century AD, torture was used only on slaves (with a few exceptions). After this point it began to be extended to all members of the lower classes. A slave's testimony was admissible *only* if extracted by torture, on the assumption that slaves could not be trusted to reveal the truth voluntarily." (WK 2013r; E. Peters 1985)

In fact, "modern scholars find the concept of torture to be compatible with society's concept of Justice during the time of Jesus Christ. Romans, Jews, Egyptians and many others cultures during that time included torture as part of their justice system. Romans had crucifixion, Jews had stoning and Egyptians had desert sun death. All these acts of torture were considered necessary (as to deter others) or good (as to punish the immoral)." (WK 2013r)

(b) Middle Ages

In the Middle Ages, "European courts used torture, depending on the crime of the accused and his or her social status. Torture was deemed a legitimate means to extract confessions or to obtain the names of accomplices or other information about a crime. It was permitted by law only if there was already half-proof against the accused. Often, defendants already sentenced to death would be tortured to force them to disclose the names of accomplices. Torture in the Medieval Inquisition began in 1252 with a papal bull Ad Extirpanda and ended in 1816 when another papal bull forbade its use." (WK 2013r; J. Franklin 2001)

Even though "secular courts often treated suspects ferociously, Will and Ariel Durant argued in *The Age of Faith* that many of the most vicious procedures were inflicted upon pious heretics by even more pious friars. The Dominicans gained a reputation as some of the most fearsomely innovative torturers in medieval Spain." (WK 2013r)

In general, "torture was usually conducted in secret, in underground dungeons. By contrast, torturous executions were typically public, and woodcuts of English prisoners being hanged, drawn and quartered show large crowds of spectators, as do paintings of Spanish auto-da-fé executions, in which heretics were burned at the stake." (WK 2013r)

(c) Early Modern Period

In the early modern period, "the torture of witches took place," but "in England the trial by jury developed considerable freedom in evaluating evidence and condemning on circumstantial evidence, making torture to extort confessions unnecessary. For this reason in England a regularized system of judicial torture never existed and its use was limited to political cases. Torture was in theory not permitted under English law, but in Tudor and early Stuart times, under certain conditions, torture was used in England." (WK 2013r)

Later, "European states abolished torture from their statutory law in the late 18th and early 19th centuries. Sweden and Prussia were the first to do so in 1722 and 1754 respectively; Denmark abolished torture in 1770, Russia in 1774, Austria in 1776, France in 1780, and the Netherlands in 1798. Bavaria abolished torture in 1806 and Württemberg in 1809. In Spain the Napoleonic conquest put an end to torture in 1808. Norway abolished it in 1819 and Portugal in 1826. The Swiss cantons abolished torture in the first half of the 19th century." (WK 2013r)

(d) Recent Times

In recent times, "from 10 December 1948, when the United Nations General Assembly adopted the Universal Declaration of Human Rights"—"sensibilities have been shaped by a profound reaction to the war crimes and crimes against humanity committed by the Axis Powers and Allied Powers in the Second World War, which have led to a sweeping international rejection of most if not all aspects of the practice. Even as many states engage in torture, few wish to be described as doing so, either to their own citizens or to the international community. A variety of devices bridge this gap, including state denial, 'secret police,' 'need to know,' a denial that given treatments are torturous in nature, appeal to various laws (national or international), the use of jurisdictional argument and the claim of 'overriding need.'" (WK 2013r; E. Lauterpacht 2002)

However, the practice of torture returned later on; "according to scholar Ervand Abrahamian, although there were several decades of prohibition of torture that spread from Europe to most parts of the world, by the 1980s, the taboo against torture was broken and torture 'returned with a vengeance,' propelled in part by television and an opportunity to break political prisoners and broadcast the resulting public recantations of their political beliefs for 'ideological warfare, political mobilization, and the need to win...hearts and minds....' According to professor Darius Rejali [2007], although dictatorships may have used tortured 'more, and more indiscriminately,' it was modern democracies, 'the United States, Britain, and France' who 'pioneered and exported techniques that have become the lingua franca of modern torture: methods that leave no marks.'" (WK 2013r)

Worse, "torture still occurs in liberal democracies despite several international treaties such as the International Covenant on Civil and Political Rights and the UN Convention Against Torture making torture illegal. Despite such international conventions, torture cases continue to arise such as the 2004 Abu Ghraib torture and prisoner abuse scandal committed by military police personnel of the United States Army." (WK 2013r)

Uses of Torture

Torture can be used in two ways, that is, (a) torture perpetrators and (b) torture by proxy, as explained below (and summarized in *Table 3.6*).

(a) Torture Perpetrators

The use of torture by perpetrators refers to "torture...inflicted by or at the instigation of or with the consent or acquiescence of a public official or other person acting in an official capacity. Those most likely to be involved in torture include persons" such as the following: (WK 2013r)

- Ex: "prison officers/detention staff"
- Ex: "the police"
- Ex: "criminals"
- Ex: "the military"
- Ex: "paramilitary forces"
- Ex: "state-controlled contra-guerilla forces"

However, others can involve too, as shown below: (WK 2013r)

- Ex: “health professionals”
- Ex: “legal professionals”
- Ex: “co-detainees acting with the approval or on the orders of public officials”
- Ex: “death squads”

Even more broadly, “in the context of armed conflicts, torture and other forms of ill-treatment could also be inflicted” by the following: (WK 2013r)

- Ex: “opposition forces”
- Ex: “the general population (in a civil war situation)”

Besides “torture perpetrators”—there is also “torture by proxy.”

(b) Torture by Proxy

For example, “in 2003, Britain's Ambassador to Uzbekistan, Craig Murray, made accusations that information was being extracted under extreme torture from dissidents in that country, and that the information was subsequently being used by Western, democratic countries that officially disapproved of torture.” (WK 2013r; R. Gedye 2004)

But “the accusations did not lead to any investigation by his employer, the Foreign and Commonwealth Office, and he resigned after disciplinary action was taken against him in 2004. No misconduct by him was proven. The National Audit Office is investigating the Foreign and Commonwealth Office because of accusations of victimisation, bullying, and intimidating its own staff.” (WK 2013r; R. Winnett 2005)

Later, “Murray...stated that he felt that he had unwittingly stumbled upon what others called 'torture by proxy' and with the euphemism of 'extraordinary rendition.' He thought that Western countries moved people to regimes and nations knowing that torturers would extract and disclose information. Murray alleged that this practice circumvented and violated international treaties against torture. If a country participated in torture by proxy and had signed the UN Convention Against Torture, that country would be in specific breach of Article 3 of that convention.” (WK 2013r; A. Davidson 2005)

Methods of Torture

Over the centuries, different methods to torture have been developed. For illustration, consider the following four major ones (as summarized in *Table 3.6*).

(a) Physical Torture

"Physical torture" refers to methods that "have been used throughout recorded history and can range from a beating with nothing more than fist and boot, through to the use of sophisticated custom designed devices such as the rack." (WK 2013r)

In fact, "remarkable ingenuity has been shown in the invention of instruments and techniques of physical torture, exploiting medical knowledge of the vulnerabilities of the human body (e.g., the sensitivity of the nail beds to pressure, or of the soles of the feet to heat). Other types of torture can include sensory or sleep deprivation, restraint or being held in awkward or damaging positions, uncomfortable extremes of heat and cold, loud noises or any other means that inflicts severe physical or mental pain." (WK 2013r)

(b) Psychological Torture

"Psychological torture" refers to "non-physical methods that cause psychological suffering. Its effects are not immediately apparent unless they alter the behavior of the tortured person. Since there is no international political consensus on what constitutes psychological torture, it is often overlooked, denied, and referred to by different names." (WK 2013r)

Hence, "psychological torture is less well known than physical torture and tends to be subtle and much easier to conceal....Physical torture is the inflicting of severe pain or suffering on a person. In contrast, psychological torture is directed at the psyche with calculated violations of psychological needs, along with deep damage to psychological structures and the breakage of beliefs underpinning normal sanity. Torturers often inflict both types of torture in combination to compound the associated effects." (WK 2013r)

In addition, "psychological torture...includes deliberate use of extreme stressors and situations such as mock execution, shunning, violation of deep-seated social or sexual norms and taboos, or extended solitary confinement. Because psychological torture needs no physical violence to be effective, it is possible to induce severe psychological pain, suffering, and trauma with no externally visible effects." (WK 2013r)

(c) Medical Torture

Unlike physical and psychological torture—"medical practitioners use torture to judge what victims can endure, to apply treatments that enhance torture, or act as torturers in their own right. Josef Mengele and Shirō Ishii were infamous during and after World War II for their involvement in medical torture and murder." (WK 2013r; M. Schreiber 2001)

(d) Pharmacological Torture

And "pharmacological torture is the use of drugs to produce psychological or physical pain or discomfort. HI Tickle torture is an unusual form of torture which nevertheless has been documented, and can be both physically and psychologically painful." (WK 2013r; G. Yamey 2011)

Arguments against Torture

Therefore, it is no wonder that there have been arguments against torture. Consider, for illustration, the following three main ones (as summarized in *Table 3.6*).

(a) Humanitarian

The first argument against torture is "humanitarian," in that "torture has been criticized on humanitarian...grounds...that evidence extracted by torture is unreliable, and because torture corrupts institutions that tolerate it. Besides degrading the victim, torture debases the torturer: American advisors alarmed at torture by their South Vietnamese allies early in the Vietnam War concluded that 'if a commander allowed his officers and men to fall in to these vices [they] would pursue then for their own sake, for the perverse pleasure they drew from them.' The consequent degeneracy destroyed discipline and morale: '[a] soldier had to learn that he existed to uphold law and order, not to undermine it.'" (WK 2013r; N. Sheehan 1988; BBC 2007)

Therefore, "organizations like Amnesty International argue that the universal legal prohibition is based on a universal philosophical consensus that torture and ill-treatment are repugnant, abhorrent, and immoral." (WK 2013r; AMN 2007)

(b) Utilitarian

The second argument against torture is "utilitarian," in that "there is simply no scientific evidence supporting its effectiveness. The lack of scientific basis for the effectiveness of torture as an interrogation techniques is summarized in a 2006 Intelligence Science Board report titled 'EDUCING INFORMATION, Interrogation: Science and Art, Foundations for the Future.'" (WK 2013r; NDIC 2006)

(c) Religious

And the third argument against torture is "religious," as shown by the change of the Catholic Church's views on torture in modern times, "which are generally associated with the Enlightenment. Thus, the Catechism of the Catholic Church (published in 1994) condemns the use of torture as a grave violation of Human Rights. In No. 2297-2298 it states: 'Torture, which uses physical or moral violence to extract confessions, punish the guilty, frighten opponents, or satisfy hatred is contrary to respect for the person and for human dignity....In times past, cruel practices were commonly used by legitimate governments to maintain law and order, often without protest from the Pastors of the Church, who themselves adopted in their own tribunals the prescriptions of Roman law concerning torture. Regrettable as these facts are, the Church always taught the duty of clemency and mercy. She forbade clerics to shed blood. In recent times it has become evident that these cruel practices were neither necessary for public order, nor in conformity with the legitimate rights of the human person. On the contrary, these practices led to ones even more degrading. It is necessary to work for their abolition. We must pray for the victims and their tormentors.'" (WK 2013r)

Problems with the Studies on Torture

However, for the critics, these studies on physical health, torture, and culture has some major problems. Consider, for illustration, a few examples below (as summarized in *Table 3.6*).

Firstly, one main criticism of the studies on physical health, torture, and culture is that there is a divide among different countries on torture.

For instance, in a report, "there was a clear divide between those countries with strong rejection of torture (such as Italy, where only 14% supported torture) and nations where rejection was less strong. Often this lessened rejection is found in countries severely and frequently threatened by terrorist attacks. E.g., Israel, despite its Supreme Court outlawing torture in 1999, showed 43% supporting torture...." (WK 2013r; BBC 2006)

Secondly, another main criticism of the studies on physical health, torture, and culture is that there is a divide between the secularists and the religiously affiliated.

For instance, "in a 2005 U.S. survey 72% of American Catholics supported the use of torture in some circumstances compared to 51% of American secularists. A Pew survey in 2009 similarly found that the religiously unaffiliated are the least likely (40 percent) to support torture, and that the more a person *claims* to attend church, the more likely he or she is to condone torture; among racial/religious groups, white evangelical Protestants were far and away the most likely (62 percent) to support inflicting pain as a tool of interrogation." (WK 2013r; L. Pitts 2009; T. Carney 2006)

Thirdly, still another main criticism of the studies on physical health, torture, and culture is that torture can work in some cases.

For instance, "those favoring torture have however pointed to some specific cases where torture has elicited true information," even if the cases were rather rare. (WK 2013r; J. Franklin 2009)

Fourthly, an additional main criticism of the studies on physical health, torture, and culture is that the definitions of torture are problematic.

For instance, for the critics, in regard to the definition by the 1984 United Nations Convention Against Torture, "this definition was restricted to apply only to nations and to government-sponsored torture and clearly limits the torture to that perpetrated, directly or indirectly, by those acting in an official capacity. It appears to exclude: (a) torture perpetrated by gangs, hate groups, rebels or terrorists who ignore national or international mandates; (b) random violence during war; and (c) punishment allowed by national laws, even if the punishment uses techniques similar to those used by torturers such as mutilation or whipping when practiced as lawful punishment. Some professionals in the torture rehabilitation field believe that this definition is too restrictive and that the definition of politically motivated torture should be broadened to include all acts of organized violence." (WK 2013r; J. Jaranson 1998)

And fifthly, another additional main criticism of the studies on physical health, torture, and culture is that all the prohibitions against torture have not prevented its practice from reemerging in history time and again.

For instance, for the critics, "in some instances, whole societies can be more or less traumatized....In general, after years of repression, conflict and war, regular support networks and structures have often been broken or destroyed." (WK 2013r; IRCT 2011) And "shortly after the September 11, 2001 attacks...some people, such as Alan M. Dershowitz and Mirko Bagaric [2005], have argued the need for information outweighs the moral and ethical arguments against torture." (WK 2013r Alibhai-Brown, Yasmin. 2005) Therefore, nowadays, "torture still occurs in liberal democracies despite several international treaties such as the International Covenant on Civil and Political Rights and the UN Convention Against Torture making torture illegal." (WK 2013r)

Beyond Torture

These criticisms of the studies on physical health, torture, and culture, however, do not imply a total rejection of their usefulness but serve to show us the two opposing sides of the debate, such that the possibility (or impossibility) and desirability (or undesirability) of physical health (from the perspective of culture with the studies on physical health, torture, and culture as a case study here) are not to the extent that the respective defenders would like us to believe.

In addition, the analysis of the studies on physical health, torture, and culture is to teach us something valualble about the ontological principles in existential dialectics, and good examples include the formalness-informalness principle, the absoluteness-relativeness principle, the partiality-totality principle, the predictability-unpredictability principle, the explicability-inexplicability principle, the fiction-reality principle, the cognitiveness-noncognitiveness principle, the finiteness-transfiniteness principle, the preciseness-vagueness principle, the simpleness-complicatedness principle, the openness-hiddenness principle, the denseness-emptiness principle, the prototypicality-variation principle, the change-constancy principle, the order-chaos principle, the slowness-quickness principle, the expansion-contraction principle, the optimality-nonoptimality principle, the theory-praxis principle, the convention-novelty principle, the evolution-transformation principle, the symmetry-asymmetry principle, the softness-hardness principle, the seriousness-playfulness principle, the activeness-inactivess principle, the selfness-otherness principle, the regression-progression principle, the same-difference principle, the stability-reaction principle, the functionality-nonfunctionality principle, and the intentionality-nonintentionality principle.

For instance, in relation to the formalness-informalness principle, if there is formalness (e.g., the formal logical requirement of soundness, completeness, and consistency in a system of ideas, as in the studies on torture), there is informalness (e.g., the non-formal existence of unsoundness, incompleteness, and inconsistency in the studies on torture, as shown in the criticisms that there is a divide among different countries on torture, that there is a divide between the secularists and the religiously affiliated, that torture can work in some cases, that the definitions of torture are problematic, and that all the prohibitions against torture have not prevented its practice from reemerging in history time and again). And the reverse direction also holds true.

In relation to the absoluteness-relativeness principle, if there is absoluteness (e.g., the absolute view against torture by the opponents), there is relativeness (e.g., what is right for the opponents against torture is not necessarily so for the critics such as Alan M. Dershowitz and Mirko Bagaric [2005], who "have argued the need for information outweighs the moral and ethical arguments against torture"). And the reverse direction also holds true.

In relation to the partiality-totality principle, if there is partiality (e.g., the partial view on torture by its supporters like Alan M. Dershowitz and Mirko Bagaric), there is totality (e.g., the more holistic view on torture, such that the whole is not the sum of its parts, that is, it cannot be reduced to the sum of opposing views by the proponents, the opponents, the researchers, etc., since there will emerge new views in the future not yet known today, just as there are already alternative views nowadays which do not side exclusively with any of them, as is the analysis here). And the reverse direction also holds true.

In relation to the predictability-unpredictability principle, if there is predictability (e.g., the predictable tendency of the supporters of Alan M. Dershowitz and Mirko Bagaric to argue that "the need for information outweighs the moral and ethical arguments against torture"), there is unpredictability (e.g., the more difficult task to predict exactly the extent to which a particular practice of torture will be effective on a particular future occasion, since, for the critics, "there is simply no scientific evidence supporting its effectiveness"). And the reverse direction also holds true.

In relation to the explicability-inexplicability principle, if there is explicability (e.g., the explanation, by Alan M. Dershowitz and Mirko Bagaric, of the desirability of torture on the basis that "the need for information outweighs the moral and ethical arguments against torture"), there is inexplicability (e.g., the lack of sufficient explanation, by Alan M. Dershowitz and Mirko Bagaric, of why their argument for torture is necessarily convincing, since "others including Robert Mueller, FBI Director since 5 July 2001,...do not believe that evidence gained by the U.S. government through what supporters of the techniques call 'enhanced interrogation' has disrupted a single attack and no one has come up with a documented example of lives saved thanks to these techniques"). (WK 2013r; D. Rose 2008; D. Froomkin 2007) And the reverse direction also holds true.

In relation to the fiction-reality principle, if there is fiction (e.g., the fictional aspect of torture, insofar as the critics like "Robert Mueller, FBI Director since 5 July 2001,...do not believe that evidence gained by the U.S. government through what supporters of the techniques call 'enhanced interrogation' has disrupted a single attack and no one has come up with a documented example of lives saved thanks to these techniques"), there is reality (e.g., the realistic aspect of torture, insofar as "torture still occurs in liberal democracies [nowadays] despite several international treaties such as the International Covenant on Civil and Political Rights and the UN

Convention Against Torture making torture illegal"). (WK 2013r) And the reverse direction also holds true.

In relation to the cognitiveness-noncognitiveness principle, if there is cognitiveness (e.g., a view of things on the basis of reason and evidences, as shown in the empirical finding that "throughout history and today, many states have engaged in torture," as discussed earlier), there is noncognitiveness (e.g., a view of things on the basis of non-cognitive factors like envy, jealousy, power, nationality, race, gender, age, class, greed, lust, status, faith, anger, sadness, joy, fear, wish, etc., as shown in the politics of "denial" by "many states" which "engage in torture" but "few wish to be described as doing so, either to their own citizens or to the international community," so they resort to "state denial," "secret police," "need to know," etc. to cover up their practice). And the reverse direction also holds true.

In relation to the finiteness-transfiniteness principle, if there is finiteness (e.g., the finite number of the methods of torture used in history, like "physical," "psychological," "medical," "pharmacological," etc.), there is transfiniteness (e.g., the transfinite number of all the individuals in history who have ever experienced, or conversely who have practiced, torture, regardless of the methods of torture used). And the reverse direction also holds true.

In relation to the preciseness-vagueness principle, if there is preciseness (e.g., the precise identification of 3 arguments against torture in the article aforecited), there is vagueness (e.g., the vagueness in the identification of the 3 arguments against torture in the article aforecited, since it is not clear why there must be only these 3, not 5, 8, 11, 14, 16, and so on). And the reverse direction also holds true.

In relation to the simpleness-complicatedness principle, if there is simpleness (e.g., the relatively simple analysis of the need to torture by the advocates), there is complicatedness (e.g., the relatively more complicated analysis of the need to torture, by challenging the claims and assumptions, as shown in the problems pointed out by the critics as cited). And the reverse direction also holds true.

In relation to the openness-hiddenness principle, if there is openness (e.g., the open exploration of a different definition of "torture" by the 1984 United Nations Convention Against Torture), there is hiddenness (e.g., the hidden bias in the definition by the 1984 United Nations Convention Against Torture, since this definition exclude: [i] torture perpetrated by gangs, hate groups, rebels or terrorists who ignore national or international mandates, [ii] random violence during war, and [iii] punishment allowed by national laws, even if the punishment uses techniques similar to those used by torturers such as mutilation or whipping when practiced as lawful punishment"). And the reverse direction also holds true.

In relation to the denseness-emptiness principle, if there is denseness (e.g., the relatively denser concentration of concerns with "the need for information" by the supporters of torture like Alan M. Dershowitz and Mirko Bagaric), there is emptiness (e.g., the relatively less dense, or more empty, concentration of concerns with "humanitarian grounds" by the supporters of torture like Alan M. Dershowitz and Mirko Bagaric). And the reverse direction also holds true.

In relation to the prototypicality-variation principle, if there is prototypicality (e.g., the prototype, like the example about the original "Universal Declaration of Human Rights" by the United Nations in 1948, with Article 5 against torture), there is variation (e.g., different variants of the protoptye, as shown in many works since the 1948 "Universal Declaration of Human Rights," like the later ones such as the subsequent "United Nations Convention Against Torture," "the Geneva Conventions III and IV," etc., though each with its own variation and contribution). And the reverse direction also holds true.

In relation to the change-constancy principle, if there is change (e.g., the ever new ways to use torture, as shown in the 4 different methods aforedescribed), there is constancy (e.g., the ever constant existence of different problems with the ever new ways to use torture, as shown in the problems with the 4 different methods pointed out by the critics). And the reverse direction also holds true.

In relation to the order-chaos principle, if there is order (e.g., the more or less orderly view on torture, if looked from the sole vantage point of the advocates like Alan M. Dershowitz and Mirko Bagaric, who simply argued that "the need for information outweighs the moral and ethical arguments against torture"), there is chaos (e.g., the more or less chaotic view on torture, if looked from the multiple, conflicting vantage points of the advocates, the critics, the researchers, etc., as discussed earlier, such that they do not add up much to anything). And the reverse direction also holds true.

In relation to the slowness-quickness principle, if there is slowness (e.g., the relatively slower speed of those exceptional torture victims, "such as Admiral James Stockdale, Medal of Honor recipient, who refused to provide information under torture" or simply resisted as much as they could until the ever end), there is quickness (e.g., the relatively quicker speed of ordinary torture victims to "say or do anything to escape the situation, including untrue 'confessions' and implication of others without genuine knowledge," in accordance to "one well documented effect of torture"). (WK 2013r) And the reverse direction also holds true.

In relation to the expansion-contraction principle, if there is expansion (e.g., the relative spread of psychological torture, especially after 1980s and, of course, after September 11, 2011 attacks, by "modern democracies" like "the United States, Britain, and France" who "pioneered and exported techniques that have become the lingua franca of modern torture: methods that leave no marks," according to Darius Rejali), there is contraction (e.g., the relative decline of physical torture for "several decades...from Europe to most parts of the world" in the second half of the 20th century, according to scholar Ervand Abrahamian). (WK 2013r) And the reverse direction also holds true.

In relation to the optimality-nonoptimality principle, if there is optimality (e.g., the search for highly favorable options, like the quest for the most effective part of the body to be tortured, like "the feet," so as "to cause carefully controllable agony without endangering the prisoner's life," and "this is clearly accomplished by staying as far as possible from the brain and the vital [viz., abdominal] organs," so "the only body part that satisfies this twin criterion is the foot"), there is nonoptimality (e.g., the existence of non-optimal alternatives to optimality, like the argument for more realistic studies by the critics, who pointed out that "there is simply no scientific evidence supporting its effectiveness"). (WK 2013mm) And the reverse direction also holds true.

In relation to the theory-praxis principle, if there is theory (e.g., the theoretical construction of "utilitarianism" in philosophy), there is praxis (e.g., the practical application of utilitarianism" in philosophy to the field of public policy, like the utilitarian argument against torture). And the reverse direction also holds true.

In relation to the convention-novelty principle, if there is convention (e.g., the conventional wisdom about "torture" which "was sanctioned" historically in different societies in antiquity), there is novelty (e.g., the alternative novel challenge to the conventional wisdom about "torture" which "was sanctioned" historically in different societies in antiquity, by the new idea of the "Article 5 of the UN Universal Declaration of Human Rights" in 1948, which prohibits torture for the first time "under international law and the domestic laws of most countries"). And the reverse direction also holds true.

In relation to the evolution-transformation principle, if there is evolution (e.g., the natural evolution of humans to "inflict...severe physical pain and possibly injury" on others in the state of nature), there is transformation (e.g., the technical transformation of human ability to "inflict...severe physical pain and possibly injury" on others by the invention of different systematic "methods" over the centuries aforediscussed). And the reverse direction also holds true.

In relation to the symmetry-asymmetry principle, if there is symmetry (e.g., the co-existence of different methods of torture, be they "physical" or "psychological"), there is asymmetry (e.g., "psychological torture is less well known than physical torture and tends to be subtle and much easier to conceal"). And the reverse direction also holds true.

In relation to the softness-hardness principle, if there is softness (e.g., the defense of torture by the advocates like Alan M. Dershowitz and Mirko Bagaric), there is hardness (e.g., the critique of torture, as shown in the problems pointed out by the critics as cited). And the reverse direction also holds true.

In relation to the seriousness-playfulness principle, if there is seriousness (e.g., the serious business of those states that have tried to punish some individuals with torture), there is playfulness (e.g., the playful part of those states that have tried to punish some individuals with torture, when they play around with different "methods" over the centuries aforediscussed). (WK 2013r & 2013mm) And the reverse direction also holds true.

In relation to the activeness-inactivess principle, if there is activeness (e.g., the relative activeness of those ordinary individuals who have never been tortured physically or have not suffered from any other physical problems, so they can engage fully in life activities), there is inactiveness (e.g., the relative inactiveness of those torture victims who have been seriously tortured, especially though not exclusively on their feet, so that they can no longer engage fully in life activities).

In relation to the selfness-otherness principle, if there is selfness (e.g., the tendency to be mostly centered on one's self or group, as shown in those states that practice torture against some individuals for "ideological warfare, political mobilization, and the need to win 'hearts and minds'"), there is otherness (e.g., the tendency to be mostly centered on others, as shown in those advocates of the UN Universal Declaration of Human Rights" to care about torture victims). (WK 2013r) And the reverse direction also holds true.

In relation to the regression-progression principle, if there is regression (e.g., the regression made by the campagin against torture, as shown in the problems pointed out by the critics), there is progression (e.g., the progress made by the campagin against torture, as shown in the contribution to the prohbition of torture, at least nominally, "under international law and the domestic laws of most countries"). And the reverse direction also holds true.

In relation to the same-difference principle, if there is similarity in outcome (e.g., the contribution to the molding and control of beliefs, values, and behaviors, regardless of whether this be done by way of the Catechism of the Catholic Church, or by way of utilitarianism, in the campaign against torture), there is difference in outcome (e.g., the contribution to the molding and control of beliefs, values, and behaviors by way of the Catechism of the Catholic Church, in the campaign against torture, for a relatively more religious lifeworld—but the contribution to the molding and control of beliefs, values, and behaviors by way of utilitarianism, in the campaign against torture, for a relatively more secular lifeworld). And the reverse direction also holds true.

In relation to the stability-reaction principle, if there is stability (e.g., the relatively more stable condition of using physical torture in antiquity), there is reaction (e.g., using physical torture in antiquity then led to further changes later on, when nowadays, according to Darius Rejali, "modern democracies, 'the United States, Britain, and France,...pioneered and exported techniques that have become the lingua franca of modern torture: methods that leave no marks," like psychological torture and other methods). And the reverse direction also holds true.

In relation to the functionality-nonfunctionality principle, if there is functionality (e.g., the presence of action for which something or someone is fitted, as shown in the use of "medical torture" by Josef Mengele and Shirō Ishii during...World War II," which served the function of Nazi and Imperial Japan militarism at the time against the subjugated), there is nonfunctionality (e.g., the relative lack of action for which something or someone is fitted, as shown in the "Article 5 of the UN Universal Declaration of Human Rights" in 1948, which prohibits torture for the first time "under international law and the domestic laws of most countries," such that "medical torture" by Josef Mengele and Shirō Ishii during...World War II" is no longer functional in our time). And the reverse direction also holds true.

In relation to the intentionality-nonintentionality principle, if there is intentionality (e.g., the planning or design of something for a certain outcome, as shown in the original intention of some supporters of torture like Alan M. Dershowitz and Mirko Bagaric, who "have argued the need for information outweighs the moral and ethical arguments against torture"), there is nonintentionality (e.g., the relative absence of planning or design of something for a certain outcome, such that the outcome can even be counter-intentional in being the opposite of what was originally planned, as shown in "one well documented effect of torture," which showed that "its victims will say or do anything to escape the situation, including untrue 'confessions' and implication of others without genuine knowledge"—contrary to the original intention of some supporters of torture like Alan M. Dershowitz and Mirko Bagaric, who "have argued the need for information outweighs the moral and ethical arguments against torture"). And the reverse direction also holds true.

And in relation to the survivability-nonsurvivability principle, if there is survivability (e.g., the relative survival of "the UN Universal Declaration of Human Rights" nowadays), there is non-survivability (e.g., the relative non-survival of the "medical torture" as practiced by Josef Mengele and Shirō Ishii during...World War II" nowadays). And the reverse direction also holds true.

Physical Health, Medical Practice, and Ethics

Another way to evaluate the possibility (or impossibility) and desirability (or undesirability) of physical health from the perspective of culture concerns physical health, medical practice, and ethics.

An argument in the literature is that there are certain "moral principles" (in medical ethics) that need to be applied to "the practice of medicine" for health care, especially in the context of the practitioner-patient relationship. (WK 2013nn)

And the term "medical ethics" here refers to "a system of moral principles that apply values and judgments to the practice of medicine. As a scholarly discipline, medical ethics encompasses its practical application in clinical settings as well as work on its history, philosophy, theology, and sociology." (WK 2013nn)

History of Medical Ethics

Historically, in the Western world, "medical ethics may be traced to guidelines on the duty of physicians in antiquity, such as the Hippocratic Oath, and early rabbinic and Christian teachings." (WK 2013nn)

For instance, "the first code of medical ethics, *Formula Comitis Archiatrorum*, was published in the 5th century, during the reign of the Ostrogothic king Theodoric the Great. In the medieval and early modern period, the field is indebted to Muslim medicine such as Ishaq bin Ali Rahawi (who wrote the *Conduct of a Physician*, the first book dedicated to medical ethics) and Muhammad ibn Zakariya ar-Razi (known as Rhazes in the West), Jewish thinkers such as Maimonides, Roman Catholic scholastic thinkers such as Thomas Aquinas, and the case-oriented analysis (casuistry) of Catholic moral theology. These intellectual traditions continue in Catholic, Islamic and Jewish medical ethics." (WK 2013nn)

Later, in the early modern era, that is, "by the 18th and 19th centuries, medical ethics emerged as a more self-conscious discourse. In England, Thomas Percival, a physician and author, crafted the first modern code of medical ethics. He drew up a pamphlet with the code in 1794 and wrote an expanded version in 1803, in which he coined the expressions 'medical ethics' and 'medical jurisprudence.'" (WK 2013nn)

By 1815, "the Apothecaries Act was passed by the Parliament of the United Kingdom. It introduced compulsory apprenticeship and formal qualifications for the apothecaries of the day under the license of the Society of Apothecaries. This was the beginning of regulation of the medical profession in the UK." (WK 2013nn)

A few decades later, "in 1847, the American Medical Association adopted its first code of ethics, with this being based in large part upon Percival's work. While the secularized field borrowed largely from Catholic medical ethics, in the 20th century a distinctively liberal Protestant approach was articulated by thinkers such as Joseph Fletcher. In the 1960s and 1970s, building upon liberal theory and procedural justice, much of the discourse of medical ethics went through a dramatic shift and largely reconfigured itself into bioethics." (WK 2013nn; J. Walter 2003)

More recently, "since the 1970s, the growing influence of ethics in contemporary medicine can be seen in the increasing use of Institutional Review Boards to evaluate experiments on human subjects, the establishment of hospital ethics committees, the expansion of the role of clinician ethicists, and the integration of ethics into many medical school curricula." (WK 2013nn; S. Lakhan 2009)

And the field of medical ethics now has quite a number of influential cases at its disposal, after all these centuries of development; some good examples are shown below: (WK 2013nn)

- Ex: "Albert Kligman's dermatology experiments"
- Ex: "deep sleep therapy"
- Ex: "human radiation experiments"
- Ex: "*Moore v. Regents of the University of California*"
- Ex: "medical experimentation on Black Americans"
- Ex: "Milgram experiment"
- Ex: "Tuskegee syphilis experiment"
- Ex: "*Greenberg v. Miami Children's Hospital Research Institute*"

Surely, there can be other cases, so the ones above are illustrative.

Values in Medical Ethics

With this introductory history mind—"a common framework used in the analysis of medical ethics is the 'four principles' approach postulated by Tom Beauchamp and James Childress in their textbook *Principles of Biomedical Ethics*. It recognizes four basic moral principles, which are to be judged and weighed against each other, with attention given to the scope of their application," and the four principles are described below (and summarized in *Table 3.7*). (WK 2013nn)

(a) Autonomy

The first moral principle in medical ethics concerns "autonomy," in that "the patient has the right to refuse or choose their treatment. (*Voluntas aegroti suprema lex.*)." (WK 2013nn)

This principle of autonomy is to "recognize...the rights of individuals to self-determination. This is rooted in society's respect for individuals' ability to make informed decisions about personal matters. Autonomy has become more important as social values have shifted to define medical quality in terms of outcomes that are important to the patient rather than medical professionals. The increasing importance of autonomy can be seen as a social reaction to a 'paternalistic' tradition within healthcare....Respect for autonomy is the basis for informed consent and advance directives." (WK 2013nn)

The value of autonomy is in fact "a general indicator of health. Many diseases are characterised by loss of autonomy, in various manners. This makes autonomy an indicator for both personal well-being, and for the well-being of the profession. This has implications for the consideration of medical ethics: 'is the aim of health care to do good, and benefit from it?'; or 'is the aim of health care to do good to others, and have them, and society, benefit from this?.'" (WK 2013nn)

In this way, "by considering autonomy as a gauge parameter for (self) health care, the medical and ethical perspective both benefit from the implied reference to health." (WK 2013nn)

In fact, "psychiatrists and clinical psychologists are often asked to evaluate a patient's capacity for making life-and-death decisions at the end of life....[P]ersons who have the mental capacity to make end-of-life decisions have the right to refuse treatment and choose an early death if that is what they truly want. In such cases, psychiatrists and psychologists are typically part of protecting that right." (WK 2013nn; C. Ryan 2010)

(b) Beneficience

The second moral principle in medical ethics concerns "beneficience," in that "a practitioner should act in the best interest of the patient. (*Salus aegroti suprema lex.*)" (WK 2013nn)

The term "beneficence" here refers to "actions that promote the well being of others. In the medical context, this means taking actions that serve the best interests of patients. However, uncertainty surrounds the precise definition of which practices do in fact help patients." (WK 2013nn)

Indeed, "some scholars, such as Edmund Pellegrino, argue that beneficence is the only fundamental principle of medical ethics. They argue that healing should be the sole purpose of medicine, and that endeavors like cosmetic surgery, contraception and euthanasia fall beyond its purview." (WK 2013nn)

(c) Non-Maleficience

The third moral principle in medical ethics concerns "non-maleficience," in that "'first, do no harm' (*primum non nocere*)." (WK 2013nn)

Some scholars "consider that should be the main or primary consideration (hence primum): that it is more important not to harm your patient, than to do them good. This is partly because enthusiastic practitioners are prone to using treatments that they believe will do good, without first having evaluated them adequately to ensure they do no (or only acceptable levels of) harm. Much harm has been done to patients as a result, as in the saying, 'The treatment was a success, but the patient died.' It is not only more important to do no harm than to do good; it is also important to know how likely it is that your treatment will harm a patient. So a physician should go further than not prescribing medications they know to be harmful—he or she should not prescribe medications (or otherwise treat the patient) unless s/he knows that the treatment is unlikely to be harmful; or at the very least, that patient understands the risks and benefits, and that the likely benefits outweigh the likely risks." (WK 2013nn)

However, "in practice,...many treatments carry some risk of harm. In some circumstances, e.g. in desperate situations where the outcome without treatment will be grave, risky treatments that stand a high chance of harming the patient will be justified, as the risk of not treating is also very likely to do harm. So the principle of *non-maleficence* is not absolute, and balances against the principle of *beneficence* (doing good), as the effects of the two principles together often give rise to a *double effect*...." (WK 2013nn)

(d) Justice

And the four moral principle in medical ethics concerns "justice," in that it "concerns the distribution of scarce health resources, and the decision of who gets what treatment (fairness and equality)." (WK 2013nn)

This concern arises especially in cases which have to do with discrimination, be it racial, ethnic, gender-based, or else.

Problems with Medical Ethics

However, for the critics, this study of physical health, medical practice, and ethics has some major problems. Consider, for illustration, a few examples below (as summarized in *Table 3.7*).

Firstly, one main criticism of the study of physical health, medical practice, and ethics is that medical ethics focuses too much on "curing," at the expense of alternative ethical concerns (e.g., "caring" in "nursing ethics").

For example, for the critics, "although much of nursing ethics can appear similar to medical ethics, there are some factors that differentiate it....For example, a concern to promote beneficence may be expressed in traditional medical ethics by the exercise of paternalism, where the health professional makes a decision based upon a perspective of acting in the patient's best interests. However, it is argued by some that this approach acts against important values found in nursing ethics. Nursing theory seeks a collaborative relationship with the person in care. Brier-Mackie suggests that nurses' focus on care and nurture rather than cure of illness results in a distinctive ethics....The distinction can be examined from different theoretical angles. Despite the move toward more deontological themes by some, there continues to be an interest in virtue ethics in nursing ethics and some support for an ethic of care. This is considered by its advocates to emphasise relationships over abstract principles and therefore to reflect the caring relationship in nursing more accurately than other ethical views." (WK 2013oo; V. Tschudin 2003; G. Rumbold 1999; S. Breier-Mackie 2006; A. Armstrong 2007)

Secondly, another main criticism of the study of physical health, medical practice, and ethics is that there is cultural bias in medical ethics.

For instance, for the critics, "culture differences can create difficult medical ethics problems. Some cultures have spiritual or magical theories about the origins of disease, for example, and reconciling these beliefs with the tenets of Western medicine can be difficult." (WK 2013nn) And "some cultures do not place a great emphasis on informing the patient of the diagnosis, especially when cancer is the diagnosis." (WK 2013nn)

Thirdly, still another main criticism of the study of physical health, medical practice, and ethics is that there are "conflicts of interest" in medical ethics, so that the values are not necessarily followed in practice.

For instance, "research has shown that conflicts of interests are very common among both academic physicians and physicians in practice....For example, doctors who receive income from referring patients for medical tests have been shown to refer more patients for medical tests....Studies show that doctors can be influenced by drug company inducements, including gifts and food....Sexual relationships between doctors and patients can create ethical conflicts, since sexual consent may conflict with the fiduciary responsibility of the physician....In the early 1990s, it was estimated that 2-9% of doctors had violated this rule." (WK 2013nn; J. Bekelman 2003; J. Ross 2007; A. Swedlow 1992; D. Güldal 2000; N. Gartrell 1992)

Fourthly, an additional main criticism of the study of physical health, medical practice, and ethics is that there is no consensus on medical ethics even within a given tradition.

For instance, for the critics, even within the Western tradition, not everyone agrees with "the 'four principles' approach postulated by Tom Beauchamp and James Childress" (aforediscussed). Instead, other scholars proposed "other values" such as "respect for persons—the patient (and the person treating the patient) have the right to be treated with dignity" and "truthfulness and honesty —the concept of informed consent has increased in importance since the historical events of the Doctors' Trial of the Nuremberg trials and Tuskegee syphilis experiment." (WK 2013nn)

Fifthly, another additional main criticism of the study of physical health, medical practice, and ethics is that the values in medical ethics are not necessarily valuable.

For instance, for the critics, "some have questioned whether the backlash against historically excessive paternalism in favor of patient autonomy has inhibited the proper use of soft paternalism to the detriment of outcomes for some patients." (WK 2013nn) In addition, "persons with a psychiatric condition such as delirium or clinical depression may not have the capacity to make end-of-life decisions. Therefore, for these persons, a request to refuse treatment may be taken in consideration of their condition and not followed." (WK 2013nn)

Sixthly, still another additional main criticism of the study of physical health, medical practice, and ethics is that scholars disagree over the priority (or ranking) of the values in medical ethics, so the conclusions can be inconsistent with each other.

For instance, "some scholars, such as Edmund Pellegrino, argue that beneficence is the only fundamental principle of medical ethics. They argue that healing should be the sole purpose of medicine"—but other scholars instead suggested that non-maleficience "should be the main or primary consideration (hence primum): that it is more important not to harm your patient, than to do them good." (WK 2013nn)

And seventhly, one last main criticism of the study of physical health, medical practice, and ethics is that nations differ in regard to their regulations concerning medical ethics.

For instance, for the critics, "depending on the cultural consensus conditioning (expressed by its religious, political and legal social system) the legal definition of non-maleficence differs. Violation of non-maleficence is the subject of medical malpractice litigation. Regulations therefore differ over time, per nation." (WK 2013nn)

Beyond Medical Ethics

These criticisms of the study of physical health, medical practice, and ethics, however, should not be misunderstood as a total rejection of its usefulness but serve to show us the two opposing sides of the debate, such that the possibility (or impossibility) and desirability (or undesirability) of physical health (from the perspective of culture with physical health, medical practice, and ethics as a case study here) are not to the extent that the respective defenders would like us to believe.

Moreover, the analysis of physical health, medical practice, and ethics constitutes a didactic lesson about the ontological principles in existential dialectics, and good examples include the formalness-informalness principle, the absoluteness-relativeness principle, the partiality-totality principle, the predictability-unpredictability principle, the explicability-inexplicability principle, the fiction-reality principle, the cognitiveness-noncognitiveness principle, the finiteness-transfiniteness principle, the preciseness-vagueness principle, the simpleness-complicatedness principle, the openness-hiddenness principle, the denseness-emptiness principle, the prototypicality-variation principle, the change-constancy principle, the order-chaos principle, the slowness-quickness principle, the expansion-contraction principle, the optimality-nonoptimality principle, the theory-praxis principle, the convention-novelty principle, the evolution-transformation principle, the symmetry-asymmetry principle, the softness-hardness principle, the seriousness-playfulness principle, the activeness-inactivess principle, the selfness-otherness principle, the regression-progression principle, the same-difference principle, the stability-reaction principle, the functionality-nonfunctionality principle, and the intentionality-nonintentionality principle.

For instance, in relation to the formalness-informalness principle, if there is formalness (e.g., the formal logical requirement of soundness, completeness, and consistency in a system of ideas, as in the study on medical ethics), there is informalness (e.g., the non-formal existence of unsoundness, incompleteness, and inconsistency in the study on medical ethics, as shown in the criticisms that medical ethics focuses too much on "curing," at the expense of alternative ethical concerns [e.g., "caring" in "nursing ethics"], that there is cultural bias in medical ethics, that there are "conflicts of interest" in medical ethics so that the values are not necessarily followed in practice, that there is no consensus on medical ethics even within a given tradition, that the values in medical ethics are not necessarily valuable, that scholars disagree over the priority [or ranking] of the values in medical ethics so the conclusions can be inconsistent with each other, and that nations differ in regard to their regulations concerning medical ethics). And the reverse direction also holds true.

In relation to the absoluteness-relativeness principle, if there is absoluteness (e.g., the absolute view on "curing" by those in medical ethics), there is relativeness (e.g., what is right for those in medical ethics in regard to "curing" is not necessarily so for those in nursing ethics in regard to "caring" instead). And the reverse direction also holds true.

In relation to the partiality-totality principle, if there is partiality (e.g., the partial view on the "four principles" in medical ethics by Tom Beauchamp and James Childress), there is totality (e.g., the more holistic view on the "four principles" in medical ethics, such that the whole is not the sum of its parts, that is, it cannot be reduced to the sum of opposing views by the advocates, the critics, the reseachers, etc., since there will emerge new views in the future not yet known today, just as there are already alternative views nowadays which do not side exclusively with any of them, as is the analysis here). And the reverse direction also holds true.

In relation to the predictability-unpredictability principle, if there is predictability (e.g., the predictable tendency of the Western tradition to focus on the "four principles" in medical ethics by Tom Beauchamp and James Childress nowadays), there is unpredictability (e.g., the more difficult task to predict exactly the extent to which the "four principles" in medical ethics by Tom Beauchamp and James Childress will remain dominant in a particular distant future era, since, for the critics, there are different problems with the principles aforediscussed). And the reverse direction also holds true.

In relation to the explicability-inexplicability principle, if there is explicability (e.g., the explanation, by some scholars like Edmund Pellegrino, of the desirability of "beneficence" on the basis that it is "the only fundamental principle of medical ethics"), there is inexplicability (e.g., the lack of sufficient explanation, by some scholars like Edmund Pellegrino, of why "beneficence" is necessarily "the only fundamental principle of medical ethics," since, for other scholars, "non-maleficience "should be the main or primary consideration [hence primum]: that it is more important not to harm your patient, than to do them good"). And the reverse direction also holds true.

In relation to the fiction-reality principle, if there is fiction (e.g., the fictional aspect of the "four principles" in medical ethics, insofar as there are "conflicts of interest" in medical ethics so that the values are not necessarily followed in practice, and the values in medical ethics are not necessarily valuable either, as discussed earlier), there is reality (e.g., the realistic aspect of the "four principles" in medical ethics, insofar as "these do not give answers as to how to handle a particular situation, but provide a useful framework for understanding conflicts"). (WK 2013kk) And the reverse direction also holds true.

In relation to the cognitiveness-noncognitiveness principle, if there is cognitiveness (e.g., a view of things on the basis of reason and evidences, as shown in the scholarly analysis of medical ethics in terms of the "four principles" by Tom Beauchamp and James Childress), there is noncognitiveness (e.g., a view of things on the basis of non-cognitive factors like envy, jealousy, power, nationality, race, gender, age, class, greed, lust, status, faith, anger, sadness, joy, fear, wish, etc., as shown in the politics of the "conflicts of interest," so that the values are not followed in practice, even though the physicians know that they "should not allow a conflict of interest to influence medical judgment"). (WK 2013kk) And the reverse direction also holds true.

In relation to the finiteness-transfiniteness principle, if there is finiteness (e.g., the finite number of the values in medical ethics, like the "four principles" and other alternative values aforecited), there is transfiniteness (e.g., the transfinite number of all the individual physicians and patients in history who have ever been affected, in one way or the other, however trivial and informal, by different values in medical practice). And the reverse direction also holds true.

In relation to the preciseness-vagueness principle, if there is preciseness (e.g., the precise identification of the "four principles" in medical ethics by Tom Beauchamp and James Childress in the article aforecited), there is vagueness (e.g., the vagueness in the identification of the "four principles" in medical ethics by Tom Beauchamp and James Childress in the article aforecited, since it is not clear why there must be only these 4, not 5, 7, 9, 11, and so on, as shown by alternative values aforecited). And the reverse direction also holds true.

In relation to the simpleness-complicatedness principle, if there is simpleness (e.g., the relatively simple analysis of the "four principles" in medical ethics by Tom Beauchamp and James Childress), there is complicatedness (e.g., the relatively more complicated analysis of the "four principles" in medical ethics, by challenging the claims and assumptions, as shown in the problems pointed out by the critics as cited). And the reverse direction also holds true.

In relation to the openness-hiddenness principle, if there is openness (e.g., the open exploration of different moral principles in medical ethics by Tom Beauchamp and James Childress), there is hiddenness (e.g., the hidden bias in the moral principles in medical ethics by Tom Beauchamp and James Childress, since, for the critics, they focus too much on "curing," at the expense of alternative ethical concerns [e.g., "nursing ethics"], there is cultural bias in them, there are "conflicts of interest" in medical ethics so that the values are not necessarily followed in practice, there is no consensus on medical ethics even within a given tradition, the values in medical ethics are not necessarily valuable, scholars disagree over the priority [or ranking] of the values in medical ethics, and nations differ in regard to their regulations concerning medical ethics). And the reverse direction also holds true.

In relation to the denseness-emptiness principle, if there is denseness (e.g., the relatively denser concentration of concerns with "curing" by those in medical ethics), there is emptiness (e.g., the relatively less dense, or more empty, concentration of concerns with "caring" by those in medical ethics). And the reverse direction also holds true.

In relation to the prototypicality-variation principle, if there is prototypicality (e.g., the prototype, like the example about the original "guidelines on the duty of physicians in antiquity, such as the Hippocratic Oath, and early rabbinic and Christian teachings"), there is variation (e.g., different variants of the protoptye, as shown in many studies since the original "guidelines on the duty of physicians in antiquity, such as the Hippocratic Oath, and early rabbinic and Christian teachings"—like the contemporary ones by the "four principles" in medical ethics by Tom Beauchamp and James Childress and the discourse on caring by those in nursing ethics, though each later version with its own variation, contribution, and disagreement). And the reverse direction also holds true.

In relation to the change-constancy principle, if there is change (e.g., the ever new ways to understand ethics, as shown in the study on medical ethics), there is constancy (e.g., the ever constant existence of different problems with the ever new ways to understand ethics, as shown in the problems with the study on medical ethics pointed out by the critics). And the reverse direction also holds true.

In relation to the order-chaos principle, if there is order (e.g., the more or less orderly view on medical ethics, if looked from the vantage point of the priority [or ranking] of the values in medical ethics by Edmund Pellegrino, who argued that "beneficence is the only fundamental principle of medical ethics"), there is chaos (e.g., the more or less chaotic view on medical ethics, if looked from the multiple, conflicting vantage points of the advocates, the critics, the researchers, etc., as shown in the numerous disagreements aforediscussed, such that they do not add up to much of anything). And the reverse direction also holds true.

In relation to the slowness-quickness principle, if there is slowness (e.g., the relatively slower speed for those patients "with a psychiatric condition such as delirium or clinical depression...to make end-of-life decisions" which are to be reasonable and sound in regard to "their best interests"), there is quickness (e.g., the relatively quicker speed for those patients who do not suffer from "psychiatric condition such as delirium or clinical depression" and others "to make end-of-life decisions" which are to be reasonable and sound in regard to "their best interests"). And the reverse direction also holds true.

In relation to the expansion-contraction principle, if there is expansion (e.g., the relatively more developed ability of those in medical ethics to deal with "curing"), there is contraction (e.g., the relatively less developed ability of those in medical ethics to deal with "caring"). And the reverse direction also holds true.

In relation to the optimality-nonoptimality principle, if there is optimality (e.g., the search for highly favorable options, like the quest for "the main or primary consideration [hence primum]" in medical ethics, which is, for these scholars, "non-maleficience," since "it is more important not to harm your patient, than to do them good"), there is nonoptimality (e.g., the existence of non-optimal alternatives to optimality, like the argument for more realistic studies by the critics, who pointed out that there is cultural bias in medical ethics, that there is no consensus on medical ethics even within a given tradition, and that scholars disagree over the priority [or ranking] of the values in medical ethics). And the reverse direction also holds true.

In relation to the theory-praxis principle, if there is theory (e.g., the theoretical construction of "autonomy" in ethics), there is praxis (e.g., the practical application of "autonomy" in ethics to the field of medicine, like "respect for autonomy" by physicians). And the reverse direction also holds true.

In relation to the convention-novelty principle, if there is convention (e.g., the conventional wisdom about the "four principles" in medical ethics by Tom Beauchamp and James Childress), there is novelty (e.g., the alternative novel challenge to the conventional wisdom about the "four principles" in medical ethics by Tom Beauchamp and James Childress, by the new idea of different values like "respect for persons" and "truthfulness and honesty" as suggested by the critics aforediscussed). And the reverse direction also holds true.

In relation to the evolution-transformation principle, if there is evolution (e.g., the natural evolution of humans to get sick at times and look for cure in the state of nature in a primitive way), there is transformation (e.g., the technical transformation of human ability to deal with the business of curing by the invention of "medical ethics" with its principles). And the reverse direction also holds true.

In relation to the symmetry-asymmetry principle, if there is symmetry (e.g., the co-existence of different moral principles, be they "autonomy," "caring"), there is asymmetry (e.g., "caring" is more important in nursing ethics than in medical ethics). And the reverse direction also holds true.

In relation to the softness-hardness principle, if there is softness (e.g., the defense of the focus on "curing" by those in medical ethics), there is hardness (e.g., the critique of the focus on "curing" by those in nursing ethics). And the reverse direction also holds true.

In relation to the seriousness-playfulness principle, if there is seriousness (e.g., the serious business of those who try to come up with different principles for medical ethics), there is playfulness (e.g., the playful part of those who try to come up with different principles for medical ethics, when they play around with different possible principles over the centuries, like "autonomy," "beneficience," "non-maleficience," "justice," "respect for persons," "truthfulness and honesty," "relationship," etc.). And the reverse direction also holds true.

In relation to the activeness-inactivess principle, if there is activeness (e.g., the relative activeness of those patients who do not suffer from "a psychiatric condition such as delirium or clinical depression" or any other mental problems, so that they can "make end-of-life decisions" which are reasonable and sound in regard to "their best interests"), there is inactiveness (e.g., the relative inactiveness of those patients who severely suffer from "a psychiatric condition such as delirium or clinical depression," so that they cannot "make end-of-life decisions" which are reasonable and sound in regard to "their best interests"). And the reverse direction also holds true.

In relation to the selfness-otherness principle, if there is selfness (e.g., the tendency to be mostly centered on one's self or group, as shown in the principle of "autonomy" stressed by a patient, in that "the patient has the right to refuse or choose their treatment"), there is otherness (e.g., the tendency to be mostly centered on others, as shown in the principle of "relationship" to be followed by a nurse, in that nurses "focus on care and nurture" vis-à-vis their patients). (WK 2013nn & 2013oo) And the reverse direction also holds true.

In relation to the regression-progression principle, if there is regression (e.g., the regression made by the principles in medical ethics, as shown in the problems pointed out by the critics aforecited), there is progression (e.g., the progress made by the principles in medical ethics, as shown in the contribution to "a useful framework for understanding conflicts" aforecited). And the reverse direction also holds true.

In relation to the same-difference principle, if there is similarity in outcome (e.g., the contribution to the molding and control of beliefs, values, and behaviors, regardless of whether this be done by way of medical ethics, or by way of nursing ethics), there is difference in outcome (e.g., the contribution to the molding and control of beliefs, values, and behaviors by way of medical ethics for a relatively more deontological lifeworld in the context of "deontological ethics"—but the contribution to the molding and control of beliefs, values, and behaviors by way of nursing ethics for a relatively more virtue-ethical lifeworld in the context of "virtue ethics"). And the reverse direction also holds true.

In relation to the stability-reaction principle, if there is stability (e.g., the relatively more stable condition of the "guidelines on the duty of physicians in antiquity, such as the Hippocratic Oath, and early rabbinic and Christian teachings" in the Western tradition), there is reaction (e.g., the "guidelines on the duty of physicians in antiquity, such as the Hippocratic Oath, and early rabbinic and Christian teachings" in the Western tradition then led to further changes later on, when nowadays, there are the "four principles" in medical ethics by Tom Beauchamp and James Childress, as well as alternative values). And the reverse direction also holds true.

In relation to the functionality-nonfunctionality principle, if there is functionality (e.g., the presence of action for which something or someone is fitted, as shown in the "four principles" in medical ethics by Tom Beauchamp and James Childress, which serve the function of promoting the tradition of "cure of illness" in medical practice), there is nonfunctionality (e.g., the relative lack of action for which something or someone is fitted, as shown in the alternative perspective of nursing ethics for "care and nurture" in a "collorative relationship," such that the "four principles" in medical ethics for "cure of illness" is not as much functional in the community of nurses). And the reverse direction also holds true.

In relation to the intentionality-nonintentionality principle, if there is intentionality (e.g., the planning or design of something for a certain outcome, as shown in the original intention of Tom Beauchamp and James Childress to use the "four principles" in medical ethics as "a useful framework for understanding conflicts" in medical practice), there is nonintentionality (e.g., the relative absence of planning or design of something for a certain outcome, such that the outcome can even be counter-intentional in being the opposite of what was originally planned, as shown in the criticisms by the critics nowadays, in that medical ethics focuses too much on "curing," at the expense of alternative ethical concerns [e.g., "nursing ethics"], that there is cultural bias in medical ethics, that there are "conflicts of interest" in medical ethics so that the values are not necessarily followed in practice, that there is no consensus on medical ethics even within a given tradition, that the values in medical ethics are not necessarily valuable, that scholars disagree over the priority [or ranking] of the values in medical ethics so the conclusions can be inconsistent with each other, and that nations differ in regard to their regulations concerning medical ethics—contrary to the original intention of Tom Beauchamp and James Childress to use the "four principles" in medical ethics as "a useful framework for understanding conflicts" in medical practice). And the reverse direction also holds true.

And in relation to the survivability-nonsurvivability principle, if there is survivability (e.g., the relative survival, nowadays, of the "four principles" in medical ethics), there is non-survivability (e.g., the relative non-survival, nowadays, of the claim by Edmund Pellegrino, who argued that "beneficence is the only fundamental principle of medical ethics"). And the reverse direction also holds true.

The Misuse of Physical Health

This comprehensive analysis of the possibility (or impossibility) and desirability (or undesirability) of physical health in the context of health care, from the perspectives of the mind, nature, society, and culture, is important to show us the different ways in which physical health is both possible and desirable, but not to the extent that the spokespersons from each side would like us to believe.

Physical health thus has its use, just as it has its misuse too, as the other side of the same coin.

And the other part of a larger story concerns mental health, the other concern in health care, which was already addressed in the last chapter (Chapter Two).

These dual analyses should not be underestimated, because those on the side of mental health often downgrade physical health merely as the other concern in health care without really appreciating it from the vantage point of physical health too—and vice versa.

Now that we have reached the end of this long intellectual journey, what then can be concluded about the future of health care? To answer this question, we now turn to the concluding chapter, Chapter Four, on the future of health care and its post-human fate.

Table 3.1. Physical Health and its Ambivalence

- **Physical Health and the Mind**
  —Ex: physical health, exercise, and effects
  —Ex: physical health, abuse, and children

- **Physical Health and Nature**
  —Ex: physical health, astral travel, and higher dimensions
  —Ex: physical health, infectious disease, and animals

- **Physical Health and Society**
  —Ex: physical health, drug use, and the law
  —Ex: physical health, domestic violence, and society

- **Physical Health and Culture**
  —Ex: physical health, torture, and culture
  —Ex: physical health, medical practice, and ethics

Notes: The examples in the categories are solely illustrative (not exhaustive), and the comparison is relative (not absolute), nor are they necessarily mutually exclusive. And some can be easily re-classified elsewhere. As generalities, they allow exceptions.
Source: A summary of Ch.3 of *FPHHC*

Table 3.2. Physical Health, Exercise, and Effects

- **Types of Physical Exercise**
  —Ex: "flexibility exercises"
  —Ex: "aerobic exercises"
  —Ex: "anaerobic exercises"

- **Categories of Physical Exercise**
  —Ex: "strength"
  —Ex: "balance"
  —Ex: "speed"
  —Ex: "accuracy"

- **Health Effects of Physical Exercise**
  —Ex: "cardiovascular system"
  —Ex: "immune system"
  —Ex: "brain function"
  —Ex: "depression"
  —Ex: "sleep"

- **Problems with Physical Exercise**
  —Firstly, vigorous exercise can have its downside.
  —Secondly, some individuals can be exercise-resistant.
  —Thirdly, the findings are inconsistent.
  —Fourthly, there is often "insufficient evidence" for any firm conclusion.
  —Fifthly, there are alternative categories of physical exercise.
  —And sixthly, some effects of physical exercise remain unknown.

Notes: The examples in the categories are solely illustrative (not exhaustive), and the comparison is relative (not absolute), nor are they necessarily mutually exclusive. And some can be easily re-classified elsewhere. As generalities, they allow exceptions.
Source: From *Sec. 3.2.1* of *FPHHC*. See book for citations.

Table 3.3. Physical Health, Abuse, and Children

• **Types of Child Abuse**
—Ex: "physical abuse"
—Ex: "sexual abuse"
—Ex: "psychological/emotional abuse"
—Ex: "neglect"

• **Causes of Child Abuse**
—Ex: "parents who physically abuse their spouses are more likely than others to physically abuse their children." (WK 2013ee)
—Ex: "children resulting from unintended pregnancies are more likely to be abused or neglected…." (WK 2013ee)
—Ex: "substance abuse can be a major contributing factor to child abuse." (WK 2013ee; J. Murphy 1991)
—Ex: "unemployment and financial difficulties are associated with increased rates of child abuse." (WK 2013ee)

• **Effects of Child Abuse**
—Ex: "psychological effects"
—Ex: "physical effects"

• **Problems with the Study of Child Abuse**
—Firstly, scholars disagree over what constitutes child abuse.
—Secondly, the alleged causes of child abuse can be questionable.
—Thirdly, the long-term effects of child abuse remains unknown.
—Fourthly, the alleged causes do not determine the often cited consequences.
—Fifthly, the prevention of child abuse can be limited.
—And sixthly, there is cultural bias in the studies.

Notes: The examples in the categories are solely illustrative (not exhaustive), and the comparison is relative (not absolute), nor are they necessarily mutually exclusive. And some can be easily re-classified elsewhere. As generalities, they allow exceptions.
Source: From *Sec. 3.2.2* of *FPHHC*. See book for citations.

Table 3.4. Physical Health, Infectious Disease, and Animals

- **Examples of Carriers**
  —Ex: "apes"
  —Ex: "birds"
  —Ex: "cats"
  —Ex: "fish"
  —Ex: "mice"
  —Ex: "snails"

- **Types of Agents**
  —Ex: "parasites"
  —Ex: "fungi"
  —Ex: "bacteria"
  —Ex: "viruses"

- **Cases of Zoonoses**
  —Ex: "anthrax"
  —Ex: "cholera"
  —Ex: "HIV"
  —Ex: "plague"

- **Problems with the Research on Zoonotic Diseases**
  —Firstly, zoonotic diseases can be historically contingent.
  —Secondly, there are infectious diseases which can go in the opposite direction.
  —Thirdly, the causes of zoonotic diseases can be more complicated than previously thought.
  —And fourthly, the acceptance of the findings in zoonotic research can be based on the politics of social impact.

Notes: The examples in the categories are solely illustrative (not exhaustive), and the comparison is relative (not absolute), nor are they necessarily mutually exclusive. And some can be easily re-classified elsewhere. As generalities, they allow exceptions.
Source: From *Sec. 3.3.2* of *FPHHC*. See book for citations.

Table 3.5. Physical Health, Domestic Violence, and Society

- **Definitions of Domestic Violence**
  —Ex: "government definitions"
  —Ex: "dynamics classification"

- **Forms of Domestic Violence**
  —Ex: "physical"
  —Ex: "sexual"
  —Ex: "emotional"
  —Ex: "economic"

- **Causes of Domestic Violence**
  —Ex: "biological"
  —Ex: "psychological"
  —Ex: "behavioral"
  —Ex: "social"

- **Effects of Domestic Violence**
  —Ex: "physical"
  —Ex: "psychological"
  —Ex: "financial"

- **Problems with the Study on Domestic Violence**
  —Firstly, there are competing defintions of "domestic violence."
  —Secondly, there is too much attention to domestic violence by men against women, but not by women against men.
  —Thirdly, the theories are "disputed."
  —Fourthly, each approach is limited to itself.
  —Fifthly, the prevention of domestic violence is not as successful as claimed.
  —Sixthly, the prevention of domestic violence may only be temporary.
  —And seventhly, the call for the prevention of domestic violence is culturally relative.

Notes: The examples in the categories are solely illustrative (not exhaustive), and the comparison is relative (not absolute), nor are they necessarily mutually exclusive. And some can be easily re-classified elsewhere. As generalities, they allow exceptions.
Source: From *Sec. 3.4,2* of *FPHHC*. See book for citations.

Table 3.6. Physical Health, Torture, and Culture

- **Uses of Torture**
  —Ex: "torture perpetrators"
  —Ex: "torture by proxy"

- **Methods of Torture**
  —Ex: "physical"
  —Ex: "psychological"
  —Ex: "medical"
  —Ex: "pharmacological"

- **Arguments against Torture**
  —Ex: "humanitarian"
  —Ex: "utilitarian"
  —Ex: "religious"

- **Problems with the Studies on Torture**
  —Firstly, one main criticism of the studies on physical health, torture, and culture is that there is a divide among different countries on torture.
  —Secondly, another main criticism of the studies on physical health, torture, and culture is that there is a divide between the secularists and the religiously affiliated.
  —Thirdly, still another main criticism of the studies on physical health, torture, and culture is that torture can work in some cases.
  —Fourthly, an additional main criticism of the studies on physical health, torture, and culture is that the definitions of torture are problematic.
  —And fifthly, another additional main criticism of the studies on physical health, torture, and culture is that all the prohibitions against torture have not prevented its practice from reemerging in history time and again.

Notes: The examples in the categories are solely illustrative (not exhaustive), and the comparison is relative (not absolute), nor are they necessarily mutually exclusive. And some can be easily re-classified elsewhere. As generalities, they allow exceptions.
Source: From *Sec. 3.5.1* of *FPHHC*. See book for citations.

Table 3.7. Physical Health, Medical Practice, and Ethics

• **Values in Medical Ethics**
—Ex: "autonomy"
—Ex: "beneficience"
—Ex: "non-maleficience"
—Ex: "justice"

• **Problems with Medical Ethics**
—Firstly, one main criticism of the study of physical health, medical practice, and ethics is that medical ethics focuses too much on "curing," at the expense of alternative ethical concerns (e.g., "caring" in "nursing ethics").
—Secondly, another main criticism of the study of physical health, medical practice, and ethics is that there is cultural bias in medical ethics.
–Thirdly, still another main criticism of the study of physical health, medical practice, and ethics is that there are "conflicts of interest" in medical ethics, so that the values are not necessarily followed in practice.
—Fourthly, an additional main criticism of the study of physical health, medical practice, and ethics is that there is no consensus on medical ethics even within a given tradition.
–Fifthly, another additional main criticism of the study of physical health, medical practice, and ethics is that the values in medical ethics are not necessarily valuable.
–Sixthly, still another additional main criticism of the study of physical health, medical practice, and ethics is that scholars disagree over the priority (or ranking) of the values in medical ethics, so the conclusions can be inconsistent with each other.
–And seventhly, one last main criticism of the study of physical health, medical practice, and ethics is that nations differ in regard to their regulations concerning medical ethics.

Notes: The examples in the categories are solely illustrative (not exhaustive), and the comparison is relative (not absolute), nor are they necessarily mutually exclusive. And some can be easily re-classified elsewhere. As generalities, they allow exceptions.
Source: From *Sec. 3.5.2* of *FPHHC*. See book for citations.

• Part Four •

Conclusion

CHAPTER 4
CONCLUSION—THE FUTURE OF HEALTH CARE

Health is a state of complete physical, mental and social well-being, and not merely the absence of disease or infirmity"
__Unknown (TE 2013)

Beyond Mind and Body

The analyses of mental health (in Chapter Two) and physical health (in Chapter Three) show the extent of their possibility (or impossibility) and desirability (or undesirability) in the study of health care (and related fields).

These two analyses are valuable for the evaluation of the opposing views on health care (and other views as already introduced in *Sec. 1.5* and the rest of the book), such that health care (in relation to both mental health and physical health) are neither possible (or impossible) nor desirable (or undesirable) to the extent that the respective ideologues (on different sides) would like us to believe.

As already indicated in *Sec.1.1*, this questioning of the opposing views on health care does not suggest that the study of health care is worthless, or that those fields (related to health care) like medicine, chiropractic, health system, dentistry, health info tech, nursing, palliative care, psychiatrics, clinical psychology, occupational therapy, pharmacy, allied health, and so on are unimportant. Needless to say, neither of these extreme views is reasonable.

Instead, this book offers an alternative (better) way to understand the future of health care, especially in regard to the dialectic relationshp between mental health and physical health in the context of mind and body—while learning from different approaches in the literature but without favoring any one of them (nor integrating them, since they are not necessarily compatible with each other).

More specifically, this book offers a new theory (that is, *the interconnected theory of health care*) to go beyond the existing approaches in a novel way.

My *interconnected theory of health care* has four major distinct features.

Firstly, my theory makes good use of all theoretical approaches to health care in relation to mental health and physical health (in the context of mind and body), be they about the mental argument, the natural argument, the societal argument, or the cultural argument—especially from the most comprehensive combined perspectives of the mind, nature, society, and culture (as already dealt with in Chapter Two and Chapter Three).

Secondly, just like many other theories of mine in my previous books, my theory here does not heavily favor any specific theory over others in the literature, nor trying to integrate them (as they are not necessarily compatible with each other).

Thirdly, my theory treats the issue of health care in the distinctive dialectic context of no mental health without physical health, and vice versa—to be eventually transcended altogether later.

And fourthly, it contains thirty-three major theses, namely, (a) the first thesis: the formalness-informalness principle, (b) the second thesis: the absoluteness-relativeness principle, (c) the third thesis: the partiality-totality principle, (d) the fourth thesis: the predictability-unpredictability principle, (e) the fifth thesis: the explicability-inexplicability principle, (f) the sixth thesis: the fiction-reality principle, (g) the seventh thesis: the cognitiveness-noncognitiveness principle, (h) the eighth thesis: the finiteness-transfiniteness principle, (i) the ninth thesis: the preciseness-vagueness principle, (j) the tenth thesis: the simpleness-complicatedness principle, (k) the eleventh thesis: the openness-hiddenness principle, (l) the twelfth thesis: the denseness-emptiness principle, (m) the thirteenth thesis: the prototypicality-variation principle, (n) the fourteenth thesis: the change-constancy principle, (o) the fifteenth thesis: the order-chaos principle, (p) the sixteenth thesis: the slowness-quickness principle, (q) the seventeenth thesis: the expansion-contraction principle, (r) the eighteenth thesis: the optimality-nonoptimality principle, (s) the nineteenth thesis: the theory-praxis principle, (t) the twentieth thesis: the convention-novelty principle, (u) the twenty-first thesis: the evolution-transformation principle, (v) the twenty-second thesis: the symmetry-asymmetry principle, (w) the twenty-third thesis: the softness-hardness principle, (x) the twenty-fourth thesis: the seriousness-playfulness principle, (y) the twenty-fifth thesis: the activeness-inactiveness principle, (z) the twenty-sixth thesis: the selfness-otherness principle, (aa) the twenty-seventh thesis: the regression-progression principle, (bb) the twenty-eighth thesis: the sameness-difference principle, (cc) the twenty-ninth thesis: the stability-reaction principle, (dd) the thirtieth thesis: the functionality-nonfunctionality principle, (ee) the thirty-first thesis: the intentionality-nonintentionality principle, (ff) the thirty-second thesis: the survivability-non-survivability principle, and (gg) the thirty-third thesis: the post-human interconnection—to be elaborated in this chapter.

Because of the last thesis on "the post-human interconnection," the word "interconnective" in the title of my theory is suggestive, because it refers to the different relationships between mental health and physical health (in the context of mind and body) in health care, in the face of changing circumstances over time—which then require a multi-faceted inquiry of the dialectic relationship between mental health and physical health, as well as an understanding of the different views regarding the dialectic relationship in health care (together with other debates as already discussed in the book)—and in the end it calls for a need to transcend them by future advanced humans and later post-humans in the context of the great transformations of health care in the future worlds (as will be discussed in this chapter).

With this clarification in mind—the seminal project will fundamentally change the way that we think about mental health and physical health (in the context of mind and body) from the combined perspectives of the mind, nature, society, and culture, with enormous implications for the human future and what I originally called its "post-human" fate.

In Relation to Method

The first seven theses are in relation to method in existential dialectics, as shown below.

1st Thesis: The Formalness-Informalness Principle

The first thesis refers to the formalness-informalness principle (on the formal requirements of logical systems) in the category of "method" in existential dialectics, which was first proposed in *FPHML* (and later, *FPHH*, *FPHGAM*, *FPHSEM*, and other books of mine), in that the formal requirements of a logical system (e.g., consistency, soundness, and completeness) have both usefulness and non-usefulness, to the extent that, if there are formal systems requiring them, there are alternative ones which do not.

The formalness-informalness principle reveals something interesting in existential dialectics, in that it goes beyond both classical and non-classical logics (while learning something from both).

Thus, it does *not* exclude classical logics but simply goes beyond both classical and non-classical logics, while learning something from each. There is no formalness without informalness—and vice versa.

For illustration, existential dialectics can make use of both classical logics under certain conditions (e.g., especially, though not exclusively, when they are clear-cut, etc.) and non-classical logics under alternative conditions (especially, though not exclusively, when they are "unknown," "irrelevant," "ambiguous," "possible," with "different degrees of truth," empirically inconsistent in a desirable way, etc.). (WK 2008u)

For instance, on the one hand, there is formalness (e.g., formal logical requirement of soundness, completeness, and consistency in a system of ideas, as in the argument for psychotherapy, in *Sec. 2.2.1*; the formal logical requirement of soundness, completeness, and consistency in a system of ideas, as in the argument on subjective well-being and genetics, in *Sec. 2.2.2*; the formal logical requirement of soundness, completeness, and consistency in a system of ideas, as in the argument on mental health, evolutionary adaptedness, and the environment, in *Sec. 2.3.1*; the formal logical requirement of soundness, completeness, and consistency in a system of ideas, as in the research on zoophilia, in *Sec. 2.3.2*; the formal logical requirement of soundness, completeness, and consistency in a system of ideas, as in the argument for the reduction of income inequality, in *Sec. 2.4.1*; the formal logical requirement of soundness and completeness in a system of ideas, as in the argument on the use of technology for mental health, in *Sec. 2.4.2*; the formal logical requirement of soundness, completeness, and consistency in a system of ideas, as in the argument for alternative medicine, in *Sec. 2.5.1*; the formal logical requirement of soundness, completeness, and consistency in a system of ideas, as in the argument for mindfulness-based therapy, in *Sec. 2.5.2*; the formal logical requirement of soundness, completeness, and consistency in a system of ideas, as in the argument on physical health, exercise, and effects, in *Sec. 3.2.1*; the formal logical requirement of soundness, completeness, and consistency in a system of ideas, as in the argument on child abuse, in *Sec. 3.2.2*; the formal logical requirement of soundness, completeness, and consistency in a system of ideas, as in the claims on astral travel, in *Sec. 3.3.1*; the formal logical requirement of soundness and completeness in a system of ideas, as in the argument on zoonotic diseases, in *Sec. 3.3.2*; the formal logical requirement of soundness, completeness, and consistency in a system of ideas, as in the debate on drug prohibition, in *Sec. 3.4.1*; the formal logical requirement of soundness, completeness, and consistency in a system of ideas, as in the studies on domestic violence, in *Sec. 3.4.2*; the formal logical requirement of soundness, completeness, and consistency in a system of ideas, as in the studies on torture, in *Sec. 3.5.1*; and the formal logical requirement of soundness, completeness, and consistency in a system of ideas, as in the study on medical ethics, in *Sec. 3.5.2*).

On the other hand, there is also informalness (e.g., the non-formal existence of unsoundness, incompleteness, and inconsistency in the argument for psychotherapy, as shown in the criticisms that "there is considerable controversy about which form of psychotherapy is most effective," that the dropout rate of psychotherapeutic patients is quite high, that psychotherapy is dispensable, that psychotherapy lacks adequate explanatory power, and that psychotherapy can be undesirable to the health of the patients, etc., in *Sec. 2.2.1*; the non-formal existence of unsoundness, incompleteness, and inconsistency in the argument on subjective well-being and genetics, as shown in the criticisms that it ignores the "objective" conditions of well-being, that the findings are not consistent across studies and across histories, that much remains uncertain about the nature of SWB, that SWB can be detrimental to health, that it neglects social factors, and that it does not give sufficient attention to cultural variations, in *Sec. 2.2.2*; the non-formal existence of unsoundness, incompleteness, and inconsistency in the argument on mental health, evolutionary adaptedness, and the environment, as shown in the criticisms that there are "non-genetic and non-adaptive explanations" which are not adequately considered, that there is the controversial issues about testability and uncertainty, that it runs the risk of committing "the naturalistic fallacy," that it is reductionistic, and that there are disagreements on the "modularity of the mind," in *Sec. 2.3.1*; the non-formal existence of unsoundness, incompleteness, and inconsistency in the defense of zoophilia, as shown in the criticisms that there is "self-selection bias" in the research on zoophilia, that the findings are inconsistent, that it commits the naturalistic fallacy, that there are health and safety concerns in zoophilia, that there are disagreements about zoophilia across cultures, that the practice can result in violent consequences, and that the practice is no longer condoned in our time," in *Sec. 2.3.2*; the non-formal existence of unsoundness, incompleteness, and inconsistency in the argument for the reduction of income inequality, as shown in the criticisms that the work constitutes a very narrow view of social stratification in relation to health care, that it provides no verification of the claim, that there is no general agreement on the desirability of income equality or its reduction, that the correlation between health and income level does not always hold, and that equality can lead to a conformist society, in *Sec. 2.4.1*; the non-formal existence of unsoundness and incompleteness in the argument on the use of technology for mental health, as shown in the criticisms that technologies do not necessarily benefit everyone, that there are "cultural" barriers, that there are "regulatory" barriers, that there are "financial" barriers, that there are "technical" barriers, and that virtual reality has its dark side, in *Sec. 2.4.2*; the non-formal existence of unsoundness, incompleteness, and inconsistency in the argument for alternative medicine, as shown in the criticisms that altnerative medicine is not scientific, that its practice is unethical, that alternative medicine often uses "ambiguous" words to mislead, that alternative medicine is not effective as claimed, and that its practice is manipulative, that its practitioners play trick on patients, in *Sec. 2.5.1*; the non-formal existence of unsoundness, incompleteness, and inconsistency in the argument for mindfulness-based therapy, as shown in the criticisms that the research works are often incomplete, that the practices are not so effective, that its terms are often not clearly defined and can mean different things, that the idea of "mindfulness" in mindfulness-based therapy programs deviates significantly from the original Buddhist version, and that because of its connection with alternative medicine, mindfulness-based therapy programs have been criticized as not being scientific, in *Sec. 2.5.2*; the non-formal existence of unsoundness, incompleteness, and inconsistency in the argument on physical health, exercise, and effects, as shown in the criticisms that vigorous exercise can have its downside, that some individuals can be exercise-resistant, that the findings are inconsistent, that there is often "insufficient evidence" for any firm conclusion, that there are alternative categories of physical exercise, and that some effects of physical exercise remain unknown, in *Sec. 3.2.1*; the non-formal existence of unsoundness, incompleteness, and inconsistency in the argument on child abuse, as shown in the criticisms that scholars disagree over what constitutes child abuse, that the alleged causes of child abuse can be questionable, that the long-term effects of child abuse remains unknown, and that the alleged causes do not determine the often cited consequences, that the prevention of child abuse can be limited, and that there is cultural bias in the studies, in *Sec. 3.2.2*; the non-formal existence of unsoundness, incompleteness, and inconsistency in the claims on astral travel, as shown in the criticisms that the experience is subjective, that there are competing interpretations of astral travel, that the claims are "contrary to the limits of science," and that the claims are not accurate, in *Sec. 3.3.1*; the non-formal existence of unsoundness and incompleteness in the argument on zoonotic diseases, as shown in the criticisms that zoonotic diseases can be historically contingent, that there are infectious diseases which can go in the opposite direction, that the causes of zoonotic diseases can be more complicated than previously thought, and that the acceptance of the findings in zoonotic research can be based on the politics of social impact, in *Sec. 3.3.2*; the non-formal existence of unsoundness, incompleteness, and inconsistency in the debate on drug prohibition, as shown in the different disagreements by both sides on 7 contentious issues aforedescribed, in *Sec. 3.4.1*; the non-formal existence of unsoundness, incompleteness, and inconsistency in the studies on domestic violence, as shown in the criticisms that there are competing defintions of "domestic violence," that there is too much attention to domestic violence by men against women [but not by women against men too], that the theories are "disputed," that each approach is limited to itself, that the prevention of domestic violence is not as successful as claimed, that the prevention of domestic violence may only be temporary, and the call for the prevention of domestic violence is culturally relative, in *Sec. 3.4.2*; the non-formal existence of unsoundness, incompleteness, and inconsistency in the studies on torture, as shown in the criticisms that there is a divide among different countries on torture, that there is a divide between the secularists and the religiously affiliated, that torture can work in some cases, that the definitions of torture are problematic, and that all the prohibitions against torture have not prevented its practice from reemerging in history time and again, in *Sec. 3.5.1*; and the non-formal existence of unsoundness, incompleteness, and inconsistency in the study on medical ethics, as shown in the criticisms that medical ethics focuses too much on "curing," at the expense of alternative ethical concerns [e.g., "caring" in "nursing ethics"], that there is cultural bias in medical ethics, that there are "conflicts of interest" in medical ethics so that the values are not necessarily followed in practice, that there is no consensus on medical ethics even within a given tradition, that the values in medical ethics are not necessarily valuable, that scholars disagree over the priority [or ranking] of the values in medical ethics so the conclusions can be inconsistent with each other, and that nations differ in regard to their regulations concerning medical ethics, in *Sec. 3.5.2*).

And the reverse direction also holds true.

However, it should be stressed (as this is something that I regularly did in my previous books, *almost verbatim*) that there are different shades of gray (or different degrees of truth) in the two opposites, and the classification is not necessarily mutually exclusive either. In fact, even when some combinations of the two occur, they only end up sharing the same dialectic relationship, but in a different degree.

Also, there are some other relationships (as a kind of family resemblance) which have something in common with the principle, but they are not exactly the same but only more or less comparable, which varies from case to case.

Good examples of family resemblance in relation to the principle are logicalness-nonlogicalness, rationality-nonrationality, etc.

2nd Thesis: The Absoluteness-Relativeness Principle

The second thesis refers to the absoluteness-relativeness principle (on the multiplicity of things) in the category of "method" in existential dialectics, which was first proposed in *FPHK*, in that there is the multiplicity of things in reality, be they about entities, qualities (or properties), and relationships. If there is something absolute, there is likewise something relative. And there is no absoluteness without relativeness—and vice versa.

Both absoluteness and relativeness here are also relevant to different modalities often cited in the literature on ontology, such as possibility (e.g., something "can" happen) and its opposite (e.g., impossibility) in alethic modalities, probability (e.g., something "will" happen) and its opposite (e.g., improbability) in temporal modalities, and necessity (e.g., something "should" happen) and its opposite (e.g., contingency) in alethic modalities.

For instance, on the one hand, there is absoluteness (e.g., the absolute view on the treatment of mental problems by Freud on the basis of "psychological causes originating in childhood experiences and the unconscious mind," in *Sec. 2.2.1*; the absolute concern with the "subjective" aspects of well-being by the advocates of SWB, in *Sec. 2.2.2*; the absolute view on psychological adaptations by those in EP, in *Sec. 2.3.1*; the absolute view on the accpetance of bestiality in some North American and Middle Eastern indigenous cultures in the older days, in *Sec. 2.3.2*; the absolute view on social stratification by Wilkinson and Pickett, because they "relied too heavily on income inequality over other forms of inequality," in *Sec. 2.4.1*; the absolute view on the use of technology for mental health by the advocates, in *Sec. 2.4.2*; the absolute view on "like cures like" and the "law of the minimum dose" by the advocates of "homeopathy," in *Sec. 2.5.1*; the absolute view on

Mindfulness-Based Stress Reduction program by Jon Kabat-Zinn "for the treatment of a variety of conditions in people both healthy and unhealthy," in *Sec. 2.5.2*; the absolute view on physical exercise and health effects by the advocates, in *Sec. 3.2.1*; the absolute view on child abuse by the abusers, in *Sec. 3.2.2*; the absolute view on astral travel by the advocates like Ingo Swann, in *Sec. 3.3.1*; the absolute view on zoonotic diseases by those in the public, based on the politics of social impact, in *Sec. 3.3.2*; the absolute view on the idea of social order by the affirmative side in the debate on drug prohibition, in *Sec. 3.4.1*; what is right for the affirmative side in regard to the idea of social order is not necessarily so for the negative side in the debate on drug prohibition, in *Sec. 3.4.2*; the absolute view on domestic violence by men against women by the feminists, in *Sec. 3.5.1*; the absolute view against torture by the opponents, in *Sec. 3.5.2*; and the absolute view on "curing" by those in medical ethics, in *Sec. 3.5.2*).

On the other hand, there is relativeness (e.g., what is right for Freud to treat mental problems on the basis of "psychological causes originating in childhood experiences and the unconscious mind" is not necessarily so for Skinner, who advocated instead "behavioral therapy approaches relied on principles of operant conditioning, classical conditioning and social learning theory to bring about therapeutic change" in patients, in *Sec. 2.2.1*; what is right for the advocates of SWB to focus on the "subjective" aspects of well-being is not necessarily so for the critics, who call for the need to include "objective conditions such as material conditions or health," and so on, in *Sec. 2.2.2*; what is right for those in EP to focus on psychological adaptations is not necessarily so for the critics, who argued that it suffers from "genetic reductionism," in *Sec. 2.3.1*; what is right for some North American and Middle Eastern indigenous cultures in the older days to accept bestiality is not necessarily so for Europe during "the Middle Ages, when "zoophilic activity was met with execution, typically burning, and death," in *Sec. 2.3.2*; what is right for Wilkinson and Pickett to focus on "income inequality" is not necessarily so for the critic like John Goldthorpe, who argued for a broader understanding of social stratification by including other forms of inequality too like "broader economic inequality" and others, in *Sec. 2.4.1*; what is right for the advocates to champion the use of technology for mental health is not necessarily so for the critics, who pointed out a lot of different problems afore-described, in *Sec. 2.4.2*; what is right for the advocates of "homeopathy" to claim "like cures like" and the "law of the minimum dose" is not necessarily so for the critcs, who consider "homeopathy…to be quackery," in *Sec. 2.5.1*; what is right for Jon Kabat-Zinn in regard to his Mindfulness-Based Stress Reduction program is not necessarily so for the critics, who pointed out different problems associated with mindfulness-based therapy aforediscussed, in *Sec. 2.5.2*; what is right for the advocates in regard to physical exercise and health effects is not necessarily so for the critics, who pointed out the different problems aforedescribed, in *Sec. 3.2.1*; what is right for the abusers in regard to child abuse is not necessarily so for the child victims, with subsequent health problems aforecited, in *Sec. 3.2.2*; what is right for the advocates like Ingo Swann in regard to the alleged ability to astral travel is not necessarily so for the critics, who pointed out that the experience is subjective, that there are competing interpretations of astral travel, that the claims are "contrary to the limits of science," and that the claims are not accurate, in *Sec. 3.3.1*; what is right for those in the public, based on the politics of social impact, is not necessarily so for the critics, who pointed out that "actual cases [like SARS or HIV/AIDS]...resonate more powerfully with the public than the more abstract explanations of environmental and health issues," but then this public perception of the cases is distorted, in *Sec. 3.3.2*; what is right for the affirmative side in regard to the idea of social order is not necessarily so for the negative side in the debate on drug prohibition, in *Sec. 3.4.1*; what is right for the feminists in regard to their obsession with domestic violence by men against women is not necessarily so for the critcs, who pointed out that "modern research into predictors of injury from domestic violence finds that the strongest predictor of injury by domestic violence is participation in reciprocal domestic violence, and that this pattern of domestic violence is more often initiated by the female in the relationship," in *Sec. 3.4.2*; what is right for the opponents against torture is not necessarily so for the critics such as Alan M. Dershowitz and Mirko Bagaric [2005], who "have argued the need for information outweighs the moral and ethical arguments against torture," in *Sec. 3.5.1*; and what is right for those in medical ethics in regard to "curing" is not necessarily so for those in nursing ethics in regard to "caring" instead, in *Sec. 3.5.2*).

And the reverse direction also holds true.

However, it should be stressed (as this is something that I regularly did in my previous books, *almost verbatim*) that there are different shades of gray (or different degrees of truth) in the two opposites, and the classification is not necessarily mutually exclusive either. In fact, even when some combinations of the two occur, they only end up sharing the same dialectic relationship, but in a different degree.

Also, there are some other relationships (as a kind of family resemblance) which have something in common with the principle, but they are not exactly the same but only more or less comparable, which varies from case to case.

Good examples of family resemblance in relation to the principle are internalness-externalness, immanence-transcendence, independence-dependence, isolatedness-interconnectiveness, internality-externality, autonomy-interdependency, universalness-relativeness, and so forth.

3rd Thesis: The Partiality-Totality Principle

The third thesis refers to the partiality-totality principle (on the relationships between whole and parts) in the category of "method" in existential dialectics, which was first proposed in *FC* and later *FPHGEOL*, based on earlier works like *FHC* and *FPHC*), in that any analysis of a phenomenon in the world requires both the examination of the individual parts and the whole of them (with the whole as being not the sum of its parts), without privileging the whole as more important than the parts, or vice-versa (that is, the parts as more important than the whole).

In fact, this principle targets two kinds of misleading methodologies as used over the ages, that is, again in the absence of better words, what I called (in *FHC*, *FPHC* and *FC*) "reductionism" and its opposite, "reverse-reductionism," which can take four major forms in relation to concept, theory, methodology, and ontology (as summarized in *Sec. 1.8*).

Thus, reductionism and reverse-reductionism can be (i) conceptual, (ii) theoretical, (iii) methodological, and (iv) ontological. And the whole is not the sum of its parts, and there is no partiality without totality—and vice versa.

Works on emergence (as in *FC*), gestalt psychology (as in *FPHGEOL*), and the hermeneutic circle (as in *FPHDA*), just to name a few of them, have contributed to the understanding of whole and parts.

For instance, on the one hand, there is partiality (e.g., the partial view on health problems by those in Freudian psychoanalysis, in *Sec. 2.2.1*; the partial view on the nature of well-being by the advocates of SWB, in *Sec. 2.2.2*; the partial view on mental health and psychological adaptations by those in EP, in *Sec. 2.3.1*; the partial view on zoophilia by some North American and Middle Eastern indigenous cultures in the older days for its acceptance, in *Sec. 2.3.2*; the partial view on social stratification by Wilkinson and Pickett, in *Sec. 2.4.1*; the partial view on the use of technology for mental health by the advocates, in *Sec. 2.4.2*; the partial view on alternative medicines by the advocates, in *Sec. 2.5.1*; the partial view on mindfulness-based therapy by the advocates, in *Sec. 2.5.2*; the partial view on physical exercise and health effects by the advocates, in

Sec. 3.2.1; the partial view on child abuse by the abusers, in *Sec. 3.2.2*; the partial view on astral travel by the advocates, in *Sec. 3.3.1*; the partial view on zoonotic diseases by the practitioners, in *Sec. 3.3.2*; the partial view on deterrence by the affirmative side, in *Sec. 3.4.1*; the partial view on domestic violence by men against women by the feminists, in *Sec. 3.4.2*; the partial view on torture by its supporters like Alan M. Dershowitz and Mirko Bagaric, in *Sec. 3.5.1*; and the partial view on the "four principles" in medical ethics by Tom Beauchamp and James Childress, in *Sec. 3.5.2*).

On the other hand, there is also totality (e.g., the more holistic view on health problems, such that the whole is not the sum of its parts, that is, it cannot be reduced to the sum of opposing views like Freudian psychoanalysis, gestalt therapy, positive psychotherapy, group psychotherapy, behavior therapy, body-oriented psychotherapy, etc., since there will emerge new views in the future not yet known today, just as there are already alternative views nowadays which do not side exclusively with any of them, as is the analysis here, in *Sec. 2.2.1*; the more holistic view on the nature of well-being, such that the whole is not the sum of its parts, that is, it cannot be reduced to the sum of opposing views like the advocates of SWB, the advocates for the study of the objective conditions of well-being, etc., since there will emerge new views in the future not yet known today, just as there are already alternative views nowadays which do not side exclusively with any of them, as is the analysis here, in *Sec. 2.2.2*; the more holistic view on mental health and psychological adaptations, such that the whole is not the sum of its parts, that is, it cannot be reduced to the sum of opposing views by those for EP, those focusing on "the complexity of individual development and experience," those for social learning theory, those for social constructionism, etc., since there will emerge new views in the future not yet known today, just as there are already alternative views nowadays which do not side exclusively with any of them, as is the analysis here, in *Sec. 2.3.1*; the more holistic view on zoophilia, such that the whole is not the sum of its parts, that is, it cannot be reduced to the sum of opposing views like the acceptance of zoophilia in some North American and Middle Eastern indigenous cultures in the older days, the rejection of zoophilia by those in Europe during "the Middle Ages, and so on, since there will emerge new views in the future not yet known today, just as there are already alternative views nowadays which do not side exclusively with any of them, as is the analysis here, in *Sec. 2.3.2*; the more holistic view on social stratification, such that the whole is not the sum of its parts, that is, it cannot be reduced to the sum of opposing views like the one by Wilkinson and Pickett on income inequality, the one by

Goldthorpe on "broader economic inequality," etc., since there will emerge new views in the future not yet known today, just as there are already alternative views nowadays which do not side exclusively with any of them, as is the analysis here, in *Sec. 2.4.1*; the more holistic view on the use of technology for mental health, such that the whole is not the sum of its parts, that is, it cannot be reduced to the sum of opposing views by the advocates, by the critics, etc., since there will emerge new views in the future not yet known today, just as there are already alternative views nowadays which do not side exclusively with any of them, as is the analysis here, in *Sec. 2.4.2*; the more holistic view on alternative medicines, such that the whole is not the sum of its parts, that is, it cannot be reduced to the sum of opposing views by the advocates, the critics, etc., since there will emerge new views in the future not yet known today, just as there are already alternative views nowadays which do not side exclusively with any of them, as is the analysis here, in *Sec. 2.5.1*; the more holistic view on mindfulness-based therapy, such that the whole is not the sum of its parts, that is, it cannot be reduced to the sum of opposing views by the advocates, by the critics, etc., since there will emerge new views in the future not yet known today, just as there are already alternative views nowadays which do not side exclusively with any of them, as is the analysis here, in *Sec. 2.5.2*; the more holistic view on physical exercise and health effects, such that the whole is not the sum of its parts, that is, it cannot be reduced to the sum of opposing views by the advocates, the critics, and so on, since there will emerge new views in the future not yet known today, just as there are already alternative views nowadays which do not side exclusively with any of them, as is the analysis here, in *Sec. 3.2.1*; the more holistic view on child abuse, such that the whole is not the sum of its parts, that is, it cannot be reduced to the sum of opposing views by the child abusers, the child victims, the child abuse researchers, etc., since there will emerge new views in the future not yet known today, just as there are already alternative views nowadays which do not side exclusively with any of them, as is the analysis here, in *Sec. 3.2.2*; the more holistic view on astral travel, such that the whole is not the sum of its parts, that is, it cannot be reduced to the sum of opposing views by the advocates, the critics, the in-between researchers, etc., since there will emerge new views in the future not yet known today, just as there are already alternative views nowadays which do not side exclusively with any of them, as is the analysis here,in *Sec. 3.3.1*; the more holistic view on zoonotic diseases, such that the whole is not the sum of its parts, that is, it cannot be reduced to the sum of opposing views by the practitioners, the critcs, the public, etc., since there will emerge new views in the future not yet known today, just as there are already alternative views nowadays which do not side exclusively with any of them, as is the analysis here, in *Sec. 3.3.2*; the more holistic view on deterrence, such that the whole is not the sum of its parts, that is, it cannot be reduced to the sum of opposing views by the affirmative side, the negative side, etc., since there will emerge new views in the future not yet known today, just as there are already alternative views nowadays which do not side exclusively with any of them, as is the analysis here, in *Sec. 3.4.1*; the more holistic view on domestic violence, such that the whole is not the sum of its parts, that is, it cannot be reduced to the sum of opposing views by the feminists, the masculinists, the critics, etc., since there will emerge new views in the future not yet known today, just as there are already alternative views nowadays which do not side exclusively with any of them, as is the analysis here, in *Sec. 3.4.2*; the more holistic view on torture, such that the whole is not the sum of its parts, that is, it cannot be reduced to the sum of opposing views by the proponents, the opponents, the researchers, etc., since there will emerge new views in the future not yet known today, just as there are already alternative views nowadays which do not side exclusively with any of them, as is the analysis here, in *Sec. 3.5.1*; and the more holistic view on the "four principles" in medical ethics, such that the whole is not the sum of its parts, that is, it cannot be reduced to the sum of opposing views by the advocates, the critics, the reseachers, etc., since there will emerge new views in the future not yet known today, just as there are already alternative views nowadays which do not side exclusively with any of them, as is the analysis here, in *Sec. 3.5.2*).

And the reverse direction also holds true.

However, it should be stressed (as this is something that I regularly did in my previous books, *almost verbatim*) that there are different shades of gray (or different degrees of truth) in the two opposites, and the classification is not necessarily mutually exclusive either. In fact, even when some combinations of the two occur, they only end up sharing the same dialectic relationship, but in a different degree.

Also, there are some other relationships (as a kind of family resemblance) which have something in common with the principle, but they are not exactly the same but only more or less comparable, which varies from case to case.

Good examples of family resemblance in relation to the principle are individualisticness-holisticness, partness-wholeness, analysis-synthesis, and the like.

4th Thesis: The Predictability-Unpredictability Principle

The fourth thesis is called the predictability-unpredictability principle (on the occurrence of events) in the category of "method" in existential dialectics (which was first proposed in *FC* and, later, other books of mine), in that both predictability and unpredictability have a major role to play in the occurrence of things, so that neither determinism nor indeterminism wins the centuries-old fight. There is no predictability without unpredictability—and vice versa.

There are events which are predictable, just as there are those which are not. Or what is regarded as unpredictable at one point in time may turn out to be predictable later, and, conversely, what is deemed as predictable may turn out to not be so predictable. Even in predictability, outcomes are subject to uncertainty, the degree of which varies from case to case.

Works on ecological uncertainty (as in *BNR*), complexity theory (as in *FC*), quantum mechanics (as in *FPHST* and *FPHG*), frequency probability, subjective (or Bayesian) probability (as in *FPHPROB*), "special causes" (as in *FPHGAM*), and measurement uncertainty (as in *FPHPROB*), just to name a few of them, have contributed to the understanding of uncertainity.

The predictability-unpredictability principle is not to be confused with the absoluteness-relativeness principle; although both can address the issue of probability, the former is concerned with the extent of certainty in prediction, whereas the latter focuses on the relativity of viewpoints.

For instance, on the one hand, there is predictability (e.g., the predictable tendency that the dropout rate of psychotherapeutic patients is "quite high," in *Sec. 2.2.1*; the predictable tendency of some correlation between SWB and health by the advocates of SWB, in *Sec. 2.2.2*; the predictable tendency of those in EP to single out the role of psychological adaptation, in *Sec. 2.3.1*; the predictable tendency of the political correctness in the foreseeable future that zoophilia "is not explicitly condoned anywhere," in *Sec. 2.3.2*; the predictable tendency of the correlation between health and lesser income inequality, according to Wilkinson and Pickett, in *Sec. 2.4.1*; the predictable tendency of the increasing use of technology for mental health in the foreseeable future, in *Sec. 2.4.2*; the predictable tendency of more or less "50% of people in developed countries" to "use some kind of complementry and alternative medicine other than prayer for health" in the foreseeable future, in *Sec. 2.5.1*; the predictable tendency by the advocates, of the working of the mindfulness-based therapy for the "elevation of positive emotions and outcomes," in *Sec. 2.5.2*; the predictable tendency of the relationship between physical exercise and improved "immune system," as pointed out by the advocates aforecited, in *Sec. 3.2.1*; the predictable tendency of child abuse to have certain causes in accordance to the studies aforecited, in *Sec. 3.2.2*; the predictable tendency of the advocates like Ingo Swann to claim the alleged ability to astral travel, in *Sec. 3.3.1*; the predictable tendency of those working on zoonotic diseases to link human health with infectious diseases from animals, in *Sec. 3.3.2*; the predictable tendency of "The United States Drug Enforcement Administration [DEA]...to suggest that illegal drugs are 'far more deadly than alcohol'" for drug prohibition, in *Sec. 3.4.1*; the predictable tendency of the advocates of "the...psychological theories [about the causes of domestic violence]" to focus on such issues like "mental illness" and "marital conflict disorder," in *Sec. 3.4.2*; the predictable tendency of the supporters of Alan M. Dershowitz and Mirko Bagaric to argue that "the need for information outweighs the moral and ethical arguments against torture," in *Sec. 3.5.1*; and the predictable tendency of the Western tradition to focus on the "four principles" in medical ethics by Tom Beauchamp and James Childress nowadays in *Sec. 3.5.2*).

On the other hand, there is unpredictability (e.g., the more difficult task to predict exactly the extent to which a particular psychotherapeutic patient will stay or drop out on a particular future occasion in *Sec. 2.2.1*; the more difficult task to predict exactly the extent to which the specific aspects of the correlation between SWB and health are, since the critics pointed out that "how durable the effects of mood and emotions on health are remains unclear," "whether some types of subjective well-being predict health independently of others is also unclear," and so on, in *Sec. 2.2.2*; the more difficult task to predict exactly the extent to which psychological adaptation may apply in a particular individual case, since, for the critics, "evolutionary psychology does not address the complexity of individual development and experience," among other problems aforecited, in *Sec. 2.3.1*; the more difficult task to predict exactly the extent to which form the defense of zoophilia will take in a particular farther future era, in light of the changing history of reacting to zoophilia in the past, in *Sec. 2.3.2*; the more difficult task to predict exactly the extent to which the correlation between health and lesser income inequality will hold on a particular future occasion, since, for the critics, for example, "Americans live no longer on average [about 77 years in 2004] than Greeks [78 years] or New Zealanders [78], though the USA is almost twice as rich," in *Sec. 2.4.1*; the more difficult task to predict exactly which forms, and to what extent, the use of technology for mental health will take in a particular future era, in light of different barriers and problems in the past afore-described, in *Sec. 2.4.2*; the more difficult task to predict exactly which particular types, and to what extent, alternative medicines will take in a particular future era, in light of its controversical past history with different problems aforediscussed, in *Sec. 2.5.1*; the more difficult task to predict exactly the extent to which the mindfulness-based therapy on the "elevation of positive emotions and outcomes" will necessarily work on a particular future occasion, since, for the critics, "the study did not address specific differences between the interventions, and how these differences may relate to well-being," and, in addition, "the effects of these meditations may become nonexistent once practice ceases," in *Sec. 2.5.2*; the more difficult task to predict exactly the extent to which physical exercise will improve "immune system" on a particular future occasion, since, for the critics, "another study did not find the effect," in that "immune cell functions are impaired following acute sessions of prolonged, high-intensity exercise, and some studies have found that athletes are at a higher risk for infections....Athletes may have slightly elevated natural killer cell count and cytolytic action, but these are unlikely to be clinically significant," in *Sec. 3.2.1*; the more difficult task to predict exactly the extent to which that the causal relationship in regard to child abuse will hold on a particular future occasion, since, for the critics, the alleged causes of child abuse can be questionable, the long-term effects of child abuse remains unknown, and the alleged causes do not determine the often cited consequences, in *Sec. 3.2.2*; the more difficult task to predict exactly the extent to which a claim about astral travel will be like in a particular distant future era, since some critics already pointed out that there are competing interpretations of astral travel over time, depending on different historical traditions, etc., in *Sec. 3.3.1*; the more difficult task to predict exactly the extent to which the causes of zoonotic diseases and their effects are on a particular future occasion, since the critics are quick to point out that "the environmental causes of health problems are complex, global, and poorly understood," such that the causes and effects of zoonotic diseases can be more complicated than previously thought, in *Sec. 3.3.2*; the more difficult task to predict exactly the extent to which the health statistics by DEA will be accurate on a particular future occasion, because of the tendency of DEA to engage in "misleading health statistics," in that "the DEA's use of such figures is questionable," for example, in *Sec. 3.4.1*; the more difficult task to predict exactly the extent to which "the...psychological theories" are appropriate on a particular future occasion, since the critic like Gelles showed that "psychological theories are limited" and that "only 10% [or less] fit this psychological profile," in *Sec. 3.4.2*; the more difficult task to predict exactly the extent to which a particular practice of torture will be effective on a particular future occasion, since, for the critics, "there is simply no scientific evidence supporting its effectiveness," in *Sec. 3.5.1*; and the more difficult task to predict exactly the extent to which the "four principles" in medical ethics by Tom Beauchamp and James Childress will remain dominant in a particular distant future era, since, for the critics, there are different problems with the principles aforediscussed in *Sec. 3.5.2*).

And the reverse direction also holds true.

Again, it should be stressed, however, that there are different shades of gray (or different degrees of truth) in the two opposites, and the classification is not necessarily mutually exclusive either. In fact, even when some combinations of the two occur, they only end up sharing the same dialectic relationship, but in a different degree.

Also, there are some other relationships (as a kind of family resemblance) which have something in common with the principle, but they are not exactly the same but only more or less comparable, which varies from case to case.

Good examples of family resemblance in relation to the principle are sureness-arbitrariness, deterministicness-randomness, likeliness-riskiness, sureness-doubtfulness, deterministicness-indeterministicness, certainty-uncertainty, reliability-unreliability, and so forth.

5th Thesis: The Explicability-Inexplicability Principle

The fifth thesis is called the explicability-inexplicability principle (on the underlying mechanisms of things) in the category of "method" in existential dialectics (which was proposed in *FPHU* and other books of mine), in that both explicability and inexplicability are part of the understanding of things. There is no explicability without inexplicability—and vice versa.

This principle tells us the dual nature of the research dilemma, in that, if reality can be explained in some ways, it also has its other ways which are not quite explainable, at a given point in time.

For instance, on the one hand, there is explicability (e.g., the explanation, by the practitioners of psychotherapy that psychotherapy can "increase the individual's sense of his/her own well-being" by employing "a range of techniques based on experiential relationship building, dialogue, communication and behavior change," in *Sec. 2.2.1*; the explanation by the advocates of SWB that positive SWB can contribute to better health, as shown in the finding that "people who rate their general health as 'good' or 'excellent' tend to experience better SWB compared to those who rate their health as 'fair' or 'poor,'" in *Sec. 2.2.2*; the explanation, by those in EP, of emotion and cognition on the basis of "evolved psychological mechanisms," in *Sec. 2.3.1*; the explanation, by the defenders of zoophilia, of the extent of its occurrence on the basis of location, in that it was 40–50% in people living near farms," according to "the Kinsey reports," in *Sec. 2.3.2*; the explanation, by Wilkinson and Pickett, of the desirability of lesser income inequality on the basis of its positive effects aforecited, in *Sec. 2.4.1*; the explanation, by the advocates, of the desirability of the use of technology for mental health on the basis of being "a supplement to mainstream therapies for mental disorders," in *Sec. 2.4.2*; the explanation, by the critics of alternative medicines, that they are undesirable because of the criticisms that altnerative medicine is not scientific, that its practice is unethical, that alternative medicine often uses "ambiguous" words to mislead, that alternative medicine is not effective as claimed, and that its practice is manipulative, that its practitioners play trick on patients, etc., in *Sec. 2.5.1*; the explanation, by the advocates, of the desirability of the scientific research on mindfulness on the basis of its practical use for therapy, in *Sec. 2.5.2*; the explanation, by the advocates, of the desirability of physical exercise on the basis of its positive effects on physical health, in *Sec. 3.2.1*; the explanation, by a child abuser, of the desirability of child abuse on the basis of "sexual stimulation" and so on, in *Sec. 3.2.2*; the explanation, by those advocates like Ingo Swann to claim the alleged ability to astral travel travel on the basis of his account of "Jupiter and observe details of the planet," in *Sec. 3.3.1*; the explanation, by the advocates, of the occurrence of zoonotic diseases on the basis of "infectious diseases…transmitted…from animals," in *Sec. 3.3.2*; the explanation, by those in the DEA, of the desirability of drug prohibition, on the ground that "compared to the social costs of drug abuse and addiction—whether in taxpayer dollars or in pain and suffering—government spending on drug control is minimal," in *Sec. 3.4.1*; the explanation, by the advocates of the "strict 'patriarchal violence' model," that "all violence in the home and elsewhere has a male perpetrator and female victim," in *Sec. 3.4.2*; the explanation, by Alan M. Dershowitz and Mirko Bagaric, of the desirability of torture on the basis that "the need for information outweighs the moral and ethical arguments against torture," in *Sec. 3.5.1*; and the explanation, by some scholars like Edmund Pellegrino, of the desirability of "beneficence" on the basis that it is "the only fundamental principle of medical ethics, in *Sec. 3.5.2*).

On the other hand, there is inexplicability (e.g., the lack of sufficient explanation, by the practitioners of psychotherapy of why it is necessarily explainable, since the critic like Bruce Wampold in *The Great Psychotherapy Debate* argued that "we do not know why psychotherapy works," in *Sec. 2.2.1*; the lack of convincing explanation, by the advocates of SWB, of why SWB is necessarily desirable for health, since the critics had pointed out that, in the case of "survival," there is "evidence" which "suggests happiness may actually be sometimes detrimental" to health, in *Sec. 2.2.2*; the lack of sufficient explanation, by those in EP, of why "evolved psychological mechanisms" is necessarily useful, since, for the critics, "evolutionary psychology…fails to explain the influence of genes on behavior in individual cases," among other problems aforecited, in *Sec. 2.3.1*; the lack of sufficient explanation, by the defenders of zoophilia, of why the factor of location necessarily has much explanatory power for the extent of its occurrence, since, for the critics, in a different report, "people who 'grew up in the country around animals were no more likely to become zoophiles than those who grew up in the city without them,'" in *Sec. 2.3.2*; the lack of sufficient explanation, by Wilkinson and Pickett, of why lesser income inequality is necessarily desirable, since the critics pointed out that the work constitutes a very narrow view of social stratification in relation to health care, that it provides no verification of the claim, that there is no general agreement on the desirability of income equality or its reduction, that the correlation between health and income level does not always hold, and that equality can lead to a conformist society, in *Sec. 2.4.1*; the lack of sufficient explanation, by the advocates, of why the use of technology for mental health is necessarily desirable, since, for the critics, there are already different barriers and problems afore-described, in *Sec. 2.4.2*; the lack of sufficient explanation, by the critics of of alternative medicines, of why "alternative medicine can be on the rise 'in countries where Western science and scientific method generally are accepted as the major foundations for healthcare" and this anomaly "has been described as an 'enigma' in the Medical Journal of Australia," in *Sec. 2.5.1*; the lack of sufficient explanation, by the advocates, of why the scientific research on mindfulness is necessarily desirable, since, for the critics, it suffers from the problems that the research works are often incomplete, that the practices are not so effective, that its terms are often not clearly defined and can mean different things, and that because of its connection with alternative medicine, mindfulness-based therapy programs have been criticized as not being scientific, in *Sec. 2.5.2*; the lack of sufficient explanation, by the advocates, of why physical exercise is necessarily desirable, since, for the critics, vigorous exercise can have its downside, besides other problems aforecited, in *Sec. 3.2.1*; the lack of sufficient explanation, by a child abuser, of why child abuse is necessarily desirable, since, for the victims, there are negative health effects aforedescribed, in *Sec. 3.2.2*; the lack of sufficient explanation, by those advocates like Ingo Swann to claim the alleged ability to astral travel on the basis of his account of "Jupiter and observe details of the planet," of why the claims are necessarily true, since the critics were quick to reveal that the claims are not accurate, as they are merely "neuroanatomy, human belief, imagination and prior knowledge to provide prosaic explanations," in *Sec. 3.3.1*; the lack of sufficient explanation, by the advocates, of the more complicated nature of the causes and effects of zoonotic diseases, since, for the critics, "the environmental causes of health problems are complex, global, and poorly understood," in *Sec. 3.3.2*; the lack of sufficient explanation, by those in the DEA, of why their calculation of "cost" in the enforcement of drug prohibition is accurate, since, for the critics, "these numbers only include direct prohibition enforcement expenditures, and as such only represent part of the total cost of prohibition," but "rise...dramatically once other issues, such as the economic impact of holding 400,000 prisoners on prohibition violations, are factored in" and "the war on drugs is extremely costly to such societies that outlaw drugs in terms of taxpayer money, lives, productivity, the inability of law enforcement to pursue mala in se crimes, and social inequality," in *Sec. 3.4.1*; the lack of sufficient explanation, by the advocates of the "strict 'patriarchal violence' model," of why this model is necessarily valid, since, for the critics, "modern research into predictors of injury from domestic violence finds that the strongest predictor of injury by domestic violence is participation in reciprocal domestic violence, and that this pattern of domestic violence is more often initiated by the female in the relationship," in *Sec. 3.4.2*; the lack of sufficient explanation, by Alan M. Dershowitz and Mirko Bagaric, of why their argument for torture is necessarily convincing, since "others including Robert Mueller, FBI Director since 5 July 2001,...do not believe that evidence gained by the U.S. government through what supporters of the techniques call 'enhanced interrogation' has disrupted a single attack and no one has come up with a documented example of lives saved thanks to these techniques," in *Sec. 3.5.1*; and the lack of sufficient explanation, by some scholars like Edmund Pellegrino, of why "beneficence" is necessarily "the only fundamental principle of medical ethics," since, for other scholars, "non-maleficience "should be the main or primary consideration [hence primum]: that it is more important not to harm your patient, than to do them good," in *Sec. 3.5.2*).

And the reverse direction also holds true.

Once more, it should be stressed, however, that there are different shades of gray (or different degrees of truth) in the two opposites, and the classification is not necessarily mutually exclusive either. In fact, even when some combinations of the two occur, they only end up sharing the same dialectic relationship, but in a different degree.

Also, there are some other relationships (as a kind of family resemblance) which have something in common with the principle, but they are not exactly the same but only more or less comparable, which varies from case to case.

Good examples of family resemblance in relation to the principle are underlyingness-regularness, causation-regularity, causation-correlation, explanation-description, explanation-narration, explanation-interpretation, and so forth.

6th Thesis: The Fiction-Reality Principle

The sixth thesis is called the fiction-reality principle (on the different faces of reality) in the category of "method" in existential dialectics (as first proposed in *FPHLIT*), in that both fiction and reality co-exist. There is no reality without fiction—and vice versa.

This principle tells us the different categories of reality, in that, if there is reality, there is also some fiction in it—just as, if there is fiction, there is also some reality in it.

For instance, on the one hand, there is fiction (e.g., the fictional aspect of psychotherapy, insofar as, "in one of the earliest studies of psychotherapy treatment, Hans Eysenck reported that two thirds of therapy patients improved significantly or recovered on their own within two years, whether or not they received psychotherapy," in *Sec. 2.2.1*; the fictional aspect of "heritability studies," insofar as "they describe long-term SWB in a sample of people in a modern western society but may not be applicable to more extreme environments that might influence SWB and do not provide absolute indicators of genetic effects" and, in addition, "heritability estimates are inconsistent across studies," in *Sec. 2.2.2*; the fictional aspect of EP, insofar as there are "non-genetic and non-adaptive explanations" which are not adequately considered, in *Sec. 2.3.1*; the fictional aspect of the research on zoophilia, insofar as there is "self-selection bias" afore-discussed, in *Sec. 2.3.2*; the fictional aspect of the claim about the correlation between health and lesser income inequality, insofar as there is the counter-example that "Americans live no longer on average [about 77 years in 2004] than Greeks [78 years] or New Zealanders [78], though the USA is almost twice as rich," in *Sec. 2.4.1*;

the fictional aspect of the argument about the use of technology for mental health, insofar as "one size does not fit all and some technologies may not be suitable for certain people," as pointed out by the critics, in *Sec. 2.4.2*; the fictional aspect of alternative medicine, insofar as "academic proponents…sometimes recommend misleading patients by using known placebo treatments in order to achieve a placebo effect," in *Sec. 2.5.1*; the fictional aspect of mindfulness-based therapy, insofar as, for the critics, "the effects of these meditations may become nonexistent once practice ceases," and "Diener, Lucas, and Scollon claimed that emotional techniques used successfully in the lab may not translate to life outside of the lab…," in *Sec. 2.5.2*; the fictional aspect of physical exercise on health, insofar as vigorous exercise can have its downside, some individuals can be exercise-resistant, etc., in *Sec. 3.2.1*; the fictional aspect of the studies on child abuse, insofar as scholars disagree over what constitutes child abuse, the alleged causes of child abuse can be questionable, and the alleged causes do not determine the often cited consequences, in *Sec. 3.2.2*; the fictional aspect of astral travel, insofar as the claims by the advocates like Ingo Swann are not accurate, based on "neuroanatomy, human belief, imagination and prior knowledge" pointed out by the critics, in *Sec. 3.3.1*; the fictional aspect of the perception of zoonotic diseases, insofar as there is the politics of social impact aforedescribed, in *Sec. 3.3.2*; the fictional aspect of the figures on "drug-induced deaths" in 2000 povided by the Centers for Disease Control and Prevention, insofar as the actual "number deaths caused by alcohol in year 2000" was "85,000—over four and a half times greater than the DEA's preferred figure," according to "the Journal of the American Medical Association," in *Sec. 3.4.1*; the fictional aspect of the "model" of power and control, insofar as "it ignores research linking domestic violence to substance abuse and psychological problems," in *Sec. 3.4.2*; the fictional aspect of torture, insofar as the critics like "Robert Mueller, FBI Director since 5 July 2001,…do not believe that evidence gained by the U.S. government through what supporters of the techniques call 'enhanced interrogation' has disrupted a single attack and no one has come up with a documented example of lives saved thanks to these techniques," in *Sec. 3.5.1*; and the fictional aspect of the "four principles" in medical ethics, insofar as there are "conflicts of interest" in medical ethics so that the values are not necessarily followed in practice, and the values in medical ethics are not necessarily valuable either, as discussed earlier, in *Sec. 3.5.2*).

On the other hand, there is reality (e.g., the realistic aspect of psychotherapy, insofar as "psychoanalytic psychotherapy has been found to be as effective as Cognitive Behavioral Therapy for immediate relief" of panic disorders, in *Sec. 2.2.1*; the realistic aspect of "heritability studies," insofar as "findings from numerous personality studies show that genetics account for 50% of the variance in Five-Factor Model and the variance in subjective well-being is also heritable," in *Sec. 2.2.2*; the realistic aspect of EP, insofar as it addresses the role of "evolved psychological mechanisms" in certain relevant cases, in *Sec. 2.3.1*; the realistic aspect of the research on zoophilia, insofar as "exclusive desire for animals rather than humans is considered a rare paraphilia," in *Sec. 2.3.2*; the realistic aspect of the claim about some correlation between health and lesser income inequality, insofar as "the most consistent finding in cross-national research on homicides has been that of a positive association between income inequality and homicides," in *Sec. 2.4.1*; the realistic aspect of the argument about the use of technology for mental health, insofar as the use of technology for mental health can be used, under certain circumstances, "as a supplement to mainstream therapies for mental disorders," in *Sec. 2.4.2*; the realistic aspect of alternative medicine, insofar as a small percentage of alternative treatments were found effective, although the rest, 95%, were not, according to the study by Ernst, in *Sec. 2.5.1*; the realistic aspect of mindfulness-based therapy, insofar as the study by "Brown [2003] found declines in mood disturbance and stress following mindfulness interventions," under certain conditions, in *Sec. 2.5.2*; the realistic aspect of physical exercise on health, insofar as "epidemiological evidence suggests that moderate exercise has a beneficial effect on the human immune system," in *Sec. 3.2.1*; the realistic aspect of the studies on child abuse, insofar as, in an estimate by the [American] National Committee to Prevent Child Abuse, "in 1997 neglect represented 54% of confirmed cases of child abuse, physical abuse 22%, sexual abuse 8%, emotional maltreatment 4%, and other forms of maltreatment 12%," in *Sec. 3.2.2*; the realistic aspect of astral travel, insofar as there are different historical sources to offer details about astral travel aforecited, although this does not imply that the claims must be true, in *Sec. 3.3.1*; the realistic aspect of the perception of zoonotic diseases, insofar as there were in fact "actual cases" like "SARS or HIV/AIDS," in *Sec. 3.3.2*; the realistic aspect of the figures on "drug-induced deaths" in 2000 provided by the Centers for Disease Control and Prevention, insofar as in 2000, there were quite a few thousand drug-induced deaths, in *Sec. 3.4.1*; the realistic aspect of the "model" of power and control, insofar as some cases in which "violence is posited to arise out of a need for power and control of one partner over the other" did occur, in *Sec. 3.4.2*; the realistic aspect of torture, insofar as "torture still occurs in liberal democracies [nowadays] despite several international treaties such as the International

Covenant on Civil and Political Rights and the UN Convention Against Torture making torture illegal," in *Sec. 3.5.1*; and the realistic aspect of the "four principles" in medical ethics, insofar as "these do not give answers as to how to handle a particular situation, but provide a useful framework for understanding conflicts," in *Sec. 3.5.2*).

And the reverse direction also holds true.

Once more, it should be stressed, however, that there are different shades of gray (or different degrees of truth) in the two opposites, and the classification is not necessarily mutually exclusive either. In fact, even when some combinations of the two occur, they only end up sharing the same dialectic relationship, but in a different degree.

Also, there are some other relationships (as a kind of family resemblance) which have something in common with the principle, but they are not exactly the same but only more or less comparable, which varies from case to case.

Good examples of family resemblance in relation to the principle are fiction-nonfiction, fiction-fact, imagination-fact, imagination-nonfiction, subjectivity-objectivity, inaccuracy-accuracy, and so forth.

7th Thesis: The Cognitiveness-Noncognitiveness Principle

The seventh thesis is called the cognitiveness-noncognitiveness principle (on the understanding of meaning) in the category of "method" in existential dialectics (as first proposed in *BNR*), in that, if a view of things is based on reason and evidences, it is also affected by non-cognitive factors (such that it is neither true nor false in the latter case)—and vice versa. In other words, there is no cognitiveness without noncognitiveness—and vice versa.

Noncognitive factors can come in all shapes and sizes, and good examples include envy, jealousy, power, nationality, race, gender, age, class, greed, lust, status, faith, anger, sadness, joy, fear, wish, etc.

Communication, even in its ideal type, is seldom based on reason and evidences only, as falsely assumed during the Age of the Enlightenment and its continued supporters nowadays. What is understood about something is often twisted on the basis of something else too. In these cases, what is at stake is often neither true nor false (which is something that classical logic has sidelined and ignored).

For instance, on the one hand, there is cognitiveness (e.g., a view of things on the basis of reason and evidences, as shown in the empirical research by Wampold that "psychotherapy" can be "effective," in *Sec. 2.2.1*; a view of things on the basis of reason and evidences, as shown in the research findings that "all cultures seem to value happiness," in *Sec. 2.2.2*; a view of things on the basis of reason and evidences, as shown in research findings about psychological adaptations on "topics such as infanticide, intelligence, marriage patterns, promiscuity," etc., in *Sec. 2.3.1*; a view of things on the basis of reason and evidences, as shown in the treatment of zoophilia as "a violation of Biblical edicts" during the "Church-oriented" Middle Ages in Europe, in *Sec. 2.3.2*; a view of things on the basis of reason and evidences, as shown in the research finding that "higher income inequality led to less of all forms of social, cultural, and civic participation among the less wealthy," in *Sec. 2.4.1*; a view of things on the basis of reason and evidences, as shown in the empirical problems of "technical training," "poor quality of transmitted records," and "evaluation time" in the "adoption of telemedicine in emergency and critical care units," in *Sec. 2.4.2*; a view of things on the basis of reason and evidences, as shown in empirical finding that "about 50% of people in developed countries use some kind of complementry and alternative medicine other than prayer for health," in *Sec. 2.5.1*; a view of things on the basis of reason and evidences, as shown in the empirical work by Wallace, who pointed out that "the modern description and practice of mindfulness are certainly valuable, as thousands of people have discovered for themselves through their own practice," in *Sec. 2.5.2*; a view of things on the basis of reason and evidences, as shown in the research finding that "when a person exercises, levels of both circulating serotonin and endorphins are increased," in *Sec. 3.2.1*; a view of things on the basis of reason and evidences, as shown in the existence of a debate in the U.S. during the 2000s on "the parental rights of abusive parents or caretakers with regard to their children, particularly in medical settings," in *Sec. 3.2.2*; a view of things on the basis of reason and evidences, as shown in different historical sources, be they Western, Islamic, or Eastern, to offer details about astral travel aforecited, in *Sec. 3.3.1*; a view of things on the basis of reason and evidences, as shown in the empirical findings on outbreaks of zoonotic diseases aforecited, in *Sec. 3.3.2*; a view of things on the basis of reason and evidences, as shown in the empirical finding by Scott Morgan that "there was no legitimate political support for ending the drug war" in the U.S. in 2008, in *Sec. 3.4.1*; a view of things on the basis of reason and evidences, as shown in the report that "in 2003,...one out of every three homeless women are homeless due to having left a DV relationship," in *Sec. 3.4.2*; a view of things on the basis of reason and evidences, as shown in the empirical finding that "throughout history and today, many states have engaged in torture," as discussed earlier, in *Sec. 3.5.1*; and a view of things on the basis of reason and evidences, as shown in the scholarly analysis of medical ethics in terms of the "four principles" by Tom Beauchamp and James Childress, in *Sec. 3.5.2*).

On the other hand, there is noncognitiveness (e.g., a view of things on the basis of non-cognitive factors like envy, jealousy, power, nationality, race, gender, age, class, greed, lust, status, faith, anger, sadness, joy, fear, wish, etc., as shown in the politics of power pointed out by feminist critics, in that "the therapist-client relationship always participates in society's power relations and political dynamics," in *Sec. 2.2.1*; a view of things on the basis of non-cognitive factors like envy, jealousy, power, nationality, race, gender, age, class, greed, lust, status, faith, anger, sadness, joy, fear, wish, etc., as shown in the "politics" of cultural identity, such that "individualistic versus collectivistic nations reliably differ in a variety of psychological characteristics that are related to SWB," such that this difference cannot be reconciled on the basis of reason and evidences alone, due to the politics in question, in *Sec. 2.2.2*; a view of things on the basis of non-cognitive factors like envy, jealousy, power, nationality, race, gender, age, class, greed, lust, status, faith, anger, sadness, joy, fear, wish, etc., as shown in the "politics" of "eugenics and social darwinism" in the early 20th century that were largely based on the naturalistic fallacy," because of the politics in action, in *Sec. 2.3.1*; a view of things on the basis of non-cognitive factors like envy, jealousy, power, nationality, race, gender, age, class, greed, lust, status, faith, anger, sadness, joy, fear, wish, etc., as shown in the "power" of coercion during the "Church-oriented" Middle Ages, when "some witches were accused of having congress with the devil in the form of an animal," and "as with all accusations and confessions extracted under torture in the witch trials in Early Modern Europe, their validity cannot be ascertained," in *Sec. 2.3.2*; a view of things on the basis of non-cognitive factors like envy, jealousy, power, nationality, race, gender, age, class, greed, lust, status, faith, anger, sadness, joy, fear, wish, etc., as shown in the ideological politics pointed out by Charles Moore [2010] about the claim by Wilkinson and Pickett, in that their work is "a socialist tract than an objective analysis of poverty," in *Sec. 2.4.1*; a view of things on the basis of non-cognitive factors like envy, jealousy, power, nationality, race, gender, age, class, greed, lust, status, faith, anger, sadness, joy, fear, wish, etc., as shown in the politics of "cultural" barriers, which refer to the "barriers occurring from the lack of desire, or unwillingness, of some physicians to adapt clinical paradigms for telemedicine applications," even when the new technologies have "much lower cost and apparently higher success rates," in *Sec. 2.4.2*; a view of things on the basis of non-cognitive factors like envy, jealousy, power, nationality, race, gender, age, class, greed, lust, status, faith, anger, sadness, joy, fear, wish, etc., as shown in the politics of "faith" by "alternative medicine users," who "appear to be doing so largely because 'they find these healthcare alternatives to be more congruent with their own values, beliefs, and philosophical orientations toward health and life,'" even though "95%" of alternative treatments were not effective, according to the study by Ernst, in *Sec. 2.5.1*; a view of things on the basis of non-cognitive factors like envy, jealousy, power, nationality, race, gender, age, class, greed, lust, status, faith, anger, sadness, joy, fear, wish, etc., as shown in the politics of historical revisionism in regard to how "mindfulness has been defined or represented in recent western psychology publications," which "differs in significant ways from how mindfulness was defined by the Buddha himself, and by much of Buddhist tradition," as pointed out by Wallace, in *Sec. 2.5.2*; a view of things on the basis of non-cognitive factors like envy, jealousy, power, nationality, race, gender, age, class, greed, lust, status, faith, anger, sadness, joy, fear, wish, etc., as shown in the "euphoric feeling" when someone "exercises" and his "levels of both circulating serotonin and endorphins are increased," but his improvement in mood, that is, the "euphoric feeling," does not automatically reflect an improvement of his social conditions, in *Sec. 3.2.1*; a view of things on the basis of non-cognitive factors like envy, jealousy, power, nationality, race, gender, age, class, greed, lust, status, faith, anger, sadness, joy, fear, wish, etc., as shown in the politics of "parental rights" advocated by "abusive parents or caretakers with regard to their children, particularly in medical settings," in *Sec. 3.2.2*; a view of things on the basis of non-cognitive factors like envy, jealousy, power, nationality, race, gender, age, class, greed, lust, status, faith, anger, sadness, joy, fear, wish, etc., as shown in the wishful imagination by those advocates of astral travel, whose "subjective nature of the experience permits explanations that do not rely on the existence of an 'astral' body and plane," which can be true or false but is irrelevat in this context, in *Sec. 3.3.1*; a view of things on the basis of non-cognitive factors like envy, jealousy, power, nationality, race, gender, age, class, greed, lust, status, faith, anger, sadness, joy, fear, wish, etc., as shown in the politics of social impact, such that "actual cases [like SARS or HIV/AIDS]…resonate more powerfully with the public than the more abstract explanations of environmental and health issues," regardless of whether the perception is accurate or not, in *Sec. 3.3.2*; a view of things on the basis of non-cognitive factors like envy, jealousy, power, nationality, race, gender, age, class, greed, lust, status, faith, anger, sadness, joy, fear, wish, etc., as shown in the "political calculation" by Peter Reuter and David Boyum, who in their book *An Analytic Assessment of U.S. Drug Policy* "admitted ignoring the legalization option in their analysis," because "there was no legitimate political support for ending the drug war" at the time, regardless of whether or not they personally believed in the legalization option, in *Sec. 3.4.1*; a view of things on the basis of non-cognitive factors like envy, jealousy, power, nationality, race, gender, age, class, greed, lust, status, faith, anger, sadness, joy, fear, wish, etc., as shown in the politics of feminism by some advocates of the "strict 'patriarchal violence' model," in that "all violence in the home and elsewhere has a male perpetrator and female victim," regardless of whether it is true or false, in *Sec. 3.4.2*; a view of things on the basis of non-cognitive factors like envy, jealousy, power, nationality, race, gender, age, class, greed, lust, status, faith, anger, sadness, joy, fear, wish, etc., as shown in the politics of "denial" by "many states" which "engage in torture" but "few wish to be described as doing so, either to their own citizens or to the international community," so they resort to "state denial," "secret police," "need to know," etc. to cover up their practice, in *Sec. 3.5.1*; and a view of things on the basis of non-cognitive factors like envy, jealousy, power, nationality, race, gender, age, class, greed, lust, status, faith, anger, sadness, joy, fear, wish, etc., as shown in the politics of the "conflicts of interest," so that the values are not followed in practice, even though the physicians know that they "should not allow a conflict of interest to influence medical judgment," in *Sec. 3.5.2*).

And the reverse direction also holds true.

Once more, it should be stressed, however, that there are different shades of gray (or different degrees of truth) in the two opposites, and the classification is not necessarily mutually exclusive either. In fact, even when some combinations of the two occur, they only end up sharing the same dialectic relationship, but in a different degree.

Also, there are some other relationships (as a kind of family resemblance) which have something in common with the principle, but they are not exactly the same but only more or less comparable, which varies from case to case.

Good examples of family resemblance in relation to the principle are proposition-attitude, cognition-emotion, cognition-prescription, theory-extratheory, justification-nonjustification, and so forth.

In Relation to Structure

The next five theses are in relation to structure in existential dialectics, as shown below.

8th Thesis: The Finiteness-Transfiniteness Principle

The eighth thesis is called the finiteness-transfiniteness principle (on the nature of numbers) in the category of "structure" in existential dialectics (as first proposed in *FPHG*), in that, if there are finite things, there are likewise transfinite ones—and vice versa.

To avoid confusion, my usage of the word "transfinite" here differs radically from the one used by Cantor (and other mathematicians) for "relative" infinity—and is more limited, in light of the problems confronting any attempt to understand the idea of infinity, be it by intuition, imagination, and conception (as detailedly analyzed in *Sec. 2.2.3* of *FPHG*).

Instead, by "transfinity," I allow numbers which can be many times larger—or smaller, for that matter—than the finite things that we encounter in daily life, but they do not have to be related to the idea of infinity at all (which may not exist).

Of course, there may be some *borderline* cases, in which it is not clear whether the number in question is transfinite (in my usage) or simply a mathematical convenience. A good example of a borderline case is the Planck unit of length for "the smallest space possibly measured in nature," which is "less than billionths of trillionths of trillionths of an inch" (or something like 1.6×10^{-35} meters). (P. Baofu 2006a; N. McAleer 1987: 219; WKV 2008; D. Corbett 2008a)

That said—my usage of "transfinity" can also resolve (or better, dissolve) an age-old problem in philosophy known as "Zeno's paradoxes" (as already explained in *Sec. 2.2.3* of *FPHG*).

In any event, in relation to the finiteness-transfiniteness principle, on the other hand, there is finiteness (e.g., the finite number of the categories of "resources available to a person experiencing emotional distress" like "the friendly support of friends, peers, family members, clergy contacts, personal reading, healthy exercise, research, and independent coping," in *Sec. 2.2.1*; the finite number of the components of SWB, like the 2 components aforedescribed, in *Sec. 2.2.2*; the finite number of the areas of research in EP, like "cognition" and "emotion/motivation" aforediscussed, in *Sec. 2.3.1*; the finite number of the "demographic categories" in the practice of zoophilia, such as "white, black, Asian, Mormon, Amish, Catholic, atheist, pagan, Jewish, male and female," in *Sec. 2.3.2*; the finite number of the causes of income inequality, as shown in the 10 examples aforecited, in *Sec. 2.4.1*; the finite number of the categories of mental health technologies like "email, SMS, virtual reality, computer programmes, blogs, social networks, the telephone, video conferencing, computer games, instant messaging and podcasts," in *Sec. 2.4.2*; the finite number of the categories of substances used in alternative medicines, like "herbs, foods, non-vitamin supplments and megavitmins, and minerals," as well as "seed oil or pills, and ginseng," for example, in *Sec. 2.5.1*; the finite number of the components in mindfullness, like "attention," "openness," etc., in *Sec. 2.5.2*; the finite number of the categories of cells in immune systems, like "natural killer cells," "cytotoxic T cells," etc., in *Sec. 3.2.1*; the finite number of the categories of child abuse effects, like "physical effects" and "psychological effects" in the article aforecited, in *Sec. 3.2.2*; the finite number of the categories of historical sources about astral travel, namely, Western, Islamic, and Eastern, in *Sec. 3.3.1*; the finite number of "infectious agent types," like "parasites," "fungi," "bacteria," "viruses," and "pria," in *Sec. 3.3.2*; the finite number of the categories of "natural plant drugs," namely, "opium, coca, cannabis, mescaline, and psilocybin," for example, in *Sec. 3.4.1*; the finite number of the forms of domestic violence like "hitting, kicking, biting, shoving, restraining, slapping, throwing objects, battery..., sexual abuse, emotional abuse, controlling or domineering, intimidation, stalking, passive/covert abuse," etc., in *Sec. 3.4.2*; the finite number of the methods of torture used in history, like "pharmacological," "physical," "psychological," "medical," etc., in *Sec. 3.5.1*; and the finite number of the values in medical ethics, like the "four principles" and other alternative values aforecited, in *Sec. 3.5.2*).

On the other hand, there is transfinitty (e.g., the transfinite number of all the individuals in human history who have ever existed and have used any of the resources available to cope with emotinal distress, in *Sec. 2.2.1*; the transfinite number of all the individuals in human history who have ever existed and can be described on the basis of the 2 compnents of SWB, in *Sec. 2.2.2*; the transfinite number of all the indiviudals in history who have ever existed and whose cognition, emotion, and motivation can be addressed from the standpoint of EP, in *Sec. 2.3.1*; the transfinite number of all the individuals in human history who have ever engaged in zoophilia in one form or the other, be it actual, virtual, fantasizing, etc., in *Sec. 2.3.2*; the transfinite number of all the individuals in human history who have ever existed and have different income levels with different causes, in *Sec. 2.4.1*; the transfinite number of all the individuals, equipments, exchanges, practices, etc. that have ever existed in the history of mental health technologies, in *Sec. 2.4.2*; the transfinite number of all the individual pieces of "herbs, foods, non-vitamin supplments and megavitmins, and minerals," as well as "seed oil or pills, and ginseng" that have ever existed and used for alternative medicines in history, in *Sec. 2.5.1*; the transfinite number of all the individuals in history who have ever existed and shared the traits of "attention, "openness," etc., in *Sec. 2.5.2*; the transfinite number of all the individual cells in immune systems that have ever existed in history, be they "natural killer cells," "cytotoxic T cells," etc., in *Sec. 3.2.1*; the transfinite number of all the individuals, young or old, who have ever existed in history and have been abused, in one way or the other, regardless of whether the incident of an abuse is minor or serious, in *Sec. 3.2.2*; the transfinite number of all the individual stories, individuals, incidents, etc. that have ever existed in history and are related to astral travel, in *Sec. 3.3.1*; the transfinite number of all the individual "parasites," "fungi," "bacteria," "viruses," and "pria" that have ever existed in history, in *Sec. 3.3.2*; the transfinite number of all the individual pieces of "opium, coca, cannabis, mescaline, and psilocybin" that have ever existed in history, in *Sec. 3.4.1*; the transfinite number of all the individual instances of "hitting, kicking, biting, shoving, restraining, slapping, throwing objects, battery..., sexual abuse, emotional abuse, controlling or domineering, intimidation, stalking, passive/covert abuse," etc. that have ever existed in history, in *Sec. 3.4.2*; the transfinite number of all the individuals in history who have ever experienced, or conversely who have practiced, torture, regardless of the methods of torture used, in *Sec. 3.5.1*; and the transfinite number of all the individual physicians and patients in history who have ever been affected, in one way or the other, however trivial and informal, by different values in medical practice, in *Sec. 3.5.2*).

And the reverse direction also holds true.

Once more, it should be stressed, however, that there are different shades of gray (or different degrees of truth) in the two opposites, and the classification is not necessarily mutually exclusive either. In fact, even when some combinations of the two occur, they only end up sharing the same dialectic relationship, but in a different degree.

Also, there are some other relationships (as a kind of family resemblance) which have something in common with the principle, but they are not exactly the same but only more or less comparable, which varies from case to case.

Good examples of family resemblance in relation to the principle are boundedness-quasiunboundedness, smallness-largeness, microness-macroness, boundedness-unboundedness, and the like.

9th Thesis: The Preciseness-Vagueness Principle

The ninth thesis is called the preciseness-vagueness principle (on the refinement of things) in the category of "structure" in existential dialectics (which was first out worked out in *FIA* and later, *FPHMORP*), in that both preciseness and vagueness are important, not that one is better than the other, but that both are used, in different degrees of preference, in accordance to the contextual application from the perspectives of nature, the mind, culture, and society. There is no preciseness without vagueness—and vice versa.

For illustration, in relation to taxonomy, preciseness has its taxonomic clarity, just as vagueness has its classificatory flexibility. And in relation to network, vagueness has its explorative liberty, just as preciseness has its conceptual definitiveness.

For instance, on the one hand, there is preciseness (e.g., the precise identification of 8 main approaches to psychotherapy in the article aforecited, in *Sec. 2.2.1*; the precise identification of 2 theories of the causes of SWB in the article aforecited, in *Sec. 2.2.2*; the precise identification of 4 research methods in the article aforecited, in *Sec. 2.3.1*; the precise identification of 2 main arguments for zoophilia in the article aforecited, in *Sec. 2.3.2*; the precise identification of 4 main effects of income inequality on health in the article aforecited, in *Sec. 2.4.1*; the precise identification of 3 types of telemedicine, namely, "store-and-forward," "remote monitoring," and "[real-time] interactive services" in the article aforecited, in *Sec. 2.4.2*; the precise identification of 5 types of alternative medecines in the article aforecited, in *Sec. 2.5.1*; the precise identification of 8 mindfulness-based therapy programs in the article aforecited, in *Sec. 2.5.2*; the precise identification of 5 main health effects of physical exercise in the article aforecited, in *Sec. 3.2.1*; the precise identification of 2 child abuse effects, that is, "physical effects" and "psychological effects," in the article aforecited, in *Sec. 3.2.2*; the precise identification of 3 main historical sources about astral travel, namely, Western, Islamic, and Eastern, in the article aforecited, in *Sec. 3.3.1*; the precise identification of 20 examples of carriers of zoonotic diseases in the article aforecited, in *Sec. 3.3.2*; the precise identification of 7 contentious issues in the debate on drug prohibition in the article aforecited, in *Sec. 3.4.1*; the precise identification of 4 causes of domestic violence in the article aforecited, in *Sec. 3.4.2*; the precise identification of 3 arguments against torture in the article aforecited, in *Sec. 3.5.1*; and the precise identification of the "four principles" in medical ethics by Tom Beauchamp and James Childress in the article aforecited, in *Sec. 3.5.2*).

On the other hand, there is vagueness (e.g., the vagueness in the identification of the 8 main approaches to psychotherapy in the article aforecited, since it is not clear why there must be these 8, not 16, 20, 23, 26, 30, and so on, in *Sec. 2.2.1*; the vagueness in the identification of the 2 theories of the causes of SWB in the article aforecited, since it is not clear why there must be only 2, not 3, 4, 5, 6, and so on, in *Sec. 2.2.2*; the vagueness in the identification of the 4 research methods in the article aforecited, since it is not clear why there must be only 4, not 5, 6, 7, and so on, in *Sec. 2.3.1*; the vagueness in the identification of the 2 main arguments for zoophilia in the article aforecited, since it is not clear why there must be only 2, not 5, 7, 8, 11, and so on, in *Sec. 2.3.2*; the vagueness in the identification of the 4 main effects of income inequality on health in the article aforecited, since it is not clear why there must be only 4, not 6, 7, 8, 9, 10, 11, and so on, in *Sec. 2.4.1*; the vagueness in the identification of 3 types of telemedicine in the article aforecited, since it is not clear why there must be only 3, not 4, 5, 6, and so on, in *Sec. 2.4.2*; the vagueness in the identification of the 5 types of alternative medecines in the article aforecited, since it is not clear why there must be only 5, not 6, 7, 8, and so on, in *Sec. 2.5.1*; the vagueness in the identification of the 8 mindfulness-based therapy programs in the article aforecited, since it is not clear why there must be only 8, not 10, 13, 14, 16, and so on, in *Sec. 2.5.2*; the vagueness in the identification of the 5 main health effects of physical exercise in the article aforecited, since it is not clear why there must be only 5, not 6, 10, 13, 17, and so on, in *Sec. 3.2.1*; the vagueness in the identification of the 2 child abuse effects in the article aforecited, since it is not clear why there must be only 2, not 3, 4, 5, 6, and so on, in *Sec. 3.2.2*; the vagueness in the identification of the 3 main historical sources about astral travel, namely, Western, Islamic, and Eastern, in the article aforecited, since it is not clear why there must be only 3, not 5, 7, 10, 11, 13, and so on, in *Sec. 3.3.1*; the vagueness in the identification of the 20 examples of carriers of zoonotic diseases in the article aforecited, since it is not clear why there must be only these 20 or so examples, not 40, 54, 64, 100, 143, and so on, in *Sec. 3.3.2*; the vagueness in the identification of the 7 contentious issues in the debate on drug prohibition in the article aforecited, since it is not clear why there must be only these 7, not 13, 16, 19, 21, 24, 27, and so on, in *Sec. 3.4.1*; the vagueness in the identification of the 4 causes of domestic violence in the article aforecited, since it is not clear why there must be only these 4, not 7, 10, 14, 21, and so on, in *Sec. 3.4.2*; the vagueness in the identification of the 3 arguments against torture in the article aforecited, since it is not clear why there must be only these 3, not 5, 8, 11, 14, 16, and so on, in *Sec. 3.5.1*; and the vagueness in the identification of the "four principles" in medical ethics by Tom Beauchamp and James Childress in the article aforecited, since it is not clear why there must be only these 4, not 5, 7, 9, 11, and so on, as shown by alternative values aforecited, in *Sec. 3.5.2*).

And the reverse direction also holds true.

Once more, it should be stressed, however, that there are different shades of gray (or different degrees of truth) in the two opposites, and the classification is not necessarily mutually exclusive either. In fact, even when some combinations of the two occur, they only end up sharing the same dialectic relationship, but in a different degree.

Also, there are some other relationships (as a kind of family resemblance) which have something in common with the principle, but they are not exactly the same but only more or less comparable, which varies from case to case.

Good examples of family resemblance in relation to the principle are clarity-ambiguity, directness-indirectness, quantitativeness-qualitativeness, specificity-obscurity, describability-nondescribability, concretness-abstractness, translatability-untranslatability, specificity-generality, clearcutness-transitionalness, sharpness-roughness, and the like.

10th Thesis: The Simpleness-Complicatedness Principle

The tenth thesis refers to the simpleness-complicatedness principle (on the interconnection among things) in the category of "structure" in existential dialectics (which was first out worked out in *FIA*, *FPHPROB*, nd other books), in that both simpleness and complicatedness are vital, without favoring one over the other, and each is utilized, depending on the basis of the perspectives of nature, the mind, culture, and society. There is no simpleness without complicatedness—and vice versa.

As an illustration, in relation to taxonomy, simpleness has its heuristic usefulness, just as complicatedness has its realistic representation. In relation to network, simpleness has its economical attractiveness, just as complicatedness has its practical reliability. And in relation to logic, there is the simple zeroth-order logic, just as there is the complicated higher-order logic.

For instance, on the one hand, there is simpleness (e.g., the relatively simple analysis of the effectiveness of psychotherapy by the advocates, in *Sec. 2.2.1*; the relatively simple analysis of SWB by the advocates, in *Sec. 2.2.2*; the relatively simple analysis of "evolved psychological mechanisms" by the advocates, in *Sec. 2.3.1*; the relatively simple analysis of zoophilia by the advocates, in *Sec. 2.3.2*; the relatively simple analysis of the need for lesser income inequality by the advocates, in *Sec. 2.4.1*; the relatively simple analysis of the use of technology for mental health by the advocates, in *Sec. 2.4.2*; the relatively simple analysis of alternative medicines by the advocates, in *Sec. 2.5.1*; the relatively simple analysis of mindfulness-based therapy programs by the advocates, in *Sec. 2.5.2*; the relatively simple analysis of the health effects of physical exercise by the advocates, in *Sec. 3.2.1*; the relatively simple analysis of the nature of child abuse by the advocates of child protection, in *Sec. 3.2.2*; the relatively simple analysis of astral travel by the advocates, in *Sec. 3.3.1*; the relatively simple analysis of the causes of zoonotic diseases by the practitioners, in *Sec. 3.3.2*; the relatively simple analysis of drug prohibition by the affirmative side, in *Sec. 3.4.1*; the relatively simple analysis of domestic violence by the feminists, in *Sec. 3.4.2*; the relatively simple analysis of the need to torture by the advocates, in *Sec. 3.5.1*; and the relatively simple analysis of the "four principles" in medical ethics by Tom Beauchamp and James Childress, in *Sec. 3.5.2*).

On the other hand, there is complicatedness (e.g., the relatively more complicated analysis of the effectiveness of psychotherapy, by challenging the claims and assumptions, as shown in the problems pointed out by the critics as cited, in *Sec. 2.2.1*; the relatively more complicated analysis of SWB, by challenging the claims and assumptions, as shown in the problems pointed out by the critics as cited, in *Sec. 2.2.2*; the relatively more complicated analysis of "evolved psychological mechanisms," by challenging the claims and assumptions, as shown in the problems pointed out by the critics as cited, in *Sec. 2.3.1*; the relatively more complicated analysis of zoophilia, by challenging the claims and assumptions, as shown in the problems pointed out by the critics as cited, in *Sec. 2.3.2*; the relatively more complicated analysis of the need for lesser income inequality, by challenging the claims and assumptions, as shown in the problems pointed out by the critics as cited, in *Sec. 2.4.1*; the relatively more complicated analysis of the use of technology for mental health, by challenging the claims and assumptions, as shown in the problems pointed out by the critics as cited, in *Sec. 2.4.2*; the relatively more complicated analysis of alternative medicines, by challenging the claims and assumptions, as shown in the problems pointed out by the critics as cited, in *Sec. 2.5.1*; the relatively more complicated analysis of mindfulness-based therapy programs, by challenging the claims and assumptions, as shown in the problems pointed out by the critics as cited, in *Sec. 2.5.2*; the relatively more complicated analysis of the health effects of physical exercise, by challenging the claims and assumptions, as shown in the problems pointed out by the critics as cited, in *Sec. 3.2.1*; the relatively more complicated analysis of the nature of child abuse, by challenging the claims and assumptions, as shown in the problems pointed out by the critics as cited, in *Sec. 3.2.2*; the relatively more complicated analysis of astral travel, by challenging the claims and assumptions, as shown in the problems pointed out by the critics as cited, in *Sec. 3.3.1*; the relatively more complicated analysis of the causes of zoonotic diseases, by challenging the claims and assumptions, as shown in the problems pointed out by the critics as cited, in *Sec. 3.3.2*; the relatively more complicated analysis of drug prohibition, by challenging the claims and assumptions, as shown in the problems pointed out by the negative side as cited, in *Sec. 3.4.1*; the relatively more complicated analysis of domestic violence , by challenging the claims and assumptions, as shown in the problems pointed out by the critics as cited, in *Sec. 3.4.2*; the relatively more complicated analysis of the need to torture, by challenging the claims and assumptions, as shown in the problems pointed out by the critics as cited, in *Sec. 3.5.1*; and the relatively more complicated analysis of the "four principles" in medical ethics, by challenging the claims and assumptions, as shown in the problems pointed out by the critics as cited, in *Sec. 3.5.2*).

And the reverse direction also holds true.

Again, it should be stressed, however, that there are different shades of gray (or different degrees of truth) in the two opposites, and the classification is not necessarily mutually exclusive either. In fact, even when some combinations of the two occur, they only end up sharing the same dialectic relationship, but in a different degree.

Also, there are some other relationships (as a kind of family resemblance) which have something in common with the principle, but they are not exactly the same but only more or less comparable, which varies from case to case.

Good examples of family resemblance in relation to the principle are inflexibility-flexibility, standardization-specialization, imperfectness-perfectness, superficiality-depth, shallowness-deepness, economicalness-elaboratedness, plainness-circumspection, onesidedness-multisidedness, succinctness-duplicatedness, simpleness-sophisticatedness, crudeness-subtleness, and the like.

11th Thesis: The Openness-Hiddenness Principle

The eleventh thesis refers to the openness-hiddenenss principle (on the detection of things) in the category of "structure" in existential dialectics (which was already worked out in my previous books, especially in *FPHU*), in that reality has its hidden face, just as it is open to outside view in some other ways. There is no openness without hiddenness—and vice versa.

For instance, on the one hand, there is openness (e.g., the open exploration of "uncovering psychotherapy," which "emphasizes facilitating the client's insight into the roots of their difficulties," in *Sec. 2.2.1*; the open exploration of the "subjective" aspects of well-being by the advocates of SWB, in *Sec. 2.2.2*; the open exploration of "evolved psychological mechanisms" in EP, in *Sec. 2.3.1*; the open exploration of the extent of occurrence of zoophilia in the research on zoophilia aforecited, in *Sec. 2.3.2*; the open exploration of the correlation between health and lesser income inequality by Wilkinson and Pickett, in *Sec. 2.4.1*; the open exploration of the use of technology for mental health by the advocates, in *Sec. 2.4.2*; the open exploration of the use of "a very low dose of substance that creates similar symptoms in a healthy person" to cure disease, according to those in homeopathy, in *Sec. 2.5.1*; the open exploration of using mindfulness to cure health problems, in *Sec. 2.5.2*; the open exploration of the health effects of physical exercise by the advocates, in *Sec. 3.2.1*; the open exploration of the types, causes, and effects of child abuse in the studies aforecited, in *Sec. 3.2.2*; the open exploration of "out-of-body experience" like "astral travel," in *Sec. 3.3.1*; the open exploration of the link between human health and infectious diseases from animals, in *Sec. 3.3.2*; the open exploration of the relationship between drug use and death by "The United States Drug Enforcement Administration [DEA]," in *Sec. 3.4.1*; the open exploration of domestic violence by men against women by the advocates of the "strict 'patriarchal violence' model," in *Sec. 3.4.2*; the open exploration of a different definition of "torture" by the 1984 United Nations Convention Against Torture, in *Sec. 3.5.1*; and the open exploration of different moral principles in medical ethics by Tom Beauchamp and James Childress, in *Sec. 3.5.2*).

On the other hand, there is hiddenness (e.g., the hidden bias in "uncovering psychotherapy," since it neglects the need to "strengthen…the client's defenses and…provid[e]…encouragement and advice," as in "supportive psychotherapy," in *Sec. 2.2.1*; the hidden bias in the "subjective" aspects of well-being by the advocates of SWB, since they ignore the "objective" aspects, in *Sec. 2.2.2*; the hidden bias in EP, because, for the critics, it suffers from "genetic reductionism," in *Sec. 2.3.1*; the hidden bias in the research on zoophilia aforecited, since there is "self-selection bias" as discovered by Andrea Beetz aforediscussed, in *Sec. 2.3.2*; the hidden bias in the correlation between health and lesser income inequality by Wilkinson and Pickett, since, for the critics, it constitutes a very narrow view of social stratification in relation to health care, it provides no verification of the claim, there is no general agreement on the desirability of income equality or its reduction, the correlation between health and income level does not always hold, and equality can lead to a conformist society, in *Sec. 2.4.1*; the hidden bias in the view on the use of technology for mental health by the advocates, because of the different problems aforecited, in *Sec. 2.4.2*; the hidden bias in homeopathy, since "this conflicts with fundamental concepts of physics and chemistry and there is no good evidence from reviews of research to support its use" and "within the medical community homeopathy is now considered to be quackery," in *Sec. 2.5.1*; the hidden bias in the mindfulness-based therapy programs, since, for the critics, the research works are often incomplete, the practices are not so effective, and because of its connection with alternative medicine, mindfulness-based therapy programs have been criticized as not being scientific, in *Sec. 2.5.2*; the hidden bias in the claim on the health effects of physical exercise by the advocates, since, for the critics, vigorous exercise can have its downside, some individuals can be exercise-resistant, the findings are inconsistent, there is often "insufficient evidence" for any firm conclusion, some effects of physical exercise remain unknown, etc., in *Sec. 3.2.1*; the hidden bias in the studies on child abuse, since the critics pointed out that scholars disagree over what constitutes child abuse, that the alleged causes of child abuse can be questionable, that the long-term effects of child abuse remains unknown, and that the alleged causes do not determine the often cited consequences, and that the prevention of child abuse can be limited, in *Sec. 3.2.2*; the hidden bias in the claims on "out-of-body experience" like "astral travel," because of the different problems pointed out by the critics aforecited, in *Sec. 3.3.1*; the hidden bias in the studies on the link between human health and infectious diseases from animals, since, for the critics, zoonotic diseases can be historically contingent, there are infectious diseases which can go in the opposite direction, the causes of zoonotic diseases can be more complicated than previously thought, and the acceptance of the findings in zoonotic research can be based on the politics of social impact, in *Sec. 3.3.2*; the hidden bias in the figures on drug-induced deaths by the DEA, since the critics revealed the tendency of DEA to engage in "misleading health statistics," in that "the DEA's use of such figures is questionable," for example, in *Sec. 3.4.1*; the hidden bias in the "strict 'patriarchal violence' model," since, for the critics, "modern research into predictors of injury from domestic violence finds that the strongest predictor of injury by domestic violence is participation in reciprocal domestic violence, and that this pattern of domestic violence is more often initiated by the female in the relationship," in *Sec. 3.4.2*; the hidden bias in the definition by the 1984 United Nations Convention Against Torture, since this definition exclude: [i] torture perpetrated by gangs, hate groups, rebels or terrorists who ignore national or international mandates, [ii] random violence during war, and [iii] punishment allowed by national laws, even if the punishment uses techniques similar to those used by torturers such as mutilation or whipping when practiced as lawful punishment," in *Sec. 3.5.1*; and the hidden bias in the moral principles in medical ethics by Tom Beauchamp and James Childress, since, for the critics, they focus too much on "curing," at the expense of alternative ethical concerns [e.g., "nursing ethics"], there is cultural bias in them, there are "conflicts of interest" in medical ethics so that the values are not necessarily followed in practice, there is no consensus on medical ethics even within a given tradition, the values in medical ethics are not necessarily valuable, scholars disagree over the priority [or ranking] of the values in medical ethics, and nations differ in regard to their regulations concerning medical ethics, in *Sec. 3.5.2*).

And the reverse direction also holds true.

Again, it should be stressed, however, that there are different shades of gray (or different degrees of truth) in the two opposites, and the classification is not necessarily mutually exclusive either. In fact, even when some combinations of the two occur, they only end up sharing the same dialectic relationship, but in a different degree.

Also, there are some other relationships (as a kind of family resemblance) which have something in common with the principle, but they are not exactly the same but only more or less comparable, which varies from case to case.

Good examples of family resemblance in relation to the principle are overtness-covertness, participation-obstruction, publicness-privateness, openness-closedness, surface-depth, transparency-secrecy, openness-biasedness, , exposition-illusion, and so on.

12th Thesis: The Denseness-Emptiness Principle

The twelfth thesis concerns the denseness-emptiness principle (on the distribution of entities in space) in the category of "structure" in existential dialectics, which is first proposed in *FPHUP*, in that both density and void are needed, in relation to the mind, nature, culture, and society, albeit in different ways. There is no denseness without emptiness—and vice versa.

Lest any misunderstanding occurs, the term "void" is used here only as an approximation of emptiness (depending on the degree of the lack of density), since, in physics, it is well known that "empty" space is not really empty all the way, because it can be full of energy (e.g., random quantum fluctuations at the sub-atomic level, and, for that matter, dark energy in the universe) and matter (e.g., different versions of sub-atomic particles, and, for that matter, dark matter in the universe). (F. Wilczek 2008)

For instance, on the one hand, there is denseness (e.g., the relatively denser concentration of concerns with "childhood experiences and the unconscious mind" by those in "psychoanalysis," in *Sec. 2.2.1*; the relatively denser concentration of concerns with the "genetic predisposition to be happy or unhappy" by those in the Top-down theories of SWB, in *Sec. 2.2.2*; the relatively denser concentration of concerns with "evolved psychological mechanisms" by those in EP, in *Sec. 2.3.1*; the relatively denser concentration of concerns with the issues of consent and enjoyment by those in the defense of zoophilia aforecited, in *Sec. 2.3.2*; the relatively denser concentration of concerns with income inequality by Wilkinson and Pickett, in *Sec. 2.4.1*; the relatively denser concentration of concerns with "email, SMS, virtual reality, computer programmes, blogs, social networks, the telephone, video conferencing, computer games, instant messaging and podcasts" by those advocating "new technologies" aforediscussed, in *Sec. 2.4.2*; the relatively denser concentration of concerns with "religion, tradition, superstition, belief in supernatural energies," etc. by those in alternative medicines, in *Sec. 2.5.1*; the relatively denser concentration of concerns with "attention" and "openness" by those in mindfulness-based therapy programs, in *Sec. 2.5.2*; the relatively denser concentration of concerns with flexibility, aerobics, and anaerobics by the advocates of physical exercise, in *Sec. 3.2.1*; the relatively denser concentration of concerns with "forceful parenting...in many Asian cultures, including China, Japan, Singapore, Vietnam and Korea," in *Sec. 3.2.2*; the relatively denser concentration of concerns with "out-of-body experience" by the advocates of "astral travel," in *Sec. 3.3.1*; the relatively denser concentration of "zoonotic diseases" in much of human history, in *Sec. 3.3.2*; the relatively denser concentration of concerns with supporting "the gateway hypothesis that certain drugs [such as cannabis] act as gateways to use of 'harder' drugs such as heroin" by "the US Drug Enforcement Agency's '2008 Marijuana Sourcebook,'" in *Sec. 3.4.1*; the relatively denser concentration of concerns with domestic violence by men against women by the advocates of the "strict 'patriarchal violence' model," in *Sec. 3.4.2*; the relatively denser concentration of concerns with "the need for information" by the supporters of torture like Alan M. Dershowitz and Mirko Bagaric, in *Sec.*

3.5.1; and the relatively denser concentration of concerns with "curing" by those in medical ethics, in *Sec. 3.5.2*).

On the other hand, there is emptiness (e.g., the relatively less dense, or more empty, concentration of concerns with "childhood experiences and the unconscious mind" by those in "behavioral therapy," in *Sec. 2.2.1*; the relatively less dense, or more empty, concentration of concerns with the "genetic predisposition to be happy or unhappy" by those in the bottom-up theories of SWB, in *Sec. 2.2.2*; the relatively less dense, or more empty, concentration of concerns with "evolved psychological mechanisms" by those in social constructionism, in *Sec. 2.3.1*; the relatively less dense, or more empty, concentration of concerns with the issues of health and safety by those in the defense of zoophilia aforecited, in *Sec. 2.3.2*; the relatively less dense, or more empty, concentration of concerns with other forms of inequality like "broader economic inequality" by Wilkinson and Pickett, in *Sec. 2.4.1*; the relatively less dense, or more empty, concentration of concerns with "traditional methods" like "medication, counselling, Cognitive Behavioral Therapy, exercise and a healthy diet" by those advocating "new technologies" aforediscussed, in *Sec. 2.4.2*; the relatively less dense, or more empty, concentration of concerns with "modern scientific reasoning" by those in alternative medicines, in *Sec. 2.5.1*; the relatively less dense, or more empty, concentration of concerns with "pre-judgement" and "past-centered awareness" by those in mindfulness-based therapy programs, in *Sec. 2.5.2*; the relatively less dense, or more empty, concentration of concerns with mental exercise by the advocates of physical exercise, in *Sec. 3.2.1*; the relatively less dense, or more empty, concentration of concerns with Western tolerant parenting "in many Asian cultures, including China, Japan, Singapore, Vietnam and Korea," in *Sec. 3.2.2*; the relatively less dense, or more empty, concentration of concerns with ordinary travel as a tourist by the advocates of "astral travel," in *Sec. 3.3.1*; the relatively less dense, or more empty, concentration of "epidemic diseases" in much of human history, in *Sec. 3.3.2*; the relatively less dense, or more empty, concentration of concerns with supporting "the gateway hypothesis" by the "study of drug users in Amsterdam over a 10-year period conducted by Jan van Ours of Tilburg University in the Netherlands," which "concluded that cannabis is not a stepping stone to using cocaine or heroin," in *Sec. 3.4.1*; the relatively less dense, or more empty, concentration of concerns with domestic violence by women against men by the advocates of the "strict 'patriarchal violence' model," in *Sec. 3.4.2*; the relatively less dense, or more empty, concentration of concerns with "humanitarian grounds" by the supporters of torture like Alan M. Dershowitz and Mirko Bagaric, in *Sec. 3.5.1*; and the relatively less dense, or more empty, concentration of concerns with "caring" by those in medical ethics, in *Sec. 3.5.2*).

And the reverse direction also holds true.

Again, it should be stressed, however, that there are different shades of gray (or different degrees of truth) in the two opposites, and the classification is not necessarily mutually exclusive either. In fact, even when some combinations of the two occur, they only end up sharing the same dialectic relationship, but in a different degree.

Also, there are some other relationships (as a kind of family resemblance) which have something in common with the principle, but they are not exactly the same but only more or less comparable, which varies from case to case.

Good examples of family resemblance in relation to the principle are fullness-voidness, nearness-farness, concentration-dispersion, denseness-nothingness, something-nothing, heaviness-lightness, composition-emptiness, solidness-void, presence-absence, focus-unfocus, emphasis-disemphasis, and the like.

In Relation to Process

The next six theses are in relation to process in existential dialectics, as shown below.

13th Thesis: The Prototypicality-Variation Principle

The thirteenth thesis concerns the prototypicality-variation principle (on the nature of duplication) in the category of "process" in existential dialectics, which is first proposed in *FPHMORPH*, in that, if there are prototypes, there are also variants of the copies. There is no prototypicality without variation—and vice versa.

There are the following four important aspects of the relationship between prototypess and their copies, as shown in the fields of morphology (e.g., "proto-languages" in *FPHMORP*), information architecture (e.g., "taxonomies" in *FIA*), and evolutionry biology (e.g., "mutation" and "variation" in *BNN*), just to cite three well-documented sources:

- Prototypes and their copies are not static and may change or die out over time, but new ones may emerge.
- Some copies may have multiple prototypes, not just one.

- It can be very challenging to trace some copies back to their prototypes, under certain difficult historical conditions.
- Copies are not solely identical duplications of prototypes but have their own variations (mutations).

In any event, on the one hand, there are prototypes (e.g., the prototype, like the example about the original work on psychoanalysis by Freud in the early 20th century, in *Sec. 2.2.1*; the prototype, like the example about the original "hedonic treadmill theory" which "proposed that most people return to a neutral level of SWB [i.e. neither happy nor unhappy] as they habituate to events," in *Sec. 2.2.2*; the prototype, like the example about the original evolutionary theory by Charles Darwin, in *Sec. 2.3.1*; the prototype, like the example about the term "zoophilia" first introduced by Krafft-Ebing in 1886, in *Sec. 2.3.2*; the prototype, like the example about the original work on income inequality and health by Wilkinson and Pickett in 2009, in *Sec. 2.4.1*; the prototype, like the example about the early works on VRT by Ralph Lamson, Larry Hodges, and others, in *Sec. 2.4.2*; the prototype, like the example about the original "traditional Chinese medicine" based "on a tradition of more than 2,000 years" ago, in *Sec. 2.5.1*; the prototype, like the example about the original work on "mindfulness" in "the Noble Eightfold Path taught by Siddhartha Gautama," that is, "the Buddha, who founded Buddhism almost 2,500 years ago," in *Sec. 2.5.2*; the prototype, like the example about the original work on the link "between physical health and exercise...in 1953 by a team led by Jerry Morris," in *Sec. 3.2.1*; the prototype, like the example about the original 1973 work by psychiatrist P. D. Scott on the link "between stepparents and child maltreatment," now known as "the Cinderella effect," in *Sec. 3.2.2*; the prototype, like the example about the original historical sources on astral travel, be they Western, Islamic, or Eastern, in *Sec. 3.3.1*; the prototype, like the example about the first cases of "HIV-1 and HIV-2," which "originated in non-human primates in West-central Africa and...transferred to humans...in the early 20th century," in *Sec. 3.3.2*; the prototype, like the example about the original medical uses of "natural plant drugs like opium, coca, cannabis, mescaline, and psilocybin," which can be dated "back thousands of years and through a variety of cultures" in antiquity, in *Sec. 3.4.1*; the prototype, like the example about the original work on "power and control" in the "Duluth Domestic Abuse Intervention Project," in *Sec. 3.4.2*; the prototype, like the example about the original "Universal Declaration of Human Rights" by the United Nations in 1948, with Article 5 against torture, in *Sec. 3.5.1*; and the prototype, like the example about the original "guidelines on the duty of physicians in antiquity, such as the Hippocratic Oath, and early rabbinic and Christian teachings," in *Sec. 3.5.2*).

On the other hand, there are variants (e.g., different variants of the protoptye, as shown in many studies of psychoanalysis since then, like the ones built upon Freud's psychoanlaysis by "Anna Freud, Alfred Adler, Carl Jung, Karen Horney, Otto Rank, Erik Erikson, Melanie Klein, and Heinz Kohut," for example, though each with his/er own variation, contribution, and disagreement, in *Sec. 2.2.1*; different variants of the protoptye, as shown in many further studies since then, like the "additional refinements to this theory [the original hedonic treadmill theory]" which "have shown that people do not adapt to all life events equally, as people tend to adapt rapidly to some events [e.g. imprisonment], slowly to others [e.g. the death of a loved one], and not at all to others [e.g. noise and sex]," in *Sec. 2.2.2*; different variants of the protoptye, as shown in many further studies on evolutionary theory since Darwin's original work, like the later theories on "inclusive fitness," "r/K selection," "parental investment," "life history," etc., though each with its own variation, contribution, and disagreement, in *Sec. 2.3.1*; different variants of the protoptye, as shown in many ways to define and classify "zoophilia" since the work by Krafft-Ebing, like the ones by the American Psychiatric Association, the World Health Organization, the Journal of Forensic and Legal Medicine, and so on, though each with its own variation, contribution, and disagreement, in *Sec. 2.3.2*; different variants of the protoptye, as shown in many further views about this work on income inequality by Wilkinson and Pickett since then, like the ones by "the Equality Trust's 'Equality Pledge,'" the article by Ed Miliband, the lecture by David Cameron, etc., though each with its own variation, contribution, and disagreement, in *Sec. 2.4.1*; different variants of the protoptye, as shown in many studies on VRT since the early works by by Ralph Lamson, Larry Hodges, and others, like the later ones by Skip Rizzo for DOD, Sally Merry at Auckland University, and so on, though each with his own variation, contribution, and disagreement, in *Sec. 2.4.2*; different variants of the protoptye, as shown in many further developments of "traditional Chinese medicine" since then, like the ones "modernized in the People's Republic of China so as to integrate many anatomical and pathological notions with scientific medicine," though each with its own variation, contribution, and disagreement, in *Sec. 2.5.1*; different variants of the protoptye, as shown in many studies about the Buddhist tradition since then, like the ones by Jon Kabat-Zinn, Thich Nhat Hanh, Jack Kornfield, Joseph Goldstein, Tara Brach, Alan Clements, and Sharon Salzberg,, etc., though each with his own variation, contribution, and disagreement, in *Sec. 2.5.2*; different variants of the protoptye, as shown in many studies since the original work on the link "between physical health and exercise…in 1953 by a team led by Jerry Morris," like other subsequent studies aforecited, though each with its own variation, contribution, and disagreement, in *Sec. 3.2.1*; different variants of the protoptye, as shown in many studies since the work on "the Cinderella effect" by Scott in 1973, like the subsequent ones by Martin Daly, Margo Wilson, Greg Tooley, and so on, though each with his own variation, contribution, and disagreement, in *Sec. 3.2.2*; different variants of the protoptye, as shown in many studies since the original historical sources on astral travel, like the contemporary ones by Robert Monroe, Oliver Fox, Sylvan Muldoon, Hereward Carrington, etc., though each with his own variation, contribution, and disagreement, in *Sec. 3.3.1*; different variants of the protoptye, as shown in many studies since the first cases of "HIV-1 and HIV-2" in West-central Africa—like the later findings on the cases of "AIDS" spread to the United States in the 1980s, though each with its own variation, because "HIV differs from many viruses in that it has very high genetic variability," in *Sec. 3.3.2*; different variants of the protoptye, as shown in many studies and uses of natural plant drugs since the orignal medical uses thousands of years ago, like the modern use of these drugs in American and European countries nowadays, though each country with its own variations, purposes, and regulations, in *Sec. 3.4.1*; different variants of the protoptye, as shown in many studies since the original work on "power and control" in the "Duluth Domestic Abuse Intervention Project," like the later ones by M. Twohey, M. Straus, etc., though each with his own variation, contribution, and disagreement, in *Sec. 3.4.2*; different variants of the protoptye, as shown in many works since the 1948 "Universal Declaration of Human Rights," like the later ones such as the subsequent "United Nations Convention Against Torture," "the Geneva Conventions III and IV," etc., though each with its own variation and contribution, in *Sec. 3.5.1*; and different variants of the protoptye, as shown in many studies since the original "guidelines on the duty of physicians in antiquity, such as the Hippocratic Oath, and early rabbinic and Christian teachings"—like the contemporary ones by the "four principles" in medical ethics by Tom Beauchamp and James Childress and the discourse on caring by those in nursing ethics, though each later version with its own variation, contribution, and disagreement, in *Sec. 3.5.2*).

And the reverse direction also holds true.

Again, it should be stressed, however, that there are different shades of gray (or different degrees of truth) in the two opposites, and the classification is not necessarily mutually exclusive either. In fact, even when some combinations of the two occur, they only end up sharing the same dialectic relationship, but in a different degree.

Also, there are some other relationships (as a kind of family resemblance) which have something in common with the principle, but they are not exactly the same but only more or less comparable, which varies from case to case.

Good examples of family resemblance in relation to the principle are archetypicality-descendedness, origin-descendedness, prototypicality-duplication, archetypicality-mutation, prototypicality-copyness, ancestry-descendedness, origin-reenactment, prototypicality-recreation, and the like.

14th Thesis: The Change-Constancy Principle

The fourteenth thesis concerns the change-constancy principle (on the alteration of things) in the category of "process" in existential dialectics, which is first named in *BCPC* (and were worked out in my books like *FHC*, *FCD*, and *FPHC)*, in that change occurs over time, although constancy is also allowed.

Old players fade away, and new ones emerges, with ever new causes and ever new forms—and asymmetry undergoes changes over time too, so does symmetry. There is no change without constancy—and vice versa.

For instance, on the one hand, there is change (e.g., the ever new ways to treat mental problems, as shown in psychotherapy, in *Sec. 2.2.1*; the ever new ways to understand the nature of health and well-being, as shown in the research on SWB, in *Sec. 2.2.2*; the ever new ways to mental health, as shown in the research on "evolved psychological mechanisms, in *Sec. 2.3.1*; the ever new ways to study health, as shown in the research on zoophilia and health, in *Sec. 2.3.2*; the ever new ways to understand inequality, as shown in the work by Wilkinson and Pickett, in *Sec. 2.4.1*; the ever new ways to treat mental health, as shown in the use of new technologies aforediscussed, in *Sec. 2.4.2*; the ever new ways to treat health problems, as shown in the use of alternative medicines, in *Sec. 2.5.1*; the ever new ways to understand therapy, as shown in the mindfulness-based therapy programs, in *Sec. 2.5.2*; the ever new ways to study exercise, as shown in the work on the link "between physical health and exercise," in *Sec. 3.2.1*; the ever new ways to study abuse, as shown in the research on child abuse, in *Sec. 3.2.2*; the ever new ways to travel, as shown in the claims about astral travel, in *Sec. 3.3.1*; the ever new ways to understand diseases, as shown in the work on zoonotic diseases, in *Sec.*

3.3.2; the ever new ways to understand drug use, as shown in the debate on physical health and drug use afore-discussed, in *Sec. 3.4.1*; the ever new ways to study violence, as shown in the research on domestic violence aforedescribed, in *Sec. 3.4.2*; the ever new ways to use torture, as shown in the 4 different methods aforedescribed, in *Sec. 3.5.1*; and the ever new ways to understand ethics, as shown in the study on medical ethics in *Sec. 3.5.2*).

On the other hand, there is constancy (e.g., the ever constant existence of different problems with the ever new ways to treat mental problems, as shown in the problems with psychotherapy pointed out by the critics, in *Sec. 2.2.1*; the ever constant existence of different problems with the ever new ways to understand the nature of health and well-being, as shown in the problems with the research on SWB pointed out by the critics, in *Sec. 2.2.2*; the ever constant existence of different problems with the ever new ways to study mental health, as shown in the problems with the research on "evolved psychological mechanisms" pointed out by the critics, in *Sec. 2.3.1*; the ever constant existence of different problems with the ever new ways to study health, as shown in the problems with the research on zoophilia and health pointed out by the critics, in *Sec. 2.3.2*; the ever constant existence of different problems with the ever new ways to understand inequality, as shown in the problems with the work by Wilkinson and Pickett pointed out by the critics, in *Sec. 2.4.1*; the ever constant existence of different problems with the ever new ways to treat mental health, as shown in the problems with the use of new technologies pointed out by the critics, in *Sec. 2.4.2*; the ever constant existence of different problems with the ever new ways to treat health problems, as shown in the problems with the use of alternative medicines pointed out by the critics, in *Sec. 2.5.1*; the ever constant existence of different problems with the ever new ways to understand therapy, as shown in the problems with mindfulness-based therapy programs pointed out by the critics, in *Sec. 2.5.2*; the ever constant existence of different problems with the ever new ways to study exercise, as shown in the problems with the work on the link "between physical health and exercise" pointed out by the critics, in *Sec. 3.2.1*; the ever constant existence of different problems with the ever new ways to study abuse, as shown in the problems with the research on child abuse pointed out by the critics earlier, in *Sec. 3.2.2*; the ever constant existence of different problems with the ever new ways to travel, as shown in the problems with the claims about astral travel pointed out by the critics, in *Sec. 3.3.1*; the ever constant existence of different problems with the ever new ways to understand diseases, as shown in the problems with the work on zoonotic diseases pointed out by the critics, in *Sec. 3.3.2*; the ever constant existence of different problems with the ever new ways to understand drug use, as shown in the contentious disagreements between both sides in the debate on physical health and drug use afore-discussed, in *Sec. 3.4.1*; the ever constant existence of different problems with the ever new ways to study violence, as shown in the problems with the research on domestic violence pointed out by the critics, in *Sec. 3.4.2*; the ever constant existence of different problems with the ever new ways to use torture, as shown in the problems with the 4 different methods pointed out by the critics, in *Sec. 3.5.1*; and the ever constant existence of different problems with the ever new ways to understand ethics, as shown in the problems with the study on medical ethics pointed out by the critics, in *Sec. 3.5.2*).

And the reverse direction also holds true.

Again, it should be stressed, however, that there are different shades of gray (or different degrees of truth) in the two opposites, and the classification is not necessarily mutually exclusive either. In fact, even when some combinations of the two occur, they only end up sharing the same dialectic relationship, but in a different degree.

Also, there are some other relationships (as a kind of family resemblance) which have something in common with the principle, but they are not exactly the same but only more or less comparable, which varies from case to case.

Good examples of family resemblance in relation to the principle are dynamicness-staticness, instability-stability, and the like.

15th Thesis: The Order-Chaos Principle

The fifteenth thesis is called the the order-chaos principle (on the pattern of things) in the category of "process" in existential dialectics (as first worked out in *FC*), in that both order and chaos are vital in the process of change in the world.

The preference for order is biased, since it does not give sufficient attention to the vital role of chaos in the transformation of the world (without somehow reducing it for the understanding of order). There is no order without chaos—and vice versa.

The scientific search for order in the world is often a hidden bias in its ontological obsession with order, since chaos is often treated as the "bad" guy, with order as the "good" guy (for the end goal of science).

Neither order nor chaos is the final end of the world, and one is not to be treated as the means for the other in the transformation of things. Both are fundamental in their recurrent dialectical interactions with each other over time, without reducing one for the other.

Order has its different forms (e.g., ascending vs. descending order in mathematics, and feeding vs. bleeding order in morphology), just as chaos has its own versions (e.g., as understood differently in chaos theory vs. complexity theory).

For instance, on the one hand, there is order (e.g., the more or less orderly view on treating health problems, if looked from the sole vantage point of "behavior therapy," with its focus on "modifying overt behavior and helping clients to achieve goals" by way of "operant and respondent conditioning," in *Sec. 2.2.1*; the more or less orderly view on health and SWB, if looked from the sole vantage point of the advocates of SWB, in that "SWB constructs are strongly associated with a range of personality traits," in *Sec. 2.2.2*; the more or less orderly view on health and the environment, if looked from the vantage point of "evolved psychological mechanisms" in EP, in *Sec. 2.3.1*; the more or less orderly view on zoophilia, if looked from the sole vantage point of the defenders, in terms of the issues of consent and enjoyment, in *Sec. 2.3.2*; the more or less orderly view on the relationship between lesser income inequality and health, if looked from the sole vantage point of Wilkinson and Pickett, in *Sec. 2.4.1*; the more or less orderly view on the use of new technologies for mental health, if looked from the sole vantage point of the advocates, in *Sec. 2.4.2*; the more or less orderly view on the treatment of disease, if looked from the sole vantage point of "like cures like" and the "law of the minimum dose" in homeopathy, in *Sec. 2.5.1*; the more or less orderly view on therapy, if looked from the sole vantage point of "attention" and "openness" by those in mindfulness-based therapy, in *Sec. 2.5.2*; the more or less orderly view on physical exercise, if looked from the sole vantage point of the advocates on the link "between physical health and exercise," in *Sec. 3.2.1*; the more or less orderly view on child abuse, if looked from the sole vantage point of its opponents, who simplistically pointed out its causes, effects, and prevention methods aforecited, in *Sec. 3.2.2*; the more or less orderly view on astral travel, if looked from the sole vantage point of someone like Ingo Swann about his travel "to Jupiter and observe details of the planet," in *Sec. 3.3.1*; the more or less orderly view on zoonotic diseases, if looked from the vantage point of "HIV" which predictably "infects vital cells in the human immune system such as helper T cells [specifically CD4+ T cells], macrophages, and dendritic cells," in *Sec. 3.3.2*; the more or less orderly view on physical health and drug use, if looked from the sole vantage point of the contribution to "social order" aforedescribed, in *Sec. 3.4.1*; the more or less orderly view on domestic violence, if looked from the vantage point of "a strict 'patriarchal violence' model," which presumes that "all violence in the home and elsewhere has a male perpetrator and female victim," in *Sec. 3.4.2*; the more or less orderly view on torture, if looked from the sole vantage point of the advocates like Alan M. Dershowitz and Mirko Bagaric, who simply argued that "the need for information outweighs the moral and ethical arguments against torture," in *Sec. 3.5.1*; and the more or less orderly view on medical ethics, if looked from the vantage point of the priority [or ranking] of the values in medical ethics by Edmund Pellegrino, who argued that "beneficence is the only fundamental principle of medical ethics," in *Sec. 3.5.2*).

On the other hand, there is chaos (e.g., the more or less chaotic view on treating health problems, if looked from the multiple, often conflicting, vantage points of different competing approaches to psychotherapy, each with its own claims and techniques, such that "no comparisons of different psychotherapies with long follow-up times have been done" and they do not really add up to much of anything, in *Sec. 2.2.1*; the more or less chaotic view on health and SWB, if looked from the multiple conflicting vantage points that it ignores the "objective" conditions of well-being, that the findings are not consistent across studies and across histories, that much remains uncertain about the nature of SWB, that SWB can be detrimental to health, that it neglects social factors, that it does not give sufficient attention to cultural variations, and so on, in *Sec. 2.2.2*; the more or less chaotic view on health and the environment, if looked from the vantage point of "random noise" in evolution, which is not necessarily adaptive at all, together with other conflicting vantage points as pointed out by the critics earlier, in *Sec. 2.3.1*; the more or less chaotic view on zoophilia, if looked from the numerous conflictng vantage points as shown in the criticisms from different perspectives aforecited, in *Sec. 2.3.2*; the more or less chaotic view on the relationship between lesser income inequality and health, if looked from the numerous, conflicting vantage points by different advocates and critics alike aforecited, in *Sec. 2.4.1*; the more or less chaotic view on the use of new technologies for mental health, if looked from the multiple, conflicting vantage points of different advocates and critics alike, as discussed earlier, in *Sec. 2.4.2*; the more or less chaotic view on the treatment of disease, if looked from all the multiple, conflicting vantage points of numerous types of alternative medicines and different versions of "evidence-based medicine," in *Sec. 2.5.1*; the more or less chaotic view on therapy, if looked from the multiple, conflicting vantage points of the advocates, the critics, and so on, as shown in the debates on the different problems afore-discussed, in *Sec.*

2.5.2; the more or less chaotic view on physical exercise, if looked from the multiple, conflicting vantage points of both the different advocates and the critics aforecited, in *Sec. 3.2.1*; the more or less chaotic view on child abuse, if looked from the multiple, conflicting vantage points of both the opponents and their critics alike, as shown in their disagrements aforecited, in *Sec. 3.2.2*; the more or less chaotic view on astral travel, if looked from the multiple, conflicting vantage points of different advocates and their critics alike, as shown in the different interpretations and disagreements aforecited, in *Sec. 3.3.1*; the more or less chaotic view on zoonotic diseases, if looked from the vantage point of "HIV," which "differs from many viruses in that it has very high genetic variability," in that it has "a high mutation rate of approximately 3 x 10−5 per nucleotide base per cycle of replication and recombinogenic properties of reverse transcriptase," so "this...leads to the generation of many variants of HIV in a single infected patient in the course of one day," in *Sec. 3.3.2*; the more or less chaotic view on physical health and drug use, if looked from the multiple, conflicting vantage points of both sides in the debate on social order and other contentious issues aforediscussed, in *Sec. 3.4.1*; the more or less chaotic view on domestic violence, if looked from the vantage point of "borderline personalities" with their "unusual variability and depth of moods," which are often unpredictable and correlate with the "psychological profile of men who abuse their wives," in *Sec. 3.4.2*; the more or less chaotic view on torture, if looked from the multiple, conflicting vantage points of the advocates, the critics, the researchers, etc., as discussed earlier, such that they do not add up much to anything in *Sec. 3.5.1*; and the more or less chaotic view on medical ethics, if looked from the multiple, conflicting vantage points of the advocates, the critics, the researchers, etc., as shown in the numerous disagreements aforediscussed, such that they do not add up to much of anything, in *Sec. 3.5.2*).

And the reverse direction also holds true.

Once more, it should be stressed, however, that there are different shades of gray (or different degrees of truth) in the two opposites, and the classification is not necessarily mutually exclusive either. In fact, even when some combinations of the two occur, they only end up sharing the same dialectic relationship, but in a different degree.

Also, there are some other relationships (as a kind of family resemblance) which have something in common with the principle, but they are not exactly the same but only more or less comparable, which varies from case to case.

Good examples of family resemblance in relation to the principle are lawfulness-disorder, order-disorder, pattern-chaos, linearity-nonlinearity, unity-disunity, linearity-irreversalness, etc.

16th Thesis: The Slowness-Quickness Principle

The sixteenth thesis concerns the slowness-quickness principle (on the speed of change) in the category of "process" in existential dialectics (which was first worked out in *FIA*), in that both slowness and quickness co-exist, with their own internal tension, to the extent that each fights for its own relevance with the other, in accordance to the perspectives of nature, the mind, culture, and society, without one being the victor and the other being the vanquished in the long haul. There is no slowness without quickness—and vice versa.

For instance, on the one hand, there is slowness (e.g., the relatively slower speed of a patient to cope with emotional distress if s/he refuses to make good use of "resources available to a person experiencing emotional distress—the friendly support of friends, peers, family members, clergy contacts, personal reading, healthy exercise, research, and independent coping," in *Sec. 2.2.1*; the relatively slower speed of some people who, according to some studies on the hedonic treadmill theory, "tend to adapt...slowly" to some events like "the death of a loved one," in *Sec. 2.2.2*; the relatively slower speed of someone to "develop close, trusting bonds with others" if s/he did not have "early childhood caregivers" who "could be trusted to provide reliable assistance and attention," according to EP, in *Sec. 2.3.1*; the relatively slower speed of zoophiles to risk health problems if they are not exposed much or not at all "to the semen, vaginal fluids, urine, saliva, feces and blood of animals," in *Sec. 2.3.2*; the relatively slower speed of an individual to ever suffer from "psychosocial stress and status anxiety" if he is very rich, according to Wilkinson and Pickett, in *Sec. 2.4.1*; the relatively slower speed of patients suffering from acrophobia to be cured without any VRT, as shown in the "randomized, tightly controlled, acrophobia treatment trials at Kaiser Permanente...conducted in 1993-4," in *Sec. 2.4.2*; the relatively slower speed of a patient to recover if he does not receive a "placebo" and also does not receive any treatment from any other sources, in *Sec. 2.5.1*; the relatively slower speed of those patients to recover from their health problems if they have never used "mindfulness-based therapy" or any other programs, as studied by Wallace, in *Sec. 2.5.2*; the relatively slower speed to sleep by someone, if he has "heavy exercise...shortly before bedtime, which may disturb sleep," in *Sec. 3.2.1*; the relatively slower speed for a child to suffer abuse, if he has not experienced any of the causes aforecited, in *Sec. 3.2.2*; the relatively slower speed for someone to travel to Jupiter by an ordinary spacecraft, not through "astral travel," if this were to become possible, in *Sec. 3.3.1*; the relatively slower speed for modern cities of many million individuals to ever get wiped out by infectious diseases, in *Sec. 3.3.2*; the relatively slower speed for an individual to ever get "addictive" if he consumes an extremely small dose of "opium, coca, cannabis, mescaline, and psilocybin" or none at all, in *Sec. 3.4.1*; the relatively slower speed for a woman to encounter domestic violence during her honeymoon, since "the period immediately following a marital separation is the period of greatest risk for the women," according to a study, in *Sec. 3.4.2*; the relatively slower speed of those exceptional torture victims, "such as Admiral James Stockdale, Medal of Honor recipient, who refused to provide information under torture" or simply resisted as much as they could until the ever end, in *Sec. 3.5.1*; and the relatively slower speed for those patients "with a psychiatric condition such as delirium or clinical depression…to make end-of-life decisions" which are to be reasonable and sound in regard to "their best interests," in *Sec. 3.5.2*).

On the other hand, there is quickness (e.g., the relatively quicker speed of a patient to cope with emotional distress if s/he makes good use of "resources available to a person experiencing emotional distress—the friendly support of friends, peers, family members, clergy contacts, personal reading, healthy exercise, research, and independent coping," in *Sec. 2.2.1*; the relatively quicker speed of some people who, according to some studies on the hedonic treadmill theory, "tend to adapt rapidly to some events [e.g. imprisonment]," in *Sec. 2.2.2*; the relatively quicker speed of someone to experience "the sweet taste of sugar and the pain of hitting one's knee against concrete," because they are are "the result of fairly obligate psychological adaptations," according to EP, in *Sec. 2.3.1*; the relatively quicker speed of zoophiles to risk health problems if they are exposed "to the semen, vaginal fluids, urine, saliva, feces and blood of animals," in *Sec. 2.3.2*; the relatively quicker speed of an individual to suffer from "psychosocial stress and status anxiety" if he is very poor, according to Wilkinson and Pickett, in *Sec. 2.4.1*; the relatively quicker speed of patients suffering from acrophobia to be cured if put in the "randomized, tightly controlled, acrophobia treatment trials at Kaiser Permanente," which "provided >90% effectiveness, conducted in 1993-4," in *Sec. 2.4.2*; the relatively quicker speed of a patient to recover if he receives a "placebo," especially for those who believe that "placebos can have both psychological and physical benefits," in *Sec. 2.5.1*; the relatively quicker speed of "thousands of people" to "discover...for themselves through the...practice" of mindfulness-based therapy, as studied by Wallace, in *Sec. 2.5.2*; the relatively quicker speed to sleep by someone, if he exercises "4 to 8 hours before bedtime," in *Sec. 3.2.1*; the relatively quicker speed for a child to suffer abuse, if he is unlucky enough to experience many of the causes aforecited, in *Sec. 3.2.2*; the relatively quicker speed for someone to travel to Jupiter through "astral travel," if this were to become real, in *Sec. 3.3.1*; the relatively quicker speed for "hunter-gatherers usually with fewer than 150 individuals" to "burn out after the...first run through a population" by "epidemic or pandemic diseases," in *Sec. 3.3.2*; the relatively quicker speed for an individual to get "addictive" if he consumes a lot of "opium, coca, cannabis, mescaline, and psilocybin," in *Sec. 3.4.1*; the relatively quicker speed for a woman to encounter domestic violence in "the period immediately following a marital separation," which is "the period of greatest risk for the women," according to a study, in *Sec. 3.4.2*; the relatively quicker speed of ordinary torture victims to "say or do anything to escape the situation, including untrue 'confessions' and implication of others without genuine knowledge," in accordance to "one well documented effect of torture," in *Sec. 3.5.1*; and the relatively quicker speed for those patients who do not suffer from "psychiatric condition such as delirium or clinical depression" and others "to make end-of-life decisions" which are to be reasonable and sound in regard to "their best interests," in *Sec. 3.5.2*).

And the reverse direction also holds true.

Again, it should be stressed, however, that there are different shades of gray (or different degrees of truth) in the two opposites, and the classification is not necessarily mutually exclusive either. In fact, even when some combinations of the two occur, they only end up sharing the same dialectic relationship, but in a different degree.

Also, there are some other relationships (as a kind of family resemblance) which have something in common with the principle, but they are not exactly the same but only more or less comparable, which varies from case to case.

Good examples of family resemblance in relation to the principle are inconvenience-convenience, passiveness-activenessness, gradualness-abruptness, deceleration-acceleration, difficulty-ease, nonresilience-resilience, patience-impatience, and the like.

17th Thesis: The Expansion-Contraction Principle

The seventeenth thesis is called the expansion-contraction principle in the category of "process" in existential dialectics, in that entities in the world can both expand in some ways and contract in other ones, as part of their nature. There is no expansion without contraction—and vice versa.

This principle, although not so explicitly called, was already used in my previous works on different topics (e.g., the theory of floating consciousness in *FCD* and *FPHC*, the union of the unions in *BWT*, and the cyclical progression of system fragmentation and integration in *FCD*).

For instance, on the one hand, there is expansion (e.g., the relative spread of postmodern psychotherapies in the last 2 decades, in *Sec. 2.2.1*; the relatively more developed ability of those in Western cultures to express "personal independence, a sense of personal agency, and self-expression," in *Sec. 2.2.2*; the relative increase of sons to be wanted by parents in good conditions, according to the Trivers-Willard hypothesis, because "parents in good conditions tend to invest more in sons…who are best able to take advantage of good conditions," in *Sec. 2.3.1*; the relatively more developed ability of zoophiles to have sex with animals, when they have "exclusive desire for animals rather than humans," in *Sec. 2.3.2*; the relatively more developed ability of someone to take advantage of others if he suffers from poverty, in accordance to the argument on less income inequality and health, in *Sec. 2.4.1*; the relatively more developed ability to deal with new technologies among those practitioning the use of technology to treat mental disorders, in *Sec. 2.4.2*; the relatively more developed ability of those in "evidence-based medicine" to deal with scientific methods in treating patients, in *Sec. 2.5.1*; the relatively more developed ability of those in mindfulness-based therapy to deal with "attention" and "a clear mental focus," in *Sec. 2.5.2*; the relatively more developed ability of a bus conductor to lead a physically active workstyle, in *Sec. 3.2.1*; the relatively more developed ability of "a medical professional" against the "confidentiality" of a child in child abuse cases to be able "to testify in court as to otherwise privileged evidence about suspected child abuse despite the wishes of the child and his/her family," in *Sec. 3.2.2*; the relative expansion of the belief in astral travel in the pre-modern era, when science was not as well developed, in *Sec. 3.3.1*; the relative spread of "the West Nile virus…in 1999 in the New York City area," in *Sec. 3.3.2*; the relative expansion of "the 'Just Say No' campaign, initiated under the patronage of Nancy Reagan" in the 1980s, in *Sec. 3.4.1*; the relative spread of prevention and intervention programs against domestic violence against women in the Western world nowadays, in *Sec.*

3.4.2; the relative spread of psychological torture, especially after 1980s and, of course, after September 11, 2011 attacks, by "modern democracies" like "the United States, Britain, and France" who "pioneered and exported techniques that have become the lingua franca of modern torture: methods that leave no marks," according to Darius Rejali, in *Sec. 3.5.1*; and the relatively more developed ability of those in medical ethics to deal with "curing," in *Sec. 3.5.2*).

On the other hand, there is contraction (e.g., the relative decline of Freudian psychoanalysis in the last 2 decades, in *Sec. 2.2.1*; the relatively less developed ability of those in Western cultures to express "an interdependent self that is inseparable from significant others" and "to suppress their personal desires when necessary in order to promote collective interests," in *Sec. 2.2.2*; the relative decrease of daughters to be wanted by parents in good conditions, according to the Trivers-Willard hypothesis, because "parents in good conditions tend to invest more in sons…who are best able to take advantage of good conditions," in *Sec. 2.3.1*; the relatively less developed ability of zoophiles to have sex with humans, when they have "exclusive desire for animals rather than humans," in *Sec. 2.3.2*; the relatively less developed ability of someone to trust others if he suffers from poverty, in accordance to the argument on less income inequality and health, in *Sec. 2.4.1*; the relatively less developed ability to deal with traditional methods among those practitioning the use of technology to treat mental disorders in *Sec. 2.4.2*; the relatively less developed ability of those in "evidence-based medicine" to deal with "religion, tradition, superstition,…supernatural energies," etc. in treating patients, in *Sec. 2.5.1*; the relatively less developed ability of those in mindfulness-based therapy to deal with wealth acquisition, colonial conquest, etc., in *Sec. 2.5.2*; the relatively less developed ability of a bus conductor to lead a sedentary workstyle, in *Sec. 3.2.1*; the relatively less developed ability of "a medical professional" against the "confidentiality" of a child in child abuse cases to insist the "standard requirements for confidentiality and legal privileges in instances of child abuse," in *Sec. 3.2.2*; the relative decline of the belief in astral travel in our time, when the scientific way of thinking is more dominant. especially in the scientific community, in *Sec. 3.3.1*; the relative decline of "the West Nile virus…in the New York City area" nowadays, in *Sec. 3.3.2*; the relative decline of "illicit drug use…from 14.1% in 1979 to 5.8% in 1992, a drop of 60%" after "the 'Just Say No' campaign," in *Sec. 3.4.1*; the relative decline of men who believe that "a husband is justified in hitting or beating his wife under certain circumstances" in the Western world nowadays, in *Sec. 3.4.2*; the relative decline of physical torture for "several decades…from Europe to most parts of the world" in the second half of the 20th century, according to scholar Ervand Abrahamian. in *Sec. 3.5.1*; and the relatively less developed ability of those in medical ethics to deal with "caring," in *Sec. 3.5.2*).

And the reverse direction also holds true.

Again, it should be stressed, however, that there are different shades of gray (or different degrees of truth) in the two opposites, and the classification is not necessarily mutually exclusive either. In fact, even when some combinations of the two occur, they only end up sharing the same dialectic relationship, but in a different degree.

Also, there are some other relationships (as a kind of family resemblance) which have something in common with the principle, but they are not exactly the same but only more or less comparable, which varies from case to case.

Good examples of family resemblance in relation to the principle are conquest-autarky, rise-fall, spread-shrink, extendingness-shorteningness, widening-narrowing, construction-deconstruction, expansion-destruction, construction-demolition, creation-destruction, expansion-contraction, expansion-constriction, expansion-decline, and so forth.

18th Thesis: The Optimality-Nonoptimality Principle

The eighteenth thesis concerns the optimality-nonoptimality principle (on the nature of highly favorable options) in the category of "process" in existential dialectics, which is first proposed in *FPHMORPH*, in that both optimality and non-optimality are important, in relation to the mind, nature, culture, and society, albeit in different ways. There is no optimality without nonoptimality—and vice versa.

There are five clarifications to remember, as shown in the fields of morphology (e.g., "perfection" in *FPHMORP*), data analysis (e.g., "bounded rationality" in *FPHO*, *FFHDA* and *FPHPROP*), probability (e.g., "decision making" in *FPHO* and *FPHPROP*), economics (e.g., "negative externalities" in *FCD* and *BCPC*), and technology (e.g., "post-capitalism" in *FCD*), just to cite five well-documented sources:

- Optimality (in terms of highly favorable options) is not perfect and can be realized in different degrees.
- "Maximization" does not necessarily entail "optimization," as shown in the problem of "negative externalities" in economics.

- Non-optimality can come in all shapes and sizes, in different degrees, like "maximizing" in economics vs. "satisficing" in sociology.
- Optimality can be more feasible in the longer term of technological improvement.
- Optimality should not be confused with the beauty of simplicity, since the more optimal a process is, the more complicated (not necessarily the simpler) it can be.

In any event, on the one hand, there is optimality (e.g., the search for highly favorable options, like the quest for optimality in some models of psychotherapy, like the view that "depending on the client's personality, a more supportive or more uncovering approach may be optimal," in *Sec. 2.2.1*; the search for highly favorable options, like the quest for "a person's baseline or equilibrium level of SWB," which, according to Set Point theory, is "a consequence of hereditary characteristics and therefore, almost entirely predetermined at birth," in *Sec. 2.2.2*; the search for highly favorable options, like the quest for "inclusive fitness," in that, "according to 'Hamilton's rule,' a self-sacrificing behavior can evolve if it helps close relatives so much that it more than compensates for the individual animal's sacrifice," in *Sec. 2.3.1*; the search for highly favorable options, like the quest for the acceptance of zoophilia on maximal utilitarian ground by "utilitarian philosopher and animal liberation author Peter Singer" who "argues that zoophilia is not unethical so long as it involves no harm or cruelty to the animal," in *Sec. 2.3.2*; the search for highly favorable options, like the quest for reducing income inequality by "Islington's Fairness Commission," following in the footsteps of Wilkinson and Pickett, in *Sec. 2.4.1*; the search for highly favorable options, like the quest for ">90% effectiveness" in the "randomized, tightly controlled, acrophobia treatment trials at Kaiser Permanente…in 1993-4," in *Sec. 2.4.2*; the search for highly favorable options, like the quest for effective scientific treatments by the National Science Foundation when it advocated only "evidence-based medicine" and dismissed "alternative medicine" as "all treatments that had not been proven effective using scientific methods," in *Sec. 2.5.1*; the search for highly favorable options, like the quest by Jon Kabat-Zinn for "the Mindfulness-Based Stress Reduction program," which can treat "a variety of conditions in people both healthy and unhealthy," in *Sec. 2.5.2*; the search for highly favorable options, like the quest for "the optimum time to exercise," by those who studied physical exercise, as they claimed that it "may be 4 to 8 hours before bedtime, though exercise at any time of day is beneficial," in *Sec. 3.2.1*; the search for highly favorable options, like the quest for "optimal caregiving" to prevent "child abuse" by researchers like Baumrind and others, in *Sec. 3.2.2*; the search for highly favorable options, like the quest for some preferred "levels or sub-planes" in astral travel, like "heavens" over "hells," in *Sec. 3.3.1*; the search for highly favorable options, like the understanding of the optimal conditions of infectious agents to survive and cause damage to human populations, in that "a biological pathogen had to be a chronic infection, stay alive in the host for long periods, or have a non-human reservoir in which to live while waiting for new hosts to pass by," in *Sec. 3.3.2*; the search for highly favorable options, like the quest for the most effective deterrence against drug use, in that, as explained by Gil Kerlikowske, Director of the US ONDCP, "controls and prohibitions help to keep prices higher, and higher prices help keep use rates relatively low, since drug use, especially among young people, is known to be sensitive to price," in *Sec. 3.4.1*; the search for highly favorable options, like the research on "the period immediately following a marital separation," which was found to be "the period of greatest risk for the women," according to a study, in *Sec. 3.4.2*; the search for highly favorable options, like the quest for the most effective part of the body to be tortured, like "the feet," so as "to cause carefully controllable agony without endangering the prisoner's life," and "this is clearly accomplished by staying as far as possible from the brain and the vital [viz., abdominal] organs," so "the only body part that satisfies this twin criterion is the foot," in *Sec. 3.5.1*; and the search for highly favorable options, like the quest for "the main or primary consideration [hence primum]" in medical ethics, which is, for these scholars, "non-maleficience," since "it is more important not to harm your patient, than to do them good," in *Sec. 3.5.2*).

On the other hand, there is non-optimality (e.g., the existence of non-optimal alternatives to optimality, like the argument for more realistic studies by the critics, who pointed out that the search for optimal approaches are unrealistic, because of the different problems aforecited, and some critics even suggested that psychotherapy is dispensable, in *Sec. 2.2.1*; the existence of non-optimal alternatives to optimality, like the argument for more realistic studies by the critics, who pointed out other complicated factors, like "social influence," "cultural variations," "objective" aspects of well-being, Western-centric samples, etc., in *Sec. 2.2.2*; the existence of non-optimal alternatives to optimality, like the argument for more realistic studies by the critics, who pointed out that there are "non-genetic and non-adaptive explanations" which are not adequately considered, that there is the controversial issues about testability and uncertainty, that it runs the risk of committing "the naturalistic fallacy," that it is reductionistic, and that there are disagreements on the "modularity of the mind, in *Sec. 2.3.1*; the existence of non-optimal alternatives to optimality, like the argument for more realistic studies by the critics, who pointed out that "animals might be traumatized even by a non-violent, sexual approach from a human," that it is "profoundly degrading," together with other criticisms aforecited, in *Sec. 2.3.2*; the existence of non-optimal alternatives to optimality, like the argument for more realistic studies by the critics, who pointed out that the work by Wilkinson and Pickett is highly problematic, for the reasons aforediscussed, in *Sec. 2.4.1*; the existence of non-optimal alternatives to optimality, like the argument for more realistic studies by the critics, who pointed out different barriers and problems confronting the use of new technologies to treat mental health aforedescribed, in *Sec. 2.4.2*; the existence of non-optimal alternatives to optimality, like the argument for more realistic studies by the critics, who pointed out that the focus on "evidence-based medicine" is questionable, since "alternative medicine can be on the rise 'in countries where Western science and scientific method generally are accepted as the major foundations for healthcare" and this anomaly "has been described as an 'enigma' in the Medical Journal of Australia," in *Sec. 2.5.1*; the existence of non-optimal alternatives to optimality, like the argument for more realistic studies by the critics, who pointed out that the research works are often incomplete, that the practices are not so effective, that its terms are often not clearly defined and can mean different things, that the idea of "mindfulness" in mindfulness-based therapy programs deviates significantly from the original Buddhist version, and that because of its connection with alternative medicine, mindfulness-based therapy programs have been criticized as not being scientific, in *Sec. 2.5.2*; the existence of non-optimal alternatives to optimality, like the argument for more realistic studies by the critics, who pointed out the different problems with physical exercise aforedescribed, in *Sec. 3.2.1*; the existence of non-optimal alternatives to optimality, like the argument for more realistic studies by the critics, who pointed out that scholars disagree over what constitutes child abuse, that the alleged causes of child abuse can be questionable, that the long-term effects of child abuse remains unknown, and that the alleged causes do not determine the often cited consequences, that the prevention of child abuse can be limited, and that there is cultural bias in the studies, in *Sec. 3.2.2*; the existence of non-optimal alternatives to optimality, like the argument for more realistic studies by the critics, who pointed out that the experience is subjective, that there are competing interpretations of astral travel, that the claims are "contrary to the limits of science," and that the claims are not accurate, in *Sec. 3.3.1*; the existence of non-optimal alternatives to optimality, like the argument for more realistic studies by the critics, who pointed out that zoonotic diseases can be historically contingent, that there are infectious diseases which can go in the opposite direction, that the causes of zoonotic diseases can be more complicated than previously thought, and that the acceptance of the findings in zoonotic research can be based on the politics of social impact, in *Sec. 3.3.2*; the existence of non-optimal alternatives to optimality, like the argument for more realistic studies by the critics, who pointed out the negative side of the debate, against the idea of deterrence aforecited, in *Sec. 3.4.1*; the existence of non-optimal alternatives to optimality, like the argument for more realistic studies by the critics, who pointed out that there is too much attention to domestic violence by men against women [but not by women against men too], that the theories are "disputed," that each approach is limited to itself, that the prevention of domestic violence is not as successful as claimed, that the prevention of domestic violence may only be temporary, and the call for the prevention of domestic violence is culturally relative, in *Sec. 3.4.2*; the existence of non-optimal alternatives to optimality, like the argument for more realistic studies by the critics, who pointed out that "there is simply no scientific evidence supporting its effectiveness," in *Sec. 3.5.1*; and the existence of non-optimal alternatives to optimality, like the argument for more realistic studies by the critics, who pointed out that there is cultural bias in medical ethics, that there is no consensus on medical ethics even within a given tradition, and that scholars disagree over the priority [or ranking] of the values in medical ethics in *Sec. 3.5.2*).

And the reverse direction also holds true.

Again, it should be stressed, however, that there are different shades of gray (or different degrees of truth) in the two opposites, and the classification is not necessarily mutually exclusive either. In fact, even when some combinations of the two occur, they only end up sharing the same dialectic relationship, but in a different degree.

Also, there are some other relationships (as a kind of family resemblance) which have something in common with the principle, but they are not exactly the same but only more or less comparable, which varies from case to case.

Good examples of family resemblance in relation to the principle are optimality-satisfaction, optimality-maximization, optimality-heuristicness, idealness-realisticness, and the like.

In Relation to Agency

The next eight theses are in relation to agency in existential dialectics, as shown below.

19th Thesis: The Theory-Praxis Principle

The nineteenth thesis is the theory-praxis principle (on the duality of knowledge) in the category of "agency" in existential dialectics (which was first worked out in *FPHE*), in that, if there is theoretical construction, there is likewise its practical application, both technical and normative. There is no theory without praxis—and vice versa.

For instance, on the one hand, there is theory (e.g., the theoretical construction of "power relations" in feminism, in *Sec. 2.2.1*; the theoretical construction of "heritability" in genetics, in *Sec. 2.2.2*; the theoretical construction of "adaptation" in "evolutionary biology," in *Sec. 2.3.1*; the theoretical construction of "consent" in the study of human sexuality on sexual acts between humans, in *Sec. 2.3.2*; the theoretical construction of "the spirit level" by Wilkinson and Pickett, in *Sec. 2.4.1*; the theoretical construction of "virtual reality" in computer science, in *Sec. 2.4.2*; the theoretical construction of "Chinese astrology" in ancient times, in *Sec. 2.5.1*; the theoretical construction of "mindfulness" in Buddhism, in *Sec. 2.5.2*; the theoretical construction of "synaptic plasticity" in neurobiology, in *Sec. 3.2.1*; theoretical construction of "rights" in ethics, in *Sec. 3.2.2*; the theoretical construction of "heavens and hells" in different religions, in *Sec. 3.3.1*; the theoretical construction of "zoonotic diseases" in conservation medicine, in *Sec. 3.3.2*; the theoretical construction of "cost," "price," "demand," etc. in economics, in *Sec. 3.4.1*; the theoretical construction of "borderline personalities" in psychology, in *Sec. 3.4.2*; the theoretical construction of "utilitarianism" in philosophy, in *Sec. 3.5.1*; and the theoretical construction of "autonomy," in ethics in *Sec. 3.5.2*).

On the other hand, there is praxis (e.g., the practical application of "power relations" in feminism to the field of psychotherapy, as in feminist therapy, in *Sec. 2.2.1*; the practical application of "heritability" in genetics to the field of psychology, like the study on the correlation between genetics and SWB, in *Sec. 2.2.2*; the practical application of "adaptation" in "evolutionary biology" to the field of "evolutionary psychology," like the study of "evolved psychological mechanisms," in *Sec. 2.3.1*; the practical application of "consent" in the study of human sexuality to the field of zoophilia, as shown in the argument for sexual acts between humans and animals, in *Sec. 2.3.2*; the practical application of "the spirit level" by Wilkinson and Pickett to the field of public politics, as shown in the work of "Islington's Fairness Commission to look at ways of reducing income inequality in the London borough," with Wilkinson being appointed as "the chair," in *Sec. 2.4.1*; the practical application of"virtual reality" in computer science to the field of medicine, like the use of emails to treat mental disorders, in *Sec. 2.4.2*; the practical application of "Chinese astrology" in ancient times to the field of medicine, as in "traditional Chinese medicine," in *Sec. 2.5.1*; the practical application of "mindfulness" in Buddhism to the field of therapy, as shown in mindfulness-based therapy programs, in *Sec. 2.5.2*; the practical application of "synaptic plasticity" in neurobiology to the field of physical exercise, in that exercise increases "growth factors that help create new nerve cells and promote synaptic plasticity," in *Sec. 3.2.1*; the practical application of "rights" in ethics to the field of health care and the law, as shown in "the 2008 New Hampshire case of Andrew Bedner" about "the parental rights of abusive parents or caretakers with regard to their children, particularly in medical settings," in *Sec. 3.2.2*; the practical application of "heavens and hells" in different religions to the field of "out-of-body experience" like "astral travel," in *Sec. 3.3.1*; the practical application of the understanding of "zoonotic diseases" in conservation medicine to the field of public health, as shown in 2006, when "a conference held in Berlin was focusing on the issue of zoonotic pathogen effects on food safety, urging governments to intervene, and the public to be vigilant towards the risks of catching food-borne diseases from farm-to-dining table," in *Sec. 3.3.2*; the practical application of "cost," "price," "demand," etc. in economics to the field of drug prohibition, as shown in the debate on "cost," in *Sec. 3.4.1*; the practical application of "borderline personalities" in psychology to the field of "domestic violence" for causal explanations, in *Sec. 3.4.2*; the practical application of utilitarianism" in philosophy to the field of public policy, like the utilitarian argument against torture, in *Sec. 3.5.1*; and the practical application of "autonomy" in ethics to the field of medicine, like "respect for autonomy" by physicians, in *Sec. 3.5.2*).

And the reverse direction also holds true.

Again, it should be stressed, however, that there are different shades of gray (or different degrees of truth) in the two opposites, and the classification is not necessarily mutually exclusive either. In fact, even when some combinations of the two occur, they only end up sharing the same dialectic relationship, but in a different degree.

Also, there are some other relationships (as a kind of family resemblance) which have something in common with the principle, but they are not exactly the same but only more or less comparable, which varies from case to case.

Good examples of family resemblance in relation to the principle are discovery-application, knowledge-action, invention-innovation, theory-intentionality, discourse-action, knowledge-interest, knowledge-motivation, universality-particularity, potentiality-actuality, theory-practice, and so forth.

20th Thesis: The Convention-Novelty Principle

The twentieth thesis is the convention-novelty principle (on the nature of creative thinking) in the category of "agency" in existential dialectics (which was first worked out in *FPHCT*), in that, if there is conventional wisdom, there is likewise novel challenge, to the extent that both convergent and divergent thinking are part of life. There is no convention without novelty—and vice versa.

As srummarized from *FPHCT* (almost verbatim here), there are (a) "creative techniques" and (b) "creative traits," which, when satisfied—in relation to the larger context of the mind, nature, society, and culture—can be used to enhance creative works.

In addition, creative thinking has its own possibilities and limits (in relation to invention), just as it has its own promises and pitfalls (in relation to innovation)— as already analyzed in *FPHCT*).

In the end, creative thinking has its own desirability and dark sides (as also already analyzed in *FPHCT*).

With these clarifications in mind—there are good empirical examples for the convention-novelty princple.

For instance, on the one hand, there is convention (e.g., the conventional wisdom about "uncovering psychotherapy," which "emphasizes facilitating the client's insight into the roots of their difficulties," in *Sec. 2.2.1*; the conventional wisdom about the correlation between health and SWB, in *Sec. 2.2.2*; the conventional wisdom about "evolved psychological mechanisms" in EP, in *Sec. 2.3.1*; the conventional wisdom against zoophilia, as shown in the tendency of "some people [to] express knee-jerk concern or disapproval of sexual interest in non-human animals, sometimes very strongly," in *Sec. 2.3.2*; the conventional wisdom about laissez-faire capitalism to stress competition between individuals among those on the right wing of the political spectrum, in *Sec. 2.4.1*; the conventional wisdom about using "medication, counselling, Cognitive Behavioral Therapy, exercise and a healthy diet" to treat mental problems, in *Sec. 2.4.2*; the conventional wisdom about "traditional Chinese medicine" in ancient times, in *Sec. 2.5.1*; the conventional wisdom about "mindfulness" in Buddhism, in *Sec. 2.5.2*; the conventional wisdom about the link "between physical health and exercise," in *Sec. 3.2.1*; the conventional wisdom about protecting child victims from abuse, in *Sec. 3.2.2*; the conventional wisdom about astral travel "in classical philosophy and in various myths and religious scriptures," in *Sec. 3.3.1*; the conventional wisdom about the link between human health and infectious diseases from animals, in *Sec. 3.3.2*; the conventional wisdom about drug prohibition for "social order," in *Sec. 3.4.1*; the conventional wisdom about domestic violence by men against women by the feminists, in *Sec. 3.4.2*; the conventional wisdom about "torture" which "was sanctioned" historically in different societies in antiquity, in *Sec. 3.5.1*; and the conventional wisdom about the "four principles" in medical ethics by Tom Beauchamp and James Childress, in *Sec. 3.5.2*).

On the other hand, there is novelty (e.g., the alternative novel challenge to the conventional wisdom about "uncovering psychotherapy," by the new idea of "feminist, constructionist and discursive sources," which suggest instead that "the therapist-client relationship...participates in society's power relations and political dynamics," in *Sec. 2.2.1*; the alternative novel challenge to the conventional wisdom about the correlation between health and SWB, by the new idea that, "in the case of "survival," there is "evidence" which "suggests happiness may actually be...detrimental" to health, in *Sec. 2.2.2*; the alternative novel challenge to the conventional wisdom about "evolved psychological mechanisms" in EP, by the new idea that EP suffers from "genetic reductionism," in *Sec. 2.3.1*; the alternative novel challenge to the conventional wisdom against zoophilia, by the new idea of defending it on the basis of "consent" and "enjoyment" aforediscussed, in *Sec. 2.3.2*; the alternative novel challenge to the conventional wisdom about laissez-faire capitalism to stress compeition between individuals, by the new idea of Wilkinson and Pickett to reduce income inequality for health and other reasons, in *Sec. 2.4.1*; the alternative novel challenge to the conventional wisdom about using "medication, counselling, Cognitive Behavioral Therapy, exercise and a healthy diet" to treat mental problems, by the new idea of new technologies for mental health aforecited, in *Sec. 2.4.2*; the alternative novel challenge to the conventional wisdom about traditional Chinese medicine" in ancient times, by the new idea nowadays that "many of its assumptions, including the model of the body, or concept of disease, are not supported by modern evidence-based medicine," in *Sec. 2.5.1*; the alternative novel challenge to the conventional wisdom about "mindfulness" in Buddhism, by the new idea of using it for therapy, as proposed by Jon Kabat-Zinn and others, in *Sec. 2.5.2*; the alternative novel challenge to the conventional wisdom about the link "between physical health and exercise," by the new idea that vigorous exercise can have its downside, or that some individuals can be exercise-resistant, in *Sec. 3.2.1*; the alternative novel challenge to the conventional wisdom about protecting child victims from abuse, by the new idea of "the 2008 New Hampshire case of Andrew Bedner" about "the parental rights of abusive parents or caretakers with regard to their children, particularly in medical settings," in *Sec. 3.2.2*; the alternative novel challenge to the conventional wisdom about astral travel "in classical philosophy and in various myths and religious scriptures," by the new idea of science nowadays that the claims are "contrary to the limits of science" and that the claims are not accurate, in *Sec. 3.3.1*; the alternative novel challenge to the conventional wisdom about the link between human health and infectious diseases from animals, by the new idea that zoonotic diseases can be historically contingent, that there are infectious diseases which can go in the opposite direction, that the causes of zoonotic diseases can be more complicated than previously thought, and that the acceptance of the findings in zoonotic research can be based on the politics of social impact, in *Sec. 3.3.2*; the alternative novel challenge to the conventional wisdom about drug prohibition for "social order," by the new idea that "prohibition protects the drug cartel insofar as it keeps the distribution in the black market and creates the risk that makes smuggling profitable," in *Sec. 3.4.1*; the alternative novel challenge to the conventional wisdom about domestic violence by men against women, by the new idea of "modern research into predictors of injury from domestic violence," which "finds that the strongest predictor of injury by domestic violence is participation in reciprocal domestic violence, and that this pattern of domestic violence is more often initiated by the female in the relationship," in *Sec. 3.4.2*; the alternative novel challenge to the conventional wisdom about "torture" which "was sanctioned" historically in different societies in antiquity, by the new idea of the "Article 5 of the UN Universal Declaration of Human Rights" in 1948, which prohibits torture for the first time "under international law and the domestic laws of most countries," in *Sec. 3.5.1*; and the alternative novel challenge to the conventional wisdom about the "four principles" in medical ethics by Tom Beauchamp and James Childress, by the new idea of different values like "respect for persons" and "truthfulness and honesty" as suggested by the critics aforediscussed, in *Sec. 3.5.2*).

And the reverse direction also holds true.

Again, it should be stressed, however, that there are different shades of gray (or different degrees of truth) in the two opposites, and the classification is not necessarily mutually exclusive either. In fact, even when some combinations of the two occur, they only end up sharing the same dialectic relationship, but in a different degree.

Also, there are some other relationships (as a kind of family resemblance) which have something in common with the principle, but they are not exactly the same but only more or less comparable, which varies from case to case.

Good examples of family resemblance in relation to the principle are convergence-divergence (or convergent thinking vs. divergent thinking), normalness-nonnormalness, conformity-nonconformity, familiarity-freshness, inertia-newness, equilibrium-disturbance, and so on.

21st Thesis: The Evolution-Transformation Principle

The twenty-first thesis refers to the evolution-transformation principle (on the multiple kinds of agency). in the category of "agency" in existential dialectics (which was first worked out in *FAE* and then in other books of mine).

This principle—and the symmetry-asymmetry principle, for instance—are both about agency. More precisely, the word "agency," in a formal definition, refers to "a person or thing through which power is exerted or an end is achieved." (MWD 2007) It therefore does not have to necessarily involve an intelligent lifeform.

Because of this dual meaning in agency, the evolution-transformation principle is more concerned with *the kind of agency*, that is, both about the *evolution* in the state of nature (e.g., an object of natural beauty) and the *transformation* in the world of intelligent lifeforms (e.g., a work of art). There is no evolution without transformation—and vice versa.

In classical Darwinian evolutionary theory (as more detailedly analyzed in *BNN*), evolution is "blind." But in the human world, change often takes place because of the conscious intervention of humans in transforming society and culture, just to cite two instances.

And the transformative part of the principle precisely refers to the other dimension in the dual meaning of agency, in giving technology (as invented by intelligent lifeforms like humans and, soon, post-humans) a major role to play in the change of the world, which is something that I extensively analyzed in *FHC* in the context of the technophilic lifeworld, espeically though not exclusively since modern times. The same theme is also elaborated in many other books of mine.

For instance, on the one hand, there is evolution (e.g., the natural evolution of humans to "deal...with crises, navigat[e]...severe social problems and find...solutions to life problems" in the state of nature, in *Sec. 2.2.1*; the natural evolution of humans to experience SWB like "affect balance" and "life satisfaction" in the state of nature in a primitive way, in *Sec. 2.2.2*; the natural evolution of humans to adapt in the state of nature, in *Sec. 2.3.1*; the natural evolution of humans to have sex with each other or, in some cases, with animals, in the state of nature, in *Sec. 2.3.2*; the natural evolution of humans to compete and copperate with each other in the state of nature, in *Sec. 2.4.1*; the natural evolution of humans to sometimes suffer from mental problems in the state of nature, in *Sec. 2.4.2*; the natural evolution of humans to sometimes get sick in the state of nature in *Sec. 2.5.1*; the natural evolution of humans to suffer from health problems at times in the state of nature, in *Sec. 2.5.2*; the natural evolution of humans to walk, run, jump, etc. in the state of nature, in *Sec. 3.2.1*; the natural evolution of humans to treat each other, which can "result...in harm, potential for harm, or threat of harm to a child," in the state of nature, in *Sec. 3.2.2*; the natural evolution of humans to wander to different places in the state of nature in a primitive way, in *Sec. 3.3.1*; the natural evolution of humans to suffer from infectious diseases at times in the state of nature in a primitive way, in *Sec. 3.3.2*; the natural evolution of humans to consume plants, including "natural plant drugs," in the state of nature, in *Sec. 3.4.1*; the natural evolution of humans to be violent towards each other at times in the state of nature, in *Sec. 3.4.2*; the natural evolution of humans to "inflict...severe physical pain and possibly injury" on others in the state of nature, in *Sec. 3.5.1*; and the natural evolution of humans to get sick at times and look for cure in the state of nature in a primitive way, in *Sec. 3.5.2*).

On the other hand, there is transformation (e.g., the technical transformation of human ability to deal...with crises, navigat[e]...severe social problems and find...solutions to life problems" by the invention of different approaches to psychotherapy, in *Sec. 2.2.1*; the technical transformation of human ability to understand SWB like "affect balance" and "life satisfaction" by the invention of "positive psychology" for the systematic study of SWB, in *Sec. 2.2.2*; the technical transformation of human ability to understand adaptation by the invention of EP for the systematic study of "evolved psychological mechanisms," in *Sec. 3.2.1*; the technical transformation of human ability to understand sex with each other or, in some cases, with animals by the invention of the field of zoophilia for a systematic study of its practice, in *Sec. 2.3.2*; the technical transformation of human ability to understand competition and cooperation by the invention of the idea of "the spirit level" for the reduction of income inequality, in *Sec. 2.4.1*; the technical transformation of human ability to treat mental problems by the invention of VRT and telemedicine, in *Sec. 2.4.2*; the technical transformation of human ability to cure sickness by the invention of "alternative medicines," in *Sec. 2.5.1*; the technical transformation of human ability to deal with health problems by the invention of mindfulness-based therapy, in *Sec. 2.5.2*; the technical transformation of human ability to walk, run, jump, etc. by the invention of physical exercise for the systematic study of its types, categories, effects, etc., in *Sec. 3.2.1*; the technical transformation of human ability to treat each other by the invention of ethics and jurisprudence, like "the 2008 New Hampshire case of Andrew Bedner" about "the parental rights of abusive parents or caretakers with regard to their children, particularly in medical settings," in *Sec. 3.2.2*; the technical transformation of human ability to wander to different places by the invention of the idea of astral travel "in classical philosophy and in various myths and religious scriptures," in *Sec. 3.3.1*; the technical transformation of human ability to deal with infectious diseases by the invention of "conservation medicine" to deal largely with "zoonoses," in *Sec. 3.3.2*; the technical transformation of human ability to deal with plants, including "natural plant drugs," by the invention of the knowledge discourse on different contentious issues about drug prohibition, in *Sec. 3.4.1*; the technical transformation of human ability to to be violent towards each other by the invention of different "prevention and intervention" programs against domestic violence, in *Sec. 3.4.2*; the technical transformation of human ability to "inflict...severe physical pain and possibly injury" on others by the invention of different systematic "methods" over the centuries aforediscussed, in *Sec. 3.5.1*; and the technical transformation of human ability to deal with the business of curing by the invention of "medical ethics" with its principles, in *Sec. 3.5.2*).

And the reverse direction also holds true.

Again, it should be stressed, however, that there are different shades of gray (or different degrees of truth) in the two opposites, and the classification is not necessarily mutually exclusive either. In fact, even when some combinations of the two occur, they only end up sharing the same dialectic relationship, but in a different degree.

Also, there are some other relationships (as a kind of family resemblance) which have something in common with the principle, but they are not exactly the same but only more or less comparable, which varies from case to case.

Good examples of family resemblance in relation to the principle are inorganicness-volition, naturalness-technologicalness, naturalness-nonnaturalness, nonwillingness-willingness, inorganicness-motivation, evolution-creation, naturalness-artificialness, and so on.

22nd Thesis: The Symmetry-Asymmetry Principle

The twenty-second thesis is labeled as the symmetry-asymmetry principle (on the relationships among existents) in the category of "agency" in existential dialectics (which was also already worked out in my previous books), in that there is no asymmetry without symmetry—and vice versa.

For instance, the Same can be symmetric and asymmetric towards the Others. But in case of asymmetry (as analyzed in *BDPD*), oppression and self-oppression can occur. So, when the Same is asymmetric towards the Others, the Same can also be relatively asymmetric towards itself in self-oppression, just as the Others can be likewise towards themselves. The subsequent oppressiveness is dualistic, as much by the Same against the Others and itself, as by the Others against the Same and themselves. Both oppression and self-oppression can be achieved by way of downgrading differences between the Same and the Others and of accentuating them.

This is true, even though not all forms of asymmetry have to be about oppression and self-oppression.

In addition, from Chapter Three of *FPHG*, symmetry is not perfect, to be understood in an approximate sense under many life circumstances. With this clarification in mind, hereafter are some empirical examples.

For instance, on the one hand, there is symmetry (e.g., the co-existence of different individuals in psychotherapy, like a therapist and a client, in *Sec. 2.2.1*; the co-existence of different events that can affect people, like "imprisonment," "the death of a loved one," etc., in *Sec. 2.2.2*; the co-existence of different traits in humans, in *Sec. 2.3.1*; the co-existence of different lifeforms, like animals and humans, in *Sec. 2.3.2*; the co-existence of different groups in society, in *Sec. 2.4.1*; the co-existence of different agents in the world of using new technologies for mental health, like practitioners and regulatory agencies, in *Sec. 2.4.2*; the co-existence of different types of medicines, be they "evidence-based" or "alternative," in *Sec. 2.5.1*; the co-existence of different agents in a mindfulness-based therapy relationship, like a Buddhist teacher and his patient, in *Sec. 2.5.2*; the co-existence of different individuals in society who try to exercise, in *Sec. 3.2.1*; the co-existence of different entities in a social relationship, like a child and an adult, in *Sec. 3.2.2*; the co-existence of different ways to understand astral travel, in *Sec. 3.3.1*; the co-existence of different directions for infectoius diseases to spread, that is, from humans to animals and from animals to humans, in *Sec. 3.3.2*; the co-existence of different agents in regard to drug prohibition, like drug users and law enforcement authorities, in *Sec. 3.4.1*; the co-existence of different views about domestic violence in the world, in *Sec. 3.4.2*; the co-existence of different methods of torture, be they "physical" or "psychological," in *Sec. 3.5.1*; and the co-existence of different moral principles, be they "autonomy," "caring," in *Sec. 3.5.2*).

On the other hand, there is asymmetry (e.g., according to "feminist, constructionist and discursive sources," "the therapist-client relationship...participates in society's power relations and political dynamics," with the therapist having power over the client, in *Sec. 2.2.1*; according to some studies on the hedonic treadmill theory, "people do not adapt to all life events equally, as people tend to adapt rapidly to some events [e.g. imprisonment], slowly to others [e.g. the death of a loved one], and not at all to others [e.g. noise and sex]," in *Sec. 2.2.2*; not all traits in humans are adaptations, since they "may also be exaptations," "byproducts," "random noise," etc., in *Sec. 2.3.1*; "animals don't have the same capacity for thinking as humans," so "they are unable to give full consent," even when humans use them for sex, according to those critics of zoophilia, in *Sec. 2.3.2*; income inequality between the rich and the poor in society, in *Sec. 2.4.1*; practitioners have to comply with the requirements as imposed by regulatory agencies, like "paying substantial licensure fees, passing additional oral and written examinations, and traveling for interviews," in *Sec. 2.4.2*; "evidence-based medicine" is more domiannt than "alternative medicine" in developed countries nowadays, in *Sec. 2.5.1*; the Buddhist teacher has authority over his patient in a mindfulness-based therapy relationship, in *Sec. 2.5.2*; some individuals like athletes are good in physical exercise—but some other individuals are "exercise-resistant" and "can never augment endurance" in exercise, in *Sec. 3.2.1*; an adult, on average, can abuse a child in a way that a child cannot do the same to an adult, especially when the child is dependent on the adult for caretaking. in *Sec. 3.2.2*; the scientific interpretaton of astral travel is more dominant or persuasive in the academic community nowadays than the sacred interpretation based on "various myths and religious scriptures," in *Sec. 3.3.1*; "in a systematic review of 1,415 pathogens known to infect humans," 61% were zoonotic [from animals to humans] but 39% were reverse-zoonotic [from humans to animals]), in

Sec. 3.3.2; law enforcement authorities can arrest and detain drug users under certain legal conditions, in *Sec. 3.4.1*; "in most developed countries domestic violence is considered unacceptable by most people" nowadays—but "in many regions of the world the views are different: according to a UNICEF survey, the percentage of *women* aged 15–49 who think that a husband is justified in hitting or beating his wife under certain circumstances is, for example: 90% in Jordan, 85.6% in Guinea, 85.4% in Zambia, 85% in Sierra Leone, 81.2% in Laos, 81% in Ethiopia," in *Sec. 3.4.2*; "psychological torture is less well known than physical torture and tends to be subtle and much easier to conceal," in *Sec. 3.5.1*; and "caring" is more important in nursing ethics than in medical ethics, in *Sec. 3.5.2*).

And the reverse direction also holds true.

Again, for the last time, it should be stressed, however, that there are different shades of gray (or different degrees of truth) in the two opposites, and the classification is not necessarily mutually exclusive either. In fact, even when some combinations of the two occur, they only end up sharing the same dialectic relationship, but in a different degree.

Also, there are some other relationships (as a kind of family resemblance) which have something in common with the principle, but they are not exactly the same but only more or less comparable, which varies from case to case.

Good examples of family resemblance in relation to the principle are balance-extremity, reflexiveness-unreflexiveness, equality-inequality, harmoniousness-unharrmoniousness, center-periphery, compatibility-incompatibility, proportion-disproportion, balance-unbalance, and something like that.

23rd Thesis: The Softness-Hardness Principle

The twenty-third thesis refers to the softness-hardness principle (on the force of change) in the category of "agency" in existential dialectics (which was first worked out in *ALD*), in that any change by an agent, be it organic (like humans) or non-organic (like natural objects), can occur in a forceful (aggressive) or gentle (pacific) way, which can come in all shapes and sizes, of course. There is no softness without hardness—and vice versa.

For instance, on the one hand, there is softness (e.g., the defense of psychotherapy by the advocates aforecited, in *Sec. 2.2.1*; the defense of SWB by the advocates, in *Sec. 2.2.2*; the defense of the idea of "evolved psychological mechanisms" by those in EP, in *Sec. 2.3.1*; the defense of zoophilia by the advocates, in *Sec. 2.3.2*; the defense of "the spirit level" by Wilkinson and Pickett, in *Sec. 2.4.1*; the defense of the use of new technologies for mental health by the advocates, in *Sec. 2.4.2*; the use of yoga and meditation to fight disease, in *Sec. 2.5.1*; the defense of mindfulness-based therapy by the advocates, in *Sec. 2.5.2*; the defense of physical exercise by the advocates, in *Sec. 3.2.1*; the defense of the prevention of child abuse by the advocates, in *Sec. 3.2.2*; the defense of the idea of astral travel by the advocates, in *Sec. 3.3.1*; the defense of the studies on zoonotic diseases by the advocates aforecited, in *Sec. 3.3.2*; the defense of drug prohibition for social order by the affirmative side, in *Sec. 3.4.1*; the defense of the "prevention and intervention" programs against domestic violence by the advocates, in *Sec. 3.4.2*; the defense of torture by the advocates like Alan M. Dershowitz and Mirko Bagaric, in *Sec. 3.5.1*; and the defense of the focus on "curing" by those in medical ethics, in *Sec. 3.5.2*).

On the other hand, there is hardness (e.g., the critique of psychotherapy by the critics aforecited, in *Sec. 2.2.1*; the critique of SWB by the critics, in *Sec. 2.2.2*; the critique of the idea of "evolved psychological mechanisms" by the critics aforecited, in *Sec. 2.3.1*; the critique of zoophilia by the critics, in *Sec. 2.3.2*; the critique of "the spirit level" by the critics like Goldthorpe and others, in *Sec. 2.4.1*; the critique of the use of new technologies for mental health, as shown in the problems pointed out by the critics as cited, in *Sec. 2.4.2*; the use of painful, invasive surgery to fight disease, in *Sec. 2.5.1*; the critique of mindfulness-based therapy, as shown in the problems pointed out by the critics as cited, in *Sec. 2.5.2*; the critique of physical exercise by the critics as cited, in *Sec. 3.2.1*; the critique of the studies on child abuse by the critics afore-cited, in *Sec. 3.2.2*; the critique of the idea of astral travel, as shown in the problems pointed out by the critics as cited, in *Sec. 3.3.1*; the critique of the studies on zoonotic diseases, as shown in the problems pointed out by the critics as cited, in *Sec. 3.3.2*; the critique of drug prohibition for social order, as shown in the problems pointed out by the negative side as cited, in *Sec. 3.4.1*; the critique of the "prevention and intervention" programs against domestic violence by the critics, as shown in the problems pointed out earlier, in *Sec. 3.4.2*; the critique of torture, as shown in the problems pointed out by the critics as cited, in *Sec. 3.5.1*; and the critique of the focus on "curing" by those in nursing ethics in *Sec. 3.5.2*).

And the reverse direction also holds true.

Again, it should be stressed, however, that there are different shades of gray (or different degrees of truth) in the two opposites, and the classification is not necessarily mutually exclusive either. In fact, even when some combinations of the two occur, they only end up sharing the same dialectic relationship, but in a different degree.

Also, there are some other relationships (as a kind of family resemblance) which have something in common with the principle, but they are not exactly the same but only more or less comparable, which varies from case to case.

Good examples of family resemblance in relation to the principle are peacefulness-violence, cooperation-competition, pacificity-aggression, dovishness-hawkishness, reward-punishment, peace-war, friendliness-unfriendliness, kindness-hostility, love-hatred, acceptance-discrimination, admiration-belittlement, inclusion-exclusion, like-dislike, and the like.

24th Thesis: The Seriousness-Playfulness Principle

The twenty-fourth thesis refers to the seriousness-playfulness principle (on the extent of seriousness) in the category of "agency" in existential dialectics (which is first worked out in *FPHH*), in that, if there is seriousness, there is also playfulness, especially for any agent with some kind of intelligence life, be it about humans, animals, or, later, post-humans. There is no seriousness without playfulness—and vice versa.

Lest any misunderstanding occurs, the word "playfulness" here should not be confused with other terms like "laughter," "smile," "joke," "tickleness," and "laugh-like vocalization" (in some animals), for instance.

Being playful can come in all shapes and sizes and therefore is not necessarily tied up with any of these terms, alhough it can result from any of them, or a combination of them, or something else altogether.

This principle, together with some other principles (especially though not exclusively, like the formalness-informalness principle), have important implications for what constitutes rationality, be it about "rationality of application" at the practical level or "rationality of knowledge" at the meta-theoretical level (as summarized in *Sec. 4.20* of *FPHH*).

For instance, on the one hand, there is seriousness (e.g., the serious business of those in psychotherapy who try to understand how to treat mental problems, in *Sec. 2.2.1*; the serious business of those in SWB who try to understand the causes of SWB. in *Sec. 2.2.2*; the serious business of those in EP who try to understand "evolved psychological mechanisms, in *Sec. 2.3.1*; the serious business of those who try to understand the practice of zoophilia, in *Sec. 2.3.2*; the serious business of those who try to understand income inequality in *Sec. 2.4.1*; the serious business of those who try to understand and treat mental problems, in *Sec. 2.4.2*; the serious business of those who try to understand the role of herbs to treat diseases, in *Sec. 2.5.1*; the serious business of those who try to use mindfulness in Buddhism for mindfulness-based therapy, in *Sec. 2.5.2*; the serious business of those who try to understand the nature of exercise, in *Sec. 3.2.1*; the serious business of those researchers who try to understand the nature of child abuse, in *Sec. 3.2.2*; the serious business of the advocates who try to understand the nature of astral travel, in *Sec. 3.3.1*; the serious business of those researchers who try to understand the nature of zoonotic diseases, in *Sec. 3.3.2*; the serious business of those who try to cope with the problem of drug use, in *Sec. 3.4.1*; the serious business of the researchers who work hard to understand the causes and effects of domestic violence, in *Sec. 3.4.2*; the serious business of those states that have tried to punish some individuals with torture, in *Sec. 3.5.1*; and the serious business of those who try to come up with different principles for medical ethics, in *Sec. 3.5.2*).

On the other hand, there is playfulness (e.g., the playful part of those in in psychotherapy, when they play around with different models of, and approaches to, psychotherpay over the centuries, as shown in the main examples aforedescribed, in *Sec. 2.2.1*; the playful part of those in SWB who try to understand the causes of SWB, when they play around with different theories over the decades, like the "top-down" and "bottom-up" versions, in *Sec. 2.2.2*; the playful part of those in EP who try to understand "evolved psychological mechanisms," when they play around with different explanations, like "adaptations," "exaptations," "byproducts," "random noise," etc., in *Sec. 2.3.1*; the playful part of those in who try to understand the practice of zoophilia, when they play around with different arguments for and against it over the centuries, like "consent," "enjoyment," "trauma," "degradation," "abuse," etc., in *Sec. 2.3.2*; the playful part of those in who try to understand income inequality, when they play around with different views on the causes and effects aforedescribed, in *Sec. 2.4.1*; the playful part of those who try to understand and treat mental problems, when they play around with different methods over the decades, like the use of "medication, counselling, Cognitive Behavioral Therapy, exercise and a healthy diet" as well as "email, SMS, virtual reality, computer programmes, blogs, social networks, the telephone, video conferencing, computer games, instant messaging and podcasts," in *Sec. 2.4.2*; the playful part of those who try to understand the role of herbs to treat diseases, when they play around with different options over the centuries, like "herbs, foods, non-vitamin supplments and megavitmins, and minerals," as well as "seed oil or pills, and ginseng," for example, in *Sec. 2.5.1*; the playful part of those who try to use mindfulness in Buddhism for mindfulness-based therapy, when they play around with different options over the decades, like the the 8 therapy programs afore-described, in *Sec. 2.5.2*; the playful part of those who try to understand the nature of exercise, when they play around with different types and categories aforeindicated over the decades, in *Sec. 3.2.1*; the playful part of those researchers who try to understand the nature of child abuse, when they play around with diffferent ideas in regards to its types, causes, effects, and prevention programs over the decades, in *Sec. 3.2.2*; the playful part of the advocates who try to understand the nature of astral travel, when they play around with different versions and interpretations over the centuries, as shown in different historical sources aforecited, in *Sec. 3.3.1*; the playful part of those researchers who try to understand the nature of zoonotic diseases, when they play around with different lists, examples, and interpretations over the decades aforecited, in *Sec. 3.3.2*; the playful part of those in who try to cope with the problem of drug use, when they play around with different arguments over the centuires, as shown in the debate on 7 contentious issues by both sides afore-discussed, in *Sec. 3.4.1*; the playful part of the researchers who work hard to understand the causes and effects of domestic violence, when they play around with different views and interpretations about the causes and effects over the decades aforediscussed, in *Sec. 3.4.2*; the playful part of those states that have tried to punish some individuals with torture, when they play around with different "methods" over the centuries aforediscussed, in *Sec. 3.5.1*; and the playful part of those who try to come up with different principles for medical ethics, when they play around with different possible principles over the centuries, like "autonomy," "beneficience," "non-maleficience," "justice," "respect for persons," "truthfulness and honesty," "relationship," etc., in *Sec. 3.5.2*).

And the reverse direction also holds true.

Again, it should be stressed, however, that there are different shades of gray (or different degrees of truth) in the two opposites, and the classification is not necessarily mutually exclusive either. In fact, even when some combinations of the two occur, they only end up sharing the same dialectic relationship, but in a different degree.

Also, there are some other relationships (as a kind of family resemblance) which have something in common with the principle, but they are not exactly the same but only more or less comparable, which varies from case to case.

Good examples of family resemblance in relation to the principle are seriousness-jokingness, seriousness-humorousness, seriousness-wittiness, seriousness-nonseriousness, Apollo-Dionysus, seriousness-restingness, seriousness-relaxedness, seriousness-clownishness, and so forth.

25th Thesis: The Activeness-Inactiveness Principle

The twenty-fifth thesis refers to the activeness-inactiveness principle (on the extent of activeness) in the category of "agency" in existential dialectics (which was first worked out in *FPHTRAN*), in that, if there is activeness, there is also inactiveness, especially (though not exclusively) for any agent with some kind of intelligence life, be it about humans, animals, or, later, post-humans. There is no activeness without inactiveness—and vice versa.

Being active can come in all shapes and sizes, just as a person (or an animal) can be inactive because he (or it) is tired, old, injured, sick, sleepy (or hibernating), uninterested, in a state of passive inertia (or disposition), etc.—and an object can be inactive because it is at rest, out of work (or order), etc.

This principle, together with some other principles (especially though not exclusively, like the formalness-informalness principle and seriousness-playfulness principle), have important implications for what constitutes rationality, be it about "rationality of application" at the practical level or "rationality of knowledge" at the meta-theoretical level (as summarized in *Sec. 4.20* of *FPHH*).

For instance, on the one hand, there is activeness (e.g., the relative activeness of those who can function well in life after successfully coping with life problems by way of psychotherapy, in *Sec. 2.2.1*; the relative activeness of those who can successfully cope with life problems because they often "apprais[e] events in an optimistic fashion" and "hav[e] a sense of control," according to the studies on SWB and genetics, in *Sec. 2.2.2*; the relative activeness of those who adapt to the environment and successfully cope with life challenges, in *Sec. 2.3.1*; the relative activeness of those humans who have healthy or safer sex with other humans and do not get sick, in *Sec. 2.3.2*; the relative activeness of those who are rich enough to engage fully in life activities without different health problems due to poverty, in *Sec. 2.4.1*; the relative activeness of those who get cured of acrophobia, so they can now go to high places, in *Sec. 2.4.2*; the relative activeness of those who recover from illness, with the help of alternative medicines, and can now engage in full life activities, in *Sec. 2.5.1*; the relative activeness of those who learn how to bring "a complete attention" with the help of "mindfulness-based therapy," so he can now engage in life activities better, in *Sec. 2.5.2*; the relative activeness of those who do a lot of different exercises, in *Sec. 3.2.1*; the relative activeness of those children who are lucky enough to not suffer from any child abuse and can engage both physically and psychologically in life activities in a healthy way, in *Sec. 3.2.2*; the relative activeness of those in dreams when they encounter "the out-of-body experience" like "flying or ascending" in different "higher realms," in *Sec. 3.3.1*; the relative activeness of those who are not infected with any zoonotic or non-zoonotic diseases and can engage fully in life activities, in *Sec. 3.3.2*; the relative activeness of those who do not suffer from any drug-induced problems and can fully engage in life activities, in *Sec. 3.4.1*; the relative activeness, in relation to their husbands, of those women who are not dependent at all on their spouse, so that they can leave their marriage if they want to and are therefore able to "cope with or change their spouse's behavior," according to the "power and control" model, in *Sec. 3.4.2*; the relative activeness of those ordinary individuals who have never been tortured physically or have not suffered from any other physical problems, so they can engage fully in life activities, in *Sec. 3.5.1*;and the relative activeness of those patients who do not suffer from "a psychiatric condition such as delirium or clinical depression" or any other mental problems, so that they can "make end-of-life decisions" which are reasonable and sound in regard to "their best interests," in *Sec. 3.5.2*).

On the other hand, there is inactiveness (e.g., the relative inactiveness of those who cannot function well in life, because they do not successfully cope with life problems, even after trying psychotherapy and other methods, in *Sec. 2.2.1*; the relative inactiveness of those who cannot successfully cope with life problems because they often show "cynicism" and make "negative attributions about others," so they get stuck with their life problems, according to the studies on SWB and genetics, in *Sec. 2.2.2*; the relative inactiveness of those who fail to adapt to the environment and become tired, sleepy, sick, injured, etc., in *Sec. 2.3.1*; the relative inactiveness of those humans who practice risky sex with animals and get very sick because of being exposed to "the semen, vaginal fluids, urine, saliva, feces and blood of animals," in *Sec. 2.3.2*; the relative inactiveness of those who cannot engage fully in life activities because of different health problems due to poverty, in *Sec. 2.4.1*; the relative inactiveness of those who suffer from acrophobia and never receive any VRT and other methods, so they cannot now go to high places, in *Sec. 2.4.2*; the relative inactiveness of those who do not recover from illness, even with the help of alternative medicines and other sources, so they cannot now engage in full life activities, in *Sec. 2.5.1*; the relative inactiveness of those who suffer from "attention-deficit disorder" and has not received any help from "mindfulness-based therapy" or any other source, so he cannot concentrate well on life activities, in *Sec. 2.5.2*; the relative inactiveness of those who are "exercise-resistant" and cannot engage in much of any exercise at all, in *Sec. 3.2.1*; the relative inactiveness of those children who are not lucky and have sufferred from different forms of child abuse, so that they cannot engage both physically and psychologically in life activities in a healthy way, because of the negative health effects aforecited, in *Sec. 3.2.2*; the relative inactiveness of those in dreams when they do not encounter "the out-of-body experience" like "flying or ascending" in different "higher realms" nor have any other dream related to intense activities, in *Sec. 3.3.1*; the relative inactiveness of those who are not lucky to have infected with zoonotic and/or non-zoonotic diseases, so they cannot engage fully in life activities, in *Sec. 3.3.2*; the relative inactiveness of those who suffer from drug-induced problems to the point of death, so they cannot engage fully in life activities, in *Sec. 3.4.1*; the relative inactiveness, in relation to their husbands, of those women who "are most dependent on the spouse for economic well being" and "fear the increased financial burden if they leave their marriage," so that "they have fewer options and few resources to help them cope with or change their spouse's behavior," according to the "power and control" model, in *Sec. 3.4.2*; the relative inactiveness of those torture victims who have been seriously tortured, especially though not exclusively on their feet, so that they can no longer engage fully in life activities, in *Sec. 3.5.1*; and the relative inactiveness of those patients who severely suffer from "a psychiatric condition such as delirium or clinical depression," so that they cannot "make end-of-life decisions" which are reasonable and sound in regard to "their best interests" in *Sec. 3.5.2*).

And the reverse direction also holds true.

Again, it should be stressed, however, that there are different shades of gray (or different degrees of truth) in the two opposites, and the classification is not necessarily mutually exclusive either. In fact, even when some combinations of the two occur, they only end up sharing the same dialectic relationship, but in a different degree.

Also, there are some other relationships (as a kind of family resemblance) which have something in common with the principle, but they are not exactly the same but only more or less comparable, which varies from case to case.

Good examples of family resemblance in relation to the principle are alertness-unalertness, activeness-decrepidness, alertness-sleepiness, activeness-tiredness, alertness-unwareness, alertness-uninterestedness, soberness-inactiveness, alertness-inactiveness, soberness-unawareness, awakenness-hibernatedness, and so on.

26th Thesis: The Selfness-Otherness Principle

The twenty-sixth thesis refers to the selfness-otherness principle (on the magnitude of self-centeredness) in the category of "agency" in existential dialectics (which is first worked out in *FPHCA*), in that, if there is the tendency to be mostly centered on one's self or group, there is likewise the tendency to be mostly centered on others, especially (though not exclusively) for any agent with some kind of intelligence life, be it about humans, animals, or, later, post-humans. There is no selfness without otherness—and vice versa.

Being self-centered and being other-centered do not have to be mutually exclusive, as the two can come in all shapes and sizes, or in different degrees. And other-centeredness does not entail desirability, any more than self-centeredness implies non-desirability, as both can go either way.

In addition, whether self-centeredness constitutes a moral alternative or, conversely, an alternative to morality is of course debatable (as addressed in my other book titled *Beyond Ethics to Post-Ethics*).

For instance, on the one hand, there is selfness (e.g., the tendency to be mostly centered on one's self or group, as shown in those advocates of the effectiveness of psychotherapy, even when the "critics of psychotherapy are skeptical of the healing power of a psychotherapeutic relationship," in *Sec. 2.2.1*; the tendency to be mostly centered on one's self or group, as shown in the studies which showed some "people" who "believe that money does more for happiness than it really does," so they become obsessed with money for themselves, in *Sec. 2.2.2*; the tendency to be mostly centered on one's self or group, as shown in the study in EP which showed that "mothers sometimes struggle with their children over weaning, which benefits the mother more than the child," in *Sec. 2.3.1*; the tendency to be mostly centered on one's self or group, as shown in those zoophiles who practice zoosadism against animals, in *Sec. 2.3.2*; the tendency to be mostly centered on one's self or group, as shown in those who are rich and want to preserve income inequality vis-a-vis the poor in society, in *Sec. 2.4.1*; the tendency to be mostly centered on one's self or group, as shown in DOD, which funded the project to use VRT "for the treatment of Posttraumatic Stress Disorder" suffered by American soldiers, in *Sec. 2.4.2*; the tendency to be mostly centered on one's self or group, as shown in those practitioners who have misled about "alternative medicine," to "the piont where it has become dangerous and unethical," as pointed out by Ernst [2011]," in *Sec. 2.5.1*; the tendency to be mostly centered on one's self or group, as shown in those captialists who have no problem in pursuing "greed" and other materialistic desires for themselves, in *Sec. 2.5.2*; the tendency to be mostly centered on one's self or group, as shown in those who are obsessed with physical exercise to improve health, such that they engage in "too much exercise," which "can be harmful," because "without proper rest, the chance of stroke or other circulation problems increases," for example, in *Sec. 3.2.1*; the tendency to be mostly centered on one's self or group, as shown in the abusive act of an abuser to abuse a child for his own pleasure, in *Sec. 3.2.2*; the tendency to be mostly centered on one's self or group, as shown in the exaggered claim by Ingo Swann about his alleged ability to astral travel travel on the basis of his account of "Jupiter and observe details of the planet," which were rejected by scientists as not accurate, in *Sec. 3.3.1*; the tendency to be mostly centered on one's self or group, as shown in those infectious agents like "parasites", who survive at the expense of the hosts, in *Sec. 3.3.2*; the tendency to be mostly centered on one's self or group, as shown in those illicit drug users, who in the process negatively affect others close or related to them like "children, parents, grandparents, friends, colleagues, work, victims of drugged drivers, crime victims, elder abuse, sexual victims etc.," so that "illicit drug use is no less victimless than alcoholism," in *Sec. 3.4.1*; the tendency to be mostly centered on one's self or group, as shown in "an abuser," who "use[s] various tactics of abuse [e.g., physical, verbal, emotional, sexual or financial] in order to establish and maintain control over the partner," according to the "power and control" model, in *Sec. 3.4.2*; the tendency to be mostly centered on one's self or group, as shown in those states that practice torture against some individuals for "ideological warfare, political mobilization, and the need to win 'hearts and minds,'" in *Sec. 3.5.1*; and the tendency to be mostly centered on one's self or group, as shown in the principle of "autonomy" stressed by a patient, in that "the patient has the right to refuse or choose their treatment," in *Sec. 3.5.2*).

On the other hand, there is otherness (e.g., the tendency to be mostly centered on others, as shown in "the American Psychological Association ethics code," in which "confidentiality is an integral part of the therapeutic relationship and psychotherapy in general," as "it includes protecting specific groups of people, like children, while treating private information" in a confidential way, in *Sec. 2.2.1*; the tendency to be mostly centered on others, as shown in the studies which showed some "people" who "believe that "spending money on others promotes happiness," so they become more others-oriented, in *Sec. 2.2.2*; the tendency to be mostly centered on others, as shown in the study on "inclusive fitness," when "a self-sacrificing behavior can evolve if it helps close relatives so much that it more than compensates for the individual animal's sacrifice," in *Sec. 2.3.1*; the tendency to be mostly centered on others, as shown in those defenders of animal rights against zoosadism, in *Sec. 2.3.2*; the tendency to be mostly centered on others, as shown in those who prefer to reduce income inequality between the rich and the poor, like Islington's Fairness Commission, in *Sec. 2.4.1*; the tendency to be mostly centered on others, as shown in the work at Auckland University to "develop...a computerised CBT fantasy 'serious' game to help tackle depression amongst adolescences," as an advance in the field of medicine. in *Sec. 2.4.2*; the tendency to be mostly centered on others, as shown in the call by "a group of prominent scientists," who "argued before the federal government that plausibility of interventions such as diet, relaxation, yoga and botanical remedies, should not be used to support research on implausible interventions based on superstition" and other questionable practices, for the advancement of medical knowledge, in *Sec. 2.5.1*; the tendency to be mostly centered on others, as shown in those who pursue a more spiritual lifestyle with the help of "mindfulness-based therapy" for "a clear mental focus" with "wisdom," away from "greed, hatred, and delusion," in *Sec. 2.5.2*; the tendency to be mostly centered on others, as shown in those researchers who warn others from engaging in "excessive exercise" which has its own downside, as an advancement in the knowledge of physical health, in *Sec. 3.2.1*; the tendency to be mostly centered on others, as shown in the work by The National Alliance of Children's Trust Funds and Prevent Child Abuse America to protect children from abuse, in *Sec. 3.2.2*; the tendency to be mostly centered on others, as shown in the skepticism by scientists like Bob Bruce of the Queensland Skeptics Association, when he showed that "the existence of an astral plane is contrary to the limits of science," as an advancement in the knowledge of different possible worlds, in *Sec. 3.3.1*; the tendency to be mostly centered on others, as shown in those working in conservation medicine to counter the threat of zoonotic diseases, for the advancement in human health, in *Sec. 3.3.2*; the tendency to be mostly centered on others, as shown in the argument by Aldous Huxley, and Terence McKenna, who argued that "persons should be able to do whatever they want with their bodies, including the recreational use of drugs, as long as they do not harm others," as an advancement in civil rights for all, in *Sec. 3.4.1*; the tendency to be mostly centered on others, as shown in recemt "criminal and civil justice systems" which "have created policies to hold offenders accountable and keep the victims safe," as an advancement in the prevention of domestic violence, in *Sec. 3.4.2*; the tendency to be mostly centered on others, as shown in those advocates of the UN Universal

Declaration of Human Rights" to care about torture victims, in *Sec. 3.5.1*; and the tendency to be mostly centered on others, as shown in the principle of "relationship" to be followed by a nurse, in that nurses "focus on care and nurture" vis-à-vis their patients, in *Sec. 3.5.2*).

And the reverse direction also holds true.

Again, it should be stressed, however, that there are different shades of gray (or different degrees of truth) in the two opposites, and the classification is not necessarily mutually exclusive either. In fact, even when some combinations of the two occur, they only end up sharing the same dialectic relationship, but in a different degree.

Also, there are some other relationships (as a kind of family resemblance) which have something in common with the principle, but they are not exactly the same but only more or less comparable, which varies from case to case.

Good examples of family resemblance in relation to the principle are egoisticness-altruisticness, selfishness-unselfishness, selfness-selflessness, egocentricness-othercentricness, and so on.

In Relation to Outcome

The next six theses are in relation to outcome in existential dialectics, as shown below.

27th Thesis: The Regression-Progression Principle

The twenty-seventh thesis is called the regression-progression princple (on the direction of history) in the category of "outcome" in existential dialectics (which was also already worked out in my previous books), in that neither the cyclical nor the linear views are adequate for explaining many phenomena at all levels. There is no regression without progression—and vice versa.

History progresses to more advanced forms, but with a regressive touch. Examples include no freedom without unfreedom, no equality without inequality, and no civilization without barbarity. This is not an inevitable law, but merely a highly likely empirical trend.

For instance, on the one hand, there is regression (e.g., the regression made by psychotherapy, as shown in the problems pointed out by the critics, in *Sec. 2.2.1*; the regression made by the study on SWB, as shown in the problems pointed out by the critics, in *Sec. 2.2.2*; the regression made by evolutionary psychology, as shown in the problems pointed out by the critics, in *Sec. 2.3.1*; the regression made by zoophilia, as shown in the problems pointed out by the critics, in *Sec. 2.3.2*; the regression made by the work on "the spirit level," as shown in the problems pointed out by the critics, in *Sec. 2.4.1*; the regression made by the use of new technologies for mental health, as shown in the problems pointed out by the critics, in *Sec. 2.4.2*; the regression made by alternative medicines, as shown in the problems pointed out by the critics, in *Sec. 2.5.1*; the regression made by "mindfulness-based therapy," as shown in the problems pointed out by the critics, in *Sec. 2.5.2*; the regression made by physical exercise, as shown in the problems pointed out by the critics, in *Sec. 3.2.1*; the regression made by the studies on child abuse, as shown in the problems pointed out by the critics, in *Sec. 3.2.2*; the regression made by the claims on astral travel, as shown in the problems pointed out by the critics, in *Sec. 3.3.1*; the regression made by the studies on zoonotic diseases, as shown in the problems pointed out by the critics, in *Sec. 3.3.2*; the regression made by drug prohibition, as shown in the problems pointed out by the negative side, in *Sec. 3.4.1*; the regression made by the works on domestic violence, as shown in the problems pointed out by the critics, in *Sec. 3.4.2*; the regression made by the campagin against torture, as shown in the problems pointed out by the critics, in *Sec. 3.5.1*; and the regression made by the principles in medical ethics, as shown in the problems pointed out by the critics aforecited, in *Sec. 3.5.2*).

On the other hand, there is progress (e.g., the progress made by psychotherapy, as shown in the contribution to the treatment of mental problems aforecited, in *Sec. 2.2.1*; the progress made by the study on SWB, as shown in the contribution to the understanding of the association between genetics and SWB aforecited, in *Sec. 2.2.2*; the progress made by evolutionary psychology, as shown in the contribution to the understanding of "evolved psychological mechanisms" aforecited, in *Sec. 3.2.1*; the progress made by zoophilia, as shown in the contribution to the understanding of the history of sexual relationships between humans and animals aforecited), in *Sec. 3.3.2*; the progress made by the work on "the spirit level," as shown in the contribution to the debate on the effects of income inequality on health and other problems aforecited, in *Sec. 2.4.1*; the progress made by the use of new technologies for mental health, as shown in the contribution to the treatment of acrophobia and other mental problems aforecited in *Sec. 2.4.2*; the progress made by alternative medicines, as shown in the contribution to the use of "diet, relaxation, yoga and botanical remedies" to treat health problems aforecited, in *Sec. 2.5.1*; the progress made by "mindfulness-based therapy," as shown in the contribution to the therapy for "attention" and "openness" afore-described, in *Sec. 2.5.2*; the progress made by physical exercise, as shown in the contribution to health aforecited, in *Sec. 3.2.1*; the progress made by the studies on child abuse, as shown in the contribution to the understanding of its types, causes, and effects aforecited, in *Sec. 3.2.2*; the progress made by the claims on astral travel, as shown in the contribution to the imagination of traveling to "higher realms" aforecited, in *Sec. 3.3.1*; the progress made by the studies on zoonotic diseases, as shown in the contribution to the understanding of the carriers and agents of zoonotic diseases aforecited, in *Sec. 3.3.2*; the progress made by drug prohibition, as shown in the positive effects pointed out by the affirmative side, in *Sec. 3.4.1*; the progress made by the works on domestic violence, as shown in the contribution to its prevention aforecited, in *Sec. 3.4.2*; the progress made by the campagin against torture, as shown in the contribution to the prohbition of torture, at least nominally, "under international law and the domestic laws of most countries," in *Sec. 3.5.1*; and the progress made by the principles in medical ethics, as shown in the contribution to "a useful framework for understanding conflicts" aforecited in *Sec. 3.5.2*).

And the reverse direction also holds true.

Again, it should be stressed, however, that there are different shades of gray (or different degrees of truth) in the two opposites, and the classification is not necessarily mutually exclusive either. In fact, even when some combinations of the two occur, they only end up sharing the same dialectic relationship, but in a different degree.

Also, there are some other relationships (as a kind of family resemblance) which have something in common with the principle, but they are not exactly the same but only more or less comparable, which varies from case to case.

Good examples of family resemblance in relation to the principle are undesirability-desirability, risk-opportunity, badness-goodness, cost-benefit, dysfunctionality-functionality, cyclicity-linearity, and so on.

28th Thesis: The Same-Difference Principle

The twenty-eighth thesis refers to the same-difference principle (on the metamorphosis of change) in the category of "outcome" in existential dialectics (which was worked out in *ALD* and other books of mine), in that an entity, as it evolves over time, can be both different from and similar to its opposing alternatives and does not have to be solely more different from them over time. There is no similarity without difference—and vice versa.

Opposites are not absolute in a black-or-white fashion; so, an entity can become relatively more similar to (or more different from) its opposite over time.

This is further constrained by another principle, that is, the symmetry-asymmetry principle about the relationships among existents under the category about agency in existential dialectics, in that if there is symmetry (equality) between two entities, there is likewise asymmetry (inequality) emerging in a different way.

For instance, on the one hand, there is similarity in outcome (e.g., the contribution to the molding and control of beliefs, values, and behaviors, regardless of whether this be done by way of positive psychotherpay, or by way of feminist therapy, in *Sec. 2.2.1*; the contribution to the molding and control of beliefs, values, and behaviors, regardless of whether this be done by way of the study on the five factor model and genetics, or by way of the Framingham Heart Study on social influences, in *Sec. 2.2.2*; the contribution to the molding and control of beliefs, values, and behaviors, regardless of whether this be done by way of evolutionary psychology, or by way of social constructionism, in *Sec. 2.3.1*; the contribution to the molding and control of beliefs, values, and behaviors, regardless of whether this be done by way of the medieval sanction against zoophilia in Europe, or by way of the contemporary sanction against zoophilia by the Humane Society of the United States on the ground of the lack of "the same capacity for thinking as humans," in *Sec. 2.3.2*; the contribution to the molding and control of beliefs, values, and behaviors, regardless of whether this be done by way of laissez-faire capitalism, or by way of the "spirit level," in *Sec. 2.4.1*; the contribution to the molding and control of beliefs, values, and behaviors, regardless of whether this be done by way of medication, counselling, exercise and a healthy diet to treat mental health problems, or by way of virtual reality therapy, in *Sec. 2.4.2*; the contribution to the molding and control of beliefs, values, and behaviors, regardless of whether this be done by way of "evidence-based medicine," or by way of "alternative medicine," in *Sec. 2.5.1*; the contribution to the molding and control of beliefs, values, and behaviors, regardless of whether this be done by way of the Mindfulness-Based Stress Reduction program, or by way of the Noble Eightfold Path taught by the Buddha, in *Sec. 2.5.2*; the contribution to the molding and control of beliefs, values, and behaviors, regardless of whether this be done by way of bus driving, or by way of bus conducting, in *Sec. 3.2.1*; the contribution to the molding and control of beliefs, values, and behaviors, regardless of whether this be done by way of child abuse, or by way of child protection. in *Sec. 3.2.2*; the contribution to the molding and control of beliefs, values, and behaviors, regardless of whether this be done by way of the defense of "astral travel," or by way of the critique of "astral travel," in *Sec. 3.3.1*; the contribution to the molding and control of beliefs, values, and behaviors, regardless of whether this be done by way of zoonosis, or by way of reverse-zoonosis, in *Sec. 3.3.2*; the contribution to the molding and control of beliefs, values, and behaviors, regardless of whether this be done by way of appealing to the argument on cost, or by way of appealing to the argument on social order, in *Sec. 3.4.1*; the contribution to the molding and control of beliefs, values, and behaviors, regardless of whether this be done by way of feminism, or by way of patriarchalism, in regard to domestic violence, in *Sec. 3.4.2*; the contribution to the molding and control of beliefs, values, and behaviors, regardless of whether this be done by way of the Catechism of the Catholic Church, or by way of utilitarianism, in the campaign against torture, in *Sec. 3.5.1*; and the contribution to the molding and control of beliefs, values, and behaviors, regardless of whether this be done by way of medical ethics, or by way of nursing ethics, in *Sec. 3.5.2*).

On the other hand, there is difference in outcome (e.g., the contribution to the molding and control of beliefs, values, and behaviors by way of positive psychotherpay for a relatively more scientific worldview—but the contribution to the molding and control of beliefs, values, and behaviors by way of.feminist therapy for a relatively more social-constructionist worldview in *Sec. 2.2.1*; the contribution to the molding and control of beliefs, values, and behaviors by way of the study on the five factor model and genetics for a relatively more biological worldview—but the contribution to the molding and control of beliefs, values, and behaviors by way of the Framingham Heart Study for a relatively more social worldview, in *Sec. 2.2.2*; the contribution to the molding and control of beliefs, values, and behaviors by way of evolutionary psychology for a relatively more genetic-reductionistic worldview—but the contribution to the molding and control of beliefs, values, and behaviors by way of social constructionism for a relatively more social-reductionistic worldview, in *Sec. 2.3.1*; the contribution to the molding and control of beliefs, values, and behaviors by way of the medieval sanction against zoophilia in Europe for a relatively more religious lifeworld—but the contribution to the molding and control of beliefs, values, and behaviors by way of the medieval sanction against zoophilia in Europe, or by way of the contemporary sanction against zoophilia by the Humane Society of the United States for a relatively more secular lifeworld, in *Sec. 2.3.2*; the contribution to the molding and control of beliefs, values, and behaviors by way of laissez-faire capitalism for a relatively more right-wing worldview—but the contribution to the molding and control of beliefs, values, and behaviors by way of the "spirit level" for a relatively more left-wing worldview, in *Sec. 2.4.1*; the contribution to the molding and control of beliefs, values, and behaviors by way of medication, counselling, exercise and a healthy diet to treat mental health problems for a relatively more traditional lifeworld—but the contribution to the molding and control of beliefs, values, and behaviors by way of virtual reality therapy for a relatively more imaginative lifeworld, in *Sec. 2.4.2*; the contribution to the molding and control of beliefs, values, and behaviors by way of "evidence-based medicine" for a relatively more scientific lifeworld—but the contribution to the molding and control of beliefs, values, and behaviors by way of "alternative medicine" for a relatively more traditional lifeworld, in *Sec. 2.5.1*; the contribution to the molding and control of beliefs, values, and behaviors by way of the Mindfulness-Based Stress Reduction program for a relatively more secular-therapeutic lifeworld—but the contribution to the molding and control of beliefs, values, and behaviors by way of the Noble Eightfold Path taught by the Buddha for a relatively more spiritual lifeworld, in *Sec. 3.5.2*; the contribution to the molding and control of beliefs, values, and behaviors by way of bus driving for a relatively more sedentary work life—but the contribution to the molding and control of beliefs, values, and behaviors by way of bus conducting for a relatively more active work life, in *Sec. 3.2.1*; the contribution to the molding and control of beliefs, values, and behaviors by way of child abuse for a relatively more amoral lifeworld—but the contribution to the molding and control of beliefs, values, and behaviors by way of child protection for a relatively more moral lifeworld, in *Sec. 3.2.2*; the contribution to the molding and control of beliefs, values, and behaviors by way of the defense of "astral travel" for a relatively more mystical or religious worldview—but the contribution to the molding and control of beliefs, values, and behaviors by way of the critique of "astral travel" for a relatively more scientific worldview, in *Sec. 3.3.1*; the contribution to the molding and control of beliefs, values, and behaviors by way of zoonosis for a relatively more animal-centric lifeworld—but the contribution to the molding and control of beliefs, values, and behaviors by way of reverse-zoonosis for a relatively more human-centric lifeworld, in *Sec. 3.3.2*; the contribution to the molding and control of beliefs, values, and behaviors by way of appealing to the argument on cost for a relatively more economic worldview—but the contribution to the molding and control of beliefs, values, and behaviors by way of appealing to the argument on social order for a relatively more political worldview, in *Sec. 3.4.1*; the contribution to the molding and control of beliefs, values, and behaviors by way of feminism, in regard to domestic violence, for a relatively more egalitarian lifeworld—but the contribution to the molding and control of beliefs, values, and behaviors by way of patriarchalism, in regard to domestic violence, for a relatively more inegalitarian lifeworld, in *Sec. 3.4.2*; the contribution to the molding and control of beliefs, values, and behaviors by way of the Catechism of the Catholic Church, in the campaign against torture, for a relatively more religious lifeworld—but the contribution to the molding and control of beliefs, values, and behaviors by way of utilitarianism, in the campaign against torture, for a relatively more secular lifeworld, in *Sec. 3.5.1*; and the contribution to the molding and control of beliefs, values, and behaviors by way of medical ethics for a relatively more deontological lifeworld in the context of "deontological ethics"—but the contribution to the molding and control of beliefs, values, and behaviors by way of nursing ethics for a relatively more virtue-ethical lifeworld in the context of "virtue ethics," in *Sec. 3.5.2*).

And the reverse direction also holds true.

Again, it should be stressed, however, that there are different shades of gray (or different degrees of truth) in the two opposites, and the classification is not necessarily mutually exclusive either. In fact, even when some combinations of the two occur, they only end up sharing the same dialectic relationship, but in a different degree.

Also, there are some other relationships (as a kind of family resemblance) which have something in common with the principle, but they are not exactly the same but only more or less comparable, which varies from case to case.

Good examples of family resemblance in relation to the principle are homogeneity-heterogeneity, we-they, similarity-contrast, and so forth.

29th Thesis: The Stability-Reaction Principle

The twenty-ninth thesis is called the stability-reaction princple (on the feedback mechanism for further changes) in the category of "outcome" in existential dialectics (which was first worked out in *FPHCHEM*), in that once an outcome becomes stabilized over time (which varies from case to case), it will undergo further changes in its multifaceted interactions with the outside world (e.g., with other entities, energy, space, and so on).

There is no stability without reaction for further changes—and vice versa.

Works on chemical reactions (as in *FPHCHEM*) and feedback mechanisms for learning in adaptive management (as in *BNR*), just to name a few of them, have contributed to the understanding of stability and reaction.

For instance, on the one hand, there is stability in outcome (e.g., the relatively more stable condition of the idealized view on the therapist-client relationship in the older days when "we think of therapy only as a helping relation" by a therapist for a client, in *Sec. 2.2.1*; the relatively more stable condition of the popular research on the relationship between genetics and SWB, in *Sec. 2.2.2*; the relatively more stable condition of EP in regard to its idea of "evolved psychological mechanisms," in *Sec. 2.3.1*; the relatively more stable condition of zoophilia in antiquity, when "bestiality was widespread," in *Sec. 2.3.2*; the relatively more stable condition of laissez-faire capitalism in the older days, in *Sec. 2.4.1*; the relatively more stable condition of traditional methods in the older days, when "medication, counselling, Cognitive Behavioral Therapy, exercise and a healthy diet" were used to treat mental problems, in *Sec. 2.4.2*; the relatively more stable condition of alternative medicines in the older days, in *Sec. 2.5.1*; the relatively more stable condition of the Buddhist tradition as shown in the Noble Eightfold Path taught by the Buddha in the older days, in *Sec. 2.5.2*; the relatively more stable condition of the belief about the link between physical health and exercise in the older days, in *Sec. 3.2.1*; the relatively more stable condition of "the Soviet period," when there was "the emphasis on equality within the sexes" in regard to child care, in *Sec. 3.2.2*; the relatively more stable condition of some "twentieth century publications on astral projection," which are "widely cited," like the works by Robert Monroe, Oliver Fox, Sylvan Muldoon and Hereward Carrington," for example, in *Sec. 3.3.1*; the relatively more stable condition of "zoonotic pathogens causing foodborne diseases" like "*Escherichia coli* O157:H7, *Campylobacter*, *Caliciviridae*, and *Salmonella*," in *Sec. 3.3.2*; the relatively more stable condition of using "natural plant drugs like opium, coca, cannabis, mescaline, and psilocybin" for medical uses in antiquity, in *Sec. 3.4.1*; the relatively more stable condition of the pre-1800 era, when "most legal systems accepted wife beating as a valid exercise of a husband's authority over his wife," in *Sec. 3.4.2*; the relatively more stable condition of using physical torture in antiquity, in *Sec. 3.5.1*; and the relatively more stable condition of the "guidelines on the duty of physicians in antiquity, such as the Hippocratic Oath, and early rabbinic and Christian teachings" in the Western tradition in *Sec. 3.5.2*).

On the other hand, there is reaction in outcome (e.g., the idealized view on the therapist-client relationship in the older days then led to further changes later on, when nowadays, according to "feminist, constructionist and discursive sources,...the therapist-client relationship always participates in society's power relations and political dynamics," in *Sec. 2.2.1*; the popular research on the relationship between genetics and SWB then led to further changes later on, when nowadays there are new criticisms that it ignores the "objective" conditions of well-being, that the findings are not consistent across studies and across histories, that much remains uncertain about the nature of SWB, that SWB can be detrimental to health, that it neglects social factors, and that it does not give sufficient attention to cultural variations, in *Sec. 2.2.2*; the established idea of "evolved psychological mechanisms" in EP then led to further changes later on, when nowadays, it receives different criticisms, including the view that it commits "the naturalistic fallacy," in *Sec. 2.3.1*; the stable condition of zoophilia in antiquity then led to further changes later on, when nowadays, "sex with animals...is not explicitly condoned anywhere," in *Sec. 2.3.2*; laissez-faire capitalism in the older days then led to further changes later on, when nowadays, there is the socialist tract of "the spirit level" to argue for lesser income inequality, in *Sec. 2.4.1*; traditional methods in the older days then led to further changes later on, when nowadays new technologies are used instead, like "email, SMS, virtual reality, computer programmes, blogs, social networks, the telephone, video conferencing, computer games, instant messaging and podcasts," in *Sec. 2.4.2*; alternative medicines in the older days then led to further changes later on, when nowadays, they are challenged by "evidence-based medicine," in *Sec. 2.5.1*; the Buddhist tradition in the older day then led to further changes later on, when nowadays, it is revised for "mindfulness-based therapy" instead, in *Sec. 2.5.2*; the belief about the link between physical health and exercise in the older days then led to further changes later on, when nowadays "a number of studies of both rodents and humans have demonstrated that individual differences in both ability and propensity for exercise [i.e., voluntary exercise] have some genetic basis," and vigorous exercise can have its downside, in *Sec. 3.2.1*; "the Soviet period" then led to further changes later on, when, nowadays in the post-Soviet period, "controlling parenting may be less of a concern," but "financial difficulty, unemployment, and substance abuse" are the "dominating factors in child abuse throughout Eastern Europe," in *Sec. 3.2.2*; some "twentieth century publications on astral projection" then led to further changes later on, when, nowadays, the critics are quick to point out that the experience is subjective, that there are competing interpretations of astral travel, that the claims are "contrary to the limits of science," and that the claims are not accurate, in *Sec. 3.3.1*; "zoonotic pathogens causing foodborne diseases" then led to further changes later on, when “in 2006, a conference held in Berlin was focusing on the issue of zoonotic pathogen effects on food safety, urging governments to intervene, and the public to be vigilant towards the risks of catching food-borne diseases from farm-to-dining table,” in *Sec. 3.3.2*; using “natural plant drugs like opium, coca, cannabis, mescaline, and psilocybin” for medical uses in antiquity then led to further changes later on, when nowadays in the U.S., there are regulations concerning drug use, in *Sec. 3.4.1*; the pre-1800 era, when “most legal systems accepted wife beating as a valid exercise of a husband's authority over his wife,” then led to further changes later on, when “modern attention to domestic violence began in the women's movement of the 1970s, particularly within the contexts of feminism and women's rights, as concern about wives being beaten by their husbands gained attention” in the Western world, in *Sec. 3.4.2*; using physical torture in antiquity then led to further changes later on, when nowadays, according to Darius Rejali, “modern democracies, 'the United States, Britain, and France,...pioneered and exported techniques that have become the lingua franca of modern torture: methods that leave no marks,” like psychological torture and other methods, in *Sec. 3.5.1*; and the “guidelines on the duty of physicians in antiquity, such as the Hippocratic Oath, and early rabbinic and Christian teachings” in the Western tradition then led to further changes later on, when nowadays, there are the “four principles” in medical ethics by Tom Beauchamp and James Childress, as well as alternative values, in *Sec. 3.5.2*).

And the reverse direction also holds true.

Again, it should be stressed, however, that there are different shades of gray (or different degrees of truth) in the two opposites, and the classification is not necessarily mutually exclusive either. In fact, even when some combinations of the two occur, they only end up sharing the same dialectic relationship, but in a different degree.

Also, there are some other relationships (as a kind of family resemblance) which have something in common with the principle, but they are not exactly the same but only more or less comparable, which varies from case to case.

Good examples of family resemblance in relation to the principle are stability-forwardness, normalcy-feedback, balance-forwardness, balance-reaction, consolidation-modification, normalcy-feedback, stability-breakup, rest-motion, and the like.

30th Thesis: The Functionality-Nonfunctionality Principle

The thirtieth thesis is called the functionality-nonfunctionality princple (on the presence of function) in the category of "outcome" in existential dialectics (which is first worked out in *FPHCA*), in that, if there is the presence of action for which something or someone is fitted, there is likewise the relative lack of action for which something or someone is fitted. There is no functionality without nonfunctionallity—and vice versa.

A *function* should not be confused with an *alternative function,* which is just another kind of function, just as *nonfunction* should not be confused with *dysfunction* (which has more to do with malfunction and is thus related more to the regression-progression principle).

In addition, being functional (or useful) and being nonfunctional (or useless) do not have to be mutually exclusive, as the two can come in all shapes and sizes, or in different degrees. And what is functional at one time may become nonfunctional at another time, and vice-versa.

For instance, on the one hand, there is functionality in outcome (e.g., the presence of action for which something or someone is fitted, as shown in the research by Bruce Wampold who showed that psychotherapy could be effective, which served the function of treating mental prolems in patients, in *Sec. 2.2.1*; the presence of action for which something or someone is fitted, as shown in the popular research on the relationship between genetics and SWB, which serves the function of providing a biological interpretation of human well-being, in *Sec. 2.2.1*; the presence of action for which something or someone is fitted, as shown in some traits which are "adaptive," as shown by the example of "toddlers' ability to learn to talk with minimal instruction." according to those in EP, in *Sec. 3.2.1*; the presence of action for which something or someone is fitted, as shown in the widespread practice of bestiality in antiquity, which served the function of incorporating it "into religious ritual" at that time, in *Sec. 2.3.2*; the presence of action for which something or someone is fitted, as shown in social darwinism in the older days, when it served the function of supporting the ideology of laissez-faire capitalism and other things, in *Sec. 2.4.1*; the presence of action for which something or someone is fitted, as shown in the use of"medication, counselling, Cognitive Behavioral Therapy, exercise and a healthy diet" to treat mental problems in the older days, which served the function of supporting traditional methods for a relatively less advanced technological society, in *Sec. 2.4.2*; the presence of action for which something or someone is fitted, as shown in the widespread use of alternative medicines in the older days, which served the function of maintaining the world of "religion, tradition, and superstition" at that time, in *Sec. 2.5.1*; the presence of action for which something or someone is fitted, as shown in the Noble Eightfold Path taught by the Buddha in the older days, which served the function of advocating the spiritual life away from "greed, hatred, and delusion" at that time, in *Sec. 2.5.2*; the presence of action for which something or someone is fitted, as shown in the link between physical health and exercise, which serves the function of "increasing the blood and oxygen flow to the brain," "increasing growth factors that help create new nerve cells," etc., in *Sec. 3.2.1*; the presence of action for which something or someone is fitted, as shown in "the emphasis on equality within the sexes" during the Soviet period, which served the ideological function of championing Communist ideals at that time, in *Sec. 3.2.2*; the presence of action for which something or someone is fitted, as shown in the widespread belief in astral travel in the older days, like the different historical sources aforedescribed, which served the function of maintaining the old-fashioned worldview of "witchcraft and shamanism" as well as "classical philosophy and...various myths and religious scriptures" at that time, in *Sec. 3.3.1*; the presence of action for which something or someone is fitted, as shown in the infection, by HIV, of "vital cells in the human immune system such as helper T cells [specifically CD4+ T cells], macrophages, and dendritic cells," which serves the function of spreading zoonotic diseases, in *Sec. 3.3.2*; the presence of action for which something or someone is fitted, as shown in the use of "natural plant drugs like opium, coca, cannabis, mescaline, and psilocybin" in antiquity, which served the function of medical and other uses at that time, in *Sec. 3.4.1*; the presence of action for which something or someone is fitted, as shown in domestic violence by men against women due to jealousy, which, according to "an evolutionary psychology explanation," serves the "male attempts to control female reproduction and ensure sexual exclusivity through violence or the threat of violence," in *Sec. 3.4.2*; the presence of action for which something or someone is fitted, as shown in the use of "medical torture" by Josef Mengele and Shirō Ishii during...World War II," which served the function of Nazi and Imperial Japan militarism at the time against the subjugated, in *Sec. 3.5.1*; and the presence of action for which something or someone is fitted, as shown in the "four principles" in medical ethics by Tom Beauchamp and James Childress, which serve the function of promoting the tradition of "cure of illness" in medical practice, in *Sec. 3.5.2*).

On the other hand, there is nonfunctionality in outcome (e.g., the relative lack of action for which something or someone is fitted, as shown in the studies in which, according to "feminist, constructionist and discursive sources,...clients are persuaded—both inside and outside the consulting room—to understand themselves and their difficulties in ways that are consistent with therapeutic ideas," so "alternative ideas...are...implicitly undermined," such that psychotherapy is no longer perceived as functional in treating mental problems nowadays among postmodern therapists, even though it used to be falsely assumed by the advocates in the older days in *Sec. 2.2.1*; the relative lack of action for which something or someone is fitted, as shown in the criticisms by the critics that the argument on genetics and SWB does not give sufficient attention to social factors and cultural variations, such that the argument is no longer functional nowadays among the critics, who ask for a more balanced approach to take into account of social and cultural factors, in *Sec. 2.2.2*; the relative lack of action for which something or someone is fitted, as shown in some traits which are "non- adaptive," as shown by the example of "within-sex variations in voice pitch," according to those in EP, in *Sec. 2.3.1*; the relative lack of action for which something or someone is fitted, as shown in the changing condition in our time, when "sex with animals...is not explicitly condoned anywhere," such that the use of bestiality for "religious ritual" is no longer much functional in our itme, in *Sec. 2.3.2*; the relative lack of action for which something or someone is fitted, as shown in the work of "the spirit level" nowadays, which promotes the reduction of income inequality between the rich and the poor, such that the older right-wing ideas like laissez-faire capitalism, social Darwinism, etc. are no longer functional in our time, in *Sec. 2.4.1*; the relative lack of action for which something or someone is fitted, as shown in the use of new technologies to treat mental problems nowadays, such that the traditional methods in the older days are no longer much functional in our time, with its relatively more advanced technological environment, in *Sec. 2.4.2*; the relative lack of action for which something or someone is fitted, as shown in the rise of "evidence-based medicine" nowadays, such that the world of "religion, tradition, and superstition" in the older days is no longer functional in our time, with its relatively more scientific expectations, in *Sec. 2.5.1*; the relative lack of action for which something or someone is fitted, as shown in the use of the Buddhist tradition for "mindfulness-based therapy," such that the Noble Eightfold Path taught by the Buddha in the older days is no longer functional in the contemporary Western psychotherapeutic community, whose "modern understanding departs significantly from the Buddha's own account of sati," in *Sec. 2.5.2*; the relative lack of action for which something or someone is fitted, as shown in the critique of physical exercise, in that it can become non-functional too, since "a number of studies of both rodents and humans have demonstrated that individual differences in both ability and propensity for exercise [i.e., voluntary exercise] have some genetic basis," such that some individuals are in fact exercise-resistant, in *Sec. 3.2.1*; the relative lack of action for which something or someone is fitted, as shown in the post-Soviet period, when "financial difficulty, unemployment, and substance abuse" are the "dominating factors in child abuse throughout Eastern Europe," which reflect the transitional period to a more market-oriented open society nowadays, such that the older Communist ideals are no longer functional, in *Sec. 3.2.2*; the relative lack of action for which something or someone is fitted, as shown in the relatively more skeptical reception of the claims on astral travel nowadays, such that the old-fashioned worldview of "witchcraft and shamanism" as well as "classical philosophy and...various myths and religious scriptures" is no longer much functional in our relatively more advanced scientific age, especially in the scientific community, in *Sec. 3.3.1*; the relative lack of action for which something or someone is fitted, as shown in the adoption of different "prevention strategies" nowadays, such that HIV is no longer functional in causing zoonotic diseases to the extent as seen in the older daysin *Sec. 3.3.2*; the relative lack of action for which something or someone is fitted, as shown in the "political calculation" by Peter Reuter and David Boyum, who in their book *An Analytic Assessment of U.S. Drug Policy* "admitted ignoring the legalization option in their analysis," because "there was no legitimate political support for ending the drug war," such that the old-fashioned use of "natural plant drugs like opium, coca, cannabis, mescaline, and psilocybin" in antiquity is no longer functional in contemporary American society, in *Sec. 3.4.1*; the relative lack of action for which something or someone is fitted, as shown in "the women's movement of the 1970s, particularly within the contexts of feminism and women's rights, as concern about wives being beaten by their husbands gained attention," such that the old-fashioned domestic violence by men against women due to jealousy in the older days is no longer functional in the Western world nowadays, in *Sec. 3.4.2*; the relative lack of action for which something or someone is fitted, as shown in the "Article 5 of the UN Universal Declaration of Human Rights" in 1948, which prohibits torture for the first time "under international law and the domestic laws of most countries," such that "medical torture" by Josef Mengele and Shirō Ishii during...World War II" is no longer functional in our time, in *Sec. 3.5.1*; and the relative lack of action for which something or someone is fitted, as shown in the alternative perspective of nursing ethics for "care and nurture" in a "collorative relationship," such that the "four principles" in medical ethics for "cure of illness" is not as much functional in the community of nurses, in *Sec. 3.5.2*).

And the reverse direction also holds true.

Again, it should be stressed, however, that there are different shades of gray (or different degrees of truth) in the two opposites, and the classification is not necessarily mutually exclusive either. In fact, even when some combinations of the two occur, they only end up sharing the same dialectic relationship, but in a different degree.

Also, there are some other relationships (as a kind of family resemblance) which have something in common with the principle, but they are not exactly the same but only more or less comparable, which varies from case to case.

Good examples of family resemblance in relation to the principle are usefulness-nonusefulness, valueness-nonvalueness, usefulness-uselessness, and the like.

31st Thesis: The Intentionality-Nonintentionality Principle

The thirty-first thesis is called the intentionality-nonintentionality princple (on the planning for outcomes) in the category of "outcome" in existential dialectics (which is first worked out in *FPHW*), in that, if there is the planning or design of something for a certain outcome, there is likewise the relative absence of planning or design of something for a certain outcome. There is no intentionality without nonintentionallity—and vice versa.

An intention for an outcome does not have to be certain, so the outcome can even be counter-intentional in being the opposite of what was originally planned. In this sense, counter-intentionality is a special case of non-intentionality; in other words, there are unintented consequences which can be just the opposite of what was originally planned.

An intention for an outcome is mostly relevant to intelligent life, but there are non-intelligent life and non-living matter in the universe too, so nonintentionality is also important.

In addition, an intention does not have to be obvious or straightforward, as William Shakspeare once famously said: "I must be cruel only to be kind."

In any event, on the one hand, there is intentionality in outcome (e.g., the planning or design of something for a certain outcome, as shown in the original intention of conventional psychotherapists to treat mental problems in patients, in *Sec. 2.2.1*; the planning or design of something for a certain outcome, as shown in the original intention of Seligman and

Csikszentmihalyi to study SWB in the context of "personality/genetics," such that "changing one's external circumstances tends to have only a temporary effect on SWB," in *Sec. 2.2.2*; the planning or design of something for a certain outcome, as shown in the original intention of the advocates of EP to use evolutionary theory for the explanation of psychological phenomena like "evolved psychological mechanisms," in *Sec. 2.3.1*; the planning or design of something for a certain outcome, as shown in the original intention of some legal scholars and philosophers to use the idea of "consent" to identify "rape" in human sexual practice, in *Sec. 2.3.2*; the planning or design of something for a certain outcome, as shown in the original intention of Wilkinson and Pickett to show the close relationship between income inequality and health problems, in *Sec. 2.4.1*; the planning or design of something for a certain outcome, as shown in the original intention of the early pioneers like Ralph Lamson, Larry Hodges, and others to use VRT for the treatment of mental disorders, in *Sec. 2.4.2*; the planning or design of something for a certain outcome, as shown in the original intention of the advocates of traditional Chinese Medicine in ancient times to use "Chinese astrology as in acupuncture" to treat health problems, in *Sec. 2.5.1*; the planning or design of something for a certain outcome, as shown in the original intention of the Buddha to teach the Noble Eightfold Path so as to strive for the spiritual life away from "greed, hatred, and delusion," in *Sec. 2.5.2*; the planning or design of something for a certain outcome, as shown in the original intention in 1953 of a team led by Jerry Morris, who showed "the link between physical health and exercise," so as to encourage people to exercise more for health benefits, in *Sec. 3.2.1*; the planning or design of something for a certain outcome, as shown in the original intention of the Eastern European leaders in the Soviet era to uphold "equality within the sexes" in regard to child care, as part of their Communist propaganda at the time, in *Sec. 3.2.2*; the planning or design of something for a certain outcome, as shown in the original intention of the historical sources of astral travel to propound the possibility of "out-of-body experience," in *Sec. 3.3.1*; the planning or design of something for a certain outcome, as shown in the original intention of those working in conservation medicine to successfully cope with the threat of zoonotic diseases, in *Sec. 3.3.2*; the planning or design of something for a certain outcome, as shown in the original intention of those pushing for laws to prohibit drug use, so as to get rid of organized crime associated with it, since the US Drug Enforcement Administration argued that "crime, violence and drug use go hand in hand," in *Sec. 3.4.1*; the planning or design of something for a certain outcome, as shown in the original intention of the advocates to campaign for "law enforcement" against domestic violence, in *Sec. 3.4.2*; the planning or design of something for a certain outcome, as shown in the original intention of some supporters of torture like Alan M. Dershowitz and Mirko Bagaric, who "have argued the need for information outweighs the moral and ethical arguments against torture," in *Sec. 3.5.1*; and the planning or design of something for a certain outcome, as shown in the original intention of Tom Beauchamp and James Childress to use the "four principles" in medical ethics as "a useful framework for understanding conflicts" in medical practice, in *Sec. 3.5.2*).

On the other hand, there is nonintentionality in outcome (e.g., the relative absence of planning or design of something for a certain outcome, such that the outcome can even be counter-intentional in being the opposite of what was originally planned, as shown in the critique by "feminist, constructionist and discursive sources," in that, "while it is seldom intended, the therapist-client relationship always participates in society's power relations and political dynamics"—contrary to the original intention of conventional psychotherapists to treat mental problems in patients, in *Sec. 2.2.1*; the relative absence of planning or design of something for a certain outcome, such that the outcome can even be counter-intentional in being the opposite of what was originally planned, as shown in the new studies nowadays which show the importance and persistence of "social influences" and "cultural variations" in SWB—contrary to the original intention of Seligman and Csikszentmihalyi to study SWB in the context of "personality/genetics," in *Sec. 2.2.2*; the relative absence of planning or design of something for a certain outcome, such that the outcome can even be counter-intentional in being the opposite of what was originally planned, as shown in the critique by the critics of EP, in that it suffres from "genetic reductionism," among other damaging criticisms aforecited—contrary to the original intention of the advocates of EP to use evolutionary theory for the explanation of psychological phenomena, in *Sec. 2.3.1*; the relative absence of planning or design of something for a certain outcome, such that the outcome can even be counter-intentional in being the opposite of what was originally planned, as shown in the use of "consent" by the defenders of zoophilia to justify human sexual contacts with animals instead—contrary to the original intention of legal scholars and philosophers to use the idea of "consent" to identify "rape" in human sexual practice, in *Sec. 2.3.2*; the relative absence of planning or design of something for a certain outcome, such that the outcome can even be counter-intentional in being the opposite of what was originally planned, as shown in the criticisms by the critics, who pointed out that the work by Wilkinson and Pickett constitutes a very narrow view of social stratification in relation to health care, that it provides no verification of the claim, that there is no general agreement on the desirability of income equality, that the correlation between health and income level does not really hold, and that equality can lead to a conformist society—contrary to the original intention of Wilkinson and Pickett to show the close relationship between income inequality and health problems, in *Sec. 2.4.1*; the relative absence of planning or design of something for a certain outcome, such that the outcome can even be counter-intentional in being the opposite of what was originally planned, as shown in the current decision of "the VA [the U.S. Department of Veterans Affairs]" to "continue…to emphasize traditional PET [prolonged exposure therapy] as the treatment of choice, and VR-based therapies have gained only limited adoption, despite active promotion by DOD [even though]…VRT having much lower cost and apparently higher success rates"—contrary to the original intention of the early pioneers to use VRT for the treatment of mental disorders, in *Sec. 2.4.2*; the relative absence of planning or design of something for a certain outcome, such that the outcome can even be counter-intentional in being the opposite of what was originally planned, as shown in the rejection of "many of its assumptions, including the model of the body, or concept of disease" which "are not supported by modern evidence-based medicine"—contrary to the original intention of the advocates of traditional Chinese Medicine in ancient times to use "Chinese astrology as in acupuncture" to treat health problems, in *Sec. 2.5.1*; the relative absence of planning or design of something for a certain outcome, such that the outcome can even be counter-intentional in being the opposite of what was originally planned, as shown in the use of the Buddhist tradition for "mindfulness-based therapy" nowadays to enhance "attention" and "openness"—contrary to the original intention of the Buddha to teach the Noble Eightfold Path so as to strive for the spiritual life away from "greed, hatred, and delusion" instead, in *Sec. 2.5.2*; the relative absence of planning or design of something for a certain outcome, such that the outcome can even be counter-intentional in being the opposite of what was originally planned, as shown in more recent findings that vigorous exercise can have its downside, that some individuals can be exercise-resistant, that the findings are inconsistent, that there is often "insufficient evidence" for any firm conclusion, and that some effects of physical exercise remain unknown—contrary to the original intention of Jerry Morris and his team, who encouraged people to exercise more for health benefits, in *Sec. 3.2.1*; the relative absence of planning or design of something for a certain outcome, such that the outcome can even be counter-intentional in being the opposite of what was originally planned, as shown in the changes in Eastern Europe nowadays, when "there is a new openness and acceptance regarding parenting styles and close relationships with children," and, although "controlling parenting may be less of a concern, financial difficulty, unemployment, and substance abuse still remain to be dominating factors in child abuse throughout Eastern Europe"—contrary to the original intention of the Eastern European leaders in the Soviet era to uphold "equality within the sexes" as part of their Communist propaganda at the time, in *Sec. 3.2.2*; the relative absence of planning or design of something for a certain outcome, such that the outcome can even be counter-intentional in being the opposite of what was originally planned, as shown in the relatively more skeptical reception of the claims on astral travel in the scientific community nowadays—contrary to the original intention of the historical sources of astral travel to propound the possibility of "out-of-body experience," in *Sec. 3.3.1*; the relative absence of planning or design of something for a certain outcome, such that the outcome can even be counter-intentional in being the opposite of what was originally planned, as shown in the realization nowadays by the critics of conservation medicine that "the environmental causes of health problems are complex, global, and poorly understood," such that the causes and effects of zoonotic diseases can be more complicated than previously thought—contrary to the original intention of those working in conservation medicine to successfully cope with the threat of zoonotic diseases, in *Sec. 3.3.2*; the relative absence of planning or design of something for a certain outcome, such that the outcome can even be counter-intentional in being the opposite of what was originally planned, as shown in the unintended consequence of "drug prohibition," which ends up protecting "the drug cartel insofar as it keeps the distribution in the black market and creates the risk that makes smuggling profitable"—contrary to the original intention of those pushing for laws to prohibit drug use, so as to get rid of organized crime associated with it, in *Sec. 3.4.1*; the relative absence of planning or design of something for a certain outcome, such that the outcome can even be counter-intentional in being the opposite of what was originally planned, as shown in some recent findings about "law enforcement," in that "arrest seemed to help in the short run in certain cases, but those arrested experienced double the rate of violence over the course of one year," and "criminologists do not fully understand the reasons why deterrent effects do not last over time"—contrary to the original intention of the advocates to campaign for "law enforcement" against domestic violence, in *Sec. 3.4.2*; the relative absence of planning or design of something for a certain outcome, such that the outcome can even be counter-intentional in being the opposite of what was originally planned, as shown in "one well documented effect of torture," which showed that "its victims will say or do anything to escape the situation, including untrue 'confessions' and implication of others without genuine knowledge"—contrary to the original intention of some supporters of torture like Alan M. Dershowitz and Mirko Bagaric, who "have argued the need for information outweighs the moral and ethical arguments against torture," in *Sec. 3.5.1*; and the relative absence of planning or design of something for a certain outcome, such that the outcome can even be counter-intentional in being the opposite of what was originally planned, as shown in the criticisms by the critics nowadays, in that medical ethics focuses too much on "curing," at the expense of alternative ethical concerns [e.g., "nursing ethics"], that there is cultural bias in medical ethics, that there are "conflicts of interest" in medical ethics so that the values are not necessarily followed in practice, that there is no consensus on medical ethics even within a given tradition, that the values in medical ethics are not necessarily valuable, that scholars disagree over the priority [or ranking] of the values in medical ethics so the conclusions can be inconsistent with each other, and that nations differ in regard to their regulations concerning medical ethics—contrary to the original intention of Tom Beauchamp and James Childress to use the "four principles" in medical ethics as "a useful framework for understanding conflicts" in medical practice, in *Sec. 3.5.2*).

And the reverse direction also holds true.

Again, it should be stressed, however, that there are different shades of gray (or different degrees of truth) in the two opposites, and the classification is not necessarily mutually exclusive either. In fact, even when some combinations of the two occur, they only end up sharing the same dialectic relationship, but in a different degree.

Also, there are some other relationships (as a kind of family resemblance) which have something in common with the principle, but they are not exactly the same but only more or less comparable, which varies from case to case.

Good examples of family resemblance in relation to the principle are purposiveness-nonpurposiveness, intention-accidentalness, design-randomness, etc.

32nd Thesis: The Survivability-Nonsurvivability Principle

The thirty-second thesis is called the survivability-nonsurvivability princple (on the survival of things) in the category of "outcome" in existential dialectics (which is first worked out in *FPHPROB*), in that, if there are some entities which survive at certain times, there are likewise other entities which do not survive. There is no survivability without nonsurvivability—and vice versa.

In nature, for illustration, there are some animals which survive in hard times, whereas others do not—and this is true, not just among different species but also among different members of the same species (and the phenomenon of "selection" in evolutionary biology has much to say on this, as already addressed in *BNN*).

Of course, the principle is not restricted solely to the animal world, since it can be used to other cases concerning non-animals too (e.g., trees, lakes, etc. in the natural world—or empires, companies, etc. in the human world).

But one should not confuse this principle with the expansion-contraction principle, since those entities which survive, say, can still expand or contract over time (e.g., those animals which survive can be more capable in some activities but not in others, for instance).

Nor should this principle be confused with the stability-reaction principle, in that the condition of survivability or non-survivability may lead to further changes later on (as shown in the emergence of new species after the extinction of some old ones, as already explained in *BNR*).

In any event, on the one hand, there is survivability in outcome (e.g., the relative survival, nowadays, of "resources available to a person experiencing emotional distress—the friendly support of friends, peers, family members, clergy contacts, personal reading, healthy exercise, research, and independent coping," in *Sec. 2.2.1*; the relative survival of those patients who "take their symptoms" serioiusly and "seek treatment" early, according to a study by Diener [2008] and his colleagues, in *Sec. 2.2.2*; the relative survival, nowadays, of EP, in *Sec. 2.3.1*; the relative survival, nowadays, of the idea that "sex with animals…is not explicitly condoned anywhere," in *Sec. 2.3.2*; the relative survival of the idea of "the spirit level" nowadays, in *Sec. 2.4.1*; the relative survival, nowadays, of using high technologies like "telenursing," "telepharmacy," "telepsychiatry," etc. to treat health problems, in *Sec. 2.4.2*; the relative survival, nowadays, of "evidence-based medicine" in developed countries, in *Sec. 2.5.1*; the relative survival, nowadays, of using the Buddhist tradition for "mindfulness-based therapy" to cope with health problems like "chronic pain," "stress," "anxiety and depression," "substance abuse," and "recurrent suicidal behavior" in the contemporary Western psychotherapeutic community, in *Sec. 2.5.1*; the relative survival, nowadays, of the belief in the link between physical health and exercise, in

Sec. 3.2.1; the relative survival of the post-Soviet period nowadays, in regard to the fact that "financial difficulty, unemployment, and substance abuse" are the "dominating factors in child abuse throughout Eastern Europe," in *Sec. 3.2.2*; the relative survival, nowadays, of the skeptical reception of the claims on astral travel in the scientific community, in *Sec. 3.3.1*; the relative survival of those individuals who suffer from infectious diseases but are benefited from different "prevention strategies" to fight them, in *Sec. 3.3.2*; the relative survival of those minimal drug users who do not suffer much from drug-induced problems, let alone death, in *Sec. 3.4.1*; the relative survival of "the women's movement" against domestic violence in the Western world nowadays, in *Sec. 3.4.2*; the relative survival of "the UN Universal Declaration of Human Rights" nowadays, in *Sec. 3.5.1*; and the relative survival, nowadays, of the "four principles" in medical ethics, in *Sec. 3.5.2*).

On the other hand, there is non-survivability in outcome (e.g., the non-survival, nowadays, of the unquestioned, "idealized" view about the "healing power of a psychotherapeutic relationship," in *Sec. 2.2.1*; the relative non-survival of those patients, who "tend to be optimistic, leading them to take their symptoms too lightly, seek treatment too late, and/or follow the doctor's instructions half-heartedly," according to a study by Diener [2008] and his colleagues, in *Sec. 2.2.2*; the relative non-survival, nowadays, of "eugenics and social darwinism," in *Sec. 2.3.1*; the relative non-survival, nowadays, of the European medieval practice of punishing zoophiles with "execution, typically burning," in *Sec. 2.3.2*; the relative non-survival of social Darwinism nowadays, in *Sec. 2.4.1*; the relative non-survival, nowadays, of using "smoke signals to warn people to stay away…in case of serious disease," in *Sec. 2.4.2*; the relative non-survival, nowadays, of homeopathy in developed countries, because "within the medical community homeopathy is now considered to be quackery," in *Sec. 2.5.1*; the relative non-survival, nowadays, of using the Buddhist tradition for a spiritual life to cope with health problems like "greed," "pleasures of the flesh," etc. in the contemporary Western psychotherapeutic community, in *Sec. 2.5.2*; the relative non-survival, nowadays, of "physically demanding work" which requries a lot of people to be physically active, since "worldwide there has been a large shift towards less physically demanding work" in our time, in *Sec. 3.2.1*; the relative non-survival of "the emphasis on equality within the sexes" in Eastern Europe nowadays, though it was the case in the Soviet period, in *Sec. 3.2.2*; the relative non-survival of the claim by Ingo Swann about the alleged ability to astral travel on the basis of his account of "Jupiter and observe details of the planet," which is now discredited as being not quite accurate by the critics aforedescribed, in *Sec. 3.3.1*; the relative non-survival of those unlucky individuals who suffer from infectious diseases, when "the human is actually an accidental victim and a dead-end host," in *Sec. 3.3.2*; the relative non-survival of those heavy drug users who died due to drug-induced deaths, in *Sec. 3.4.1*; the relative non-survival, nowadays in the Western world, of the practice often found in the pre-1800 era, when "most legal systems accepted wife beating as a valid exercise of a husband's authority over his wife," in *Sec. 3.4.2*; the relative non-survival of the "medical torture" as practiced by Josef Mengele and Shirō Ishii during…World War II" nowadays, in *Sec. 3.5.1*; and the relative non-survival, nowadays, of the claim by Edmund Pellegrino, who argued that "beneficence is the only fundamental principle of medical ethics," in *Sec. 3.5.2*).

And the reverse direction also holds true.

Again, it should be stressed, however, that there are different shades of gray (or different degrees of truth) in the two opposites, and the classification is not necessarily mutually exclusive either. In fact, even when some combinations of the two occur, they only end up sharing the same dialectic relationship, but in a different degree.

Also, there are some other relationships (as a kind of family resemblance) which have something in common with the principle, but they are not exactly the same but only more or less comparable, which varies from case to case.

Good examples of family resemblance in relation to the principle are survival-extinction, existence-nonexistence, life-death, etc.

33rd Thesis: The Post-Human Interconnection

And the thirty-third thesis is about the role of "post-humans," which I originally proposed in my previous books, starting with the first book titled *The Future of Human Civilization* in 2000 and all others afterwards.

As already pointed out in *Sec. 1.8*, I need to emphasize, as this is something that I used to repeat (*almost verbatim*) from my previous books, two clarifications here about the term "post-human" as a neologism in my works.

Firstly, the word "post-human" here should *not* be confused with another term which looks similar but has a totally different meaning in the literature of postmodernism, namely, "post-humanism"—which constitutes a critique of "humanism" as tradionally understood (especially, though not exclusively, in relation to the idea of progress in science and reason in the Enlightenment project). (WK 2008)

My works reject the project of "postmodernism" and propose the future world of what I orignally called "after-postmodernity" in *FHC* and *FCD*, for instance.

And secondly, the word "post-human" here should also *not* be confused with a similar term which is used to champion the ideology of technology for the future co-existence between humans and cyborgs in "trans-humanism." (WK 2008a)

Instead, my term "post-human" in relation to "posthuman-ism" also rejects "transhumanism" (especially, though not exclusively, in relation to the promises of technology) and refers to something else altogether, that is, the future extinction of humans and its post-human successors in deep space and beyond unto multiverses.

My critique of "transhumanism" was more extensively elabroated in *Sec. 2.4.1* of *BEPE*—just as my critique of different futuristic scenarios of fictional artificial intelligence in science fiction was given in *Sec. 3.5.2* of *FPHCOM.*

With these two clarifications in mind (as summarized in *Table 1.31*)—the post-human interconnection in health care can be addressed in relation to five main directions, based on my *interconnected theory of health care*, as analysed in this book (together with my visions as already worked out in my previous books).

Firstly, the post-human interconnection in health care will learn from my interconnected theory of health care, in relation to the dialectic context of no analysis of mental health without that of physical health (and vice versa), to be later transcended altogether, in the context of health care.

Secondly, the post-human interconnection in health care will learn from my interconnected theory of health care in relation to the four perspectives of the mind, nature, society, and culture.

Thirdly, the post-human interconnection in health care will learn from my interconnected theory of health care in relation to the non-privilege of any specific theory over others in the literature and the non-integration of them all (as they are not necessarily compatible with each other).

Fourthly, the post-human interconnection will have to confront the new challenges as posed by the long-term civilizational development of intelligent life in the distant future, both here on this planet Earth and elsewhere in deep space until multiverses.

As this is something that I regularly pointed out in my previous books for background information (and summarize here, *almost verbatim*, with some updates), I already worked out, in my numerous books, what these new challenges will be and provide different original visions to meet them—especially in regard to the following future evolutions:

- of the mind (e.g., "supersession computing," "metamorphic humor," "contrarian personality," "hyper-martial body," "hyper-sexual body," "floating consciousness," "hyper-spatial consciousness," "thinking machines," "unfolding unconsciousness," "thinking robots," "genetically altered superior beings," "cyborgs," and others)
- of nature (e.g., "resilient natural resources," "transdisciplinary architecture," "creational chemistry," "multilateral sound," "resettlement geology," "post-cosmology," "the alteration of space-time," "the creation of new matter-energy," "selective geometry," and the like)
- of society (e.g., "post-capitalism," "post-democracy," "authoritarian liberal democracy," "transfigurative waste," "panoramic transportation," "cyclical-progressive migration," "reflective criminology," "interventive-reshaping geography," "detached gambling," "heterodox education," "multifaceted war and peace," "virtual organizations," the movement of "cyclical progression" at both structural and systemic levels, "ambivalent technology," and so forth)
- of culture (e.g., "fusional morphology," "modificative sports," "inquisitive culinary art," "interactive semantics," "transdisciplinary performing arts," "comparative-impartial literature," "post-human mind games," "comparative-substitutive religion," "post-ethics," "post-civilization," "transformative aesthetic experience," "contrastive mathematical-logic," and the whatnot)
- in history (e.g., "multifold history," the age of "after-postmodernity," etc.)
- in methodology (e.g., "sophisticated methodologial holism," "critical-dialectic formal science," "complex data analysis," "interpretivist probability," etc.)
- in ontology (e.g., "existential dialectics," "contrastive rationality," etc.)

Of course, the examples (as listed above) are not exhaustive but illustrative, since my numerous books have worked out many other visions (as already roughly summarized in *Sec.1.8* and *Sec. 1.9*). Many, though not all, of my visions on the mind, nature, society, culture, history, methodology, and ontology (as cited above) are summarized in the tables as shown in Chapter One and Chapter Four (especially in *Table 4.43* about my original theories on numerous topics).

And finally, or fifthly, the post-human interconnection in health care will learn from my interconnected theory of health care in regard to the need to go beyond mind and body (or beyond mental health and physical health)—to be further elaborated in the next section.

Towards the Post-Human Interconnection

This "post-human" interconnection to transcend both mind and body (or mental health and physical health in health care) can be understood in terms of nine great future transformations of health care, in relation to the mind, nature, society, and culture—as explained below (and summarized in *Table 1.2*).

Nine Great Future Transformations of Health Care

The nine great future transformations of health care (in relation to the mind, nature, society, and culture) can be explained hereafter, with the caveat, however, that the classification in terms of nine is solely illustrative, as there is no objective basis that it must be classified in term of nine (as this is something that I often stressed and repeated in my previous books, albeit in the context of different topics).

The First Great Future Transformation of Health Care

The first great future transformation of health care in the post-human era concerns what I originally call *new goals,* in relation to the mind.

This search for "new goals" will give future advanced humans and later their successors, namely, the post-humans, the capacity to be motivated to provide health care in a way that current humans cannot.

There are already some indications that the future of health care is moving toward this direction.

Consider, for illustration, the different "goals" as already seen in the history of health care, such as the quest for mental health (*Sec. 2.2.1*), the quest for subjective well-being (*Sec. 2.2.2*), the quest for evolutionary adaptedness (*Sec. 2.3.1*), the quest for alternative sexuality (*Sec. 2.3.2*), the quest for the spirit level (*Sec. 2.4.1*), the quest for virtual reality therapy (*Sec. 2.4.2*), the quest for alternative medicine (*Sec. 2.5.1*), the quest for mindfulness (*Sec. 2.5.2*), the quest for physical fitness (*Sec. 3.2.1*), the quest for child abuse prevention (*Sec. 3.2.2*), the quest for astral travel (*Sec. 3.3.1*), the quest for conservation medicine (*Sec. 3.3.2*), the quest for drug prohibition (*Sec. 3.4.1*), the quest for domestic violence management (*Sec. 3.4.2*), the quest for torture ban (*Sec. 3.5.1*), and the quest for medical ethics (*Sec. 3.5.2*), for instance.

More importantly, this future quest for new goals should also be understood in relation to my previous works on the future "post-human" supersession of the human mind from the combined perspectives of the mind, nature, society, and culture—with good examples like "supersession computing," "metamorphic humor," "contrarian personality," "hyper-martial body," "hyper-sexual body," "floating consciousness," "hyper-spatial consciousness," "unfolding unconsciousness," "thinking robots," "thinking machines," "genetically altered superior beings," "cyborgs," and others.

In any event, all these are just some illustrative (relatively primitive) examples in our time, of course, but the important point to remember here is that the search for different new goals will further transform health care at the more advanced level in the post-human future that the human world has never known.

The Second Great Future Transformation of Health Care

The second great future transformation of health care in the post-human era concerns what I originally call *new means,* in relation to the mind.

This quest for "new means" will give future advanced humans and later their successors, namely, the post-humans, the capacity to find novel options to achieve the goals in regard to health care in a way that current humans cannot.

There are already some indications that the future of health care is moving toward this direction.

Consider, for illustration, the different "means" as already seen in the history of health care, such as different approaches to psychotherapy (*Sec. 2.2.1*), positive thinking for well-being (*Sec. 2.2.2*), the study of emotion and motivation to understand evolved pscyhological mechanisms (*Sec. 2.3.1*), zoophilic fantasies as a way to achieve zoophilia (*Sec. 2.3.2*), lesser income inequality for public health (*Sec. 2.4.1*), the use of technology for mental health (*Sec. 2.4.2*), yoga to achieve better health (*Sec. 2.5.1*), Gestalt therapy to achieve mindfulness (*Sec. 2.5.2*), aerobics for physical fitness (*Sec. 3.2.1*), cognitive behavioral therapy for child abuse prevention (*Sec. 3.2.2*), the study of ancient Hindu scriptures to learn how to do astral travel (*Sec. 3.3.1*), the study of veterinary medicine to fight zoonoses (*Sec. 3.3.2*), cannabis as gateways to use of harder drugs (*Sec. 3.4.1*), law enforcement to fight domestic violence (*Sec. 3.4.2*), the Catechism of the Catholic Church as a way to argue against torture (*Sec.*

3.5.1), and the four principles as a framework for understanding conflicts (*Sec. 3.5.2*), for instance.

All these are just some illustrative (relatively primitive) examples in our time, of course, but the important point to remember here is that the search for different new means will further transform heatlh care at the more advanced level in the post-human future that the human world has never known.

The Third Great Future Transformation of Health Care

The third great future transformation of health care in the post-human era concerns what I originally call *new comparisons*, in relation to nature.

This search for "new comparisons" will give future advanced humans and later their successors, namely, the post-humans, the ability to learn from animals, plants, and the universe, through comparison and contrast, about health care in a way that current humans cannot.

There are already some indications that the future of health care is moving toward this direction.

Consider, for illustration, the different forms of comparison and contrast, such as as already seen in the history of health care, such as evolved mechanisms for both humans and animals (*Sec. 2.3.1*), sexual similarities and differences between humans and animals (*Sec. 2.3.2*), the knowledge of "vital force" from nature for health (*Sec. 2.5.1*), the comparison of the individual as an microcosm of the universe (*Sec. 3.3.1*), and the comparison and contrast between zoonosis and reverse-zoonosis (*Sec. 3.3.2*), for instance.

All these are just some illustrative (relatively primitive) examples in our time, of course, but the important point to remember here is that the search for different new comparisons will further transform health care at the more advanced level in the post-human future that the human world has never known.

The Fourth Great Future Transformation of Health Care

The fourth great future transformation of heatlh care in the post-human era concerns what I originally call *new integrations*, in relation to nature.

This search for "new integrations" will give future advanced humans and later their successors, namely, the post-humans, the ability to live and interact with nature for health care in a way that current humans cannot.

There are already some indications that the future of health care is moving toward this direction.

Consider, for illustration, the different integrations as already seen in the history of health care, such as the sexual relationship between humans and animals (*Sec. 2.3.2*), the integration of herbs in nature with the maintenance of human health *Sec. 2.5.1*), the integration with higher realms in astral travel (*Sec. 3.3.1*), the integration of human medicine with veterinary medicine (*Sec. 3.3.2*), for instance.

More importantly, this future quest for new integrations should also be understood in relation to my previous works on the future "post-human" adventures into different dimensions of space-time unto multiverses from the combined perspectives of the mind, nature, society, and culture—with good examples like "the alteration of space-time" (*Table 1.3* and *Table 1.4*), "multiverses" (*Table 1.7* and *Table 1.8*), "hyperspace" (*Table 1.9* and *Table 1.25*), "time travel" (*Table 1.10* and *Table 1.11*), and others.

In addition, in my previous book titled *The Future of Post-Human Geology* (2010), I already envisioned the three great future transformations of geology, namely, "solar geology," "galactic geology," and "cosmic geology," in the context of my "resettlement theory of geology," in that humans and later post-humans will explore and migrate to other planets, solar systems, galaxies, and cosmos in the long haul.

Then, in another book of mine titled *The Future of Post-Human Geography* (2011), I linked the two books together, since geography has much to learn from geology (as in "physical geography," which, as already introduced in *Sec. 1.3* of *FPHGEOG*, relies heavily on the earth sciences) and discussed the search for "new explorations" in the context of the three forms of environments outside the planet Earth, namely, what I originally called "solar geography," "galactic geography," and "cosmic geography"—as a further elaboration of the three great future transformations of geology (in *FPHGEOL*).

Later, in still another book of mine titled *The Future of Post-Human Migration* (2012), I envisioned the future integrations in different forms, namely, what I originally called "solar migration," "galactic migration," "clustery migration," "cosmic migration," and "multiversal migration."

And then, in an additional book of mine titled *The Future of Post-Human Transportation* (2012), I envisioned the future integrations in different forms, namely, what I originally called "solar transportation," "galactic transportation," "clustery transportation," "cosmic transportation," and "multiversal transportation."

This extension is consistent with my other theory, namely, "the theory of the cyclical progression of system integration and fragmentation" in

FCD (2002)—at the social-systemic level (as already clarified in *Sec. 1.8* and shown below):

Local → Regional → Global →Solar →
Galactic → Clustery…→ Multiversal

All these are just some illustrative (relatively primitive) examples in our time, of course, but the important point to remember here is that the search for different new integrations will further transform health care at the more advanced level in the post-human future that the human world has never known.

The Fifth Great Future Transformation of Health Care

The fifth great future transformation of health care in the post-human era concerns what I originally call *new praxes*, in relation to society.

This search for "new praxes" will give future advanced humans and later their successors, namely, the post-humans, the ability to engage in practice (like activism, politics, personal experience, etc.) for the future of heatlh care in a way that current humans cannot.

There are already some indications that the future of heatlh care is moving toward this direction.

Consider, for illustration, the different praxes as already seen in history of health care like the practical application of feminism to the field of psychotherapy (*Sec. 2.2.1*), the practical application of genetics to the field of psychology (*Sec. 2.2.2*), the practical application of evolutionary theory to the field of psychology (*Sec. 2.3.1*), the practical application of consent in the study of human sexuality to the field of zoophilia (*Sec. 2.3.2*), the practical application of the spirit level to the field of public politics (*Sec. 2.4.1*), the practical application of computer science to the field of medicine (*Sec. 2.4.2*), the practical application of astrology to the field of medicine (*Sec. 2.5.1*), the practical application of Buddhism to the field of therapy (*Sec. 2.5.2*), the practical application of neurobiology to the field of physical exercise (*Sec. 3.2.1*), the practical application of ethics to the field of health care and the law (*Sec. 3.2.2*), the practical application of different religions to the field of "out-of-body experience" (*Sec. 3.3.1*), the practical application of conservation medicine to the field of public health (*Sec. 3.3.2*), the practical application of economics to the field of drug prohibition (*Sec. 3.4.1*), the practical application of psychology to the field of domestic violence (*Sec. 3.4.2*), the practical application of utilitarianism to the field of public policy (*Sec. 3.5.1*), and the practical application of ethics to the field of medicine (*Sec. 3.5.2*), for instance.

All these are just some illustrative (relatively primitive) examples in our time, of course, but the important point to remember here is that the search for different new praxes will further transform health care at the more advanced level in the post-human future that the human world has never known.

The Sixth Great Future Transformation of Health Care

The sixth great future transformation of health care in the post-human era concerns what I originally call *new technologies*, in relation to society.

This search for "new technologies" will give future advanced humans and later their successors, namely, the post-humans, the ability to come up with different techniques, materials, and experiments for health care in a way that current humans cannot.

There are already some indications that the future of health care is moving toward this direction.

Consider, for illustration, the use of different technologies as already seen in the history of health care, such as techniques of psychotherapy (*Sec. 2.2.1*), techniques of modeling SWB (*Sec. 2.2.2*), research methods of evolutionary psychology (*Sec. 2.3.1*), techniques of zoosexual acts (*Sec. 2.3.2*), techniques to measure income inequality (*Sec. 2.4.1*), technologies for mental health (*Sec. 2.4.2*), techniques of acupuncture (*Sec. 2.5.1*), research methods for mindfulness (*Sec. 2.5.2*), research techniques to measure exercise levels for public health (*Sec. 3.2.1*), techniques to treat child-abuse victims (*Sec. 3.2.2*), Taoist alchemical technique for astral travel (*Sec. 3.3.1*), research methods in conservation medicine to incorporate multiple disciplines (*Sec. 3.3.2*), Gallup poll techniques to measure public opinion on drug laws (*Sec. 3.4.1*), research methods to understand the social causes of domestic violence (*Sec. 3.4.2*), torture methods (*Sec. 3.5.1*), and the research method of the Milgram experiment (*Sec. 3.5.2*), for instance.

For instance, most advanced forms of future intelligent life in deep space until multiverses will make good use of their technological prowess to discover the genetic basis of health (as discussed in *Sec. 2.2.2*), to treat mental health (as discussed in *Sec. 2.4.2*), to come up with new techniques for torture (as discussed in *Sec. 3.5.1*), and others in the distant future.

All these are just some illustrative (relatively primitive) examples in our time, of course, but the important point to remember here is that the search for new technologies will further transform health care at the more advanced level in the post-human future that the human world has never known.

The Seventh Great Future Transformation of Health Care

The seventh great future transformation of health care in the post-human era concerns what I originally call *new stratifications*, in relation to society.

This emergence of "new stratifications" will lead future advanced humans and later their successors, namely, the post-humans, to face new inequalities in health care in a way that current humans cannot.

There are already some indications that the future of health care is moving toward this direction.

Consider, for illustration, the different inequalities as already seen in the history of health care, such as the therapist vs. the client (*Sec. 2.2.1*), the adaptation of an individual to different life events unequally (*Sec. 2.2.2*), solving everyday practical problems vs. solving abstract problems (*Sec. 2.3.1*), humans vs. animals (*Sec. 2.3.2*), the rich vs. the poor (*Sec. 2.4.1*), physical reality vs. virtual reality (*Sec. 2.4.2*), mainstream Western medicine vs. alternative medicine (*Sec. 2.5.1*), Bishop's view on mindfulness vs. the Buddha's view on mindfulness (*Sec. 2.5.2*), exercise-tolerant individuals vs. exercise-resistant individuals (*Sec. 3.2.1*), child abusers vs. child-abuse victims (*Sec. 3.2.2*), the believers vs. the skeptics (*Sec. 3.3.1*), humans vs. animals (*Sec. 3.3.2*), drug users vs. law enforcement authorities (*Sec. 3.4.1*), men vs. women (*Sec. 3.4.2*), torturers vs. torture victims (*Sec. 3.5.1*), and caring vs. curing (*Sec. 3.5.2*), for instance.

All these are just some illustrative (relatively primitive) examples in our time, of course, but the important point to remember here is that the emergence of new stratifications will further transform health care at the more advanced level in the post-human future that the human world has never known.

The Eighth Great Future Transformation of Health

The eighth great future transformation of health care in the post-human era concerns what I originally call *new sub-fields*, in relation to culture.

This search for "new sub-fields" will give future advanced humans and later their successors, namely, the post-humans, the ability to explore new specialties (or new games) for health care in a way that current humans cannot.

There are already some indications that the future of health care is moving toward this direction.

Consider, for illustration, the different sub-fields as already seen in the history of health care, such as psychotherapy (*Sec. 2.2.1*), positive psychology (*Sec. 2.2.2*), evolutionary psychology (*Sec. 2.3.1*), zoophilia (*Sec. 2.3.2*), wealth disparity (*Sec. 2.4.1*), virtual reality therapy (*Sec. 2.4.2*), alternative medicine (*Sec. 2.5.1*), mindfulness-based therapy (*Sec. 2.5.2*), physical fitness (*Sec. 3.2.1*), child abuse (*Sec. 3.2.2*), astral travel (*Sec. 3.3.1*), conservation medicine (*Sec. 3.3.2*), drug policy (*Sec. 3.4.1*), domestic violence (*Sec. 3.4.2*), torture policy (*Sec. 3.5.1*), and medical ethics (*Sec. 3.5.2*), for instance.

All these are just some illustrative (relatively primitive) examples in our time, of course, but the important point to remember here is that the search for new sub-fields will further transform health care at the more advanced level in the post-human future that the human world has never known.

The Ninth Great Future Transformation of Health Care

And the ninth great future transformation of health care in the post-human era concerns what I originally call *new interpretations*, in relation to culture.

This search for "new interpretations" will give future advanced humans and later their successors, namely, the post-humans, the ability to come up with different evaluations and views about health care in a way that current humans cannot.

There are already some indications that the future of health care is moving toward this direction.

Consider, for illustration, the different interpretations as already seen in the history of health care, such as the interpretation of uncovering psychotherapy (*Sec. 2.2.1*), the argument for the correlation between genetics and SWB (*Sec. 2.2.2*), the view of evolved psychological mechanisms (*Sec. 2.3.1*), the interpretation of consent for zoophilia (*Sec. 2.3.2*), the argument for lesser income inequality (*Sec. 2.4.1*), the argument for telemedicine (*Sec. 2.4.2*), the argument for homeopathy (*Sec. 2.5.1*), the interpretation of mindfulness based on Buddhism (*Sec. 2.5.2*), the argument for positive exercise effects on the human immune system (*Sec. 3.2.1*), the argument for children's rights (*Sec. 3.2.2*), the Islamic interpretation of astral travel (*Sec. 3.3.1*), the interpretation of the importance of zoonoses to the history of human development (*Sec. 3.3.2*), the gateway hypothesis (*Sec. 3.4.1*), the biological interpretation of domestic violence (*Sec. 3.4.2*), utilitarian arguments against torture (*Sec.

3.5.1), and the interpretation of caring as an alternative value in medicine (*Sec. 3.5.2*), for instance.

All these are just some illustrative (relatively primitive) examples in our time, of course, but the important point to remember here is that the search for new interpretations will further transform health care at the more advanced level in the post-human future that the human world has never known.

Enormous Implications

These nine great future transformations of health care have enormous implications for some soul-searching questions which have challenged some of the finest minds in the history of health care (in the context of mental health and physical health).

For illustration, consider the following questions in the history of health care:

- Ex: to what extent does positive thinking really enhance health, or can it impede it instead?
- Ex: how is human well-being to be understood and measured correctly?
- Ex: to what extent is health genetic in nature?
- Ex: how exactly are the health relations between humans and animals linked?
- Ex: is astral projection possible for human health?
- Ex: to what extent can technologies be used to treat diseases?
- Ex: does social equality really promote health?
- Ex: how are abuse and violence to be addressed in a way which is fair to all?
- Ex: to what extent are alternative medicines effective?

Questions and disagreements like this will receive new answers in the future history of health care in the advanced human and later post-human eras, at least in two fundamental ways.

The first fundamental way is to examine the relationships between mental health and physical health—such that their possibility (or impossibility) and desirability (or undesirability) are not to the extent that the respective defenders would like us to believe.

The different views about health care, as already addressed in *Sec. 1.1*, *Sec. 1.5*, and the rest of the book, are just different ways to understand health care and its future, with each from its own vantage point.

Each view has its own merits and defects and is preferred over others by different proponents with their own different interests, but none of them is possible (or impossible) and desirable (or undesirable) to the extent that its respective advocates would like us to believe.

And the second fundamental way is to inquire about, and then transcend, in the long haul, the debate about mental health and physical health, such that it will be shifted to different directions, as shown in the nine great future transformations that I have envisioned and outlined above. To transcend them all is to move into these different directions, in conjunction with the various visions of my previous books (as already summarized in *Sec. 1.8* and also earlier in this chapter, with the further help of the tables at this end of Chapter One and this chapter).

Nine good examples can be summarized below:

- to create new psychological approaches to well-being
- to come up with new types and categories of physical exercise
- to understand better the genetic basis of health
- to explore new health relations between different forms of intelligent life (e.g., animals, humans, and, later, post-humans)
- to adventure into different dimensions of space-time
- to discover new technologies for the treatment of diseases
- to create new social institutions to deal with health problems
- to search new ways to deal with abuse and violence which are fair to all sides (e.g., men vs. women, physicians vs. clients, etc.)
- to look into new types of alternative medicines

Of course, these examples are illustrative, not exhaustive, as there are other issues as already discussed in the rest of the book.

Lest any misunderstanding occurs, one must remember that these nine great future transformations of health care will bring neither utopia nor dystopia, regardless of some optimistic expectations about the use of hi-tech in our time, just to cite an obvious example—as this is something that I have warned time and again in all of my previous books, *almost verbatim*.

In any event, as I so often stressed in my previous books, it is not up to us current humans to decide whether or not, or to what extent, the post-human future of health care will be for better and for worse, because it will be judged by the values and beliefs of future post-humans on earth and in deep space unto multiverses—in a way that the entire history of the human world has never known.

Thus is the future of health care—and of its post-human fate.

Table 4.1. Sophisticated Methodological Holism (Part I)

• "My methodological holism implies the partiality-totality principle in the ontology of existential dialectics (see the table on the partiality-totality principle for summary), which is against the varieties of (a) reductionism and (b) reverse-reductionism, in relation to (i) concept, (ii) theory, (iii) methodology, and (iv) ontology." (*FC*)

• "[M]y methodological holism here is not opposed to methodological individualism but includes it (and, for that matter, other methodologies too)…." (*FPHC*) For this reason (and others too, as summarized hereafter), my version of methodological holism is sophisticated—not vulgar as sometimes used by inapt scholars using the same term. (*FC*)

• "[M]y methodological holism does not democratically presume that all levels are equally valid, as all levels are not created equal. In other words, in relation to issue X, level A may be more relevant than level B, but in relation to Y, level B can be more relevant than level A instead." (*FPHC*) One excellent example of this vulgar democratic presumption is what I called in *BNN* "the compromise fallacy." (*FC*)

• My methodological holism does not presume that a lower level of analysis is more important than a higher level, solely because the former serves as the foundation for the latter—and vice versa, for that matter. One excellent example of this reductionistic presumption is what I called in *FPHST* "the foundation fallacy." (*FPHST*, *FC*)

(continued on next page)

Table 4.1. Sophisticated Methodological Holism (Part II)

• "[M]y methodological holism does not make any a-priori postulation that there must be a definite (and, for that matter, indefinite) number of levels" in any analysis. (*FPHC*) Nor does it dogmatically require that there must be a certain combination of levels of analysis in a given inquiry. (*FC*)

• "[M]ethodological holism, in my usage, does not assume that all levels...can necessarily be integrated, since methodological holism is not aimed to search for the holy grail of 'an integral theory...' (as is the case for Wilber). In other words, it allows that sometimes some levels may experience irreducible gaps between them, to be understood, at best, as empirical correlations, not as causal relations...." (*FPHC*)

• "[D]ifferent levels may overlap and even interact with each other in a given context (but sometimes may not), and the fact that I even proposed different ways of re-classifying the levels (whenever needed) in *FDC* reinforces this point....The dual danger here is either forcefully making different levels interact when they are just different (or, metaphorically speaking, apples and oranges) or inappropriately ignoring their interactions when some situations instead require them." (*FPHC*)

• "[T]o understand different levels from their own (unique) perspectives (as required by my methodological holism) is not the same as trying to reduce them to a preferred level in the process of learning from other levels. This second kind of multidisciplinary work is not genuine and does no justice to the unique complexities and merits inherent at each level." (*FPHC*)

(continued on next page)

Table 4.1. Sophisticated Methodological Holism (Part III)

• "[My] methodological holism walks a fine line between the artificial classification (separation) of levels and the simultaneous incorporation of them, if only for the sake of human scholarly endeavor. It should be reminded that nature does not impose upon itself the academic classification of the levels of analysis as humans have. The enterprise of classification is therefore anthropocentric." (*FPHC*)

• "[M]y methodological holism advocates neither epistemic subjectivism nor epistemic non-subjectivism (e.g., realism, idealism, and historicism), neither epistemic relativism (e.g., subjectivism, historicism) nor epistemic absolutism (e.g., realism, positivism), neither epistemic reductionism nor epistemic emergencism, and neither epistemic objectivism (e.g., realism, idealism) nor epistemic historicism....Neither does methodological holism, in my usage, accept the false meta-conceptual dichotomy between nominalism and realism....These false dichotomies...are to be transcended. In other words, methodological holism does not fully accept epistemic realism, positivism (a form of epistemic idealism), historicism, subjectivism, and reductionism in epistemology and philosophy of science but learns from the strengths and weaknesses of all of the opposing approaches without siding with any of them...." (*FPHC*)

• "Sophisticated methodological holism is subject to the constraints as imposed by the syntax of existential dialectics (e.g., the partiality-totality principle and the predictability-unpredictability principle). Even in predictability, outcomes are subject to uncertainty, the degree of which varies from case to case." (*FC*)

(continued on next page)

Table 4.1. Sophisticated Methodological Holism (Part IV)

- "Sophisticated methodological holism—when applied, especially though not exclusively, as illustrated in my numerous works—can enrich the understanding of reality in some distinctive ways. Here are three examples (as revealed in each of my books)." (*FPHCT*; *FPHL*)
  - —"Firstly, it provides a comprehensive analysis of a subject matter, from which much can be learned about reality," "both in relation to the perspectives of the mind, nature, society, and culture and also in relation to a new classification of the subject matter."
  - —"Secondly, it suggests some visions of the future in relation to the subject matter in question."
  - —"And thirdly, it proposes some insights on meta-theory (e.g., methodology and ontology) in general—with the clear understanding, however, of the dilemma of specific vs. general ontology (as shown in the table on the syntax of existential dialectics in the context of the dilemma of ontology). For this very reason, all of these ways are important, without reducing one into the analysis of another."
- "In the end, my meta-theory (both sophisticated methodological holism and existential dialectics) serves as a foundation to unify all domains of knowledge into *an unified theory of everything* (by way of some ontological principles and the comprehensive perspectives of the mind, nature, society, and culture). This is so, without commiting the sins of reductionism and reverse-reductionism (as often seen in many holistic approaches, with the fad of sysems approach—be it about systems theory, chaos theory, complexity theory, or else—as a most recent notorious example, which I debunked in *The Future of Complexity* and also in *The Future of Post-Human Formal Science*). My distinctive approach makes good use of different schools of thought without favoring any of them nor trying to integrate them (as they are not necessarily compatible with each other), so as to adjust for subjectivity, diversity, conflict, and complexity, for example. In this sense, the word "unified" does not have to mean integrative approach, in a narrow sense, nor systems approach, in a broad one, both of which I reject while learning from them." (*FPHFS*; *FPHS*)

Sources: A summary of *Sec.1.2* in *FPHC*—and also from *BNN*, *FPHST*, *ALD*, *FC*, *FPHCT*, and the rest of all other books of mine. See the books for more detail.

Table 4.2. On Reductionism and Reverse-Reductionism (Part I)

- **The Partiality-Totality Principle**
  —The partiality-totality principle in the ontology of existential dialectics targets against the varieties of reductionism and reverse-reductionism (as already worked out in my previous books).

- **Against the Varieties of Reductionism**
  —*Conceptual Reductionism*
    - Some illustrative instances involve myriad dualities like mind vs. body, self vs. world, democracy vs. non-democracy, and the like (as already addressed in *FHC*, *FPHC*, and *BDPD*, for instance).

  —*Theoretical Reductionism*
    - A fascinating case study concerns what I originally called "the foundation fallacy" in *FPHST*, in any attempt to naively understand space-time from the physical perspective as the foundation and, consequently, to dangerously dismiss other perspectives.
    - In *FAE*, I elaborated further these versions of reductionism in the literature on aesthetics (e.g., form vs. content, representation vs. expression, critics vs. artists, and externalism vs. internalism).
    - In *FIA*, I revealed other forms of reductionism in the literature on information architecture (e.g., the constructivist argument).
    - In *FPHU*, I showed the persistent legacy of reductionism, this time, in the literature on anomalous experience (e.g., the obsession with physics, chemistry, and biology for explaining anomalous experience).
    - In *FPHE*, I examined another case of reductionism in action, in the context of engineering (e.g., technical constraints vs. normative constraints).
    - In *FPHMM*, I elaborated one more version of reductionism, in relation to the three domains of communication (e.g., the competing views on sending, connecting, and receiving).
    - In *FPHCT*, I explored another version of reductionism, in relation to invention and innovation (e.g., the bio-psychological argument vs. the socio-cultural arguments).

(continued on next page)

Table 4.2. On Reductionism and Reverse-Reductionism (Part II)

- **Against the Varieties of Reductionism** ***(cont'd)***
  - —*Theoretical Reductionism (cont'd)*
    - In *FPHG*, I identify another version of reductionism, in relation to infinity, symmetry, and dimensionality (e.g., the Euclidean argument vs. the non-Euclidean arguments).
    - In *FPHUP*, I analyzed another version of reductionism, in relation to density and void (e.g., the engineering argument and the ecology argument).
    - In *FPHL*, I examined another version of reductionism, in relation to structure and context (e.g., the structuralist argument and the contextualist argument).
    - In *PFHO*, I explored another version of reductionism, in relation to communcation, decision-making, and leadership (e.g., the rational-system argument vs. the natural-system argument).
    - In *PFHMA*, I revealed another version of reductionism, in relation to the martial body and spirit (e.g., the spiritual argument vs. the materialist argument vs. the defensive argument).
    - In *PFHS*, I analyzed another version of reductionism, in relation to the sexual body and spirit (e.g., the naturalist argument vs. the constructivist argument).
    - In *PFHLAW*, I examined another version of reductionism, in relation to law (e.g., the necessity argument vs. the contengency argument).
    - In *FPHWP*, I showed another version of reductionism, in relation to war and peace (e.g., the aggressivist argument vs. the pacifist argument).
    - In *BEPE*, I analyzed another version of reductionism, in relation to morality and immorality (e.g., the objectivist argument vs. the non-objectivist argument vs. the skeptical argument).
    - In *BCOS*, I examined another version of reductionism, in relation to the contested beginnings and speculative ends of the universe (e.g., the scientific argument vs. the religious argument vs. the esoteric argument vs. the metaphysical argument).
    - In *FPHP*, I show another version of reductionism, in relation to normality and abnormality (e.g., the natural argument vs. the social argument vs. the cultural argument vs. the mental argument).

(continued on next page)

Table 4.2. On Reductionism and Reverse-Reductionism (Part III)

- **Against the Varieties of Reductionism** ***(cont'd)***
  - *—Theoretical Reductionism (cont'd)*
    - In *FPHGEOL*, I scrutinized another version of reductionism, in relation to statics and dynamics (e.g., the catastrophe argument vs. the uniformity argument vs. the revision argument).
    - In *FPHCHESS*, I showed another version of reductionism, in relation to tactics and strategy (e.g., the natural argument vs. the social argument vs. the cultural argument vs. the mental argument).
    - In *FPHR*, I revealed another version of reductionism, in relation to secularness and sacredness (e.g., the critical argument vs. the skeptical argument vs. the theist argument).
    - In *FPHEDU*, I examined another version of reductionism, in relation to teaching and learning (e.g., the teacher-centered argument vs. the student-centered argument vs. the balanced argument).
    - In *FPHH*, I explored another version of reductionism, in relation to joking and laughing (e.g., the natural argument vs. the social argument vs. the cultural argument vs. the mental argument).
    - In *FPHA*, I proposed another version of reductionism, in relation to sound and silence (e.g., the natural argument vs. the social argument vs. the cultural argument vs. the mental argument).
    - In *FPHGAM*, I proposed another version of reductionism, in relation to risk and caution (e.g., the natural argument vs. the social argument vs. the cultural argument vs. the mental argument).
    - In *FPHCOM*, I worked out another version of reductionism, in relation to hardware and software (e.g., the natural argument vs. the social argument vs. the cultural argument vs. the mental argument).
    - In *FPHLIT*, I proposed another version of reductionism, in relation to fiction and non-fiction (e.g., the natural argument vs. the social argument vs. the cultural argument vs. the mental argument).
    - In *FPHCHEM*, I proposed another version of reductionism, in relation to substances and their changes (e.g., the natural argument vs. the social argument vs. the cultural argument vs. the mental argument).

(continued on next page)

Table 4.2. On Reductionism and Reverse-Reductionism (Part IV)

- **Against the Varieties of Reductionism** ***(cont'd)***
  —*Theoretical Reductionism (cont'd)*
    - In *FPHDA*, I proposed another version of reductionism, in relation to quantitative and qualitative research (e.g., the natural argument vs. the social argument vs. the cultural argument vs. the mental argument).
    - In *FPHGEOG*, I proposed another version of reductionism, in relation to environments and their interactions (e.g., the natural argument vs. the social argument vs. the cultural argument vs. the mental argument).
    - In *FPHPA*, I proposed another version of reductionism, in relation to the body and its presence (e.g., the natural argument vs. the social argument vs. the cultural argument vs. the mental argument).
    - In *FPHSEM*, I proposed another version of reductionism, in relation to internality and externality (e.g., the natural argument vs. the social argument vs. the cultural argument vs. the mental argument).
    - In *FPHARCH*, I proposed another version of reductionism, in relation to form and function (e.g., the natural argument vs. the social argument vs. the cultural argument vs. the mental argument).
    - In *FPHCRIM*, I proposed another version of reductionism, in relation to heroes and villains (e.g., the natural argument vs. the social argument vs. the cultural argument vs. the mental argument).
    - In *FPHHIST*, I proposed another version of reductionism, in relation to universality and relativity (e.g., the natural argument vs. the social argument vs. the cultural argument vs. the mental argument).
    - In *FPHMIG*, I proposed another version of reductionism, in relation to Sameness, Otherness, and identity (e.g., the natural argument vs. the social argument vs. the cultural argument vs. the mental argument).

(continued on next page)

Table 4.2. On Reductionism and Reverse-Reductionism (Part V)

- **Against the Varieties of Reductionism *(cont'd)***
  —*Theoretical Reductionism (cont'd)*
    - In *FPHTRAN*, I proposed another version of reductionism, in relation to networks and operations (e.g., the natural argument vs. the social argument vs. the cultural argument vs. the mental argument).
    - In *FPHCA*, I proposed another version of reductionism, in relation to ingredients and techniques (e.g., the natural argument vs. the social argument vs. the cultural argument vs. the mental argument).
    - In *FPHW*, I proposed another version of reductionism, in relation to uselessness and usefulness (e.g., the natural argument vs. the social argument vs. the cultural argument vs. the mental argument).
    - In *BNR*, I proposed another version of reductionism, in relation to diversity and discontinuity (e.g., the natural argument vs. the social argument vs. the cultural argument vs. the mental argument).
    - In *FPHSPORT*, I proposed another version of reductionism, in relation to training and winning (e.g., the natural argument vs. the social argument vs. the cultural argument vs. the mental argument).
    - In *FPHPROB*, I proposed another version of reductionism, in relation to objectivity and subjectivity (e.g., the natural argument vs. the social argument vs. the cultural argument vs. the mental argument).
    - In *FPHMORP*, I proposed another version of reductionism, in relation to typologies and rules (e.g., the natural argument vs. the social argument vs. the cultural argument vs. the mental argument).
    - And in *FPHHC*, I propose another version of reductionism, in relation to mind and body (e.g., the natural argument vs. the social argument vs. the cultural argument vs. the mental argument).

(continued on next page)

Table 4.2. On Reductionism and Reverse-Reductionism (Part VI)

- **Against the Varieties of Reductionism** ***(cont'd)***
  —*Methodological Reductionism*
    - A good instance concerns the debate between different versions of qualitative and quantitative methods (as already analyzed in *FC* and also *FHC*). In *FPHML*, I examined similar reductionism, this time, in the literature on mathematical logic (e.g., the obsession with consistency, soundness, and completeness). And in *FPHFS*, I also explored the problems of reductionism in the context of formal science (e.g., the analytical argument).

  —*Ontological Reductionism*
    - An excellent example is the debate between emergentism and reductionism in complexity theory and also in psychology (as elaborated in *FPHC*, in the context of Being and Becoming).

- **Against the Varieties of Reverse-Reductionism**
  —*Conceptual Reverse-Reductionism*
    - Any concept of "art" (e.g., fine art, cave art, outsider art, junk art) is deemed acceptable in postmodernism (as already addressed in Ch.4 of *FHC*).

  —*Theoretical Reverse-Reductionism*
    - There are numerous art and literary theories co-exist. Take the case of literary studies, as there are now Literary Structuralism, Marxist Literary Criticism, New Criticism, Phenomenology, Hermeneutics, Language-Game Literary Criticism, Feminist Literary Criticism, Reception Theory, Reader Response Criticism, Poststructuralism, Semiotics, Pyschoanalytic Literary Criticism, just to cite some well-known ones, with no one being said to be better than any others (as detailedly analyzed in Ch.4 of *FHC*). (S. Raman 1997) In *BNN*, I even introduced "the compromise fallacy" as another good illustration of theoretical reverse-reductionism, in misleadingly treating both genetic and environmental approaches as equally valid.

(continued on next page)

Table 4.2. On Reductionism and Reverse-Reductionism (Part VII)

- **Against the Varieties of Reverse-Reductionism *(cont'd)***
  —*Methodological Reverse-Reductionism*
  - There is the "anything-goes" mentality in postmodernism (e.g., doing art without praxis, doing art with praxis, and doing art by sublation), as analyzed in Ch.4 of *FHC*. And in *FPHFS*, I also exposed the problems of reverse-reductionism in the context of formal science in relation to systems theory.

  —*Ontological Reverse-Reductionism*
  - There are likewise no privileged ontology, and the door is open for anything in postmodernism (e.g., the equal status of the ontology of Being vs. that of Becoming, as already addressed in Ch.4 of *FHC*—and also in *FPHC)*. In *FAE*, I also introduced another version of reverse-reductionism, that is, "the pluralist fallacy," in the context of understanding aesthetic experience, for instance—although this fallacy has been committed not exclusively in relation to the ontological level (but also at the conceptual, theoretical, and methodological ones).

Sources: From my previous books.

Table 4.3. The Concepton of Existential Dialectics (Part I)

- **Sets and Elements**
  - —Sets
    - Ex: the Same
    - Ex: the Others
  - —Elements
    - Ex: whites in 20th century America (in the set of "the Same")
    - Ex: Iraq during the U.S. invasion in 2003 (in the set of "the Others")

- **Relations, Operations, Functions**
  - —Relations (e.g., "belongs," "equals to," "is greater than")
    - Ex: symmetric interactions within the Same (or the Others)
    - Ex: asymmetric interactions between the Same and the Others
  - —Operations (e.g., "and," "or," "not," "if…then")
    - Ex: if the Same oppresses the Others, it will also oppress itself.
    - Ex: the Same is not the Others.
  - —Functions (e.g., goals)
    - Ex: the Same is hegemonic in relation to the Others.

- **Truth Values**
  - —"1" if True (in Symbolic Logic)
    - Ex: the proposition that imperial Japan was hegemonic to China during WWII
  - —"0" if False (in Symbolic Logic)
    - Ex: the proposition that Grenada invaded France in 2003
  - —"1" & "0" if Both True and False (in Dialectic Logic)
    - Ex: the proposition that the rabbit-duck picture refers to a duck
  - —"~1" & "~0" if Neither True Nor False (or N/A, in Dialectic Logic)
    - Ex: the proposition that God really exists

(continued on next page)

Table 4.3. The Conception of Existential Dialectics (Part II)

- **Axioms and Postulates**
  —Axioms
    - Ex: the reflexive axiom—"any quantity is equal to itself"
  —Postulates
    - Ex: the SSS postulate—"if the three sides of a triangle are congruent to their corresponding parts, then the triangles are congruent"

- **Theorems and Principles**
  —Theorems (and Principles) in Existential Dialectics
    - *In Relation to Method*
      –#32: The formalness-informalness principle
      –#31: The absoluteness-relativeness principle
      –#30: The partiality-totality principle
      –#29: The predictability-unpredictability principle
      –#28: The explicability-inexplicability principle
      –#27: The fiction-reality principle
      –#26: The cognitiveness-noncognitiveness principle
    - *In Relation to Structure*
      –#25: The finiteness-transfiniteness principle
      –#24: The preciseness-vagueness principle
      –#23: The simpleness-complicatedness principle
      –#22: The openness-hiddenness principle
      –#21: The denseness-emptiness principle
    - *In Relation to Process*
      –#20: The prototypicality-variation principle
      –#19: The change-constancy principle
      –#18: The order-chaos principle
      –#17: The slowness-quickness principle
      –#16: The expansion-contraction principle
      –#15: The optimality-nonoptimality principle

(continued on next page)

Table 4.3. The Conception of Existential Dialectics (Part III)

- **Theorems and Principles (*cont'd*)**
  —Theorems (and Principles) in Existential Dialectics
  - *In Relation to Agency*
    –#14: The theory-praxis principle
    –#13: The convention-novelty principle
    –#12: The evolution-transformation principle
    –#11: The symmetry-asymmetry principle
    –#10: The softness-hardness principle
    –#9: The seriousness-playfulness principle
    –#8: The activeness-inactiveness principle
    –#7: The selfness-otherness principle
  - *In Relation to Outcome*
    –#6: The regression-progression principle
    –#5: The same-difference principle
    –#4: The stability-reaction principle
    –#3: The functionality-nonfunctionality principle
    –#2: The intentionality-nonintentionality principle
    –#1: The survivability-nonsurvivability principle

Notes: The categories and examples in each are solely illustrative (not exhaustive). The comparison is also relative (not absolute), nor are they mutually exclusive. As generalities, they allow exceptions.
Sources: Starting from Ch.6 of *BCPC* and also from other books of mine

Table 4.4. The Syntax of Existential Dialectics I:
The Principles
(Part I)

- **In Relation to Method**

—*The Formalness-Informalness Principle*

(On the Formal Requirements of Logical Systems)

- The formal requirements of a logical system (e.g., consistency, soundness, and completeness) have both usefulness and non-usefulness, to the extent that, if there are formal systems requiring them, there are alternative ones which do not. Thus, it does *not* exclude classical logics but simply goes beyond both classical and non-classical logics, while learning something from each. There is no formalness without informalness—and vice versa.
- For instance, existential dialectics can make use of both classical logics under certain conditions (e.g., especially, though not exclusively, when they are clear-cut, etc.) and non-classical logics under alternative conditions (especially, though not exclusively, when they are "unknown," "irrelevant," "ambiguous," "possible," with "different degrees of truth," empirically inconsistent in a desirable way, etc.). (WK 2008u)
- Family resemblance: e.g., logicalness-nonlogicalness, rationality-nonrationality, etc.
- Sources: From *FPHML*, *FPHH*, *FPHGAM*, *FPHSEM*, and my later books.

(continued on next page)

Table 4.4. The Syntax of Existential Dialectics I: The Principles (Part II)

- **In Relation to Method *(cont'd)***
  - *—The Absoluteness-Relativeness Principle*
    (On the Multiplicity of Things)
    - There is the multiplicity of things in reality, be they about entities, qualities (or properties), and relationships, such that what is acceptable from one standpoint may not be so from another. For instance, if there is something absolute, there is likewise something relative. There is no absoluteness without relativeness—and vice versa.
    - Both absoluteness and relativeness here are also relevant to different modalities often cited in the literature on ontology, such as possibility (e.g., something "can" happen) and its opposite (e.g., impossibility) in alethic modalities, probability (e.g., something "will" happen) and its opposite (e.g., improbability) in temporal modalities, and necessity (e.g., something "should" happen) and its opposite (e.g., contingency) in alethic modalities.
    - Family resemblance: e.g., independence-dependence, isolatedness-interconnectiveness, universalness-relativeness, immanence-transcendence, autonomy-interdependency, internalness-externalness, etc.
    - Sources: From *FPHK*. See also my later books.

(continued on next page)

Table 4.4. The Syntax of Existential Dialectics I: The Principles (Part III)

- **In Relation to Method *(cont'd)***
  —*The Partiality-Totality Principle*
  (On the Relationships between Whole and Parts)
  - The whole is not the sum of the parts. There is no partiality without totality—and vice versa.
  - Any inquiry about a phenomenon in the work is to guard against the varieties of (a) reductionism and (b) reverse-reductionism.
  - Reductionism and reverse-reductionism can be (i) conceptual, (ii) theoretical, (iii) methodological, and (iv) ontological.
  - Works on emergence (as in *FC*), gestalt psychology (as in *FPHGEOL*), the hermeneutic circle (as in *FPHDA*), and mental language (as in *FPHSEM*), to name just a few of them, have contributed to the understanding of whole and parts.
  - Family resemblance: e.g., individualisticness-holisticness, partness-wholeness, analysis-synthesis, etc.
  - Sources: Especially from *FC* & *FPHGEOL*. See also my later books.

(continued on next page)

Table 4.4. The Syntax of Existential Dialectics I: The Principles (Part IV)

- **In Relation to Method** ***(cont'd)***

  —*The Predictability-Unpredictability Principle*

  (On the Occurrence of Events)

  - Both predictability and unpredictability have a major role to play in the occurrence of things, so that neither determinism nor indeterminism wins the centuries-old fight. There is no predictability without unpredictability—and vice versa.
  - There are events which are predictable, just as there are those which are not. Or what is regarded as unpredictable at one point in time may turn out to be predictable later, and, conversely, what is deemed as predictable may turn out to not be so predictable. Even in predictability, outcomes are subject to uncertainty, the degree of which varies from case to case.
  - Works on complexity theory (as in *FC*), quantum mechanics (as in *FPHST* and *FPHG*), frequency probability, subjective (or Bayesian) probability (as in *FPHPROB*), "special causes" (as in *FPHGAM*), and measurement uncertainty (as in *FPHPROB*), just to name a few of them, have contributed to the understanding of uncertainity.
  - The predictability-unpredictability principle is not to be confused with the absoluteness-relativeness principle; although both can address the issue of probability, the former is concerned with the extent of certainty in prediction, whereas the latter focuses on the relativity of viewpoints.
  - Family resemblance: e.g., sureness-arbitrariness, certainty-uncertainty, deterministicness-indeterministicness, sureness-doubtfulness, likeliness-riskiness, deterministicness-randomness, reliability-unreliability, etc.
  - Sources: Especially from *FC* & *FPHGAM*. See also my later books.

(continued on next page)

Table 4.4. The Syntax of Existential Dialectics I: The Principles (Part V)

- **In Relation to Method *(cont'd)***
  - —*The Explicability-Inexplicability Principle (On the Underlying Mechanisms of Things)*
    - Both explicability and inexplicability are part of the understanding of things. There is no explicability without inexplicability—and vice versa.
    - This principle tells us the duality of the research dilemma, in that, if reality can be explained in some ways, it also has its other ways which are not quite explainable, at a given point in time.
    - Family resemblance: e.g., underlyingness-regularness, causation-regularness, causation-correlation, explanation-description, explanation-narration, explanation-interpretation, etc.
    - Sources: Especially from *FPHU*—and also *FPHC*. See also my later books.
  - —*The Fiction-Reality Principle (On the different faces of Reality)*
    - If there is reality, there is also fiction, especially for any agent with some kind of intelligence life, be it about humans, animals, or, later, post-humans. There is no reality without fiction—and vice versa.
    - The distinction between reality and fiction is not absolute, since there can be a mixture of both. Fiction can have non-fictional elements, just as non-fiction can have fictional ones. So, the distinction is in degree, not in kind.
    - Family resemblance: e.g., fiction-nonfiction, fiction-fact, imagination-fact, subjectivity-objectivity, imagination-nonfiction, inaccuracy-accuracy, etc.
    - Sources: First from *FPHLIT*.

(continued on next page)

Table 4.4. The Syntax of Existential Dialectics I: The Principles (Part VI)

- **In Relation to Method *(cont'd)***
  —The Cognitiveness-Noncognitiveness Principle
  (On the Understanding of Meaning)
  - If a view of things is based on reason and evidences, it is also affected by non-cognitive factors (such that it is neither true nor false in the latter case)—and vice versa. In other words, there is no cognitiveness without noncognitiveness—and vice versa.
  - Noncognitive factors can come in all shapes and sizes, and good examples include envy, jealousy, power, nationality, race, gender, age, class, greed, lust, status, faith, anger, sadness, joy, fear, wish, etc.
  - Communication, even in its ideal type, is seldom solely based reason and evidences, as falsely assumed during the Age of the Enlightenment and its continued supporters nowadays. What is understood about something is often twisted on the basis of something else too. In these cases, what is at stake is often neither true nor false (which is something that classical logic has sidelined and ignored).
  - Family resemblance: e.g., proposition-attitude, cognition-emotion, cognition-prescription, justification-nonjustification, theory-extratheory, etc.
  - Sources: First from *BNR*.

(continued on next page)

Table 4.4. The Syntax of Existential Dialectics I: The Principles (Part VII)

- **In Relation to Structure**
  —*The Finiteness-Transfiniteness Principle*
  (On the Nature of Numbers)
  - If there are finite things, there are likewise transfinite ones. There is no finiteness without transfiniteness—and vice versa.
  - To avoid confusion, my usage of the word "transfinite" here differs radically from the one used by Cantor (and other mathematicians) for "relative" infinity—and is more limited, in light of the problems confronting any attempt to understand the idea of infinity, be it by intuition, imagination, and conception (as detailedly analyzed in *Sec. 2.2.3* of *FPHG*).
  - Instead, by "transfinity," I allow numbers which can be many times larger—or smaller, for that matter—than the finite things that we encounter in daily life, but they do not have to be related to the idea of infinity at all (which may not exist).
  - Of course, there may be some *borderline* cases, in which it is not clear whether the number in question is transfinite (in my usage) or simply a mathematical convenience. A good example of a borderline case is the Planck unit of length for "the smallest space possibly measured in nature," which is "less than billionths of trillionths of trillionths of an inch" (or something like 1.6×10^{-35} meters).
  - That said—my usage of "transfinity" can also resolve (or better, dissolve) an age-old problem in philosophy known as "Zeno's paradoxes" (as already explained in *Sec. 2.2.3* of *FPHG*).
  - Family resemblance: e.g., boundedness-quasiunboundedness, smallness-largeness, boundedness-unboundedness, etc.
  - Source: From *FPHG*. See also my later books.

(continued on next page)

**Table 4.4. The Syntax of Existential Dialectics I:
The Principles
(Part VIII)**

• **In Relation to Structure *(cont'd)***
 —*The Preciseness-Vagueness Principle*
 (On the Refinement of Things)
 • Both preciseness and vagueness are important, not that one is better than the other, but that both are used, in different degrees of preference, in accordance to the contextual application from the perspectives of nature, the mind, culture, and society. Even when both are used in a combination, the dilemma is shifted instead to one of combinational concern. There is no preciseness without vagueness—and vice versa.
 • In relation to taxonomy, preciseness has its taxonomic clarity, just as vagueness has its classificatory flexibility, for instance. And in relation to network, vagueness has its explorative liberty, just as preciseness has its conceptual definitiveness, for instance.
 • Family resemblance: e.g., clarity-ambiguity, directness-indirectness, quantitativeness-qualitativeness, describability-nondescribability, sharpness-roughness, specificity-generality, concreteness-abstractness, specificity-obscurity, translatability-untranslatability, clearcutness-transitionalness, etc.
 • Sources: Especially from *FIA* and *FPHMORP*. See also my later books.

(continued on next page)

Table 4.4. The Syntax of Existential Dialectics I: The Principles (Part IX)

- **In Relation to Structure *(cont'd)***
  —*The Simpleness-Complicatedness Principle*
  (On the Interconnection among Things)
  - Both simpleness and complicatedness are vital, without favoring one over the other, in that each is utilized, depending on the basis of the perspectives of nature, the mind, culture, and society. And even when a combination of them is preferred, the dilemma is only shifted to a combinational degree of concern. There is no simpleness without complicatedness—and vice versa.
  - For illustration, in relation to taxonomy, simpleness has its heuristic usefulness, just as complicatedness has its realistic representation, for instance. In relation to network, simpleness has its economical attractiveness, just as complicatedness has its practical reliability, for instance. And in relation to logic, there is the simple zeroth-order logic, just as there is the complicated higher-order logic.
  - Family resemblance: e.g., inflexibility-flexibility, standardization-specialization, imperfectness-perfectness, superficiality-depth, shallowness-deepness, economicalness-elaboratedness, plainness-circumspection, onesidedness-multisidedness, succinctness-duplicatedness, simpleness-sophisticatedness, crudeness-subtleness, etc.
  - Sources: Especially from *FIA* and *FPHPROB*. See also my later books.

(continued on next page)

Table 4.4. The Syntax of Existential Dialectics I:
The Principles
(Part X)

- **In Relation to Structure *(cont'd)***
  —*The Openness-Hiddenness Principle*
  (On the Detection of Things)
  - Reality has its hidden face, just as it is open to outside view in some other ways. There is no openness without hiddenness—and vice versa.
  - For instance, in the context of anomalous experience, certain aspects of reality can be open for examination (e.g., the experiment with SPECT images, the transmission of telepathemic bit, and the use of metonymies and metaphors). Other aspects, however, remain hidden, and examples include the elusive deeper nature of spiritual reality in the intangible realm, the undetectability of different branched universes, the underlying mechanisms of signals traveling between different folds of physical space-time, and the dependence on language and the bias for science and logic).
  - Family resemblance: e.g., overtness-covertness, publicness-privateness, openness-closedness, transparency-secrecy, openness-biasedness, participation-obstruction, exposition-illusion, surface-depth, etc.
  - Sources: Especially from *FPHU*. See also my later books.

(continued on next page)

Table 4.4. The Syntax of Existential Dialectics I: The Principles (Part XI)

- **In Relation to Structure *(cont'd)***
  —*The Denseness-Emptiness Principle*
  (On the Distribution of Entities in Space)
  - Both density and void are needed, in relation to the mind, nature, culture, and society, albeit in different ways. There is no denseness without emptiness—and vice versa.
  - For clarity, the term "void" is used here only as an approximation of emptiness (depending on the degree of the lack of density), since, in physics, it is well known that "empty" space is not really empty all the way, because it can be full of energy (e.g., random quantum fluctuations at the sub-atomic level, and, for that matter, dark energy in the universe) and matter (e.g., different versions of sub-atomic particles, and, for that matter, dark matter in the universe).
  - Family resemblance: e.g., fullness-voidness, nearness-farness, concentration-dispersion, denseness-nothingness, presence-absence, focus-unfocus, solidness-void, something-nothing, heaviness-lightness, composition-emptiness, emphasis-disemphasis, etc.
  - Sources: First worked out in *FPHUP*. See also my later books.

(continued on next page)

Table 4.4. The Syntax of Existential Dialectics I: The Principles (Part XII)

- **In Relation to Process**

—*The Prototypicality-Variation Principle*
(On the Nature of Duplication)

- If there are prototypes, there are also variants of the copies. There is no prototypicality without variation—and vice versa.
- Prototypes and their copies are not static and may change or die out over time, but new ones may emerge.
- Some copies may have multiple prototypes, not just one.
- It can be very challenging to trace some copies back to their prototypes, under certain difficult historical conditions.
- Copies are not solely identical duplications of prototypes but have their own variations (mutations).
- Family resemblance: e.g., archetypicality-descendedness, origin-descendedness, ancestry-descendedness, prototypicality-duplication, archetypicality-mutation, origin-reenactment, prototypicality-recreation, prototypicality-copyness, and the like.
- Sources: First worked out in *FPHMORP*. See also my later books.

—*The Change-Constancy Principle*
(On the Alteration of Things)

- Change occurs over time, although constancy is also allowed. There is no change without constancy—and vice versa.
- Asymmetry undergoes changes over time, so does symmetry.
- Old players fade away, and new ones emerges, with ever new causes and ever new forms.
- Family resemblance: e.g., dynamicness-staticness, instability-stability, etc.
- Sources: First named in *BCPC*. Especially from *FHC*, *FCD*, and *FPHC*. See also other books of mine (from that point on).

(continued on next page)

Table 4.4. The Syntax of Existential Dialectics I: The Principles (Part XIII)

- **In Relation to Process *(cont'd)***
  —*The Order-Chaos Principle*
  (On the Pattern of Things)
  - Both order and chaos are vital in the process of change in the world. The preference for order is biased, since it does not give sufficient attention to the vital role of chaos in the transformation of the world (without somehow reducing it for the understanding of order). There is no order without chaos—and vice versa.
  - The scientific search for order in the world is often a hidden bias in its ontological obsession with order, since chaos is often treated as the "bad" guy, with order as the "good" guy (for the end goal of science).
  - Neither order nor chaos is the final end of the world, and one is not to be treated as the means for the other in the transformation of things. Both are fundamental in their recurrent dialectical interactions with each other over time, without reducing one for the other.
  - Order has its different forms (e.g., ascending vs. descending order in mathematics, and feeding vs. bleeding order in morphology), just as chaos has its own versions (e.g., as understood differently in chaos theory vs. complexity theory).
  - Family resemblance: e.g., lawfulness-disorder, order-disorder, linearity-nonlinearity, linearity-irreversalness, pattern-chaos, unity-disunity, etc.
  - Sources: Especially from *FC*. See also my later books.

(continued on next page)

Table 4.4. The Syntax of Existential Dialectics I: The Principles (Part XIV)

- **In Relation to Process *(cont'd)***
  - —*The Slowness-Quickness Principle*
    (On the Speed of Change)
    - Both slowness and quickness co-exist, with their own internal tension, to the extent that each fights for its own relevance with the other, in accordance to the perspectives of nature, the mind, culture, and society, without one being the victor and the other being the vanquished in the long haul. Even when both are chosen in other cases, this dilemma is only transferred into something else with a combinational character. There is no slowness without quickness—and vice versa.
    - In relation to taxonomy, quickness has its efficient usability, just as slowness has its aesthetic appeal, for instance. And in relation to network, quickness has its adventurous readiness, just as slowness has its risk-adverse convenience, for instance.
    - Family resemblance: e.g., inconvenience-convenience, passiveness-activenessness, gradualness-abruptness, deceleration-acceleration, difficulty-ease, nonresilience-resilience, patience-impatience, etc.
    - Sources: Especially from *FIA*. See also my later books.

(continued on next page)

Table 4.4. The Syntax of Existential Dialectics I: The Principles (Part XV)

- **In Relation to Process *(cont'd)***
  —*The Expansion-Contraction Principle*
  (On the Growth of Things)
  - Entities in the world can both expand in some ways and contract in other ones, as part of their nature. There is no expansion without contraction—and vice versa.
  - For instance, in the context of anomalous experience, one of its most fascinating expressions is none other than the analysis of different causes of the slow but steady expansion (and, furthermore, if put in a different way, unfolding) of unconsciousness.
  - Family resemblance: e.g., conquest-autarky, rise-fall, spread-shrink, extendingness-shorteningness, widening-narrowing, expansion-destruction, expansion-decline, construction-demolition, creation-destruction, construction-deconstruction, expansion-contraction, expansion-constriction, etc.
  - Sources: Especially from *FPHU*. See also my later books.

(continued on next page)

Table 4.4. The Syntax of Existential Dialectics I: The Principles (Part XVI)

- **In Relation to Process *(cont'd)***
  —*The Optimality-Nonoptimality Principle*
  (On the Nature of Highly Favorable Options)
  - Both optimality and non-optimality are important, in relation to the mind, nature, culture, and society, albeit in different ways. There is no optimality without nonoptimality—and vice versa.
  - Optimality (in terms of highly favorable options) is not perfect and can be realized in different degrees.
  - "Maximization" does not necessarily entail "optimization," as shown in the problem of "negative externalities" in economics.
  - Non-optimality can come in all shapes and sizes, in different degrees, like "maximizing" in economics vs. "satisficing" in sociology.
  - Optimality can be more feasible in the longer term of technological improvement.
  - Optimality should not be confused with the beauty of simplicity, since the more optimal a process is, the more complicated (not necessarily the simpler) it can be.
  - Family resemblance: e.g., optimality-satisfaction, optimality-maximization, optimality-heuristicness, idealness-realisticness, and the like.
  - Sources: First worked out in *FPHMORP*. See also my later books.

(continued on next page)

Table 4.4. The Syntax of Existential Dialectics I: The Principles (Part XVII)

- **In Relation to Agency**
  —*The Theory-Praxis Principle*
  (On the Duality of Knowledge))
  - This has to do with the duality of knowledge in existential dialectics, in that, if there is theoretical construction, there is likewise its practical application, both technical and normative. There is no theory without praxis—and vice versa.
  - Family resemblance: e.g., discovery-application, knowledge-action, invention-innovation, knowledge-motivation, theory-intentionality, universality-particularity, discourse-action, knowledge-interest, potentiality-actuality, theory-practice, etc.
  - Source: Especially from *FPHE*. See also my later books.

(continued on next page)

Table 4.4. The Syntax of Existential Dialectics I: The Principles (Part XVIII)

- **In Relation to Agency *(cont'd)***
  —*The Convention-Novelty Principle*
  (On the Nature of Creative Thinking)
  - If there is conventional wisdom, there is likewise novel challenge, to the extent that both convergent and divergent thinking are part of life. There is no convention without novelty—and vice versa.
  - In addition, in this context of the convention-novelty principle, there are, in the absence of better words, what I want to call (a) *creative techniques* and (b) *creative traits*, which, when satisfied—in relation to the larger context of the mind, nature, society, and culture—can be used to enhance creative works. The list of creative techniques and traits (as summarized in *Table 4.1* of *FPHCT*) are not exhaustive, of course, but the examples here constitute a great beginning of understanding the structure of creative thinking.
  - Yet, lest the reader gets carried away by the euphoria about creative thinking in our time, it should be reminded that creative thinking has its own possibilities and limits (as shown in *Table 2.1* of *FPHCT* on invention), just as it has its own promises and pitfalls (as shown in *Table 3.1* of *FPHCT* on innovation). In the end, it should also be stressed that creative thinking has its own desirability and dark sides (as shown in *Table 4.2* of *FPHCT, BNN*, and *FPHMIG*).
  - This has important daily implications for an average individual, and the word "average" here allows different degrees of variation from one individual to another in a population, at any given point in history.
  - Family resemblance: e.g., normalness-nonnormalness, conformity-nonconformity, convergence-divergence, familiarity-freshness, inertia-newness, equilibrium-disturbance, etc.
  - Sources: First from *FPHCT*. See also my later books.

(*continued on next page*)

Table 4.4. The Syntax of Existential Dialectics I: The Principles (Part XIX)

- **In Relation to Agency** ***(cont'd)***

  —*The Evolution-Transformation Principle*

  (On the Multiple Kinds of Agency)

  - This principle (and the symmetry-asymmetry principle) are both about *the agency of change*. The word "agency," in a formal definition, refers to "a person or thing through which power is exerted or an end is achieved." (MWD 2007b) It therefore does not have to necessarily involve an intelligent lifeform.
  - Because of this dual meaning in agency, the evolution-transformation principle is more concerned with *the multiple kinds of agency*, that is, both about the *evolution* in the state of nature (e.g., an object of natural beauty) and the *transformation* in the world of intelligent lifeforms (e.g., a work of art, an air-conditioner, etc.). There is no evolution without transformation—and vice versa.
  - And the transformative part of the principle precisely refers to the other dimension in the dual meaning of agency, in giving technology a major role to play in the change of the world, which is something that I extensively analyzed in *FHC* in the context of the technophilic lifeworld, espeically though not exclusively since modern times. The same theme is also elaborated in other books of mine.
  - Family resemblance: e.g., nonwillingness-willingness, naturalness-technologicalness, evolution-creation, naturalness-nonnaturalness, inorganicness-volition, naturalness-artificialness, inorganicness-motivation, etc.
  - Sources: Especially from *FAE*. See also other books of mine.

(*continued on next page*)

Table 4.4. The Syntax of Existential Dialectics I: The Principles (Part XX)

- **In Relation to Agency *(cont'd)***
  —*The Symmetry-Asymmetry Principle*
  (On the Relationships among Existents)
  - There is no symmetry without asymmetry—and vice versa.
  - For instance, the Same can be symmetric and asymmetric towards the Others. But in case of asymmetry, oppression and self-oppression can occur. So, when the Same is asymmetric towards the Others, the Same can also be relatively asymmetric towards itself in self-oppression, just as the Others can be likewise towards themselves.
  - The subsequent oppressiveness is dualistic, as much by the Same against the Others and itself, as by the Others against the Same and themselves.
  - Both oppression and self-oppression can be achieved by way of downgrading differences between the Same and the Others and of accentuating them.
  - This is true, even though not all forms of asymmetry have to be about oppression and self-oppression.
  - In addition, from Chapter Three of *FPHG*, symmetry is not perfect, to be understood in an approximate sense under many life circumstances.
  - Family resemblance: e.g., balance-extremity, reflexiveness-unreflexiveness, balance-unbalance, equality-inequality, center-periphery, compatibility-incompatibility, proportion-disproportion, harmoniousness-unharrmoniousness, etc.
  - Sources: From all my books, starting with *FHC*. First named in *BCPC*. See, for instance, *FCD* for more details on the Same and the Others.

(*continued on next page*)

Table 4.4. The Syntax of Existential Dialectics I: The Principles (Part XXI)

- **In Relation to Agency** ***(cont'd)***
  —*The Softness-Hardness Principle*
  (On the Force of Change)
  - This has to do with *the force of change* under the category about agency in existential dialectics, in that any change by an agent, be it organic (like humans) or non-organic (like natural objects), can occur in a forceful (aggressive) or gentle (pacific) way, which can come in all shapes and sizes, of course. There is no softness without hardness—and vice versa.
  - Family resemblance: e.g., peacefulness-violence, cooperation-competition, acceptance-discrimination, love-hatred, peace-war, pacificity-aggression, dovishness-hawkishness, reward-punishment, kindness-hostility, admiration-belittlement, inclusion-exclusion, friendliness-unfriendliness, like-dislike, etc.
  - Sources: Especially from *ALD*. See also my later books.

(continued on next page)

Table 4.4. The Syntax of Existential Dialectics I: The Principles (Part XXII)

• **In Relation to Agency** ***(cont'd)***

—*The Seriousness-Playfulness Principle*

(On the Extent of Seriousness)

- If there is seriousness, there is also playfulness, especially for any agent with some kind of intelligence life, be it about humans, animals, or, later, post-humans. There is no seriousness without playfulness—and vice versa.
- Lest any misunderstanding occurs, the word "playfulness" here should not be confused with other terms like "laughter," "smile," "joke," "tickleness," and "laugh-like vocalization" (in some animals), for instance.
- Being playful can come in all shapes and sizes and therefore is not necessarily tied up with any of these terms, alhough it can result from any of them, or a combination of them, or something else altogether.
- This principle, together with some other principles (especially though not exclusively, like the formalness-informalness principle), have important implications for what constitutes rationality, be it about "rationality of application" at the practical level or "rationality of knowledge" at the meta-theoretical level (as summarized in *Sec. 4.20* of *FPHH*).
- Family resemblance: e.g., seriousness-jokingness, seriousness-humorousness, seriousness-wittiness, seriousness-nonseriousness, seriousness-relaxedness, seriousness-restingness, Apollo-Dionysus, etc.
- Sources: First from *FPHH* & *FPHGAM* See also my later books.

(*continued on next page*)

Table 4.4. The Syntax of Existential Dialectics I: The Principles (Part XXIII)

- **In Relation to Agency *(cont'd)***
  —*The Activeness-Inactiveness Principle*
  (On the Extent of Activeness)
  - If there is activeness, there is also inactiveness, especially (though not exclusively) for any agent with some kind of intelligence life, be it about humans, animals, or, later, post-humans. There is no activeness without inactiveness—and vice versa.
  - Being active can come in all shapes and sizes, as a person can be inactive because he is tired, old, sick, sleepy, uninterested, etc., just as an object can be inactive because it is at rest, out of work, etc.
  - This principle, together with some other principles (especially though not exclusively, like the formalness-informalness principle and seriousness-playfulness principle), have important implications for what constitutes rationality, be it about "rationality of application" at the practical level or "rationality of knowledge" at the meta-theoretical level (as summarized in *Sec. 4.20* of *FPHH*).
    - Family resemblance: e.g., alertness-unalertness, activeness-decrepidness, alertness-sleepiness, awakenness-hibernatedness, activeness-tiredness, alertness-uninterestedness, alertness-unwareness, soberness-unawareness, soberness-inactiveness, alertness-inactiveness, etc.
  - Sources: First from *FPHTRAN.*

(*continued on next page*)

Table 4.4. The Syntax of Existential Dialectics I: The Principles (Part XXIV)

- **In Relation to Agency *(cont'd)***
  - —*The Selfness-Otherness Principle*
    (On the Magnitude of Self-Centeredness)
    - If there is the tendency to be mostly centered on one's self or group, there is likewise the tendency to be mostly centered on others, especially (though not exclusively) for any agent with some kind of intelligence life, be it about humans, animals, or, later, post-humans. There is no selfness without otherness—and vice versa.
    - Being self-centered and being other-centered do not have to be mutually exclusive, as the two can come in all shapes and sizes, or in different degrees. And other-centeredness does not entail desirability, any more than self-centeredness implies non-desirability, as both can go either way.
    - In addition, whether self-centeredness constitutes a moral alternative or, conversely, an alternative to morality is of course debatable (as addressed in my other book titled *Beyond Ethics to Post-Ethics*).
    - Good examples of family resemblance in relation to the principle are egoisticness-altruisticness, selfishness-unselfishness, selfness-selflessness, egocentricness-othercentricness, and so on.
    - Source: First from *FPHCA*

(*continued on next page*)

Table 4.4. The Syntax of Existential Dialectics I: The Principles (Part XXV)

- **In Relation to Outcome**

—*The Regression-Progression Principle (On the Direction of History)*

- Neither the cyclical nor the linear views are adequate for explaining many phenomena at all levels. There is regression without progression—and vice versa.
- History progresses to more advanced forms, but with a regressive touch. Examples include no freedom without unfreedom, no equality without inequality, and no civilization without barbarity.
- This is not an inevitable law, but merely a highly likely empirical trend.
- Family resemblance: e.g., cost-benefit, undesirability-desirability, badness-goodness, risk-opportunity, dysfunctionality-functionality, cyclicity-linearity, etc.
- Sources: From all my books, starting with *FHC*. First named in *BCPC*.

—*The Same-Difference Principle (On the Metamorphosis of Change)*

- An entity, as it evolves over time, can be both different from and similar to its opposing alternatives and does not have to be solely more different from them over time. There is no similarity without difference—and vice versa.
- Opposites are not absolute in a black-or-white fashion; so, an entity can become relatively more similar to (or more different from) its opposite over time.
- Family resemblance: e.g., homogeneity-heterogeneity, we-they, similarity-contrast, etc.
- Sources: Especially from ALD. See also my later books

(*continued on next page*)

Table 4.4. The Syntax of Existential Dialectics I:
The Principles
(Part XXVI)

- **In Relation to Outcome** ***(cont'd)***
  —*The Stability-Reaction Principle*
  (On the Feedback Mechanism for Further Changes)
  - Once an outcome becomes stabilized over time (which varies from case to case), it will undergo further changes in its multifaceted interactions with the outside world (e.g., with other entities, energy, space, and so on).
  - There is no stability without reaction for further changes—and vice versa.
  - Family resemblance: e.g., stability-forwardness, balance-reaction, balance-forwardness, rest-motion, normalcy-feedback, stability-breakup, consolidation-modification, etc.
  - Sources: First from *FPHCHEM.*

(*continued on next page*)

Table 4.4. The Syntax of Existential Dialectics I: The Principles (Part XXVII)

- **In Relation to Outcome** ***(cont'd)***
  - —*The Functionality-Nonfunctionality Principle*
    (On the Presence of Function)
    - If there is the presence of action for which something or someone is fitted, there is likewise the relative lack of action for which something or someone is fitted. There is no functionality without nonfunctionallity—and vice versa.
    - A *function* should not be confused with an *alternative function,* which is just another kind of function; just as *nonfunction* should not be confused with *dysfunction* (which has more to do with malfunction and is thus related more to the regression-progression principle).
    - In addition, being functional (or useful) and being nonfunctional (or useless) do not have to be mutually exclusive, as the two can come in all shapes and sizes, or in different degrees. And what is functional at one time may become nonfunctional at another time, and vice-versa.
    - Good examples of family resemblance in relation to the principle are usefulness-nonusefulness, usefulness-uselessness, valueness-nonvalueness, and the like.
    - Source: First from *FPHCA*

(*continued on next page*)

Table 4.4. The Syntax of Existential Dialectics I: The Principles (Part XXVIII)

- **In Relation to Outcome *(cont'd)***
  —*The Intentionality-Nonintentionality Principle*
  (On the Planning for Outcomes)
  - If there is the planning or design of something for a certain outcome, there is likewise the relative absence of planning or design of something for a certain outcome. There is no intentionality without nonintentionallity—and vice versa.
  - An intention for an outcome does not have to be certain, so the outcome can even be counter-intentional in being the opposite of what was originally planned. In this sense, counter-intentionality is a special case of non-intentionality; in other words, there are unintented consequences which can be just the opposite of what was originally planned.
  - An intention for an outcome is mostly relevant to intelligent life, but there are non-intelligent life and non-living matter in the universe too, so nonintentionality is also important.
  - In addition, an intention does not have to be obvious or straightforward, as William Shakspeare once famously said: "I must be cruel only to be kind."
  - Good examples of family resemblance in relation to the principle are purposiveness-nonpurposiveness, intention-accidentalness, design-randomness, etc.
  - Source: First from *FPHW*

(*continued on next page*)

**Table 4.4. The Syntax of Existential Dialectics I:
The Principles
(Part XXIX)**

- **In Relation to Outcome** ***(cont'd)***
  —*The Survivability-Nonsurvivability Principle*
  (On the Survival of things)
  - If there are some entities which survive at certain times, there are likewise other entities which do not survive. There is no survivability without nonsurvivability—and vice versa. In nature, for illustration, there are some animals which survive in hard times, whereas others do not—and this is true, not just among different species but also among different members of the same species (and the phenomenon of "selection" in evolutionary biology has much to say on this, as already addressed in *BNN*).
  - Of course, the principle is not restricted solely to the animal world, since it can be used to other cases concerning non-animals too (e.g., trees, lakes, etc. in the natural world—or empires, companies, etc. in the human world).
  - But one should not confuse this principle with the expansion-contraction principle, since those entities which survive, say, can still expand or contract over time (e.g., those animals which survive can be more capable in some activities but not in others, for instance).
  - Nor should this principle be confused with the stability-reaction principle, in that the condition of survivability or non-survivability may lead to further changes later on (as shown in the emergence of new species after the extinction of some old ones, as already explained in *BNR*).
  - Good examples of family resemblance in relation to the principle are survival-extinction, life-death, existence-nonexistence, and the like.
  - Source: First from *FPHPROB*

Notes: The examples here are solely illustrative (not exhaustive). The comparison is also relative (not absolute), nor are they mutually exclusive. As generalities, they allow exceptions.

Table 4.5. The Syntax of Existential Dialectics II: The Principles as Short Cuts (Part I)

• The principles should be treated with caution, lest misunderstanding occurs, since they do not constitute rigid dualities (or dichotomies).

• The reason is that each pair in an ontological principle consists of two opposites, which are, however, merely short cuts both for multiple variations and degrees, as well as for different interactions with multiple other entities unlike them. In this light, each pair can end up having hundred (or even thousand, if not more) different versions, which interact with hundred (or even thousand, if not more) other entities. There are two clarifications here.

• Firstly, this conception of shortcuts is not mutually exclusive nor absolute, in that the opposites can come in all shapes and sizes, with different degrees. For instance, by analogy, just as there are different degrees of the two colors "white" and "black"—there are likewise different degrees of the opposites in each ontological pair, to the extent that there can be multiple entities (not only two) interacting with each other in each pair.

• And secondly, this conception of shortcuts do not ignore other possible entities in interacting with the two opposites (with their different versions) in each pair. For instance, by analogy, there are not only the two colors "white" and "black" as opposites, since there are other colors too besides them like "yellow," "green," "purple," or else. The same logic can be applied to each ontological pair, in that they also interact with other entities, not with only two of them (with their different versions).

• Therefore, with these two clarifications in mind—each pair in an ontological principle serves only as an abbreviation for something more complicated and, therefore, although it contains two opposites, it should not be confused as a duality (dualism).

(continued on next page)

Table 4.5. The Syntax of Existential Dialectics II: The Principles as Short Cuts (Part II)

• Existential dialectics rejects any dualism (or dichotomy) as too rigid and instead allows the multiplicity of entities, to the extent that between the two opposites in each pair exist many other alternatives to choose from. They are named in that short form for aesthetic elegance, instead of listing all possible entities between the two opposites in the title.

• To be dialectic is to go beyond any rigid dichotomy and transcend into something different altogether in the long haul. One may be tempted to call the dialectic logic here with a different name like existential "multilectics" (instead of "dialectics"), but this naming is incorrect (or even misleading), for the two reasons aforestated.

• After all, each ontological pair come in all shapes and sizes (with different degrees) and do not exist by themselves but also interact with other entities unlike them. The virtue of revealing an ontological pair is to show how they relate within themselves (in multiple versions) and also interact with others unlike them (also in multiple versions).

• This will be clear in the table on "the dialectic constraints imposed by the principles."

Source: From Ch.1 of *FPHK*

Table 4.6. The Syntax of Existential Dialectics III: The Principles as Family Resemblances

• Each ontological principle is generic, with some other comparable ontological pairs to be put in the same family (like a *family resemblance*). Ludwig Wittgenstein (1953) once suggested the idea of "family resemblance" in explaining different games classified under the same family called *games*.

• Why should, for instance, playing football and chess as playing "games," when it is well understood that football is not the same as chess? The answer is that, although each game is different and has different rules, many of them (though not all) share, more or less, some commonalites (e.g., scoring as necessary for winning).

• And this is so, even though some games share more than some others in any given selection of critieria, and no two games are exactly identical. So, his point here is that there is no essential core which is common to all games, and the best that one can look for is some characteristics which are common to many (but not all) games. (A. Biletzki 2006)

• By the same logic—in the previous section on selection criteria, the flexibility-inflexibility pair can be put in the family resemblance of the simpleness-complicatedness principle, although the two pairs are not exactly identical. Likewise, the directness-indirectness pair can be put in the family resemblance of the preciseness-vagueness principle, although, again, the two pairs are not exactly identical.

• In this sense, which specific pair in a family should be used to designate the name of the family can be at times a bit arbitrary, but with good reason.

• For illustration, in the context of method, the partiality-totality principle can take the different form like individualisticness-holisticness, just as the explicability-inexplicability principle can take the different form like underlyingness-regularness—although each two pairs are not exactly identical and have slightly different meanings and usages. A more comprehensive listing of this family resemblance for all other principles is shown in the table on the syntax of existential dialectics.

Source: From Ch.1 of *FPHK*

Table 4.7. The Syntax of Existential Dialectics IV: The Dialectic Constraints Imposed by the Principles (Part I)

- **Co-Existent and Asymmetric**

—The principles, as they constitute the syntax of existential dialectics, are dialectic in character, such that, when they are applied, they impose dialectic constraints on how reality is to be understood. Consider, say, the symmetry-asymmetry principle as an illustration here, in order to summarize two main characters of the dialectic constraints in question.

—Firstly, to be dialectic here is to go beyond the narrow dichotomies (and, for that matter, any rigid multi-dimensional classificatory scheme), be they about "self" vs. "world," "freedom" vs. "unfreedom," "barbarity" vs. "civilization," "individuality" vs. "communality," and so on.

—One way to do so (to go beyond) is to consider them all in terms of co-existence (without favoring one over the rest). For instance, my theory of "post-civilization" (to be summarized later in the section on the pragmatics of existential dialectics) is to go beyond barbarity and civilization in terms of understanding barbarity and civilization as being co-existent. And the same logic can be said in relation to my theories of "post-democracy," "post-capitalsm," and others (also to be introduced later in the section on the pragmatics of existential dialectics), in regard to freedom vs. unfreedom, equality vs. inequality, communality vs. individuality, spirituality vs. materiality, and so on.

—But to consider them all (in the dichotomies—and, for that matter, in any rigid multi-dimensional classifactory schme) as co-existent is not the same as to imply that the opposites in any classificatory scheme are all equal, since, in accordance to the symmetry-asymmetry principle (as an illustration here), if they are equal in terms of being considered as co-existent, they are asymmetric in terms of being unequal in dialectic interaction (e.g., X can be more dominant than Y in case A, or Y is more dominant than X in case B).

(continued on next page)

Table 4.7. The Syntax of Existential Dialectics IV: The Dialectic Constraints Imposed by the Principles (Part II)

—For this reason, there are different versions of "post-democracy" and "post-capitalism" in my theories. As an illustration, in version I of the theory of post-democracy, freedom is more dominant than equality, whereas in version II of the theory of post-democracy, equality is more so than freedom.

—But this "X more than Y" has to be understood in the context of dialectic logic (not in conventional logic), in that both "X" and "Y" are important in post-democracy (in the context of dialectic logic), but in an asymmetry way. By contrast, in conventional logic, it often favors one over the other—be it in regard to privileging freedom over equality in Fascism, favoring freedom relatively more than equality in Liberal Democracy, or favoring equality relatively more than freedom in Socialist Democracy. In the latter two cases (about Liberal Democracy and Socialist Democracy), the difference between dialectic logic and conventional logic can be one in degree, not in kind—in this sense, albeit not in other senses.

—The same logic can be said about the relatonships between individuality and communality, between spirituality and materiality, and between formal legalism and informal legalism in the different versions of my theory of post-capitalism.

• **Transcendent**

—Secondly, to be dialectic is to go beyond the narrow dichotomies (and, for that matter, any rigid multi-dimensional classificatory scheme) in another way, this time, in a transcendent way, that is, in exploring other possibilities or even other issues not considered within the narrow confines of narrow dichotomies (and, for that matter, any rigid multi-dimensional classificatory scheme).

(continued on next page)

Table 4.7. The Syntax of Existential Dialectics IV: The Dialectic Constraints Imposed by the Principles (Part III)

—As an analogy, to go beyond the narrow color dichotomy of "black" and "white" is not just to choose both "black" and "white" (as in the first meaning) but also to explore other color options (e.g., "green," "purple," "blue," etc.—and, alternatively, "shade," "line," "curve," etc.). By the same logic, to go beyond "democracy" is to transcend democracy (as in version III of the theory of "post-democracy") and to explore other possibilties of lifeforms (e.g., floating consciousness, hyper-spatial consciousness, etc., to live beyond the narrow obsession with freedom and equality).

—This dialectic character of the principles in existential dialectics has important implications for the pragmatics of existential dialectics (as will be clear shortly, in the section on the pragmatics of existential dialectics).

Notes: The examples here are solely illustrative (not exhaustive). The comparison is also relative (not absolute), nor are they mutually exclusive. As generalities, they allow exceptions.

Sources: First explicitly stated in *ALD*. Also from all other books of mine.

Table 4.8. The Syntax of Existential Dialectics V: Further Clarifications (Part I)

- **Pioneering**

—Firstly, the total number of ontological principles is unknown, to be discovered later, as our knowledge of the world becomes more advanced.

—Consequently, the principles as introduced in my books are not exhaustive, with new ones being added, whenever more of them are discovered in later research.

—At least, future generations can pick up where I leave off and continue the discovery.

—In this sense, my work should be treated as a pioneering effort for the development of a systematic, comprehensive analysis of a new general ontology for the future of knowledge.

- **Flexible**

—Secondly, the principles are not rigidly classified, as they can be reclassified in a different way.

—For instance, the preciseness-vagueness principle is classified under the category of "structure" but can be reclassified under the category of "method," although in so doing, it has a different meaning in the context of method.

—The same logic applies to the same-difference principle under the category of "outcome," which can be reclassified under the category of "structure," although in so doing, once more, it has a different meaning in the context of structure.

- **Mutually Constraining**

—Thirdly, the principles are to be understood together, not that each prinicple is to be analyzed independently of others. After all, the principles are mutually constraining, in that they work together as a whole.

(continued on next page)

Table 4.8. The Syntax of Existential Dialectics V: Further Clarifications (Part II)

- **Selectively Useful**
  —Fourthly, the principles are relevant to all subject matters, but some principles are more useful to some subject matters than others—as implied in the symmetry-asymmetry principle. This is true, even if different studies of the same kind can yield different views about the degree of relevance for each ontological principle, depending on the specific nature of a research in question, needless to say.

- **Anti-Reductionistic**
  —And fifthly, the principles constitute only two levels of analysis, this time, at the ontological and methodological levels—while other levels of analysis (from the perspectives of the mind, nature, society, and culture) are also needed, in order to understand reality in its totality (as explained in the section on "sophisticated methodological holism," so as to avoid the dual dangers of reductionism and reverse-reductionism).

Notes: The examples here are solely illustrative (not exhaustive). The comparison is also relative (not absolute), nor are they mutually exclusive. As generalities, they allow exceptions.
Sources: From my previous books like *FHC*, *FCD*, *FPHC*, *BDPD*, *BCPC*, *BNN*, *FC*, *FAE*, and so on.

Table 4.9. The Syntax of Existential Dialectics VI: The Dilemma of Specific vs. General Ontology (Part I)

• Ontology is often more complicated and imposes some seemingly insurmountable difficulties concerning what constitutes a kind of ontology which can be valid enough to be accepted by the wider intellectual community in question. An excellent example concerns what I want to call *the dilemma of ontology* in relation to the relationship between "specific ontology" and "general ontology." (M. Bunge 1999; R. Corazzon 2007)

• On the one hand, "general ontology," as Mario Bunge (1999) put it, "studies all existents." But, on the other hand, "special ontology studies one genus of thing or process—physical, chemical, biological, social, etc." (M. Bunge 1999; R. Corazzon 2007)

• Consequently, the relationship between the former and the latter is that, as an illustration, "whereas general ontology studies the concepts of space, time, and event, the ontology of the social investigates such general sociological concepts as those of social system, social structure, and social change." (M. Bunge 1999; R. Corazzon 2007)

• With this formal definition in mind, the relationship between the two forms of ontology only poses *the dilemma of ontology*, in that general ontology is possible to the extent that its general contructs must be broad enough to serve as the "lowest common denominator" for all disciplines, but this character of the lowest common denominator is not only hard to find but also its usefulness is limited. (WK 2008b)

• But specific ontology fares no better either, in that its specific constructs primarily serve a specific discipline in question, although other disciplines can appropriate them for their own purposes, but in a different context (especially, though not exclusively, when used as a metaphor from one field to another). For instance, the Kantian category of understanding under the heading of "quantity" constitutes a type of specific ontology, which is specific to the discipline of mathematics, although other disciplines can make use of the categories in their own context.

(continued on next page)

Table 4.9. The Syntax of Existential Dialectics VI: The Dilemma of Specific vs. General Ontology (Part II)

• A solution lies in my proposal of "sophisticated methodological holism," which requires all levels of analysis in any subject matter. See the tables on sophisticated methodological holism, and on reductionism and reverse-reductionism, for more details.

Source: From *Sec. 1.4* of *FPHK*

Table 4.10. The Syntax of Existential Dialectics VII: Types of Inappropriate Family Resemblances (Part I)

- **Inadequate Family Resemblances**
  —Ex: consistency-inconsistency: the formalness-informalenss principle
  —Ex: cognition-noncognition: the formalness-informalness principle

- **Compound Family Resemblances**
  —Ex: reality-nonreality: the formalness-informalness principles, the absoluteness-relativeness principle
  —Ex: normality-abnormality: the symmetry-asymmetry principle, the density-emptiness principle, the convention-novelty principle, the same-difference principle
  —Ex: structure-context: the simpleness-complicatedness principle, the theory-praxis principle
  —Ex: freedom-unfreedom: the expansion-contraction principle
  —Ex: morality-immorality: the denseness-emptiness principle, the symmetry-asymmetry, the same-difference principle
  —Ex: particularness-universalness: the preciseness-vagueness principle, the simpleness-complicatedness principle
  —Ex: pureness-mixedness: the absoluteness-relativeness principle, the simpleness-complicatedness principle, the same-difference principle
  —Ex: shortsightedness-foresightedness: the partiality-totality principle, the simpleness-complicatedness principle
  —Ex: shorttermness-longtermness: the partiality-totality principle, the simpleness-complicatedness principle, the slowness-quickness principle

- **One-Sided Family Resemblances**
  —Ex: sound-silence: asymmetry (in the symmetry-asymmetry principle)
  —Ex: vision-blindness: asymmetry (in the symmetry-asymmetry principle)

(continued on next page)

Table 4.10. The Syntax of Existential Dialectics VII: Types of Inappropriate Family Resemblances (Part II)

- **Vague Family Resemblances**
  —Ex: shortness-longness, narrowness-broadness, smallness-largeness, smallness-greatness, microness-macroness, and littleness-muchness: three different possibilities, namely, (a) finiteness (in the finiteness-transfiniteness principle), if both opposites are defined on a finite scale, (b) transfiniteness (in the finiteness-transfiniteness principle) if both opposites are defined on a transfinite scale, and (c) the finiteness-transfiniteness principle if one opposite is defined on a finite scale and the other opposite is defined on a transfinite scale.

- **One-Sided and Compound Family Resemblances**
  —Ex: extroversion-introversion: one-sided, in being part of the side (category) of "normality" in the normality-abnormality pair. And compounded, because the normality-abnormality pair is in turn related to the symmetry-asymmetry principle, the density-emptiness principle, the convention-novelty principle, the same-difference principle
  —Ex: organizedness-spontaneousness: one-sided, in being part of the side (category) of "normality" in the normality-abnormality pair. And compounded, because the normality-abnormality pair is in turn related to the symmetry-asymmetry principle, the density-emptiness principle, the convention-novelty principle, the same-difference principle
  —Ex: risk-caution: one-sided, in being part of the side (category) of "normality" in the normality-abnormality pair. And compounded, because the normality-abnormality pair is in turn related to the symmetry-asymmetry principle, the density-emptiness principle, the convention-novelty principle, the same-difference principle

Notes: The examples here are solely illustrative (not exhaustive). The comparison is also relative (not absolute), nor are they mutually exclusive. As generalities, they allow exceptions.
Source: First summarized in *BEPE* (and updated in later books)

Table 4.11. The Semantics of Existential Dialectics (Part I)

- **Abstract Structure vs. Specific Meanings**
  —The syntax of existential dialectics so understood in terms of ontological principles only gives us the structure of ontology in the world, in an abstract (general) sense. These principles by themselves do not tell us the specific meanings in a given context.
  —In order to grasp the specific meanings of the principles in a given context, it is necessary to study the semantics of existential dialectics. And the analysis of the ontological principles as family resemblances in the section on syntax is only a starting point (and thus overlaps a bit with the semantics of existential dialectics here).
  —With this caveat in mind, the reason that I have often gone in great lengths in my previous books on different subjects is to explain the specific meanings of the principles when applied in different contexts.

- **Specific Meanings in Specific Fields**
  —For instance, in *FPHST*, I used the first three principles (i.e., the change-constancy principle, the regression-progression principle, and the symmetry-asymmetry principle) to propose "the perspectival theory of space-time," for a better way to understand space and time—especially, though not exclusively, in relation to future post-human history (as summarized in *Table 3.6*, *Table 3.7*, *Table 3.8*, and *Table 3.9*). In so doing, I had to introduce concepts and theories specific to the field of physics and other related fields (e.g., "absolute space" and "absolute time" in "classical mechanics" and "relative space-time" in "the theory of relativity").
  —In *BNN*, I also exploited the three principles to propose the "transcendent" approach to the study of genes and memes as a new way to understand the interaction between nature and nurture. In so doing, I had to explore concepts and theories in the world of evolutionary theory (e.g., "mutation," "variation," "adaptation," "selection," and "inheritance" in Darwinian evolutionary theory) and neural biology (e.g., "chromosome," "gene," "DNA," "RNA," "protein," "neuron," "neural network," and "behavior").

(continued on next page)

Table 4.11. The Semantics of Existential Dialectics (Part II)

- **Two Types of Translation (Interpretation)**
  —In the technical jargons of semantics, these exercises in my books perform two essential functions of translation (or interpretation), namely, (a) "intensive" interpretation (about the properties or relations of the principles in existential dialectics), and (b) "extensive" interpretation (about the classes or cases to which the properties and relations of the principles in existential dialectics are applied). (WK 2011oo)

- **Limits of Translation (Interpretation)**
  —But there are limits of translation (or interpretation), and an excellent example is that "there is a problem with the 'objectivity' of translation, as it is relative to different cultural (or sub-cultural) contexts. For instance, one of the still unresolved problems in linguistics is: 'Is there an objective gauge for the quality of translation?'" (*FPHCOM* & WK 2011pp)
  —This is one serious problem about the logic of translation and interpretation that I already addressed in *Sec. 3.5.1* of *FPHCOM (*and also, for that matter, in *FHC*, in the context of hermeneutics).

Notes: The categories and examples in each are solely illustrative (not exhaustive). The comparison is also relative (not absolute), nor are they mutually exclusive. As generalities, they allow exceptions.
Sources: First explicitly stated in *ALD* (and later revised in *FPHCOM*). Also from all other books of mine.

Table 4.12. The Pragmatics of Existential Dialectics (Part I)

- **The Two-Way Street Connecting Theory and Meta-Theory**
  - —The pragmatics of existential dialectics is not a one-way street (that is, using the ontological principles for theoretical insights in praxis) but a two-way one, that is, (a) from meta-theory to theory, and (b) from theory to meta-theory.
  - —(a) On one side of the street, the ontological principles can inspire some theoretical insights in praxis, that is, in relation to some specific fields.
  - —(b) On the other (opposing) side of the street, however, the study of a subject matter in the specific fields in turn reveals some more hitherto unknown ontological principles to be discovered and identified. For this reason, three new principles were added in *FC*, one in *FAE*, and two in *ALD*, on top of the original three in *BCPC*—after some research on the specific subject matters.

- **Direct and Indirect Applications**
  - —*Direct*
    - The logic of existential dialectics can shed some theoretical insights on diverse phenomena in the world, and good instances are the pertinent use of the principles of existential dialectics for the theoretical insights on the freedom/unfreedom dialectics, the equality/inequality dialectics, and the wealth/poverty dialectics in my previous works.
    - My latest books like *FPHST* and *BNN* also use the principles to reveal some theoretical insights on the perspectives of space and time (as in *FPHST*) and of nature and nurture (as in *BNN*).
  - —*Indirect*
    - The theoretical insights can further be used to reveal other phenomena directly from them (viz., the theoretical insights) and therefore indirectly from the principles themselves. A good instance is the use of the theoretical insights on the freedom/unfreedom and equality/inequality dialectics for the understanding of the civilization/barbarity dialectics.

(continued on next page)

Table 4.12. The Pragmatics of Existential Dialectics (Part II)

- **Direct and Indirect Applications (*cont'd*)**
    - Even in indirect applications, however, a phenomenon under study can still be directly related back to the principles themselves. In the example as cited above, the civilization/barbarity dialectics can be directly related to the principles of existential dialectics without the intermediate role of the freedom/unfreedom and equality/inequality dialectics.

- **Multiple Levels of Application**

—The theoretical insights can be applied to different levels of analysis, even though in a given example, it may refer to one level only. For instance, in the example concerning the freedom/unfreedom dialectics, it can be used at the structural level (e.g., in relation to the theory of cyclical progression of hegemony), but it can be exploited as well for other levels (e.g., the theory of post-capitalism at the institutional level).

Notes: The categories and examples in each are solely illustrative (not exhaustive). The comparison is also relative (not absolute), nor are they mutually exclusive. As generalities, they allow exceptions.
Sources: From Ch.6 of *BCPC*. See also other books of mine.

Table 4.13. The Freedom-Unfreedom Dialectics (Part I)

- **On Having**
  - —*In Relation to the Technological*
    - (1) if freer from submission to Nature, then less free from ecological degradation (Deep and Social Ecology), even if in a hi-tech form
    - (2) if freer from technological inconvenience / backwardness, then less free from technological control and the loss of privacy
    - (3) if freer from technological (material) backwardness, then less free from the abusive (barbaric) maltreatment of the primitive Others
  - —*In Relation to the Everyday*
    - (1) if freer from abject poverty, then less free from artificial needs/discontents (Frankfurt School)
    - (2) if freer from sensual suppression, then less free from violent sublimation (Freud)
    - (3) if freer from the snobbishness of high culture, then less free from the shabbiness (leveling-off effect) of mass culture (Tocqueville)
    - (4) if freer from the inefficiency of traditional "compassionate economy," then less free from the bondage of a "ruthless [competitive] economy" (Keynes)
    - (5) if freer from anarchy in the state of nature (system fragmentation), then less free from government regulations and controls in system integration

---

(continued on next page)

Table 4.13. The Freedom-Unfreedom Dialectics (Part II)

- **On Belonging**
  - *—In Relation to the Good and the Just*
    - (1) if freer from disciplinary society, then less free from society of control (Foucault)
    - (2) if freer from the tyranny of one or a few, then less free from the tyranny of the majority (or sometimes, minority veto)
    - (3) if freer from elitist decision making, then less free from political gridlock/cleavage
    - (4) if freer from arbitrary (discretionary) administration, then less free from bureaucratic irrationality (Weber) and legal trickery (loopholes)

- **On Being**
  - *—In Relation to the True*
    - (1) if freer from unscientific dogmas, then less free from instrumental abyss (nihilism). Or conversely, if freer from meaninglessness, then less free from dogmas.
    - (2) if freer from the bondage of partiality/partisanship (e.g., prejudice, discrimination), then less free from the danger of impartiality and neutrality (e.g., opportunism, unrealisticness, lack of compassion, inaction)
    - (3) if freer from making generalizations, then less free from being unable to understand much of anything
  - *—In Relation to the Holy*
    - (1) if freer from collective conscience, then less free from social loneliness
    - (2) if freer from religious absoluteness, then less free from spiritual emptiness
  - *—In Relation to the Beautiful/Sublime*
    - (1) if freer from artistic non-autonomy, then less free from aesthetic disillusion (deconstruction)

(continued on next page)

Table 4.13. The Freedom-Unfreedom Dialectics (Part III)

Notes: The examples in each category are solely illustrative (not exhaustive), and the comparison is relative (not absolute), nor are they necessarily mutually exclusive. And some can be easily re-classified elsewhere. As generalities, they allow exceptions.
Sources: A reconstruction from Ch.10 of *FCD*, based on *FHC*

Table 4.14. The Equality-Inequality Dialectics (Part I)

- **On Having**
  - *In Relation to the Technological*
    - (1) if more equal in treating Nature with spiritual unity, then less equal in suppressing the dominant drive to transcend it altogether
  - *In Relation to the Everyday*
    - (1) if more equal in building social plurality, then less equal in leveling-off effects (e.g., the subsequent relative intolerance of high/intellectual ethos in mass culture industry)
    - (2) if more equal in socioeconomic distribution beyond a certain point, then less equal in efficiency (e.g. resentment, the erosion of work ethics)
    - (3) if more equal in urging an affirmative action program, then less equal in creating victim mentality (in oneself), stigma (from others), reverse discrimination (against the once privileged), and mediocracy (against the more able)

- **On Belonging**
  - *In Relation to the Good and the Just*
    - (1) if more equal in banning monarchic/oligarchic exclusion, then less equal in producing "the tyranny of the majority" or of "minority veto"
    - (2) if more equal in encouraging participatory decision making, then less equal in inducing political divisiveness (gridlock/cleavage in power blocs) and organizational oligarchy
    - (3) if more equal in institutionalizing a decentralized bureaucracy, then less equal in falling into more territorial/turf politics (intrigues)

(continued on next page)

Table 4.14. The Equality-Inequality Dialectics (Part II)

- **On Being**
  - —In Relation to the Beautiful / Sublime
    - (1) if more equal in accepting diverse styles ("anything goes" mentality), then less equal in artistic good quality (in leveling-off effects against the best)
  - —In Relation to the True
    - (1) if more equal in tolerating multiple viewpoints (no matter how extreme), then less equal in epistemic standards
  - —In Relation to the Holy
    - (1) if more equal in celebrating any cults and sects (no matter how questionable), then less equal in spiritual depth and authenticity

Notes: The examples in each category are solely illustrative (not exhaustive), and the comparison is relative (not absolute), nor are they mutually exclusive. And some can be easily reclassified elsewhere. As generalities, they allow exceptions.
Sources: A reconstruction from Ch.10 of *FCD*, based on *FHC*

Table 4.15. The Duality of Oppression in Existential Dialectics: Oppression and Self-Oppression (Part I)

- **From the Same to the Others and Itself**
  - —The Oppression by the Same against the Others
    - *By way of downgrading differences*
      - –Ex: on judiciary caprice for corporate crimes (*Sec.2.2.1.2.1*)
      - –Ex: on the deceptive politics of liberation (*Sec.3.5*)
      - –Ex: on the humanitarian mystique (*Sec.4.4*)
      - –Ex: on the fad of emotional intelligence (*Sec.5.3*)
    - *By way of accentuating differences*
      - –Ex: on the legal sophistry of self-defense (*Sec.2.3*)
      - –Ex: on the legal semantics of proportionality (*Sec.2.4*)
      - –Ex: on the tricky politics of external threat (*Sec.3.4*)
      - –Ex: on the appeal of the Far Right for democracy (*Sec.5.4*)
      - –Ex: on the democratic axis of evil (*Sec.5.5*)
      - –Ex: on the democratic way of brutality and revenge (*Sec.5.6*)
      - –Ex: on democratic autocracy (*Sec.6.4*)
  - —The Oppression by the Same against Itself
    - *By way of downgrading differences*
      - –Ex: on the politics of fear (*Sec.2.2*)
      - –Ex: on the trickery of compassionate conservatism (*Sec.3.2*)
      - –Ex: on the deceptive politics of patriotism (*Sec.3.3*)
    - *By way of accentuating differences*
      - –Ex: on the caprice of due process on domestic suspects (*Sec.2.2*)
      - –Ex: on the false security/freedom dilemma (*Sec.6.5.2*)

(continued on next page)

Table 4.15. The Duality of Oppression in Existential Dialectics: Oppression and Self-Oppression (Part II)

- **From the Others to the Same and Themselves**
  - —The Oppression by the Others against the Same
    - *By way of downgrading differences*
      - –Ex: on judiciary caprice in the reverse direction (*Sec.2.2.1.2.2*)
      - –Ex: on equal pay (*Sec.6.2.1.1*)
      - –Ex: on equal representation (*Sec.6.2.1.2*)
      - –Ex: on affirmative action program (*Sec.6.3.1.1*)
      - –Ex: on same-sex marriage (*Sec.6.3.1.2*)
    - *By way of accentuating differences*
      - –Ex: on sexual harassment (*Sec.6.2.2.1*)
      - –Ex: on physical violence (*Sec.6.2.2.2*)
      - –Ex: on sexual exploitation (*Sec.6.2.2.3*)
  - —The Oppression by the Others against Themselves
    - *By way of downgrading differences*
      - –Ex: on the reverse-class mystique (*Sec.4.2*)
      - –Ex: on the reverse-black mystique (*Sec.4.3*)
      - –Ex: on self-discrimination by downgrading (*Sec.6.3.2.2*)
    - *By way of accentuating differences*
      - –Ex: on self-discrimination by accentuating (*Sec.6.3.2.1*)

Notes: The examples are solely illustrative (not exhaustive), nor are they mutually exclusive. As generalities, they allow exceptions. Also, both forms of oppression co-exist in all of the examples, so the listing of them are only meant in a relative, not absolute, sense.
Source: A summary of the sections (as cited) in Chs.2-6 of *BDPD*. See text for more info and references.

Table 4.16. The Structure of Existential Dialectics I: The Freedom/Unfreedom and Equality/Inequality Dialectics

• Each freedom and equality produces its own unfreedom and inequality, regardless of whether the pair occurs in political society (with the nation-state), in civil society (with some autonomy from the state), or elsewhere (e.g., in the private sphere of individual homes)—and regardless of whether freedom and equality are understood as "negative" or "positive."

• Oppression is dualistic, as much by the Same against the Others and itself, as by the Others against the Same and themselves.

• Both forms of oppression and self-oppression can be achieved by way of downgrading differences (between the Same and the Others) and of accentuating them.

• The relationships are relatively asymmetric between the Same and the Others and relatively symmetric within them. This is true, even when the Same can be relatively asymmetric towards itself in self-oppression, just as the Others can be likewise towards themselves.

• Symmetry and asymmetry change over time, with ever new players, new causes, and new forms.

Notes: The examples in each category are solely illustrative (not exhaustive) nor necessarily mutually exclusive, and the comparison is relative (not absolute). As generalities, they allow exceptions. "Negative" freedom is freedom "from" (e.g., freedom from poverty), whereas "positive" freedom is freedom "to" (e.g., freedom to the state of enlightenment). "Negative" equality is "procedural" equality (e.g., equality of opportunity), while "positive" equality is "substantive" equality (e.g., equality of outcome). Existential dialectics impose constraints on freedom and equality in democracy, non-democracy, and post-democracy. There is no utopia, in the end; even should there be one, dystopia would exist within it.
Sources: From *Table 1.5* of *BDPD*—and also from *FHC*, *FCD*, and *FPHC*

Table 4.17. The Structure of Existential Dialectics II: The Wealth/Poverty Dialectics

• There is no wealth without poverty, just as there is no poverty without wealth.

• The wealth/poverty dialectics occurs in the realms of having, belonging, and being, in relation to the material, relational, and spiritual.

• The wealth/poverty dialectics also expresses itself at the multiple levels of analysis in accordance to methodological holism, be they about the micro-physical, the chemical, the biological, the psychological, the organizational, the institutional, the structural, the systemic, the cultural, and the cosmological.

• The wealth/poverty dialectics is a different manifestation of existential dialectics in general, subject to the principles in its logic of ontology—just as the freedom/unfreedom and equality/inequality dialectics are likewise.

• There is no economic utopia, in the end; even should there be one, dystopia would exist within it.

Notes: The main points here are solely illustrative (not exhaustive) nor necessarily mutually exclusive, and the comparison is relative (not absolute). As generalities, they allow exceptions.
Sources: From *BCPC*. See also *FCD* and *FHC*.

Table 4.18. The Structure of Existential Dialectics III: The Civilization/Barbarity Dialectics

- There is no civilization without barbarity.

- The civilization/barbarity dialectics applies in the four civilizing processes (e.g., the rationalizing process, the pacifying process, the stewardizing process, and the subliming process).

- The civilization/barbarity dialectics is another (different) manifestation of existential dialectics in general, subject to the principles in its logic of ontology—just as the freedom/unfreedom and equality/inequality dialectics and the wealth/poverty dialectics are likewise.

- There is no utopia, in the end; even should there be one, dystopia would exist within it.

Notes: The main points here are solely illustrative (not exhaustive) nor necessarily mutually exclusive, and the comparison is relative (not absolute). As generalities, they allow exceptions.
Sources: From *BCIV*. See also *FCD*, *FHC*, and *BDPD*.

Table 4.19. The Double Sides of Virtual Organizations (Part I)

- **Psychological**
  —Ex: virtual psychosis
  —Ex: impersonality and loneliness in quaternary social relations

- **Organizational**
  —Ex: the race for power and interests
  —Ex: the world of unequal successes
  —Ex: the bureaucratic life of its own
  —Ex: lesser accountability and transparency

- **Economic**
  —Ex: the economic divides
  —Ex: the erosive impact of commercialization

- **Political**
  —Ex: the anti-authoritarian myth
  —Ex: different power struggles among groups (e.g., Conservative, Reformist, Radical)

- **Structural**
  —Ex: different localities (e.g., climates, scenery)
  —Ex: divided domains (e.g., core, peripheral, sub-peripheral)
  —Ex: substitution effect of social capital

- **Systemic**
  —Ex: uneven advances in transportation and communications, and geographical migration

- **Cultural**
  —Ex: conflicting civilizational fabrics (e.g., Confucian, Islamic, Western)
  —Ex: the bias of the Liberal Democratic agenda
  —Ex: the addiction to moral fanaticism

(continued on next page)

Table 4.19. The Double Sides of Virtual Organizations (Part II)

Notes: These categories and examples are solely illustrative (not exhaustive), and some of the items can be reclassified somewhere else. Nor are they mutually exclusive. Since they are generalities, exceptions are expected.
Source: From Ch.7 of *FCD*

Table 4.20. Beyond the World of Titans, and the Remaking of the World Order

- **Hyper-Empires**
  —Ex: The Chinese Union
  —Ex: The Indian Union

- **Meso-Empires**
  —Ex: The European Union
  —Ex: The North American Union

- **Micro-Empires**
  —Ex: The Latin American Union
  —Ex: The Middle Eastern Union

- **The Rest of the World**
  —Odd Powers
    - Ex: Japan
    - Ex: Russia

  —The Poor Club
    - Ex: The African Union

  —Ambivalent Regions
    - Ex: Southeast Asia
    - Ex: Oceania
    - Ex: South Asia
    - Ex: Central Asia
    - Ex: Southern/Eastern Europe
    - Ex: North Africa
    - Ex: Central America
    - Ex: Others (e.g., the Korean peninsula)

Source: A summary of Chs.2-5 (of *BWT*)

Table 4.21. The Origins of Authoritarian Liberal Democracy

- **The Geopower of Nature (Ch.4 of *ALD*)**
  —Ex: Power Character and Geographical Strategy
  —Ex: Living Space and Territorial Expansion
  —Ex: Strategic Heartland and Containment

- **The Biopsychology of the Mind (Ch.5 of *ALD*)**
  —Ex: The Bell Curve and Mass Intelligence
  —Ex: Group Analysis and Mass Knowledge
  —Ex: Groupthink and Elite (Mis)calculation

- **The Disciplinary Control of Society (Ch.6 of *ALD*)**
  —Ex: Social Organizations of Ruthlessness
  —Ex: Social Institutions of Greed
  —Ex: Social Structure of Exclusion
  —Ex: Social Systems of Violence

- **The Molding Force of Culture (Ch.7 of *ALD*)**
  —Ex: The Tradition of Conquest
  —Ex: The Rationalization of Unreason

Notes: The examples in each category are solely illustrative (not exhaustive), and they are also relative (not absolute), nor are they mutually exclusive. As generalities, they allow exceptions.
Source: A summary of Chs.4-7 of *ALD*

Table 4.22. The Theory of Post-Democracy I: The Priority of Freedom over Equality (Part I)

- **Differences**
  - —*For the aggressive Lions (the strong Elitists)*
    - •Setting up rank distinctions among unequals (e.g., between inferior humans and superior post-humans, or later among inferior post-humans and superior ones, relatively speaking)
    - •Yearning for being not only distinguished from unequals, but also the first among equals (the best of the very best)
    - •Soul-searching for a high spiritual culture (not the trashy one for the masses). Mass culture is a dirty joke for them.
  - —*For the manipulative Foxes (the weak Counter-Elitists)*
    - •Seeking a gentle hegemony by way of more communitarian concerns (for inferior humans and, later, inferior post-humans)
    - •Being more sympathetic to less formal-legalistic institutions and values

- **Similarities**
  - —*For both Lions and Foxes*
    - •Exploring different spheres of non-human consciousness in the cosmos (something vastly superior than the human one)
    - •Recognizing the democratic illusions (e.g., no freedom without unfreedom, no equality without inequality, or simply no justice without injustice, and vice versa)

(continued on next page)

Table 4.22. The Theory of Post-Democracy I: The Priority of Freedom over Equality (Part II)

Notes: The two callings and examples in each category are solely illustrative (not exhaustive), since there will be many different post-human value ideals in the distant future of post-human civilization. The comparison is also relative (not absolute) towards post-democracy, so this is not just a version of free-market democracy (nor Fascism/Nazism, as shown in the table later on democracy, non-democracy, and post-democracy). Nor are they mutually exclusive. As generalities, they allow exceptions. And the specific forms of post-human post-democratic ideals need to be further developed in future after-postmodern history, as they will be different from the ones we now know. The point here is to solely give an extremely rough picture of a small part of the world to come that we have never known.
Source: From Ch.10 of *FCD*. Refer to text for more info and references.

Table 4.23. The Theory of Post-Democracy II:
The Priority of Equality over Freedom

- **Hybrid Versions of**
  —Ex: the Trans-Feminine Calling
  —Ex: the Trans-Sinitic Calling
  —Ex: the Trans-Islamic Calling
  —Ex: the Trans-Outerspace Calling

- **Qualifications**
  —These four versions of post-capitalist value ideals need not automatically be post-democratic, just as capitalism does not necessarily mean democracy. They are two different entities—though closely related.
  —But up to a certain threshold of elevating equality at the farther expense of freedom, the democratic ideals will be overcome and cease to exist.
  —The overcome will not be socialist or communist, but post-democratic with no freedom without unfreedom and no equality without inequality, subject to the constraints of existential dialectics.

Notes: The callings are solely illustrative (not exhaustive), since there will be many different post-human value ideals in the distant future of post-human lifeforms. The comparison is also relative (not absolute), nor are they mutually exclusive. As generalities, they allow exceptions. And the specific forms of post-human post-democratic ideals need to be further developed in future after-postmodern history, as they will be different from the ones we now know. The point here is to solely give an extremely rough picture of a small part of the world to come that we have never known.
Source: From Ch.10 of *FCD*. Refer to text for more info and references.

Table 4.24. The Theory of Post-Democracy III:
The Transcendence of Freedom and Equality
(Part I)

- **Transcending Freedom in Floating Existence**
  —*Freedom*: seeking an ultimate elimination of the body. Being without the body. The aim is to transcend freedom in the end into a metaphysical state (i.e., beyond the physique).
  —*Unfreedom*: yet facing difficult trade-offs. The sacrifice of bodily existence and its joyfulness. An eternal boredom in floating existence in dark deep space, though with alternative pleasures. There is no free lunch even in the state of transcending freedom.

- **Transcending Equality in the Rivalry of Cosmic Hegemony**
  —*Inequality*: competing to outlast other lifeforms in floating existence, or just marginalizing them for one's hegemonic expansiveness in the rest of the cosmos (and even beyond). Universalism is only for the mediocre.
  —*Equality*: accepting only those of one's rank as equal partners in the vast spacetime for cosmic supremacy. Even here, the aim is to transcend equality into a metaphysical state.

(continued on next page)

Table 4.24. The Theory of Post-Democracy III: The Transcendence of Freedom and Equality (Part II)

Notes: Do not confuse this transcendence of freedom and equality (as one version of post-democracy) with the naïve temptation to transcend the freedom/unfreedom and equality/inequality dialectics. Existential dialectics hold true for freedom and equality in all cultures and societies—past, present, or future (i.e., democracy, non-democracy, and post-democracy), regardless of whether freedom and equality are conventionally understood as "negative" or "positive."

Also, the two features and examples in each are solely illustrative (not exhaustive), since there will be many different post-human value ideals in the distant future of post-human lifeforms. The comparison is also relative (not absolute), nor are they mutually exclusive. As generalities, they allow exceptions. And the specific forms of post-human ideals even for these radically alien floating lifeforms (and others unknown to us) need to be further developed in future after-postmodern history, as they will likely be different from the ones herein illustrated. The point here is to solely give a very rough picture of a small part of the extremely alien world to come that we have never known.

Source: From Ch.10 of *FCD*. Refer to text for more info and references.

Table 4.25. Democracy, Non-Democracy, and Post-Democracy (Part I)

- **Democracy**
  —*Theoretical Constructs*
  •The pursuit of freedom and equality (in various degrees), regardless of whether freedom and equality can be understood as "negative" or "positive"
  (1) more equality than freedom: The relative priority of the good over the right
  (2) more freedom than equality: The relative priority of the right over the good
  —*Types*
  •Only (1): Different versions of communitarian moral universalism
  •Only (2): Different versions of liberal moral universalism
  •(1) or (2): Different versions of anarchic (non-nation-state) moral universalism
  •(1) or (2): Different versions of postmodern moral localism

- **Non-Democracy**
  —*Theoretical Constructs*
  •The focus on (1') equality or (2') freedom, but not both, regardless of whether freedom and equality can be understood as "negative" or "positive"
  —*Types*
  •Only (1'): Different versions on the Far Left (e.g., Stalinism, Robespierrianism)
  •Only (2'): Different versions on the Far Right (e.g., Nazism, absolute monarchism)

(continued on next page)

Table 4.25. Democracy, Non-Democracy, and Post-Democracy (Part II)

- **Post-Democracy**

  —*Theoretical Constructs*

  •The priority of (1'') equality over freedom, or (2'') freedom over equality, or (3'') the transcendence of freedom and equality, regardless of whether freedom and equality are "negative" or "positive." In degree, (1'') or (2'') is less than (1') or (2') but more than (1) or (2)—respectively.

  •Like democracy and non-democracy, post-democracy is also subject to the freedom/unfreedom and equality/inequality dialectics (or existential dialectics in general). Unlike them, post-democracy acknowledges the constraints of existential dialectics and no longer value freedom and equality as sacred virtues. There is no utopia, in the end; even were there one, dystopia would exist within it.

  —*Types*

  •(1''): Different versions of trans-Sinitic value ideals

  •(1''): Different versions of trans-feminine value ideals

  •(1''): Different versions of trans-Islamic value ideals

  •(1''): Different versions of trans-outerspace value ideals

  •(2''): Different versions of post-human elitist value ideals

  •(3''): Different versions of the value ideals of floating consciousness (etc.)

(continued on next page)

Table 4.25. Democracy, Non-Democracy, and Post-Democracy (Part III)

Notes: The examples are solely illustrative (not exhaustive), nor are they mutually exclusive. As generalities, they allow exceptions. "Negative" freedom is freedom "from" (e.g., freedom from poverty), whereas "positive" freedom is freedom "to" (e.g., freedom to the state of enlightenment). "Negative" equality is "procedural" equality (e.g., equality of opportunity), while "positive" equality is "substantive" equality (e.g., equality of outcome). Existential dialectics impose constraints on freedom and equality in democracy, non-democracy, and post-democracy, regardless of whether freedom and equality can be understood as "negative" or "positive" in conventional discourse. Therefore, do not confuse the transcendence of freedom and equality in (3'') with the naïve temptation to transcend existential dialectics. There is no utopia, in the end; even should there be one, it would not exist without dystopia embedded within it.
Sources: A summary, based on my previous works, especially Ch.5 of *FHC*, Chs.5-10 of *FCD*, Chs.2-4 of *FPHC*, and Chs.1 & 7 of *BDPD*. The reader should consult the books for more analysis, as this is only a summary here.

Table 4.26. Multiple Causes of the Emergence of Post-Democracy (Part I)

• **At the Micro-Physical Level**
—Ex: intelligent life without the human physical-chemical system
—Sources: Ch.7 of *FHC*; Chs.9-10 of *FCD*; Ch.1 of *FPHC*

• **At the Chemical Level**
—Ex: space radiation and toxins
—Sources: Ch.7 of *FHC*; Chs.9-10 of *FCD*

• **At the Bio-Psychological Level**
—Ex: exo-biological evolution in deep space
—Ex: genetic engineering of new beings
—Ex: limits of cognitive partiality
—Ex: illusions of emotional neutrality
—Ex: human biological inequality
—Ex: the rise of unfolding unconsciousness
—Sources: Ch.2 & Chs.9-10 of *FCD*; Ch.7 of *FHC*; Ch.4 of *BCPC*; *FPHU*

• **At the Institutional Level**
—Ex: the flawed logic of equality
—Ex: the conflicting nature of governance
—Sources: Ch. 5 of *FHC*; Chs. 6 & 10 of *FCD*; Ch. 3 of *FPHC*; Chs.2-5 of *BDPD*

• **At the Organizational Level**
—Ex: e-civic alienation
—Ex: the dark sides of formal-legalistic routines
—Sources: Ch.3 of *FHC*; Ch.7 of *FCD*; Ch.3 of *FPHC*

• **At the Structural Level**
—Ex: ever new forms of inequities, at home and abroad
—Ex: the emergence of China, women, and Islam as major actors
—Sources: Chs.5-6 of *FHC*; Chs.7, 9 & 10 of *FCD*; Chs.4-5 of *BDPD*

(continued on next page)

Table 4.26. Multiple Causes of the Emergence of Post-Democracy (Part II)

- **At the Cultural Level**
  —Ex: freedom/unfreedom dialectics
  —Ex: equality/inequality dialectics
  —Ex: system fragmentation and integration
  —Sources: Ch.5 of *FHC*; Chs. 3, 9 & 10 of *FCD*; Ch.4 of *FPHC*; Ch.1 of *BDPD*; Ch.4 of *BCPC*

- **At the Systemic Level**
  —Ex: space habitats (in zero-gravity) and colonization
  —Ex: ultra advanced future info systems
  —Ex: qualitative demography
  —Sources: Ch.7 of *FHC*; Chs.9 &10 of *FCD*

- **At the Cosmological Level**
  —Ex: the colonization of multiverses
  —Ex: the alteration of space-time and the creation of new matter-energy
  —Ex: the expansion of floating consciousness
  —Ex: the spread of hyper-spatial consciousness
  —Sources: Ch.7 of *FHC*; Chs.9 &10 of *FCD*; Ch.4 of *FPHC*; *FPHST*

Notes: The examples in each category are solely illustrative (not exhaustive), and some of the items can be reclassified somewhere else. Nor are they always mutually exclusive. Since they are generalities, exceptions are expected.
Sources: Especially from *FHC*, *FCD*, *FPHC*, *BCPC*, *BDPD*, *FPHST*, and *FPHU*. See also other books and my perspectives on civilizational holism.

Table 4.27. Some Clarifications about Post-Capitalism and Post-Democracy (Part I)

• The prefix "trans-" in the first category of post-capitalism (with its four versions) refers to something "going beyond" (not "uniting" or "combining"). Ex: *Sec.10.3.3* of *FCD*; *Sec.2.4* & *Sec.4.4* of *FPHC*; *Sec.7.2* of *BCPC*

• Such terms like "post-democracy," "post-capitalism," "post-human elitist," "trans-feminine calling," and the like as used in my works are more for our current intellectual convenience than to the liking of future humans and post-humans, who will surely invent more tasteful neologisms to call their own eras, entities, and everything else, for that matter. But the didactic point here is to use the terms to foretell what the future might be like, not that its eras and entities must be called so exactly and permanently.
Ex: *Sec.11.1* of *FCD*; *Sec.7.2* of *BCPC*

• The four versions in the first category of post-capitalist value ideals need not automatically be post-democratic, just as capitalism does not necessarily mean democracy. They are two different entities—though closely related. But up to a certain threshold of elevating equality at the farther expense of freedom, the democratic ideals will be overcome and cease to exist. The same is true for the post-human elitist calling in the second category of post-capitalism in relation to post-democracy, depending on the extent to which freedom is elevated at the expense of equality.
Ex: *Sec.10.4.3.3* of *FCD*; *Table 3.9* of *FPHC*; *Table 7.6* of *BDPD*

• The comparison in each of the three realms of existence in all forms of post-capitalism is not absolute, but relative. Examples include "communal" vs. "individualistic," and the like.
Ex: Notes in *Table 10.8*, *Table 10.9*, *Table 10.10*, & *Table 10.11* of *FCD*; Chs.2-4 of *FPHC*; *Sec.7.2* of *BCPC*

(continued on next page)

Table 4.27. Some Clarifications about Post-Capitalism and Post-Democracy (Part II)

• The emergence of post-capitalism (and post-democracy, for that matter) has multiple causes (to not be reduced to one or only a few).
Ex: Ch.10 of *FCD*, Chs.2-4 of *FPHC*; *Sec.1.3* & *Sec.7.2* of *BCPC* (or *Table 1.8* & *Table 7.11*)

• The specific forms of post-capitalism (and post-democracy, for that matter) need to be further developed in future after-postmodern history, as they will be different from the ones we now know. The point here is to solely give an extremely rough sketch of a world to come that we have never known.
Ex: *Sec.10.3.3* & *Sec.10.4.3.3* of *FCD*; *Table 10.14* & *Table 10.15* of *FCD*; *Sec.7.2* of *BCPC*

• All forms of post-capitalism are not part of a "teleological law," but of "historical trends" only. The same is also true for all forms of post-democracy.
Ex: *Sec.7.1* of *FHC*; *Sec.9.5.3.2* & *Sec.10.3.4.2* of *FCD*; *Sec.7.2* of *BCPC*

• Post-capitalism is not better than capitalism in an "absolute" sense but only fits in better, on the basis of the historical contingency of culture, society, nature, and the mind in some future eras. The same is true for post-democracy in relation to democracy. The term "better" is historically relative.
Ex: *Sec.10.3.3* of *FCD*; *Sec.1.7* of *BDPD*; *Sec.1.5* of *BCPC*

(continued on next page)

Table 4.27. Some Clarifications about Post-Capitalism and Post-Democracy (Part III)

• All forms of post-capitalism and post-democracy are subject to the constraints of existential dialectics. In the process, the dialectic direction is to go beyond the conventional "either-or" dichotomies (e.g., freedom vs. unfreedom, equality vs. inequality, freedom vs. equality, individuality vs. communality, spirituality vs. materiality, formal legalism vs. informal legalism, etc.). As is true in post-civilization, to go beyond the dichotomies is to acknowledge the co-existence of both in each dichotomy, although the degree of scaling one over the over varies from case to case (e.g., the theory of post-capitalism I, the theory of post-capitalism II, the theory of post-democracy I, the theory of post-democracy II, etc.)—but is not to be extreme in largely favoring one over the other, *on average* (all things considered). There is no utopia to be had in the end; even should there be one, dystopia would exist within it.
Ex: Ch.5 of *FHC*; *Sec.10.4.4.2* of *FCD*; *Sec.1.5* of *BDPD*; *Sec.1.3* of *BCPC*; *BCIV*

• All forms of post-capitalism, however different from each other though they are, share one common feature, in that they all inspire for a higher spiritual culture. The same is also true for post-democracy.
Ex: *Sec.10.3*, *Sec.10.4* & *Sec.10.5* of *FCD*; *Chs.2-4* of *FPHC*; *Sec.7.2* of *BCPC*

• All forms of post-capitalism try to avoid the excess in capitalist consumerism by favoring more basic than artificial needs in having, but the quality and quantity of these "basic" needs will be measured by future standards, not by our current ones. Standards are historically relative.
Ex: *Sec.10.3*, *Sec.10.4* & *Sec.10.5* of *FCD*; Ch.2 of *FPHC*; *Sec.7.2* of *BCPC*

(continued on next page)

Table 4.27. Some Clarifications about Post-Capitalism and Post-Democracy (Part IV)

• All forms of post-capitalism make use of a different degree of political authority with advanced info systems in future history and strives for higher spiritual cultures (especially in the post-human age), while acknowledging the constraints of existential dialectics and no longer valuing free market (as in capitalism) and economic control (as in non-capitalism) as sacred virtues.
Ex: *Sec.10.3.4.2*, *Sec.10.3*, *Sec.10.4* & *Sec.10.5* of *FCD*; Chs.2-4 of *FPHC*; *Sec.1.5* of *BDPD*; *Sec.7.2* of *BCPC*

Notes:: The main points here are solely illustrative (not exhaustive) nor necessarily mutually exclusive, and the comparison is relative (not absolute). As generalities, they allow exceptions. The sections as cited are only illustrative (not exhaustive).
Sources: From *FHC*, *FCD*, *FPHC*, and *BDPD*

Table 4.28. The Theory of Post-Capitalism I.1: By Group— Ex: Spiritual/Communal in the Trans-Feminine Calling

- **More Communal Than Individual**
  —*Sharing*: learning from others, as different ideas mutually enrich
  —*Cooperative*: encouraging a sense of shared leadership and teamwork

- **More Informal-Legalistic Than Formal-Legalistic**
  —*Specific*: listening more from the heart than from the head, to know a person as a concrete, not as an abstract, unit
  —*Affective*: thinking and acting with others on a more affective tone. Business can mix with an emotional touch.
  —*Ascriptive*: hiring (or firing) can be done on the basis of merit (or lack of it), but deep solidarity (sisterhood) is important too.
  —*Particularistic*: making decisions on the basis of cost-benefit analysis, but a given group relationship is vital

- **More Spiritual Than Secular**
  —*Long-Term Looking*: sharing for a long-term relationship (e.g., love, friendship), not just for a short-term gain
  —*Loving/Caring*: showing compassion for the sufferings of others, without quickly blaming and pre-judging
  —*Respectful*: showing acceptance about others' feelings (and thoughts)

Notes: The categories and examples are solely illustrative, since there can be different versions, and the comparison is relative (not absolute), nor are they mutually exclusive. As generalities, they allow exceptions. The specific forms of the trans-feminine version need to be further developed in future after-postmodern history, as they will be different from the ones we now know, since the prefix "trans-" here means going beyond or deconstructing the feminine values, while using them as the inspirational point at the beginning.
Source: From Ch.10 of *FCD*. Refer to text for more info and references.

Table 4.29. The Theory of Post-Capitalism I.2: By Nation-State— Ex: Spiritual/Communal in the Trans-Sinitic Calling

- **More Communal Than Individualistic**
  —*Centralized*: being more top-down in management
  —*Collective*: encouraging more group cooperation
  —*Social*: investing in trust and connection

- **More Informal-Legalistic Than Formal-Legalistic**
  —*Specific*: knowing more of those related or connected
  —*Affective*: behaving in a paternalistic, hierarchical way
  —*Ascriptive*: favoring family members and those related
  —*Particularistic*: building connection (guanxi) as imperative

- **More Spiritual Than Secular**
  —*Expansionist*: diffusing civilizational values (e.g., the superiority complex of civilizationalism)
  —*Holistic*: synthesizing things into a panoramic horizon
  —*Historical*: learning from the lessons of the ancient past
  —*Respectful*: deferential to elders and superiors

Notes: The categories and examples are solely illustrative, since there can be different versions, and the comparison is relative (not absolute), nor are they mutually exclusive. As generalities, they allow exceptions. The specific forms of the trans-Sinitic version need to be further developed in future after-postmodern history, as they will be different from the ones we now know, since the prefix "trans-" here means going beyond or deconstructing the Sinitic values, while using them as the inspirational point at the beginning.
Source: From Ch.10 of *FCD*. Refer to text for more info and references.

Table 4.30. The Theory of Post-Capitalism I.3: By Region— Ex: Spiritual/Communal in the Trans-Islamic Calling

- **More Communal Than Individualistic**
  —*Collective*: building the webs of relationships to bind individuals
  —*Sharing*: cultivating the established "wisdom" through common experience
  —*Cooperative*: stressing harmony, solidarity, and commonality

- **More Informal-Legalistic Than Formal-Legalistic**
  —*Specific*: making efforts to know well the participants (family and larger community) in matters of common concern
  —*Affective*: mixing work with language and ritual on explicit religious (Islamic) ideals, texts, stories, and examples
  —*Ascriptive*: privileging local history and custom on relationships among kinship groups
  —*Particularistic*: preferring an unbiased insider with ongoing connections to all parties

- **More Spiritual Than Secular**
  —*Historical*: learning from the lessons of the past as a source of stability and guidance
  —*Deferential*: showing respect for age, experience, status, and leadership in communal affairs
  —*Honorable*: emphasizing face, dignity, prestige, and fairness
  —*Compassionate*: giving mercy and charity ("Zahah") to others

Notes: The categories and examples are solely illustrative (not exhaustive), and the comparison is relative (not absolute), nor are they mutually exclusive. As generalities, they allow exceptions. The specific forms of the trans-Islamic version need to be further developed in future after-postmodern history, as they will be different from the ones we now know, since the prefix "trans-" here means going beyond or deconstructing the Islamic values, while using them as the inspirational point at the beginning.
Sources: From Ch.10 of *FCD*. Refer to text for more info and references, especially from the works by George Irani (2000) and C. Murphy (September 19, 2001).

Table 4.31. The Theory of Post-Capitalism I.4: By Universe— Ex: Spiritual/Communal in the Trans-Outerspace Calling

- **More Communal Than Individual**
  —*Cooperative*: requiring teamwork in small space habitats
  —*Sharing*: learning from, and enjoying being with, each other in a small group in outer space

- **More Informal-Legalistic Than Formal-Legalistic**
  —*Specific*: knowing more about each other to facilitate living and working together in space, both as fellow astronauts and space-mates
  —*Affective*: being friendly and social to each other as vital to working and living in small space quarters
  —*Ascriptive*: nurturing comaraderie among fellow astronauts as if they are family members over time
  —*Particularistic*: building work relationship with enduring memory in a space mission

- **More Spiritual Than Secular**
  —*Long-Term*: looking beyond selfish materialistic concerns in a precarious space environment with potential life or death
  —*Loving/Caring*: cultivating deep bondage for the success of a long term space mission
  —*Transcendent*: searching for life meaning in outer space

Notes: The calling and examples in each category are solely illustrative (not exhaustive), since there will be many different outer-space value ideals in the distant future of space colonization. The comparison is also relative (not absolute), nor are they mutually exclusive. As generalities, they allow exceptions. And the specific forms of trans-outer-space calling need to be further developed in future after-postmodern history, as they will be different from the ones we now know, since the prefix "trans-" here means going beyond or deconstructing the current outer-space values, while using them as the inspirational point at the beginning. The point here is to solely give an extremely rough picture of a small part of the world to come that we still do not know much about.
Source: From Ch.10 of *FCD*. Refer to text for more info and references.

Table 4.32. The Theory of Post-Capitalism II: Spiritual/Individualistic in the Post-Human Elitist Calling (Part I)

- **More Individualistic Than Communal**
  —Setting up rank distinctions among unequals (e.g., between inferior humans and superior post-humans, or later among inferior post-humans and superior ones, relatively speaking)
  —Yearning for being not only distinguished from unequals, but also the first among equals (the best of the very best)
  —Recognizing the constraints of equality/inequality dialectics (or existential dialectics in general)

- **More Spiritual Than Secular**
  —Soul-searching for a high spiritual culture (not the trashy one for the masses). Mass culture is a dirty joke for them.
  —Exploring different spheres of non-human consciousness in the cosmos (something vastly superior than the human one)
  —Recognizing the constraints of freedom/unfreedom dialectics (or existential dialectics in general)

- **Qualifications**
  —Although post-human elitist post-democracy is comparable to post-human elitist post-capitalism in some respects, the former does not necessarily imply the latter (post-human elitist post-capitalism), just as democracy does not have to entail capitalism. They are two different (though related) entities.
  —But up to a certain threshold of incorporating government intervention with advanced info systems in future civilizations for higher spiritual concerns at the expense of the free market and materialist pursuit, the capitalist ideal will be overcome.
  —The overcome will not be Fascist or feudalistic, but post-capitalist, subject to the constraints of existential dialectics.

(continued on next page)

Table 4.32. The Theory of Post-Capitalism II: Spiritual/Individualistic in the Post-Human Elitist Calling (Part II)

Notes: The calling and examples in each category are solely illustrative (not exhaustive). The comparison is also relative (not absolute), nor are they mutually exclusive. As generalities, they allow exceptions. And the specific forms of post-human elitist post-capitalism need to be further developed in future after-postmodern history, as they will be different from the ones we now know, while using them as the inspirational point at the beginning. The point here is to solely give an extremely rough picture of a small part of the world to come that we still do not know much about.
Sources: From Ch.10 of *FCD* (and also *FPHC*, *BDPD*, and *BCPC*). Refer to the text for more info and references.

Table 4.33. Capitalism, Non-Capitalism, and Post-Capitalism (Part I)

- **Capitalism**
  - —*Theoretical Constructs*
    - •Allocation of scarce resources among alternative wants largely by free market for competition (whose characteristics in its ideal form include, for instance, no barrier to entry or exit, homogeneity, perfect information, a large number of buyers/sellers, and perfect factor mobility)
    - •More formal-legalistic than informal-legalistic, more individualistic than communal, and more material (secular) than spiritual
    - •Either (1) minimal government or (2) relatively active government
  - —*Types*
    - •Only (1): Different versions of market capitalism (e.g., the U.S.)
    - •Only (2): Different versions of welfare capitalism (e.g., Sweden)

- **Non-Capitalism**
  - —*Theoretical Constructs*
    - •Allocation of scarce resources among alternative wants mainly by political authority for policies (which can be regulative, redistributive, symbolic, and participatory)
    - •More informal-legalistic than formal-legalistic
    - •Either (1') more individualistic (for the elites), often (though not always) for material (secular) concerns, or (2') more communal (for the masses), often (though not always) for spiritual concerns
  - —*Types*
    - •Only (1'): Different versions on the Right (e.g., Fascist corporate-state economy for the glory of the new Rome, medieval lord-vassal-serf economy for the power of the feudalistic order)
    - •Only (2'): Different versions on the Left (e.g., Soviet command economy for the creation of the New Socialist Man)

(continued on next page)

Table 4.33. Capitalism, Non-Capitalism, and Post-Capitalism (Part II)

- **Post-Capitalism**

—*Theoretical Constructs*

•Allocation of scarce resources among alternative wants largely by political authority with advanced info systems in future civilizations, subject to existential dialectics. In degree of allocating by authority, post-capitalism is more than capitalism but less than non-capitalism.

•More spiritual than secular (material)

•Either (1'') more individualistic or (2") more communal

•Like capitalism and non-capitalism, post-capitalism is also subject to the freedom/unfreedom and equality/inequality dialectics (or existential dialectics in general). There is no utopia, in the end; even were there one, dystopia would exist within it.

•Unlike capitalism and non-capitalism, post-capitalism makes use of a different degree of political authority with advanced info systems in future civilizations and strives for higher-spiritual cultures (especially in the post-human age), while acknowledging the constraints of existential dialectics and no longer valuing free market (as in capitalism) and economic control (as in non-capitalism) as sacred virtues.

—*Types*

•Only (1"): Different versions of post-human elitist value ideals

•Only (2''): Different versions of trans-Sinitic value ideals

•Only (2''): Different versions of trans-feminine value ideals

•Only (2''): Different versions of trans-Islamic value ideals

•Only (2''): Different versions of trans-outerspace value ideals

---

(continued on next page)

Table 4.33. Capitalism, Non-Capitalism, and Post-Capitalism (Part III)

Notes: The calling and examples in each category are solely illustrative (not exhaustive). The comparison is also relative (not absolute), nor are they mutually exclusive. As generalities, they allow exceptions. And the specific forms of each calling need to be further developed in future after-postmodern history, as they will be different from the ones we now know, while using them as the inspirational point at the beginning. The point here is to solely give an extremely rough picture of a small part of the world to come that we still do not know much about.
Source: From Ch.10 of *FCD*. Refer to the text for more info and references.

Table 4.34. Multiple Causes of the Emergence of Post-Capitalism (Part I)

- **At the Micro-Physical Level**
  —Ex: intelligent life without the human physical-chemical system
  —Ex: mastering of quantum mechanics, electromagnetism, and other fields for the understanding of a broad range of anomalous experiences and the application for artificial intelligence for spiritual quest
  —Sources: Ch.7 of *FHC*; Chs.9-10 of *FCD*; Ch.1 of *FPHC*

- **At the Chemical Level**
  —Ex: space radiation and toxins
  —Sources: Ch.7 of *FHC*; Chs.9-10 of *FCD*

- **At the Bio-Psychological Level**
  —Ex: exo-biological evolution in deep space
  —Ex: genetic engineering of new beings
  —Ex: limits of human cognition
  —Ex: the rise of unfolding unconsciousness
  —Sources: Ch.2 & Chs.9-10 of *FCD*; Ch.7 of *FHC*; *FPHU*

- **At the Institutional Level**
  —Ex: the flawed logic of the free market
  —Ex: the need of a post-autistic economics
  —Sources: Ch.10 of *FCD*

- **At the Organizational Level**
  —Ex: the dark sides of formal-legalistic routines
  —Sources: Ch.3 of *FHC*; Ch.7 of *FCD*; Ch.3 of *FPHC*

- **At the Structural Level**
  —Ex: ever new forms of inequities, at home and abroad
  —Ex: the emergence of China, women, and Islam as major actors
  —Sources: Chs.5-6 of *FHC*; Chs.7, 9 & 10 of *FCD*; Chs.4-5 of *BDPD*

(continued on next page)

Table 4.34. Multiple Causes of the Emergence of Post-Capitalism (Part II)

- **At the Cultural Level**
  —Ex: freedom/unfreedom dialectics
  —Ex: equality/inequality dialectics
  —Sources: Ch.5 of *FHC*; Chs.3 & 10 of *FCD*; Ch.4 of *FPHC*; Ch.1 of *BDPD*

- **At the Systemic Level**
  —Ex: space habitats (in zero-gravity) and colonization
  —Ex: ultra advanced future info systems
  —Ex: qualitative demography
  —Sources: Ch.7 of *FHC*; Chs. 9 & 10 of *FCD*

- **At the Cosmological Level**
  —Ex: the colonization of multiverses
  —Ex: the alteration of space-time and the creation of new matter-energy
  —Ex: the expansion of floating consciousness
  —Ex: the spread of hyper-spatial consciousness
  —Sources: Ch.7 of *FHC*; Chs. 9 & 10 of *FCD*; Ch.4 of *FPHC*; *FPHST*

Notes: The examples in each category are solely illustrative (not exhaustive), and some of the items can be reclassified somewhere else. Nor are they always mutually exclusive. Since they are generalities, exceptions are expected.
Sources: Especially from *FHC*, *FCD*, *FPHC*, *BCPC*, *BDPD*, *FPHST*, and *FPHU*. See also other books and my perspectives on civilizational holism.

Table 4.35. The Theoretical Debate on Civilization

- **The Progressive Theory of Civilization**
  —*Thesis*: The "civilizing" process is "good," as opposed to the "barbarizing" process as something "bad," relatively speaking.
  —*Discourse*: Especially, though not exclusively, in the Enlightenment era and a bit before. Example: Thomas Hobbes—in that the tribes in primitive societies were "savages."

- **The Romantic Theory of Barbarity**
  —*Thesis*: The "civilizing" process is "bad," as opposed to the "barbarizing" process as something "good," relatively speaking.
  —*Discourse*: Especially, though not exclusively, in the Counter-Enlightenment circle. Example: Jean-Jacques Rousseau—in that civilization "corrupts" men, and the "savages" are in fact "noble."

- **The Moderate Theory of Civilization**
  —*Thesis*: The "civilizing" process is "good," but there is a price to pay, especially in systematic (compulsive) self-control.
  —*Discourse*: Especially, though not exclusively, in some late modern and postmodern circles. Example: Norbert Elias—in that social manners become more refined in the civilizing process, but self-control also becomes more systematic.

- **The Theory of Post-Civilization**
  —*Thesis*: The civilizing process is as evil and good as barbarity, and each cannot exist without the other, to be eventually superseded by post-civilization unto the post-human age.
  —*Discourse*: Proposed by Peter Baofu. See the rest of *BCIV* for more analysis.

Source: From *BCIV* on the theoretical debate

Table 4.36. No Freedom Without Unfreedom in the Civilizing Processes (Part I)

• **The Rationalizing Process (at the Level of Culture)**
—if freer from the dominance of unreason (as in barbarism) in the civilizing process, then less free from the rationalizing process (be it in the form of the principle of either transcendence or immanence)
—if freer from the principle of immanence in the rationalizing process, then less free from the inclination to commit terror in the name of reason and the relative underdevelopment of non-reason (e.g., in relation to yoga and meditation)
—if freer from the principle of transcendence in the rationalizing process, then less free from the relative underdevelopment of reason (e.g., in relation to systematic methodology) and the occurrence of oppression in the name of non-reason

• **The Pacifying Process (at the Level of Society)**
—if freer from the dominance of pillage (as in savagery) in the civilizing process, then less free from the pacifying process (be it in the form of external control or self-control)
—if freer from self-control in the pacifying process, then less free from the temptation of expansionist oppression and rebellious mindset in external control
—if freer from external control in the pacifying process, then less free from the gruesome psychological self-torture and conformism in self-control

• **The Stewardizing Process (at the Level of Nature)**
—if freer from the dominance of nature (as in the state of nature) in the civilizing process, then less free from the stewardizing process (be it in the form of the stewardship of creation or the covenant with nature)
—if freer from the stewardship of creation in the stewardizing process, then less free from material underdevelopment, relatively speaking, and spiritual exclusion in the covenant with nature
—if freer from the covenant with nature in the stewardizing process, then less free from ecological degradation and spiritual disconnection from nature in the stewardship of creation

(continued on next page)

Table 4.36. No Freedom Without Unfreedom in the Civilizing Processes (Part II)

- **The Subliming Process (at the Level of the Mind)**
  —if freer from the dominance of spontaneity (as in the wild state of the mind) in the civilizing process, then less free from the subliming process, be it in the form of (cyclical-centric) self-refinement or (linear-centric) self-discipline
  —if freer from (cyclical-centric) self-refinement in the subliming process, then less free from the (linear-centric) self-regimen (as a form of neurosis)
  —if freer from (linear-centric) self-discipline in the subliming process, then less free from the (cyclical-centric) self-torture (equally as a form of neurosis)

Notes: The examples in each category are solely illustrative (not exhaustive), and the comparison is relative (not absolute), nor are they necessarily mutually exclusive. And some can be easily re-classified elsewhere. As generalities, they allow exceptions.
Sources: From *BCIV*. See also *FHC*, *FCD*, *FPHC*, *BDPD*, and *BCPC*.

Table 4.37. No Equality Without Inequality in the Civilizing Processes (Part I)

- **The Rationalizing Process (at the Level of Culture)**
  —if more equal for the role of rationalization in the rationalizing process (of civilizational making), then less equal for that of mythicization (as in barbarism)
  —if more equal for the principle of transcendence in (linear-centric) rationalizing process, then less equal for the principle of immanence
  —if more equal for the principle of immanence in (cyclical-centric) rationalizing process, then less equal for the principle of transcendence

- **The Pacifying Process (at the Level of Society)**
  —if more equal for pacification in civilizational making, then less equal for the institution of pillaging and others (as in savagery)
  —if more equal for external control, relatively speaking, in pacifying process, then less equal for self-control
  —if more equal for self-control, relatively speaking, in pacifying process, then less equal for external-control

- **The Stewardizing Process (at the Level of Nature)**
  —if more equal for stewardship in the stewardizing process (of civilizational making), then less equal for reverent (submissive) existence (as in barbarism)
  —if more equal for the stewardship of creation in (linear- centric) stewardizing process, then less equal for the (cyclical-centric) covenant with nature for harmonious co-existence
  —if more equal for the (cyclical-centric) covenant with nature in the stewardizing process, then less equal for the (linear-centric) stewardship of nature for domination

(continued on next page)

Table 4.37. No Equality Without Inequality in the Civilizing Processes (Part II)

- **The Subliming Process (at the Level of the Mind)**
  —if more equal for the role of reason in the subliming process, then less equal for that of unreason (as in the natural state of wildness)
  —if more equal for the primacy of reason in (linear-centric) subliming process, then less equal for other faculties (e.g., intuition, existential feelings, and analogous thinking) in cyclical-centric one
  —if more equal for the exercise of other faculties (e.g., intuition, existential feelings, and analogous thinking) in cyclical-centric subliming process, then less equal for the role of reason in linear-centric counterpart

Notes: The examples in each category are solely illustrative (not exhaustive), and the comparison is relative (not absolute), nor are they mutually exclusive. And some can be easily reclassified else-where. As generalities, they allow exceptions.
Sources: From *BCIV*. See also *FHC*, *FCD*, *FPHC*, *BDPD*, and *BCPC*.

Table 4.38. Five Theses on Post-Civilization

• Post-civilization no longer treats civilization as good and barbarity as evil (relatively speaking), nor does it nostalgically regard barbarity as good and civilization as evil (relatively speaking again). Civilization is as evil and good as barbarity.

• Post-civilization also no longer accepts the dichotomy between civilization and barbarity. Civilization cannot exist without barbarity. It is no longer necessary to preserve civilization, any more than it is imperative to destroy barbarity. To go beyond civilization and barbarity is to acknowledge the co-existence of both, although the degree of scaling one over the over varies from case to case—but is not to be extreme in largely favoring one over the other, *on average* (subject to the constraints of existential dialectics).

• Post-civilization is thus subject to the constraints of existential dialectics. There is no freedom without unfreedom, and no equality without inequality, for instance. There will be no utopia; even should there be one, there would be dystopia embedded within it.

• Post-civilization will eventually replace civilization (as a form of life settlement), to be dominated by post-capitalist and post-democratic lifeforms here on earth and in deep space (besides other alien lifeforms that we have never known), unto the post-human age in multiverses. Those few post-humans who keep civilization will live in a "post-human civilization," while the rest (the majority), who choose post-civilization, will evolve towards the state of "post-human post-civilization." One therefore should not confuse "post-human civilization" with "post-human post-civilization," as the two are not the same.

• Post-civilization will confront psychosis as a primary problem in the culture of virtuality unto the post-human age, just as civilization has neurosis as a primary one of its own (although both neurosis and psychosis are major problems in both).

Notes: The comparison in each category is relative (not absolute), nor are they necessarily mutually exclusive. And some can be easily re-classified elsewhere. As generalities, they allow exceptions.
Sources: From *BCIV*. See also *FHC*, *FCD*, *FPHC*, *BDPD*, and *BCPC*.

Table 4.39. Barbarity, Civilization, and Post-Civilization

- **The Rationalizing Process (at the Level of Culture)**
  —*Barbarity*
    - More mythicizing than rationalizing, relatively speaking

  —*Civilization*
    - More rationalizing than mythicizing, relatively speaking

  —*Post-Civilization*
    - Beyond the dichotomy, subject to existential dialectics

- **The Pacifying Process (at the Level of Society)**
  —*Barbarity*
    - More pillaging than pacifying, relatively speaking

  —*Civilization*
    - More pacifying than pillaging, relatively speaking

  —*Post-Civilization*
    - Beyond the dichotomy, subject to existential dialectics

- **The Stewardizing Process (at the Level of Nature)**
  —*Barbarity*
    - More revering than stewardizing, relatively speaking

  —*Civilization*
    - More stewardizing than revering, relatively speaking

  —*Post-Civilization*
    - Beyond the dichotomy, subject to existential dialectics

- **The Subliming Process (at the Level of the Mind)**
  —*Barbarity*
    - More impulsing than subliming, relatively speaking

  —*Civilization*
    - More subliming than impulsing, relatively speaking

  —*Post-Civilization*
    - Beyond the dichotomy, subject to existential dialectics

Notes: The comparison in each category is relative (not absolute), nor are they necessarily mutually exclusive. And some can be easily re-classified elsewhere. As generalities, they allow exceptions.
Sources: From *BCIV*. See also *FHC*, *FCD*, *FPHC*, *BDPD*, and *BCPC*.

Table 4.40. Types of Super Civilization in the Cosmos (Part I)

- **Type I**
  —a civilization which gains control of and uses the total energy output "falling on its planet from its sun for interstellar communication" (or, in general, space colonization). For N. Kardashev, who proposed the first three types, human civilization is currently Type Zero (Type O), which is below even Type I, since its present energy consumption for all purposes, let alone for interstellar communication, is still 10,000 times less.

- **Type II**
  —a civilization which gains control of and uses directly the total energy output of its sun for interstellar communication (or, in general, space colonization).

- **Type III**
  —a civilization which gains control of and uses the total energy output of its galaxy for interstellar communication (or, in general, space colonization).

- **Type IV**
  —a civilization which gains control of and uses the total energy output of its cluster of galaxies for interstellar communication (or, in general, space colonization).

- **Type V**
  —a civilization which gains control of and uses the total energy output of its supercluster of galaxies for interstellar communica-tion (or, in general, space colonization).

(continued on next page)

Table 4.40. Types of Super Civilization in the Cosmos (Part II)

- **Type…n**
  —So continues the series in what I call the cyclical progression of hegemony in the cosmos and beyond.

Notes: The Russian astrophysicist Nikolai Kardashev proposed the first three types of super civilization in terms of total energy out-put for interstellar communication. (CSM 1979) I extend his argument further to propose Type IV, Type V, Type VI, and Type…n, in the context of my claim about the cyclical progression of he-gemony in the cosmos and beyond.
Sources: From *Table 9.4* of *FCD.* See *FHC*, *FCD*, and *FPHC* for more info.

Table 4.41. The Civilizational Project from Pre-Modernity to After-Postmodernity (Part I)

	Pre-Modern	*Modern*	*Postmodern*	*After-Postmodern*
Main narratives	•Sacralness •Courtliness •Vitalism •Animism	•Freedom •Equality •Fraternity	•Multiplicity •Hybridization	•Naked contingency •Cyclical progres-sion of hegemony
Main institutions	•Monarchy •Aristocracy •Feudalism •Holy order •Primitivism	•Capitalism •Liberalism •Socialism •Nazism •Fascism	•Capitalism •Liberalism •Postmodern politics of difference	•Post-Capitalism •Post-Democracy •Others
Main techno-logical and economic revolutions	•Agricultural	•Service •Industrial	•Informational	•Biological •Material •Energy •Space •Others

(continued on next page)

Table 4.41. The Civilizational Project from Pre-Modernity to After-Postmodernity (Part II)

	Pre-Modern	*Modern*	*Postmodern*	*After-Postmodern*
Main agents	•Males •Upper strata •Mini-states	•Males •Upper strata •Whites •Empires	•Males •Upper strata •Whites •Others •Supra-states •IO's	•Post-humans •Humans •Others
Main impacts	•Local	•Inter-national	•Global	•Outer-space •Multiverse
Main outcomes	•Towards moderntiy •Rise of linear- & cyclical-centric civiliza-tions	•Towards post-modernity •Dominance of linear-centric civilization	•Towards after-post-moderntiy •Linear-centric civiliza-tion in crisis	•Towards human (& maybe post-human) extinction •Rise of post-civiliza-tion, especially in post-human forms of space-time

Notes: The examples in each category are solely illustrative (not exhaustive) nor necessarily mutually exclusive, and the comparison is relative (not absolute). As generalities, they allow exceptions.
Sources: From *Table 10.16* of *FCD*—and also from *BCIV* on post-civilization (and *FPHST*)

Table 4.42. Civilizational Holism (Part I)

- **At the Micro-Physical Theoretical Level**
  —Ex: Mastering of quantum mechanics, electromagnetism, and other fields for the understanding of a broad range of anomalous experiences and theapplication for artificial intelligence (*Sec.1.4.1* of *FPHC*)

- **At the Chemical Theoretical Level**
  —Ex: Unprecedented expansion of (and violence to) the mind through ever new forms of drugs (and virtual technologies, for that matter) (Ch.9 of *FCD*)

- **At the Biological Theoretical Level**
  —Ex: Humans are not biologically equal, on the basis of race, gender, ethnicity, age, and whatnot. (*Sec.2.6* & Ch.10 of *FCD*; *BNN*) And post-humans will experience the same fate, in an even more amazing way.

- **At the Psychological Theoretical Level**
  —Ex: Human cognitive impartiality and emotional neutrality are quite limited. (*Secs.2.4-2.5* of *FCD*)
  —Ex: Rise of Floating Consciousness (Ch.10 of *FCD*; Chs.1 & 4 of *FPHC*) and Unfolding Unconsciousness (*FPHU*)

- **At the Organizational Theoretical Level**
  —Ex: Administrative colonization of deep space, with less legal-formalism in some corners. (Chs.9-10 of *FCD*)

- **At the Institutional Theoretical Level**
  —Ex: Both capitalism and democracy will not last, to be superseded by different versions of post-capitalism and post-democracy in after-postmodernity. (Ch.10 of *FCD*)

(continued on next page)

Table 4.42. Civilizational Holism (Part II)

- **At the Structural Theoretical Level**
  —Ex: Social stratification reappears in ever new forms, also with new causes and new players in the cyclical progression of hegemony. (Chs.8-10 of *FCD*)
  —Ex: The world of hyper-empires, and the union of the unions (*BWT*)

- **At the Systemic Theoretical Level**
  —Ex: Outerspace expansion: local → regional → global → solar → galactic → clustery → multiversal (Ch.9 of *FCD*)
  —Ex: Demographic transition: human extinction, and the rise of post-humans (e.g., cyborgs, thinking machines, thinking robots, genetically altered superior beings, floating consciousness, hyper-spatial consciousness) (Ch.4 of *FPHC*; Ch.10 of *FCD*; & Ch.7 of *FHC*)
  —Ex: New technological forces in material sciences, electronic and communication sciences, energy sciences, biosciences, manufacturing and engineering sciences, and space sciences (Ch.10 of *FCD* & Ch.7 of *FHC*)
  —Ex: Systematic dominance towards nature for space colonization (Chs.9-10 of *FCD*; Chs.2 & 7 of *FHC*)

- **At the Cultural Theoretical Level**
  —Ex: The post-human transcendence of freedom and equality (Ch.10 of *FCD*)
  —Ex: Methodological Holism (Ch.1 of *FCD*; Ch.1 of *FPHC*; *Sec.2.1* & *Sec.2.5* of *BCPC*)
  —Ex: The Evolution from Barbarity to Post-Civilization (*BCIV*)

- **At the Cosmological Theoretical Level**
  —Ex: Mastering of dark matter and dark energy, and the exploration of multiverses (Ch.4 of *FPHC*; Ch.10 of *FCD*; & Ch.7 of *FHC*)
  —Ex: Alternation of space-time (*FPHST*)
  —Ex: The emergence of hyper-spatial consciousness (*FPHC*)

(continued on next page)

Table 4.42. Civilizational Holism (Part III)

- **At Other Levels**
  —Ex: Historical: pre-modernity → modernity → postmodernity → after-postmodernity (human distinction, and the rise of post-humans, including floating consciousness, hyper-spatial consciousness, and unfolding unconsciousness) (Ch.7 of *FHC*; Ch.10 of *FCD*; *FPHC*; *FPHU*)

Notes: These examples are solely illustrative (not exhaustive), and some of the items can be reclassified somewhere else. Nor are they always mutually exclusive. Since they are generalities, exceptions are expected. And the comparison is relative, not absolute.
Sources: From *Table 5.1* of *FPHC*—with details from *FHC*, *FCD*, and the rest of my books. Not every aspect in each category as discussed in all my books are presented here, since there are too many issues. For more info, also consult the table on theories on civilizational holism and, of course, the books themselves.

Table 4.43. Theories on Civilizational Holism (Part I)

I. Theories in Relation to Nature

—At the Chemical Theoretical Level

• 67. Creational Theory of Chemistry (Peter Baofu) (*FPHCHEM*)

(• 62). Resilient Theory of Natural Resources (Peter Baofu) (*BNR*)

—At the Macro-Physical (Cosmological) Theoretical Level

• 66. Resettlement Theory of Geology (Peter Baofu) (*FPHGEOL*)

• 65. Theory of Post-Cosmology (Peter Baofu) (*BCOS*)

• 64. Theory of Hyper-Spatial Consciousness (Peter Baofu) (Ch.4 of *FPHC*; *FPHG*)

(• 62). Resilient Theory of Natural Resources (Peter Baofu) (*BNR*)

(• 61). Panoramic Theory of Transportation (Peter Baofu) (*FPHTRAN*)

(• 59). Multilateral Theory of Acoustics (Peter Baofu) (*FPHA*)

(• 58). Selective Theory of Geometry (Peter Baofu) (*FPHG*)

(• 57). Perspectival Theory of Space-Time (Peter Baofu) (*FPHST*)

(• 56). Dialectic Theory of Complexity (Peter Baofu) (*FC*)

(• 31). Theory of Floating Consciousness (Peter Baofu) (Ch.10 of *FCD*; Chs.1 & 4 of *FPHC*)

• 63. Theory of the Geopower of Nature (Ch.4 of *ALD*)—refined as the Interventive-Reshaping Theory of Geography (Peter Baofu) (*FPHGEOG*)

(continued on next page)

Table 4.43. Theories on Civilizational Holism (Part II)

I. Theories in Relation to Nature (*cont'd*)

—At the Micro-Physical Theoretical Level

- 62. Resilient Theory of Natural Resources (Peter Baofu) (*BNR*)
- 61. Panoramic Theory of Transportation (Peter Baofu) (*FPHTRAN*)
- 60. Transcendent Theory of Architecture (Peter Baofu) (*FPHARCH*)
- 59. Multilateral Theory of Acoustics (Peter Baofu) (*FPHA*)
- 58. Selective Theory of Geometry (Peter Baofu) (*FPHG*)
- 57. Perspectival Theory of Space-Time (Peter Baofu) (*FPHST*)
- 56. Dialectic Theory of Complexity (Peter Baofu) (*FC*)

II. Theories in Relation to Culture

—At the Cultural Theoretical Level

- 55. Fusional Theory of Morphology (Peter Baofu) (*FPHMORP*)
- 54. Modificative Theory of Sports (Peter Baofu) (*FPHSPORT*)
- 53. Inquisitive Theory of Culinary Art (Peter Baofu) (*FPHCA*)
- 52. Interactive Theory of Semantics (Peter Baofu) (*FPHSEM*)
- 51. Transdicsiplinary Theory of Performing Arts (Peter Baofu) (*FPHPA*)
- 50. Comparative-Impartial Theory of Literature (Peter Baofu) (*FPHLIT*)

(continued on next page)

Table 4.43. Theories on Civilizational Holism (Part III)

II. Theories in Relation to Culture (*cont'd*)

—*At the Cultural Theoretical Level* (*cont'd*)

- • 49. Mediative-Variative Theory of Chess (Peter Baofu) (*FPHCHESS*)
- • 48. Theory of Post-Ethics (Peter Baofu) (*BEPE*)
- • 47. Dualistic Theory of Mass Culture (Peter Baofu) (Ch.2 of *FHC*)
- • 46. Comparative Theory of Religion—also known as the Comparative-Substitutive Theory of Religion (Peter Baofu) (Ch.3 of *FHC*; Ch.9 of *FCD*; Ch.1 of *FPHK*; *FPHR*)
- • 45. Theory of Post-Civilization (Peter Baofu) (*BCIV*)
- • 44. Theory of the Trinity of Modernity to Its After-Postmodern Counterpart (Peter Baofu) (*FHC*; Ch.10 of *FCD*)
- • 43. Transformative Theory of Aesthetic Experience (Peter Baofu) (*FAE*)
- (• 21). Theory of Post-Capitalism (Peter Baofu) (Ch.10 of *FCD*; Chs.2 & 4 of *FPHC*; *BCPC*)
- (• 20). Theory of Post-Democracy (Peter Baofu) (Ch.10 of *FCD*; Chs.3 & 4 of *FPHC*; *BDPD*)
- (• 5). Theory of Methodological Holism (Peter Baofu) (Ch.1 of *FCD*; Ch.1of *FPHC*; *Sec.2.1* & *Sec.2.5* of *BCPC*; *FC*; *FPHK*; etc.)
- (• 4). Theory of Existential Dialectics, or the Holistic Theory of Knowledge (Peter Baofu) (*FHC*; *FCD*; *FPHC*; *BDPD*; *FC*; *FAE*; *ALD; FIA; FPHK*; etc,)
- (• 3). Contrastive Theory of Rationality (Peter Baofu) (*FPHML*)

(continued on next page)

Table 4.43. Theories on Civilizational Holism (Part IV)

II. Theories in Relation to Culture (*cont'd*)

—*At the Cultural Theoretical Level* (*cont'd*)

(• 4). Theory of Existential Dialectics,
or the Holistic Theory of Knowledge (Peter Baofu)
(*FHC*; *FCD*; *FPHC*; *BDPD*; *FC*; *FAE*; *ALD; FIA; FPHK*; etc,)

(• 3). Contrastive Theory of Rationality (Peter Baofu)
(*FPHML*)

III. Theories in Relation to the Mind

—*At the Biological Theoretical Level*

• 42. Interconnected Theory of Health Care (Peter Baofu)
(*FPHHC*)

• 41. Theory of Contrastive Advantages (Peter Baofu)
(*Sec.2.6* & Ch.10 of *FCD; BNN*)

(• 31).Theory of Floating Consciousness (Peter Baofu)
(Ch.10 of *FCD*; Chs.1 & 4 of *FPHC*)

—*At the Psychological Theoretical Level*

• 40. Complex Theory of Data Analysis (Peter Baofu)
(*FPHDA*)

• 39. Supersession Theory of Computing (Peter Baofu)
(*FPHCOM*)

• 38. Metamorphic Theory of Humor (Peter Baofu)
(*FPHH*)

• 37. Contrarian Theory of Personality (Peter Baofu)
(*FPHP*)

• 36. Theory of Virtual Sexuality (Peter Baofu)
(*FPHS*)

• 35. Expansive-Contractive Theory of Martial Arts (Peter Baofu)
(*FPHMA*)

• 34. Multilogical Theory of Learning (Peter Baofu)
(*FPHL*)

• 33. Comprehensive Theory of Creative Thinking (Peter Baofu)
(*FPHCT*)

(continued on next page)

Table 4.43. Theories on Civilizational Holism (Part V)

III. Theories in Relation to the Mind (*cont'd*)

—*At the Psychological Theoretical Level* (*cont'd*)

- 32. Theory of Unfolding Unconsciousness—also known as the Unfolding Theory of Anomalous Experience (Peter Baofu) (*FPHU*)
- 31. Theory of Floating Consciousness (Peter Baofu) (Ch.10 of *FCD*; Chs.1 & 4 of *FPHC*)
- 30. Theory of Cognitive Partiality (Peter Baofu) (*Sec.2.4* of *FCD*; *Sec.4.5.1.1* of *BCPC*)
- 29. Theory of Emotional Non-Neutrality (Peter Baofu) (*Sec.2.5* of *FCD*; *Sec.4.5.2* of of *BCPC*)
- 28. Theory of Behavioral Alteration (Peter Baofu) (*Sec.4.5.3* of *BCPC*)

IV. Theories in Relation to Society

—*At the Organizational Theoretical Level*

- 27. Theory of E-Civic Alienation (Peter Baofu) (Ch.7 of *FCD*)
- 26. Combinational Theory of Organization (Peter Baofu) (*FPHO*; Ch.6 of *ALD*)

—*At the Institutional Theoretical Level*

- 25. Reflective Theory of Criminality (Peter Baofu) (*FPHCRIM*)
- 24. Detached Theory of Gambling (Peter Baofu) (*FPHGAM*)
- 23. Heterodox Theory of Education (Peter Baofu) (*FPHEDU*)
- 22. Reconstruction Theory of Law (Peter Baofu) (*FPHLAW*)
- 21. Theory of Post-Capitalism (Peter Baofu) (Ch.10 of *FCD*; Chs.2 & 4 of *FPHC*; *BCPC*)
- 20. Theory of Post-Democracy (Peter Baofu) (Ch.10 of *FCD*; Chs.3 & 4 of *FPHC*; *BDPD*)

(continued on next page)

Table 4.43. Theories on Civilizational Holism (Part VI)

IV. Theories in Relation to Society (*cont'd*)

—*At the Institutional Theoretical Level (cont'd)*

- 19. Dynamic Theory of Comparative Political Systems (Peter Baofu) (*ALD*)
- (• 9.) Theory of the Cyclical Progression of Empire-Building (Peter Baofu) (*BWT*)

—*At the Systemic Theoretical Level*

- 18. Transfigurative Theory of Waste (Peter Baofu) (*FPHW*)
- 17. Theory of the Cyclical Progression of Migration (Peter Baofu) (*FPHMIG*)
- (• 66). Resettlement Theory of Geology (Peter Baofu) (*FPHGEOL*)
- 16. Contingent Theory of Urban Planning (Peter Baofu) (*FPHUP*)
- 15. Totalistic Theory of Communication (Peter Baofu) (*FPHMM*; *FCD*; *FHC*)
- 14. Ambivalent Theory of Technology (Peter Baofu) (*FPHE*; *FCD*; *FHC*)
- 13. Multifaceted Theory of War and Peace (Peter Baofu) (Ch.9 of *FCD*; Ch.1 of *FPHK*)
- 12. Theory of Post-Humanity (Peter Baofu) (Ch.7 of *FHC*; Chs.3, & 10 of *FCD*; Chs.1, 3 & 4 of *FPHC*; and other books of mine)
- 11. Theory of the Cyclical Progression of System Integration and Fragmentation (Peter Baofu) (Chs.9-10 of *FCD*)
- 10. Synthetic Theory of Information Architecture (Peter Baofu) (*FIA*)

—*At the Structural Theoretical Level*

- 9. Theory of the Cyclical Progression of Hegemony (Peter Baofu) (Chs.9-10 of *FCD*; Chs.1, 3 & 4 of *FPHC*; *BDPD*)
- 8. Theory of the Cyclical Progression of Empire-Building (Peter Baofu) (*BWT*)

(continued on next page)

Table 4.43. Theories on Civilizational Holism (Part VII)

V. Meta-Theories (in Relation to Theories)

—*At the Methodological Meta-Theoretical Level*

(• 52).Interactive Theory of Semantics (Peter Baofu) (*FPHSEM*)

(• 40). Complex Theory of Data Analysis (Peter Baofu) (*FPHDA*)

• 7. Interpretivist Theory of Probability (Peter Baofu) (*FPHROB*)

• 6. Critical-Dialectic Theory of Formal Science (Peter Baofu) (*FPHFS*)

• 5. Theory of Methodological Holism (Peter Baofu) (Ch.1 of *FCD*; Ch.1of *FPHC*; *Sec.2.1* & *Sec.2.5* of *BCPC*; *FC*; *FPHK*; etc.)

—*At the Ontological Meta-Theoretical Level*

• 4. Theory of Existential Dialectics, or the Holistic Theory of Knowledge (Peter Baofu) (*FHC*; *FCD*; *FPHC*; *BDPD*; *FC*; *FAE*; *ALD; FIA; FPHK*; etc,)

• 3. Contrastive Theory of Rationality (Peter Baofu) (*FPHML*)

VI. Theories in Relation to the Rest

—*At the Meta-Historical Level*

• 2. Multifold Theory of History (Peter Baofu) (*FPHHIST*)

—*At the Empirical-Historical Level*

• 1. Theory of the Evolution from Pre-Modernity to After-Postmodernity (Peter Baofu) (*FHC*; Ch.9-10 of *FCD*; *FPHC*)

Notes: All these theories are my constructions, as some of the main contributions of my grant project on civilization and its future. These examples are solely illustrative (not exhaustive), and some of the items can be reclassified somewhere else. Nor are they always mutually exclusive. Since they are generalities, exceptions are expected.

Sources: From my previous books.

Table 4.44. Three Great Future Transformations of Mind Games

- **Virtual Games**
  —Ex: online chess
  —Ex: virtual experience

- **Novel Games**
  —Ex: new chess variants
  —Ex: new chess engines

- **Post-Human Mind Games**
  —Ex: the quest for broader/deeper mental benefits of chess playing
  —Ex: games designed for the evolution of the mind into different body-less forms (e.g., "floating consciousness," "hyper-spatial consciousness," "unfolding unconsciousness")

Notes: The examples in the categories are solely illustrative (not exhaustive), and the comparison is relative (not absolute), nor are they necessarily mutually exclusive. And some can be easily re-classified elsewhere. As generalities, they allow exceptions.
Sources: From *Sec. 4.16* of *FPHCHESS*. See text for more info. Also, consult *FCD* for strategy and tactics in warfare and *FPHO* for strategy and tactics in organization.

BIBLIOGRAPHY

About.com (ABO). 2006. "What is Mental Health?" (July 25). <http://mentalhealth.about.com/cs/stressmanagement/a/whatismental.htm>.

Acharya, Deepak; & Shrivastava Anshu. 2008. *Indigenous Herbal Medicines: Tribal Formulations and Traditional Herbal Practices*. Jaipur: Aavishkar Publishers Distributor.

Abbott, P. 1999. "Women, Health and Domestic Violence." *Journal of Gender Studies,* 8: 83–10. <http://www.tandfonline.com/doi/abs/10.1080/09589239 9102841>.

Adams, A. E.; C. Sullivan; D. Bybee; & M. Greeson. 2008. "Development of the Scale of Economic Abuse." *Violence Against Women*, 14 (5): 563–588. <http://vaw.sagepub.com/content/14/5/563>.

Aggrawal, Anil. 2013. "A New Classification of Zoophilia" (February 01). *Sciencedirect.com*. <http://www.sciencedirect.com/science/article/pii/S17529 28X11000102>.

_____.2009. *Forensic And Medico-legal Aspects of Sexual Crimes And Unusual Sexual Practices*. U.S.: CRC Press.

Akmatov, Manas. 2011. "Child Abuse in 28 Developing and Transitional Countries—Results from the Multiple Indicator Cluster Surveys." *Int J Epidemiol,* 40(1): 219-27. <http://www.ncbi.nlm.nih.gov/pubmed/2094 3933>.

Alberta Rural Physician Action Plan (ARPAP). 2011. "Levels of Care." <http://www.albertaphysicianlink.ab.ca/orientation_guide/levels-of-care.ht ml>.

Alibhai-Brown, Yasmin. 2005. "People Matter more than Holy Books" (May 23). *The Independent*. <http://www.independent.co.uk/columnists_a_l/yasmin_ alibhai_brown/story.jsp?story=640612>.

American Psychiatric Association (APA). 2000. "Diagnostic and Statistical Manual of Mental Disorders: DSM-IV." Washington, DC: American Psychiatric Association.

American Telemedicine Association (ATA). 2011. "Telemedicine/Telehealth Terminology." <http://www.americantelemed.org/files/public/abouttelemedi cine/Terminology.pdf>.

Amnesty International (AMN). 2007. "Torture and Ill-Treatment: The Arguments:

1. What is Torture? What is Ill-Treatment? What's the Difference?." <http://web.archive.org/web/20071205141017/http://web.amnesty.org/pages/stoptorture-arguments-eng>.

_____.2005. "Torture and Ill-Treatment in the 'War on Terror'" (November 01). <http://www.amnesty.org/en/library/info/ACT40/ 014/2005/en>.

_____.1973. "Torture in the Eighties." <http://www.amnesty.org/en/library/asset/ACT40/001/1984/en/66491fc3-a18f-4ed5-8bd5-074d0a8a9130/act400011984eng.pdf>.

Aneshensel, C. S. 1992. "Social Stress: Theory and Research." *Annual Review of Sociology*, 18: 15–38. <http://www.annualreviews.org/doi/abs/10.1146/annurev.so.18.080192.000311>.

Anthony, Kate; DeeAnna Merz Nagel; & Stephen Goss, eds. 2010. *The Use of Technology in Mental Health : Applications, Ethics and Practice*. Springfield, IL: Charles C. Thomas Publishers.

Arch, J. J., & M. Craske. 2006. "Mechanisms of Mindfulness: Emotion Regulation Following a Focused Breathing Induction." *Behaviour Research and Therapy*, 44 (12): 1849–58. <http://www.sciencedirect.com/science/article/pii/S0005796705002743>.

Archontaki, D.; G. J. Lewis; & T. C. Bates. 2012. "Genetic Influences on Psychological Well-Being: A Nationally Representative Twin Study." *Journal of* Personality.

Armstrong, Alan. 2007. *Nursing Ethics: A Virtue-Based Approach*. UK: Palgrave Macmillan.

Ascione, Frank. 2008. *The International Handbook of Animal Abuse and Cruelty: Theory, Research, and Application.* West Lafayette, IN: Purdue University Press.

Aspe.hhs.gov (ASPE). 2002. "Physical Activity Fundamental To Preventing Disease" (June 20). <http://aspe.hhs.gov/health/reports/physicalactivity/>.

Astin, J. A. 1998. "Why Patients Use Alternative Medicine: Results of a National Study." *JAMA*, 279 (19): 1548–53. <http://jama.jamanetwork.com/article.aspx?articleid=187543>.

Auckland University (AUCK). 2013. "CCBT Game" (February 03). <http://www.metia.co.nz/etherapy.htm>.

Baer, Ruth A. 2013. *Mindfulness Training as a Clinical Intervention: A Conceptual and Empirical Review*. <http://www.wisebrain.org/papers/MindfulnessPsyTx.pdf>.

Bagaric, Mirko; & Clarke Julie. 2005. "Not Enough Official Torture in the World? The Circumstances in Which Torture Is Morally Justifiable." *University of San Francisco Law Review*, 39 (3): 581-616. <http://web.archive.org/web/20080209232527/http://www.usfca.edu/lawreview/Vol39number3.htm>.

Baker, P. R.; D. Francis; J. Soares; A. Weightman; & C. Foster. 2011. "Community Wide Interventions for Increasing Physical Activity." *Cochrane Database of Systematic Reviews,* (4): CD008366. <http://onlinelibrary.wiley.com/doi/10.1002/14651858.CD008366.pub2/abstract;jsessionid=766696D63DEDDFED729708C4C263D8D1.d02t04>.

Baofu, Peter. 2013. *The Future of Post-Human Thanatology: Towards a New Theory of Death and After-Death.* Berlin, Germany: Logos Verlag Berlin.

_____.2013a. *The Future of Post-Human Health Care: Towards a New Theory of Mind and Body.* Hauppauge, NY: Nova Science Publishers, Inc.

_____.2013b. *The Future of Post-Human Morphology: Towards a New Theory of Typologies and Rules.* Hauppauge, NY: Nova Science Publishers, Inc.

_____.2013c. *The Future of Post-Human Sports: Towards a New Theory of Training and Winning.* Cambridge, England: Cambridge Scholars Publishing.

_____.2013d. *Beyond Human Resources to Post-Human Resources: Towards a New Theory of Diversity and Discontinuity.* Cambridge, England: Cambridge Scholars Publishing.

_____.2012. *The Future of Post-Human Waste: Towards a New Theory of Uselessness and Usefulness.* Cambridge, England: Cambridge Scholars Publishing.

_____.2012a. *The Future of Post-Human Culinary Art: Towards a New Theory of Ingredients and Techniques.* Cambridge, England: Cambridge Scholars Publishing.

_____.2012b. *The Future of Post-Human Transportation: A Preface to a New Theory of Networks and Operations.* Cambridge, England: Cambridge Scholars Publishing.

_____.2012c. *The Future of Post-Human Migration: A Preface to a New Theory of Sameness, Otherness, and Identity.* Cambridge, England: Cambridge Scholars Publishing.

_____.2012d. *The Future of Post-Human History: A Preface to a New Theory of Universality and Relativity.* Cambridge, England: Cambridge Scholars Publishing.

_____.2012e. *The Future of Post-Human Criminality: A Preface to a New Theory of Heroes and Villains.* Cambridge, England: Cambridge International Science Publishing, Ltd.

_____.2012f. *The Future of Post-Human Architecture: A Preface to a New Theory of Form and Function.* Cambridge, England: Cambridge International Science Publishing, Ltd.

_____.2012g. *The Future of Post-Human Semantics: A Preface to a New Theory of Internality and Externality.* Cambridge, England: Cambridge Scholars Publishing.

_____.2012h. *The Future of Post-Human Performing Arts: A Preface to a New Theory of the Body and its Presence*. Cambridge, England: Cambridge Scholars Publishing.

_____.2011. *The Future of Post-Human Geography: A Preface to a New Theory of Environments and their Interactions*. Cambridge, England: Cambridge International Science Publishing, Ltd.

_____.2011a. *The Future of Post-Human Data Analysis: A Preface to a New Theory of Quantitative and Qualitative Research*. Cambridge, England: Cambridge International Science Publishing, Ltd.

_____.2011b. *The Future of Post-Human Chemistry: A Preface to a New Theory of Substances and their Changes*. Cambridge, England: Cambridge Scholars Publishing.

_____.2011c. *The Future of Post-Human Literature: A Preface to a New Theory of Fiction and Non-Fiction*. Cambridge, England: Cambridge International Science Publishing, Ltd.

_____.2011d. *The Future of Post-Human Computing: A Preface to a New Theory of Hardware, Software, and the Mind*. Cambridge, England: Cambridge International Science Publishing, Ltd.

_____.2011e. *The Future of Post-Human Gambling: A Preface to a New Theory of Risk and Caution*. Cambridge, England: Cambridge International Science Publishing, Ltd.

_____.2011f. *The Future of Post-Human Acoustics: A Preface to a New Theory of Sound and Silence*. Cambridge, England: Cambridge International Science Publishing, Ltd.

_____.2011g. *The Future of Post-Human Humor: A Preface to a New Theory of Joking and Laughing*. Cambridge, England: Cambridge International Science Publishing, Ltd.

_____.2011h. *Beyond Ethics to Post-Ethics: A Preface to a New Theory of Morality and Immorality*. Charlotte, NC: Information Age Publishing.

_____.2011i. *The Future of Post-Human Education: A Preface to a New Theory of Teaching and Learning*. Cambridge, England: Cambridge International Science Publishing, Ltd.

_____.2010. *The Future of Post-Human Religion: A Preface to a New Theory of Spirituality*. Cambridge, England: Cambridge International Science Publishing, Ltd.

_____.2010a. *The Future of Post-Human Chess: A Preface to a New Theory of Tactics and Strategy*. Cambridge, England: Cambridge International Science Publishing, Ltd.

_____.2010b. *The Future of Post-Human Geology: A Preface to a New Theory of Statics and Dynamics*. Cambridge, England: Cambridge International Science Publishing, Ltd.

_____.2010c. *Beyond Cosmology to Post-Cosmology: A Preface to a New Theory of Different Worlds*. Cambridge, England: Cambridge International Science Publishing, Ltd.

_____.2010d. *The Future of Post-Human Personality: A Preface to a New Theory of Normality and Abnormality*. Cambridge, England: Cambridge International Science Publishing, Ltd.

_____.2010e. *The Future of Post-Human War and Peace: A Preface to a New Theory of Aggression and Pacificity*. Cambridge, England: Cambridge Scholars Publishing.

_____.2010f. *The Future of Post-Human Formal Science: A Preface to a New Theory of Abstraction and Application*. Cambridge, England: Cambridge Scholars Publishing.

_____.2010g. *The Future of Post-Human Law: A Preface to a New Theory of Necessity, Contingency, and Justice*. Cambridge, England: Cambridge Scholars Publishing.

_____.2010h. *The Future of Post-Human Sexuality: A Preface to a New Theory of the Body and Spirit of Love Makers*. Cambridge, England: Cambridge Scholars Publishing.

_____,2009. *The Future of Post-Human Martial Arts: A Preface to a New Theory of the Body and Spirit of Warriors*. Cambridge, England: Cambridge Scholars Publishing.

_____.2009a. *The Future of Post-Human Organization: A Preface to a New Theory of Communication, Decision-Making, and Leadership*. Cambridge, England: Cambridge Scholars Publishing.

_____.2009b. *The Future of Post-Human Language: A Preface to a New Theory of Structure, Context, and Learning*. Cambridge, England: Cambridge Scholars Publishing.

_____.2009c. *The Future of Post-Human Urban Planning: A Preface to a New Theory of Density, Void, and Sustainability*. Cambridge, England: Cambridge Scholars Publishing.

_____.2009d. *The Future of Post-Human Geometry: A Preface to a New Theory of Infinity, Symmetry, and Dimensionality*. Cambridge, England: Cambridge Scholars Publishing.

_____.2009e. *The Future of Post-Human Creative Thinking: A Preface to a New Theory of Invention and Innovation*. Cambridge, England: Cambridge Scholars Publishing.

_____.2009f. *The Future of Post-Human Mass Media: A Preface to a New Theory of Communication*. Cambridge, England: Cambridge Scholars Publishing.

_____.2009g. *The Future of Post-Human Engineering: A Preface to a New Theory of Technology*. Cambridge, England: Cambridge Scholars Publishing.

_____.2008. *The Future of Post-Human Mathematical Logic: A Preface to a New Theory of Rationality*. Cambridge, England: Cambridge Scholars Publishing.

_____.2008a. *The Future of Post-Human Knowledge: A Preface to a New Theory of Methodology and Ontology*. Oxford, United Kingdom: Chandos Publishing (Oxford) Ltd.

_____.2008b. *The Future of Post-Human Unconsciousness: A Preface to a New Theory of Anomalous Experience*. Cambridge, England: Cambridge Scholars Publishing.

_____.2008c. *The Future of Information Architecture: Conceiving a New Way to Understand Taxonomy, Network, and Intelligence*. Oxford, United Kingdom: Chandos Publishing (Oxford) Ltd.

_____.2007. *The Rise of Authoritarian Liberal Democracy: A Preface to a New Theory of Comparative Political Systems*. Cambridge, England: Cambridge Scholars Publishing.

_____.2007a. *The Future of Aesthetic Experience: Conceiving a Better Way to Beauty, Ugliness, and the Rest*. Cambridge, England: Cambridge Scholars Publishing.

_____.2007b. *The Future of Complexity: Conceiving a Better Way to Understand Order and Chaos*. London, United Kingdom: World Scientific Publishing Co.

_____.2007c. *Beyond the World of Titans, and the Remaking of World Order: A Preface to a New Logic of Empire-Building*. Cambridge, England: Cambridge Scholars Publishing.

_____.2006. *Beyond Nature and Nurture: Conceiving a Better Way to Understand Genes and Memes*. Cambridge, England: Cambridge Scholars Publishing.

_____.2006a. *The Future of Post-Human Space-Time: Conceiving a Better Way to Understand Space and Time*. New York: Peter Lang Publishing, Inc.

_____.2006b. *Beyond Civilization to Post-Civilization: Conceiving a Better Model of Life Settlement to Supersede Civilization*. New York: Peter Lang Publishing, Inc.

_____.2005. *Beyond Capitalism to Post-Capitalism: Conceiving a Better Model of Wealth Acquisition to Supersede Capitalism*. New York: The Edwin Mellen Press.

_____.2004. *The Future of Post-Human Consciousness*. New York: The Edwin Mellen Press.

_____.2004a. *Beyond Democracy to Post-Democracy: Conceiving a Better Model of Governance to Supersede Democracy*. Volume 1. New York: The Edwin Mellen Press.

_____.2004b. *Beyond Democracy to Post-Democracy: Conceiving a Better Model of Governance to Supersede Democracy*. Volume 2. New York: The Edwin

Mellen Press.

_____.2002. *The Future of Capitalism and Democracy*. Maryland: The University Press of America.

_____.2000. *The Future of Human Civilization*. Volume 1. New York: The Edwin Mellen Press.

_____.2000a. *The Future of Human Civilization*. Volume 2. New York: The Edwin Mellen Press.

Barden, J. C. 1987. "Marital Rape: Drive for Tougher Laws is Pressed." <http://www.nytimes.com/1987/05/13/us/marital-rape-drive-for-tougher-laws-is-pressed.html>.

Barnes, P. M., E. Powell-Griner; K. McFann; & R. Nahin. 2004. "Complementary and Alternative Medicine Use among Adults: United States, 2002." *Advance Data*, (343): 1–19. <http://www.cdc.gov/nchs/data/ad/ad343.pdf>.

Barnett, O. W. 2001. "Why Battered Women Do Not Leave, Part 2: External Inhibiting Factors--Social Support and Internal Inhibiting Factors." *Trauma, Violence, & Abuse*, 2: 3-1. <http://tva.sagepub.com/content/2/1/3>.

Barrow, John D. 1998. *Impossibility: The Limits of Science and the Science of Limits*. Oxford: Oxford University Press.

Barth, Richard. 1994. *Child Welfare Research Review*, Volume 1. NY: Columbia University Press. <http://books.google.com.pe/books?hl=en&lr=&id=OzTq7SHLlIMC&oi=fnd&pg=PA28&dq=child+abuse+cultural+norms+movement+change&ots=1R7uyr4BLg&sig=NA_diabapBmL9pT13432noel628&redir_esc=y#v=onepage&q=movement&f=true>.

BBC News (BBC). 2010. "Rise in African Children Accused of Witchcraft" (July 17). <http://www.bbc.co.uk/news/world-africa-10671790>.

_____.2007. "Consequentialist Reasons Why Torture is Wrong" (December 13). <http://web.archive.org/web/20071213004811/http://www.bbc.co.uk/religion/ethics/torture/ethics/wrong_2.shtml>.

_____.2006. "One Third Support Some Torture" (October 19). <http://news.bbc.co.uk/2/hi/6063386.stm>.

Bebchuk, Lucian; & Jesse Fried. 2004. *Pay without Performance: The Unfulfilled Promise of Executive Compensation*. Cambridge, MA: Harvard University Press.

Beetz, Andrea M. 2004. "Bestiality/Zoophilia: A Scarcely-Investigated Phenomenon between Crime, Paraphilia, and Love." *Journal of Forensic Psychology Practice*, 4 (2): 1-36. <http://www.scie-socialcareonline.org.uk/profile.asp?guid=fac3acab-5377-4f9a-a9f0-007248ee2e43>.

Bekelman, J. E.; Y. Li; & C. Gross. 2003. "Scope and Impact of Financial Conflicts of Interest in Biomedical Research: A Systematic Review." *JAMA*, 289 (4): 454–65. <http://jama.jamanetwork.com/article.aspx?articleid=195

843>.

Berman, Brian M.; Helene M. Langevin; Claudia M. Witt; & Ronald Dubner. 2010. "Acupuncture for Chronic Low Back Pain." *New England Journal of Medicine*, 2010; 363:454-461. <http://www.nejm.org/doi/full/10.1056/NEJMct0806114>.

Berrios, D. C.; & D. Grady. 1991. "Domestic Violence. Risk Factors and Outcomes." *The Western Journal of Medicine*, 155 (2): 133–135. <http://www.ncbi.nlm.nih.gov/pmc/articles/PMC1002942/>.

Besant, Annie Wood. 1897. *The Ancient Wisdom: An Outline of Theosophical Teachings*. Theosophical publishing society.

Bethea, Lesa. 1999. "Primary Prevention of Child Abuse." *American Family Physician*. <http://www.aafp.org/afp/1999/0315/p1577.html>.

Beyerstein, B. L. 2001. "Alternative Medicine and Common Errors of Reasoning." *Academic Medicine: Journal of the Association of American Medical Colleges*, 76 (3): 230–237. <http://www.ncbi.nlm.nih.gov/pubmed/11242572>.

Biletzki, Anat; & Anat Matar. 2006. "Ludwig Wittgenstein" (Nov. 17). *Stanford Encyclopedia of Philosophy*. <http://plato.stanford.edu/entries/wittgenstein/>.

Bishop, S. R.; M. Lau; S. Shapiro; L. Carlson; et al. 2004. "Mindfulness: A Proposed Operational Definition." *Clin Psychol Sci Prac*, 11:230–241. <http://www.personal.kent.edu/~dfresco/mindfulness/Bishop_et_al.pdf>.

Blackmore, Susan. 1991. "Near-Death Experiences: In or out of the body?." *Skeptical Inquirer*, 16: 34-45. <http://web.archive.org/web/20080419061634/http://www.susanblackmore.co.uk/si91nde.html>.

Blechner, M. 2007. "Approaches to Panic Attacks." *Neuro-Psychoanalysis*, 9: 93-102.

Booth, Robert. 2010. "The Spirit Level: How 'Ideas Wreckers' Turned Book into Political Punchbag" (August 13). *The Guardian*. <http://www.guardian.co.uk/books/2010/aug/14/the-spirit-level-equality-thinktanks>.

Bouchard, Claude; Ping An; Treva Rice; James S. Skinner; Jack H. Wilmore; Jacques Gagnon; Louis Perusse; Arthus S. Leon; & D. C. Rao. 1999. "Familial Aggregation of VO(2max) Response to Exercise Training: Results from the HERITAGE Family Study." *Journal of Applied Physiology*, 87 (3): 1003–1008. <http://jap.physiology.org/content/87/3/1003.abstract?ijkey=189eebcbc5a461258da582b4aef41ebcf7bec51f&keytype2=tf_ipsecsha>.

Bouchaud, J.; & M. Mezard. 2000. "Wealth Condensation in a Simple Model of Economy." *Physica A: Statistical Mechanics and its Applications*. 282 (3–4): 536. <http://adsabs.harvard.edu/abs/2000PhyA..282..536B>.

Bouchard, Thomas J., Jr.; & J. Loehlin. 2001. "Genes, Evolution, and Personality." *Behavior Genetics*, 31 (3): 243–273. <http://link.springer.com/article/10.1023

%2FA%3A1012294324713>.

Breier-Mackie, Sarah. 2006. "Medical Ethics and Nursing Ethics: Is There Really Any Difference?." *Gastroenterology Nursing*, 29 (2): 182–3. <http://www.nursingcenter.com/pdf.asp?AID=641332>.

Brewster, M. P. 2003. "Power and Control Dynamics in Prestalking and Stalking Situations." *Journal of Family Violence*, 18 (4): 207–217. <http://link.springer.com/article/10.1023%2FA%3A1024064214054>.

Briere, John. 1992. *Child Abuse Trauma*. CA: Sage.

Brown, David. 2009. "Scientists Speak Out Against Federal Funds for Research on Alternative Medicine" (March 17). *Washingtonpost*. <http://www.washingtonpost.com/wp-dyn/content/article/2009/03/16/AR2009031602139.html?hpid=sec-health>.

_____.2007. "Psychedelic Healing?." *Scientific American*. <http://www.scientificamerican.com/article.cfm?id=psychedelic-healing>.

Brown, Dennis; & Stephen Morris. 2003. *Religion and Human Experience*. Rhinegold Eeligious Studies Study Guides. London, UK: Rhinegold. <http://books.google.co.uk/books?id=7OkAqYod1CgC&lpg=PP1&pg=PA115#v=onepage&q&f=false>.

Brown, K. W.; R. Ryan. 2003. "The Benefits of Being Present: Mindfulness and its Role in Psychological Well-Being." *Journal of Personality and Social Psychology*, 84 (4): 822–48. <http://psycnet.apa.org/?&fa=main.doiLanding&doi=10.1037/0022-3514.84.4.822>.

Brown, Patricia Leigh. 2011. "In Oakland, Redefining Sex Trade Workers as Abuse Victims" (May 24). *The New York Times*. <http://www.nytimes.com/2011/05/24/us/24oakland.html?_r=0>.

Bruce, Robert. 1999. *Astral Dynamics*. Charlottesville, Virginia: Hampton Roads Publishing Company, Inc.

Bullough, Vern L.; & Bonnie Bullough. 1994. *Human Sexuality: An Encyclopedia*. New York: Garland Pub.

Bunge, Mario. 1999. *Dictionary of philosophy*. Amherst, MA: Prometheus Books.

Burfoot, Amby. 2004. "Runner's High." *Runner's World*. <http://www.runnersworld.com/runners-stories/runners-high>.

Buman, M. P.: & A. King. 2010. "Exercise as a Treatment to Enhance Sleep." *American Journal of Lifestyle Medicine*.

Buss, D. M. 2011. *Evolutionary Psychology*. Boston, MA: Pearson/A and B.

_____.2004. *Evolutionary Psychology: The New Science of the Mind*. Boston, MA: Pearson Education, Inc.

_____; M. Haselton; T. Shackelford; A. Bleske; J. Wakefield. 1998. "Adaptations, Exaptations, and Spandrels." *American Psychologist*, 53 (5): 533–548.

Byrd, Andrea. 1999. "Biology 202, Serotonin and Its Uses."

<http://serendip.brynmawr.edu/bb/neuro/neuro99/web1/Byrd.html>.

Byrne, Rhonda. 2006. *The Secret*. Chicago, IL: T.S. Production.

Calcutta News (CAL). 2009. "Half of India's Children Malnourished, says NGO Report" (October 15). <http://www.calcuttanews.net/story/554769>.

Carney, Tom. 2006. "Majority of Catholics Would Support Torture" (March 24). <http://web.archive.org/web/20080612093225/http://ncronline.org/NCR_Online/archives2/2006a/032406/032406h.htm>.

Carroll Robert Todd. 2003. *The Skeptic's Dictionary: A Collection of Strange Beliefs, Amusing Deceptions, and Dangerous Delusions*. NY: John Wiley and Sons.

Casey, Benedict. 2004. "For Psychotherapy's Claims, Skeptics Demand Proof" (August 10). *The New York Times*. <http://www.nytimes.com/2004/08/10/health/psychology/10ther.html?pagewanted=1&ei=5090&en=e6560227dc7526f7&ex=1249876800&partner=rssuserland>.

Cassileth, B. R. 1999. "Evaluating Complementary and Alternative Therapies for Cancer Patients." *CA Cancer J Clin*, 49 (6): 362–75. <http://onlinelibrary.wiley.com/doi/10.3322/canjclin.49.6.362/full>.

CBS News (CBS). 2006. "Alternative Medicine Goes Mainstream" (July 20). <http://www.cbsnews.com/stories/2006/07/20/health/webmd/main1823747.shtml>.

Cdc.gov (CDC). 2013. "How Much Physical Activity do Adults Need?." <http://www.cdc.gov/physicalactivity/everyone/guidelines/adults.html>.

Centers for Disease Control and Prevention (CDCP). 2005. "Compendium of Measures To Prevent Disease Associated with Animals in Public Settings." <http://www.cdc.gov/mmwr/PDF/

_____.2005a. "Outbreaks of Escherichia Coli O157:H7 Associated with Petting Zoos—North Carolina, Florida, and Arizona, 2004 and 2005." *MMWR*, 54 (50): 1279.

_____.2001. "Outbreaks of Escherichia Coli O157:H7 Infections among Children Associated with Farm Visits—Pennsylvania and Washington 2000." *MMWR*, 50 (15): 293–297. <http://www.cdc.gov/mmwR/preview/mmwrhtml/mm5015a5.htm>.

_____.1988. "Human Infection with Swine Influenza Virus–Wisconsin." *MMWR*, 37 (43): 661–3. <http://www.cdc.gov/MMWR/preview/mmwrhtml/00021592.htm>.

Charlton, B. G. 1996. "What is the Ultimate Cause of Socio-Economic Inequalities in Health? An Explanation in Terms of Evolutionary Psychology." *Journal of the Royal Society of Medicine*, 89 (1): 3–8. <http://www.ncbi.nlm.nih.gov/pmc/articles/PMC1295633/pdf/jrsocmed00059-0007.pdf>.

Chase, Scott. 1993. "Tachyons" (March). *Physics FAQ*. <http://math.ucr.edu/home/baez/physics/ParticleAndNuclear/tachyons.html>.

Chia, Mantak. 1989. *Fusion of the Five Elements*. Rochester, VT: Destiny Books.

Children and Family Court Advisory and Support Service (CFCASS). 2007. "Domestic Violence Assessment Policy." <http://web.archive.org/web/20071130235416/http://www.cafcass.gov.uk/English/Publications/consultation/04DecDV%20Policy.pdf>.

Cia, G. 1995. *Tongue Diagnosis in Chinese Medicine*. CA: Eastland Press.

Clarke, Peter Bernard. 2000. *Japanese New Religions: in Global Perspective*. NY: Routledge.

Clune, J.; J. Mouret; & H. Lipson. 2012. "The Evolutionary Origins of Modularity." <http://arxiv.org/pdf/1207.2743v1.pdf>.

CNN. 2010. "Court in UAE says Beating Wife, Child OK if No Marks are Left" (October 19). <http://articles.cnn.com/2010-10-19/world/uae.court.ruling_1_islamic-law-sharia-law-ruling?_s=PM:WORLD>.

Cohen, Peter; & Arjan Sas. 1994. "Cocaine Use in Amsterdam in Non-Deviant Subcultures." *Addiction Research*, 2 (1): 71-94. <http://www.cedro-uva.org/lib/cohen.cocaine.html#RTFToC19>.

Colfer, George R. 2006. "Skill-Related Fitness Necessary for Sports Success" (October 17). <http://web.archive.org/web/20110617084150/http://www.tradoc.army.mil/pao/Web_specials/H_and_PWB/013204.htm>.

Common Sense for Drug Policy (CSDP). 2007. "Economics." <http://drugwarfacts.org/cms/?q=node/38>.

_____.2007a. "Prisons, Jails and Probation–Overview." <http://drugwarfacts.org/cms/?q=node/62>.

Confer, J. C.; J. Easton; D. Fleischman; C. Goetz; D. Lewis; C. Perilloux; & D. Buss. 2010. "Evolutionary Psychology: Controversies, Questions, Prospects, and Limitations." *American Psychologist*, 65 (2): 110–126. <http://homepage.psy.utexas.edu/homepage/Group/BussLAB/pdffiles/evolutionary_psychology_AP_2010.pdf>.

Corazzon, Raul. 2007. "Definitions of Ontology: From Nicolai Hartmann to the Present Time." <http://www.formalontology.it/section_4_two.htm>.

Corbett, Dan. 2008. "Introduction to String Theory" (November 23). *ThinkQuest*. <http://library.thinkquest.org/27930/stringtheory1.htm>.

Corbin, Henri. 1969. *Creative Imagination in the Sufism of Ibn Arabi*. Ralph Mannheim, tr. NJ: Princeton University Press.

Corp, N.; A. Tsaroucha; & P. Kingston. 2008. "Human Givens Therapy: The Evidence Base." *Mental Health Review Journal*, 13 (4): 44–52. <http://www.emeraldinsight.com/products/pier/>.

Cosmides, L; & J. Tooby. 1997. "Evolutionary Psychology: A Primer." *Center for Evolutionary Psychology*. <http://www.cep.ucsb.edu/primer.html>.

Coulter, Ian D.; & Evan M Willis. 2004. "The Rise and Rise of Complementary and Alternative Medicine: A Sociological Perspective." *Medical Journal of Australia*, 180 (11): 587-589.

Crépault, C., & M. Couture. 1980. "Men's Erotic Fantasies." *Archives of Sexual Behavior*, 9 (6): 565–81.

Cron, T. 1986. "The Surgeon General's Workshop on Violence and Public Health: Review of the recommendations." *Public Health Rep.*, 101: 8-14.

CrossFit Journal (CRO). 2002. "What Is Fitness?" (October). <http://library.crossfit.com/free/pdf/CFJ-trial.pdf>.

Daszak, P.; A. Cunningham; & A. Hyatt. 2001. "Anthropogenic Environmental Change and the Emergence of Infectious Diseases in Wildlife." *Acta Trop.*, 78 (2): 103–116. <http://www.sciencedirect.com/science/article/pii/S0001706X 00001790>.

Davidson, Amy. 2005. "Q & A: Torture by Proxy" (February 14). *The New Yorker*.

DeNeve, Kristina M. 1999. "Happy as an Extraverted Clam? The Role of Personality for Subjective Well-Being." *Current Directions in Psychological Science*. 8 (5): 141–144. <http://cdp.sagepub.com/content/8/5/141.abstract>.

Diener, Ed. 2008. *Happiness: Unlocking the Mysteries of Psychological Wealth*. Malden, MA: Blackwell Pub.

_____.2000. "Subjective Well-Being: The Science of Happiness and a Proposal for a National Index." *American Psychologist*, 55 (1): 34–43.

_____.E. Suh; R. Lucas; & H. Smith. 1999. "Subjective Well-Being: Three Decades of Progress." *Psychological Bulletin*, 125 (2): 276–302. <http://www.psychology.illinois.edu/people/bwrobrts>.

_____.1984. "Subjective Well-Being." *Psychological Bulletin*, 95 (3): 542–575. <http://psycnet.apa.org/journals/bul/95/3/542/>.

Dinwiddie, S.; A. Heath; M. Dunne; K. Bucholz; P. Madden; W. Slutske; L. Bierut; D. Statham, et al. 2000. "Early Sexual Abuse and Lifetime Psychopathology: A Co-Twin-Control Study." *Psychological Medicine*, 30 (1): 41–52. <http://journals.cambridge.org/action/displayAbstract?fromPage=online&aid=26191>.

Doblin, Rick, 2004. "Exaggerating MDMA's Risks to Justify A Prohibitionist Policy." Multidisciplinary Association for Psychedelic Studies. <http://www.maps.org/mdma/rd011604.html>.

Dodd, L. W. 2009. "Therapeutic Groupwork with Young Children and Mothers who have Experienced Domestic Abuse." *Educational Psychology in Practice*, 25: 21–36. <http://www.tandfonline.com/doi/abs/10.1080/0266736 0802697571>.

Doherty, Gavin; David Coyle; & Mark Matthews. 2010. "Design and Evaluation Guidelines for Mental Health Technologies." *Interacting with Computers*, 22 (4): 243–252. <http://www.sciencedirect.com/science/article/pii/S09535438 10000238>.

Doumas, D.; G. Margolin; & R. John. 1994. "The Intergenerational Transmission of Aggression across Three Generations." *Journal of Family Violence*, 9 (2): 157. <http://link.springer.com/article/10.1007%2FBF01531961>.

Donnelly, John. 2000. "Apart From Personal Use, A Key Issue Stays Away." Globe Newspaper Company. <http://www.mapinc.org/drugnews/v00/n321/a04.html>.

DrugScience.org (DRUG). 2006. "Cannabis as a Gateway Drug." <http://www.drugscience.org/sfu/sfu_gateway.html>.

Durrant, R.; & B. Ellis. 2003. "Evolutionary Psychology." *Comprehensive Handbook of Psychology, Volume Three: Biological Psychology*. M. Gallagher & R. J. Nelson, eds. New York: Wiley & Sons.

D'Zurilla, T. J.; & A. Nezu. 1982. "Social Problem Solving in Adults." *Advances in Cognitive-Behavioral Research and Therapy*. P. C. Kendall, ed. New York: Academic Press.

de Vos, N.; N. Singh; D. Ross; T. Stavrinos, et al. 2005. "Optimal Load for Increasing Muscle Power During Explosive Resistance Training in Older Adults." *The Journals of Gerontology*, 60A (5): 638–647.

Drug Free Australia (DRA). 2010. "Arguments for Prohibition" (April 20). <http://www.drugfree.org.au/fileadmin/Media/Global/Taskforce_Arguments_for_Prohibition.pdf>.

Durrant, Joan E. 1996. "The Swedish Ban on Corporal Punishment: Its History and Effects." *Family Violence Against Children: A Challenge for Society*. Detlev Frehsee, Wiebke Horn, and Kai-D. Bussmann, eds. New York: Walter de Gruyter & Co..

Eardley, Peter; & Carl Still. 2010. *Aquinas: A Guide for the Perplexed*. London: Continuum.

Economist, the (ECON). 2011. "Alternative Medicine: Think Yourself Better" (May 21): 83–84. <http://www.economist.com/node/18710090>.

_____.2010. "Putting the Smallest First: Why India Makes a Poor Fist of Feeding the Young, and How it Could do Better" (September 23). <http://www.economist.com/node/17090948?story_id=17090948>.

Ehrenreich, Barbara. 2009. *Bright-Sided: How the Relentless Promotion of Positive Thinking Has Undermined America*. UK: MacMillan.

Eisenberg, D. M.; R. Davis; S. Ettner, et al. 1998. "Trends in Alternative Medicine Use in the United States, 1990–1997: Results of a Follow-Up National Survey. *JAMA*, 280 (18): 1569–75. <http://jama.jamanetwork.com/article.aspx?articleid=188148>.

_____; et al. 1993. "Unconventional Medicine in the United States—Prevalence, Costs, and Patterns of Use." *N Engl J Med*. 328 (4): 246–252. <http://www.nejm.org/doi/full/10.1056/NEJM199301283280406>.

Eisenberg, Leon; & Sarah Hart Brown. 1995. *The Best Intentions: Unintended Pregnancy and the Well-Being of Children and Families*. Washington, D.C: National Academy Press.

Ellis, Bruce J.; & Thomas Boyce. 2008. "Biological Sensitivity to Context." *Current Directions in Psychological Science*, 17 (3): 183–187. <http://cdp.sagepub.com/content/17/3/183>.

Emson, H. E. 1987. "Health, Disease and Illness: Matters for Definition." *CMAJ*, 136 (8): 811–3. <http://www.ncbi.nlm.nih.gov/pmc/articles/PMC1492114/>.

Ernst, Edzard. 2013. "Complementary Medicine: The Good, the Bad and the Ugly" (February 03). <http://www.healthwatch-uk.org/awardwinners/edzardernst.html>.

_____.2011. "Alternative Medicine Remains an Ethics-Free Zone" (November 08). *The Guardian*. <http://www.guardian.co.uk/science/blog/2011/nov/08/alternative-medicine-ethics-free-zone>.

_____.2005. "Complementary Medicine: The Good, the Bad and the Ugly." <http://www.healthwatch-uk.org/awardwinners/edzardernst.html>.

_____.2002. "A Systematic Review of Systematic Reviews of Homeopathy." *British Journal of Clinical Pharmacology*, 54 (6): 577-82. <http://onlinelibrary.wiley.com/doi/10.1046/j.1365-2125.2002.01699.x/abstract;jsessionid=4619E1E224F9D26264A21A96E2E06D58.d02t02>.

Evans, M. R.; & D. Gardner. 1996. "'Cryptosporidiosis' Outbreak Associated with an Educational Farm Holiday." *Commun Dis Rep CDR Rev.*, 29 6 (4): R67.

Everett, Hugh. 1957. "'Relative State' Formulation of Quantum Mechanics" (July). *Reviews of Modern Physics*, vol. 29, no.3. <http://www.univer.omsk.su/omsk/Sci/Everett/paper1957.html>.

Eysenck, Hans. 1952. "The Effects of Psychotherapy: An Evaluation." *Journal of Consulting Psychology*, 16: 319–324.

Feltham, Colin. 1997. *Which Psychotherapy?: Leading Exponents Explain their Differences*. Thousand Oaks, CA: SAGE Publication.

Field, H.; P. Young; J. Yob; J. Mills; L. Hall; & J. Mackenzie. 2001. "The Natural History of Hendra and Nipah Viruses." *Microbes and Infection*, 3 (4): 307–314.<http://www.sciencedirect.com/science/article/pii/S1286457901013843>.

Firehammer, Reginald. 2005. "Basic Principles of Ontology" (January 05). <http://usabig.com/autonomist/philosophy/ontology2.html>.

Follingstad, D. R.; D. Dehart. 2000. "Defining Psychological Abuse of Husbands Toward Wives: Contexts, Behaviors, and Typologies." *Journal of Interpersonal Violence*, 15 (9): 891. <http://jiv.sagepub.com/content/15/9/891>.

Fowler, J. H; & N. Christakis. 2008. "Dynamic Spread of Happiness in a Large Social Network: Longitudinal Analysis over 20 Years in the Framingham Heart Study" (December 4). *BMJ*, 337 (dec04 2): a2338–a2338. <http://www.bmj.com/content/337/bmj.a2338>.

Franklin, J. 2009. "Evidence Gained from Torture: Wishful Thinking, Checkability and Extreme Circumstances." *Cardozo Journal of International and Comparative Law*, 17 (2): 281–90. <http://web.maths.unsw.edu.au/~jim/torturecardozo.pdf>.

_____.2001. *The Science of Conjecture: Evidence and Probability Before Pascal*. Baltimore, MD: Johns Hopkins University Press.

Frazer, Peter. 2010. "Astral Projection? In your Dreams, say Sceptics" (September 30). *Brisbane Times.* <http://www.brisbanetimes.com.au/lifestyle/astral-projection-in-your-dreams-say-sceptics-20100929-15x6n.html>.

Friedman, Milton. 2013. "The Drug War as a Socialist Enterprise" (February 16). <http://www.druglibrary.org/special/friedman/socialist.htm>.

Froomkin, Dan. 2007. "Did Torture Work?" (December 11). *Washington Post.* <http://www.washingtonpost.com/wp-dyn/content/blog/2007/12/11/BL2007121101053.html?nav=rss_opinion/columns>.

Fuller-Thomson, E.; & S. Brennenstuhl. 2009. "Making a Link between Childhood Physical Abuse and Cancer: Results from a Regional Representative Survey." *Cancer,* 115 (14): 3341–50. <http://onlinelibrary.wiley.com/doi/10.1002/cncr.24372/abstract>.

Garland, E., et al. 2009. "The Role of Mindfulness in Positive Reappraisal." *The Journal of Science and Healing,* 5 (1): 37–44. <http://www.explorejournal.com/article/S1550-8307%2808%2900321-2/abstract>.

Garland, T., Jr.; H. Schutz; M. Chappell; B. Keeney; T. Meek; L. Copes; W. Acosta; C. Drenowatz; R. Maciel; G. van Dijk; C. Kotz; & J. Eisenmann. 2011. "The Biological Control of Voluntary Exercise, Spontaneous Physical Activity and Daily Energy Expenditure in Relation to Obesity: Human and Rodent Perspectives." *Journal of Experimental Biology,* 214: 206–229.

Garrett, Thomas A. 2010. "Income Inequality: It's Not So Bad." <http://www.stlouisfed.org/publications/itv/articles/?id=1920>.

Gartrell, N.; N. Milliken; W. Goodson; S. Thiemann; & B. Lo. 1992. "Physician-Patient Sexual Contact. Prevalence and Problems." *West J Med,* 157 (2): 139–43. <http://www.ncbi.nlm.nih.gov/pmc/articles/PMC1011231/>.

Garvey, Anne. 2004. "Depressed? Go and Clean the Kitchen" (May 4). *The Guardian.* <http://www.guardian.co.uk/lifeandstyle/2004/may/04/healthandwellbeing.mentalhealth>.

Gaulin, Steven; & Donald H. McBurney. 2003. *Evolutionary Psychology.* Upper Saddle River, NJ: Prentice Hall.

Gauthier, L.; G. Stollak; L. Messé; & J. Aronoff. 1996. "Recall of Childhood Neglect and Physical Ause as Differential Predictors of Current Psychological Functioning." *Child Abuse & Neglect,* 20 (7): 549–59. <http://www.sciencedirect.com/science/article/pii/0145213496000439>.

Gedye, Robin. 2004. "The Envoy Silenced after Telling Undiplomatic Truths" (October 23). *The Daily Telegraph.* <http://www.telegraph.co.uk/news/uknews/1474852/The-envoy-silenced-after-telling-undiplomatic-truths.html>.

Gerstein, D.; & A. Johnson. 1998. "Initiation of Use of Alcohol, Cigarettes, Marijuana, Cocaine, and Other Substances in US Birth Cohorts since 1919." *American Journal of Public Health,* 88 (1): 27. <http://www.druglibrary.org/crl/perspectives/Johnson%20&%20Gerstein%2098%20Usage%20Trends_%20AmJPubHealth.pdf>.

Gleeson, M. 2007. "Immune Function in Sport and Exercise." *J. Appl. Physiol.*, 103 (2): 693–9. <http://jap.physiology.org/content/103/2/693>.

Goetz, A. T. 2010. "The Evolutionary Psychology of Violence." *Psicothema*, 22 (1): 15–21. *PMID*. <http://www.ncbi.nlm.nih.gov/pubmed/ 20100422>.

Goldacre, Ben. 2008. "Cocaine Study that Got up the Nose of the US." <http://www.guardian.co.uk/commentisfree/2009/jun/13/bad-science-cocaine-study>.

_____.2007. "Cannabis Data Comes to the Crunch." <http://www.guardian.co.uk/ science/2007/jul/28/drugs.drugsandalcohol>.

Golden, J. A.; & W. Prather. 2009. "A Behavioral Perspective of Childhood Trauma and Attachment Issues: Toward Alternative Treatment Approaches for Children with a History of Abuse." *International Journal of Behavioral and Consultation Therapy*, 5: 56-74.

Goldrosen, M. H.; & S. Straus. 2004. "Complementary and Alternative Medicine: Assessing the Evidence for Immunological Benefits." *Nature Perspectives*, 4: 912-921. <http://www.nature.com/nri/journal/v4/n11/pdf/nri1486.pdf>.

Goldthorpe, J. 2009. "Analysing Social Inequality: A Critique of Two Recent Contributions from Economics and Epidemiology." *European Sociological Review*, 26 (6): 731-744. <http://esr.oxfordjournals.org/content/26/6/731. abstract>.

Goode, William. 1971. "Force and Violence in the Family." *Journal of Marriage and the Family (National Council on Family Relations)*, 33 (4): 624–36. <http://www.jstor.org/discover/10.2307/349435?uid=3738800&uid=2&uid=4 &sid=21101664854423>.

Goss, Stephen; & Joe Ferns. 2010. "Using Cell/Mobile Phone SMS to Enhance Client Crisis and Peer Support." *The Use of Technology in Mental Health: Applications, Ethics and Practice*. Kate Anthony, DeeAnna Merz Nagel and Stephen Goss, eds. Springfield, IL: Charles C. Thomas Pub Ltd.

Gott, J. Richard. 2002. *Time Travel in Einstein's Universe*. Boston : Houghton Mifflin.

Grinspoon, Lester; & James Bakalar. 2013. "Medical Uses of Illicit Drugs." Schaffer Library of Drug Policy <http://www.druglibrary.org/schaffer/hemp/ medical/meduse.htm>.

Grondard, Clément; et al. 2005. "Regular Exercise Prolongs Survival in a Type 2 Spinal Muscular Atrophy Model Mouse." *The Journal of Neuroscience*, 25 (33): 7615–7622. <http://www.jneurosci.org/content/25/33/7615>.

Grossman, P., L. Niemann, S. Schmidt; & H. Walach. 2004. "Mindfulness-Based Stress Reduction and Health Benefits: A Meta-Analysis." Journal *of Psychosomatic Research*, 57 (1): 35–43. <http://www.jpsychores.com/ article/S0022-3999%2803%2900573-7/abstract>.

Guilfoyle, M. 2005. "From Therapeutic Power to Resistance: Therapy and Cultural Hegemony." *Theory & Psychology*, 15 (1): 101-124.

Güldal, D.; & S. Semin. 2000. "The Influences of Drug Companies' Advertising Programs on Physicians." *Int J Health Serv*, 30 (3): 585–95. <http://baywood.metapress.com/app/home/contribution.asp?referrer=parent& backto=issue,9,13;journal,51,169;linkingpublicationresults,1:300313,1>.

Gurría, Angel. 2011. "Press Release for Divided We Stand: Why Inequality Keeps Rising (Report)" (December 05). <http://www.oecd.org/social/dividedwe standwhyinequalitykeepsrisingspeech.htm>.

Guth, Alan. 1997. *The Inflationary Universe: The Quest for a New Theory Of Cosmic Origins*. New York: Helix Books.

Hahnemann, Samuel. 1833. *The Homœopathic Medical Doctrine, or "Organon of the Healing Art"*. Dublin: W.F. Wakeman.

Haniff, David. 2007. "Mental Health Issues and Pervasive Computing." *BCS-HCI '07 Proceedings of the 21st British HCI Group Annual Conference on People and Computers: HCI...But Not as We Know it,* Volume 2. Swindon: British Computer Society.

Harris, Russ. 2008. *The Happiness Trap*. Boston, MA: Trumpeter Books.

Hart, B. L. 1988. "Biological Basis of the Behavior of Sick Animals." *Neurosci Biobehav Rev*, 12 (2): 123–137. <http://www.sciencedirect.com/science/ article/pii/S0149763488800046>.

Hathaway, J. E.; L. A. Mucci; & J. G. Silverman, et al. 2000. "Health Status and Health Care Use of Massachusetts Women Reporting Partner Abuse." *Am J Prev Med*, 19: 302–307.

Hart, W. D. 1997. "Dualism." *A Companion to the Philosophy of Mind*. S. Guttenplan, ed. Hoboken, NJ: Blackwell.

Hayes, Steven C. 2004. *Get Out of Your Mind and Into Your Life*. Oakland, CA: New Harbinger Press.

HealthyPeople.gov (HEAL). 2011. "Family Planning—Healthy People 2020" (August 18). <http://healthypeople.gov/2020/topicsobjectives2020/overview. aspx?topicid=13>.

Heimler, E. 1975. *Survival in Society*. London, UK: Weidenfeld and Nicolson.

Heindel, Max. 1911. *The Rosicrucian Mysteries*. <http://www.rosicrucian.com/ rms/rmseng02.htm#Chapter_IV>.

Hertzog, C., A. Kramer; S. Wilson; & U. Lindenberger. 2008. "Enrichment Effects on Adult Cognitive Development: Can the Functional Capacity of Older Adults Be." *Psychological Science in the Public Interest*, 9 (1): 1–65. <http://www.psychologicalscience.org/journals/pspi/pdf/PSPI_9_1%20main_ text.pdf>.

Ho, Peng Yoke. 2000. *Li, Qi, and Shu: An Introduction to Science and Civilization in China*. NY: Dover Publications

Hoffman, Hunter G. 2004. "Virtual-Reality Therapy" (July 24). *Scientific*

American. <http://www.scientificamerican.com/article.cfm?id=virtual-reality-therapy>.

Hofmann, S., G. 2011. *An Introduction to Modern CBT. Psychological Solutions to Mental Health Problems*. Chichester, UK: Wiley-Blackwell.

Hopfensperger, D. J.; et al. 1991. "Swine Influenza Virus Infections. Transmission from Ill Pigs to Humans at a Wisconsin Agricultural Fair and Subsequent Probable Person-to-Person Transmission." *JAMA*, 265 (4): 478–81. <http://jama.jamanetwork.com/article.aspx?doi=10.1001/jama.265.4.478>.

Hosin, A.A., ed. 2007. *Responses to Traumatized Children*. Basingstoke: Palgrave Macmillan.

Hu., F., J. Manson, M. Stampfer; C. Graham, et al. 2001. "Diet, Lifestyle, and the Risk of Type 2 Diabetes Mellitus in Women." *The New England Journal of Medicine*, 345(11): 790–797.

Hunsberger, J. G.; S. Newton; A. Bennett; C. Duman; D. Russell; S. Salton; & R. Duman. 2007. "Antidepressant Actions of the Exercise-Regulated Gene VGF." *Nat. Med.*, 13 (12): 1476–82. <http://www.nature.com/nm/journal/v13/n12/full/nm1669.html>.

Independent, the (IND). 2007. "Birth Rates 'Must be Curbed to Win War on Global Poverty" (January 31). <http://www.independent.co.uk/news/world/politics/birth-rates-must-be-curbed-to-win-war-on-global-poverty-434387.html>.

International Rehabilitation Council for Torture Victims (IRCT). 2011. "Rehabilitation." <http://www.irct.org/what-is-torture/rehabilitation.aspx>.

Islington Tribune (ISL). 2011. "Professor Richard Wilkinson: 'I Didn't Realise Islington was so Unequal.'" <http://www.islingtontribune.com/news/2011/jun/professor-richard-wilkinson-'i-didn't-realise-islington-was-so-unequal>.

Jain, S., et al. 2007. "A Randomised Controlled Trial of Mindfulness Meditation versus Relaxation Training: Effects on Distress, Positive States of Mind, Rumination, and Distraction." *Annals of Behavioral Medicine*, 33 (1): 11–21. <http://link.springer.com/article/10.1207%2Fs15324796abm3301_2>.

Jaranson, James. 1998. "The Science and Politics of Rehabilitating Torture Survivors." *Caring for Victims of Torture*. Michael K. Popkin, ed. Washington, DC: Amer Psychiatric Pub Inc.

Jarvis, Brooke. 2010. "Why Everyone Suffers in Unequal Societies" (March 04). <http://www.yesmagazine.org/happiness/want-the-good-life-your-neighbors-need-it-too>.

Jewkes, R. 2002. "Intimate Partner Violence: Causes and Prevention." *The Lancet*, 359 (9315): 1423–1429. <http://linkinghub.elsevier.com/retrieve/pii/S0140673602083575>.

Jha, Ap, et al. 2010. "Examining the Protective Effects of Mindfulness Training on Working Memory Capacity and Affective Experience." *Emotion*, 10 (1): 54–

64. <http://psycnet.apa.org/?&fa=main.doiLanding&doi=10.1037/a0018438>.

Johns Hopkins Medicine (JKM). 2011. "Patient Care: Tertiary Care Definition." <http://www.hopkinsmedicine.org/patient_care/pay_bill/insurance_footnotes.html>.

Johnson, R. 2002. "The Concept of Sickness Behavior: A Brief Chronological Account of Four Key Discoveries." *Veterinary Immunology and Immunopathology*, 87 (3–4): 443–450. <http://www.sciencedirect.com/science/article/pii/S0165242702000697>.

Journalist's Resource.org (JOUR). 2011. "Growing Income Inequality in OECD Countries. <http://journalistsresource.org/studies/government/international/income-inequality-in-oecd-countries/>.

Judge, William Quan. 1893. *The Ocean of Theosophy*. London, UK: Theosophical Publishing Society.

Kabat-Zinn, J. 1990. *Full Catastrophe Living: Using the Wisdom of Your Body and Mind to Face Stress, Pain, and Illness*. NY: Dell.

_____.1982. "An Out-Patient Program in Behavioral Medicine for Chronic Pain Patients based on the Practice of Mindfulness Meditation: Theoretical Considerations and Preliminary Results." *Gen. Hosp. Psychiatry*, 4 (1): 33–47. <http://www.sciencedirect.com/science/article/pii/0163834382900263>.

Kaku, Michio. 1994. *Hyperspace: A Scientific Odyssey Through Parallel Universes, Time Warps, and The Tenth Dimension*. Illustrations by Robert O'Keefe. Oxford: Oxford University Press.

Härkänen, T.; P. Knekt; E. Virtala; & O. Lindfors. 2005. "A Case Study in Comparing Therapies involving Informative Drop-Out, Non-Ignorable Non-Compliance and Repeated Measurements." *Statistics in Medicine*, 24 (24): 3773–3787. <http://onlinelibrary.wiley.com/doi/10.1002/sim.2409/abstract;jsessionid=294D629ADA8BEC6819BC3BD36414260A.d02t01>.

Hofmann, S. G.; A. Sawyer; A. Witt; & D. Oh. 2010. "The Effect of Mindfulness-Based Therapy on Anxiety and Depression: A Meta-Analytic Review." *J Consult Clin Psychol*, 78 (2): 169–83. <http://psycnet.apa.org/?&fa=main.doiLanding&doi=10.1037/a0018555>.

Johnsgard, Keith, W. 2004. *Conquering Depression and Anxiety Through Exercise*. Amherst, NY: Prometheus Books. <http://books.google.com.pe/books?id=A6oIAAAACAAJ&redir_esc=y>.

Johnson, M. P. 2006. "Conflict and Control: Gender Symmetry and Asymmetry in Domestic Violence." *Violence Against Women*, 12 (11): 1003–1018. <http://vaw.sagepub.com/content/12/11/1003>.

_____; & K. Ferraro. 2000. "Research on Domestic Violence in the 1990s: Making Distinctions." *Journal of Marriage and Family*, 62 (4): 948. <http://onlinelibrary.wiley.com/doi/10.1111/j.1741-3737.2000.00948.x/abstract;jsessionid=C44C8D95DBE8FF20E464770DB725F56B.d02t01>.

_____.1995. "Patriarchal Terrorism and Common Couple Violence: Two Forms of

Violence against Women." *Journal of Marriage and Family*, 57 (2): 283–294. <http://www.jstor.org/discover/10.2307/353683?uid=3738800&uid=2&uid=4&sid=21101664656873>.

Jones, R.; & D. Horan. 1997. "The American College of Obstetricians and Gynecologists: A Decade of Responding to Violence against Women." *International Journal of Gynaecology and Obstetrics*, 58 (1): 43–50. <http://www.ncbi.nlm.nih.gov/pubmed/9253665>.

Kay, John. 2009. "The Spirit Level." *The Financial Times*. <http://www.ft.com/cms/s/2/77b1bd26-14db-11de-8cd1-0000779fd2ac.html>.

Kelley, K. W.; R. Bluthe; R. Dantzer; J. Zhou; W. Shen; R. Johnson; & S. Broussard. 2003. "Cytokine-Induced Sickness Behavior." *Brain Behav Immun,* 17 (Suppl 1): S112–118. <http://www.sciencedirect.com/science/article/pii/S0889159102000776>.

Kemp, A. M.; F. Dunstan; & S. Harrison, et al. 2008. "Patterns of Skeletal Fractures in Child Abuse: Systematic Review." *BMJ*, 337 (oct02 1): a1518. <http://www.bmj.com/content/337/bmj.a1518?view=long&pmid=18832412>.

Kerlikowske, Gil. 2010. "Why Marijuana Legalization Would Compromise Public Health and Public Safety."

Klieman, Rikki. 2013. "Domestic Abuse: The Crime That Crosses Class and Color Lines" (February 24). <http://www.thedailybeast.com/articles/2013/02/24/the-crime-that-crosses-class-and-color-lines.html>.

Kolata, Gina. 2002. "Why Some People Won't Be Fit Despite Exercise." *The New York Times*. <http://www.nytimes.com/2002/02/12/health/why-some-people-won-t-be-fit-despite-exercise.html>.

Kuper, Simon. 2009. "The Man who Invented Exercise." *Financial Times.* <http://www.ft.com/cms/s/e6ff90ea-9da2-11de-9f4a-00144feabdc0,Authorised=false.html?_i_location=http%3A%2F%2Fwww.ft.com%2Fcms%2Fs%2F0%2Fe6ff90ea-9da2-11de-9f4a-00144feabdc0.html&_i_referer=http%3A%2F%2Fen.wikipedia.org%2Fwiki%2FPhysical_exercise#axzz2KoNrrDvK>.

Kurzban, Robert. 2011. *Why Everyone (Else) Is a Hypocrite: Evolution and the Modular Mind.* NJ: Princeton University Press.

Lakhan, S. E.; E. Hamlat; T. McNamee; & C. Laird. 2009. "Time for a Unified Approach to Medical Ethics." *Philosophy, Ethics, and Humanities in Medicine*, 4 (3): 13. <http://www.ncbi.nlm.nih.gov/pmc/articles/PMC2745426/>.

Lamson, Ralph J. 2005. "Application: VR in Psycho Therapy: Virtual Therapy of Anxiety Disorders." <http://www.cyberedge.com/info_r_a%2Bp03-lamson.html>.

Lancee, Bram; & Hermanvande Werfhorst. 2011. "Income Inequality and Participation: A Comparison of 24 European Countries." *GINI Discussion Paper,* 6 (Amsterdam Centre for Inequality Studies). <http://www.uva-aias.net/uploaded_files/publications/DP6-Lancee,vdWerfhorst-2.pdf>.

Laroche, Denis. 2004. "Context and Consequences of Domestic Violence Against

Men and Women in Canada in 2004." <http://www.stat.gouv.qc.ca/publications/conditions/pdf2008/ViolenceH_F2004_an.pdf>.

Lau, A. S.; D. Takeuchi; & M. Alegría. 2006. "Parent-to-Child Aggression among Asian American Parents: Culture, Context, and Vulnerability." *Journal of Marriage and Family*, 68 (5): 1261-1275.

Laurance, Jeremy. 2010. "Mephedrone Did not Kill Youths, Tests Reveal" (May 29). *The Independent* (UK). <http://www.independent.co.uk/news/uk/home-news/mephedrone-did-not-kill-youths-tests-reveal-1986193.html>.

Lauterpacht, Elihu; & C. J. Greenwood. 2002. *International Law Reports*. UK: Cambridge University Press.

Laws, D. Richard; & William T. O'Donohue. 2008. *Sexual Deviance*. NY: Guilford Press.

Lazenbatt, A.; & M. Thompson-Cree. 2009. "Recognizing the Co-Occurrence of Domestic and Child Abuse: A Comparison of Community- and Hospital-Based Midwives." *Health & Social Care in the Community*, 17 (4): 358. <http://onlinelibrary.wiley.com/doi/10.1111/j.1365-2524.2009.00833.x/ab stract>.

Lee, Matthew R.; & William B. Bankston. 1999. "Political Structure, Economic Inequality,and Homicide: A Cross-National Analysis." *Deviant Behavior*, 20 (1): 50.

Leeb, R. T.; L. Paulozzi; C. Melanson; T. Simon; & I. Arias. 2008. "Child Maltreatment Surveillance: Uniform Definitions for Public Health and Recommended Data Elements." Centers for Disease Control and Prevention. <http://www.cdc.gov/ViolencePrevention/index.html>.

Levitan, R. D.; N. A. Rector; T. Sheldon; & P. Goering. 2003. "Childhood Adversities Associated with Major Depression and/or Anxiety Disorders in a Community Sample of Ontario: Issues of Co-morbidity and Specificity." *Depression & Anxiety*, 17: 34–42. <http://onlinelibrary.wiley.com/doi/10.1002/da.10077/abstract>.

Linehan, Marsha. 1993. *Cognitive-Behavioral Treatment of Borderline Personality Disorder*. NY: Guilford Press.

Lykken, David; et al. 1996. "Happiness Is a Stochastic Phenomenon." *Psychological Science*, 7 (3): 186.

Lynch, Timothy. 2000. *After Prohibition. An Adult Approach to Drug Policies in the 21st Century*. Washington, DC: CATO Institute.

Lynskey, M. 2003. "Escalation of Drug Use in Early-Onset Cannabis Users vs Co-Twin Controls." *JAMA*, 289 (4): 427-433.

Lyons-Ruth, K.; & D. Jacobvitz. 1999. "Attachment Disorganization: Unresolved Loss, Relational Violence and Lapses in Behavioral and Attentional Strategies." *Handbook of Attachment*. J. Cassidy and P. Shaver, eds. New York: Guilford Pres.

Lyubomirsky, Sonja. 2001. "Why are Some Happier than Others? The Role of Cognitive and Motivational Processes in Well-Being." *American*

Psychologist, 56 (3): 239–324.

MacDonald, J. M. 1963. "The Threat to Kill." *American Journal of Psych*iatry, 120 (2): 125-30. <http://journals.psychiatryonline.org/article.aspx?articleid=149172>.

Main, M.; & E. Hesse. 1990. "Parents' Unresolved Traumatic Experiences are Related to Infant Disorganized Attachment Status." *Attachment in the Preschool Years: Theory, Research, and Intervention.* M. Greenberg; D. Ciccehetti; & E. Cummings. Chicago, Il: University of Chicago Press.

Malinosky-Rummell, R.; & D. Hansen. 1993. "Long-Term Consequences of Childhood Physical Abuse." *Psychological Bulletin*, 114 (1): 68–79. <http://psycnet.apa.org/?&fa=main.doiLanding&doi=10.1037/0033-2909.114.1.68>.

Martin, J.; J. Anderson; S. Romans; P. Mullen; & M. O'Shea. 1993. "Asking about Child Sexual Abuse: Methodological Implications of a Two Stage Survey." *Child Abuse & Neglect*, 17 (3): 383–92. <http://www.sciencedirect.com/science/article/pii/0145213493900619>.

Masson, Jeffrey Moussaieff. 1988. *Against Therapy: Emotional Tyranny and the Myth of Psychological Healing*. Canada: Common Courage Press.

Masten, A. S. 2009. "Ordinary Magic: Lessons from Research on Resilience in Human Development." *Education Canada*, 49 (3): 28–32. <http://www.cea-ace.ca/sites/default/files/EdCan-2009-v49-n3-Masten.pdf>.

Masters, R. E. L. 1962. *Forbidden Sexual Behavior and Morality*. New York, NY: Lancer Books, Inc.

McAleer, Neil. 1987. *The Mind-Boggling Universe*. New York: Doubleday & Co.

McAuley, Edward; Arthur F. Kramer; & Stanley J. Colcombe. 2004. "Cardiovascular Fitness and Neurocognitive Function in Older Adults: A Brief Review." Brain, Behavior, and Immunity, 18: 214–220. <http://web.archive.org/web/20070616225929/http://www.kch.uiuc.edu/labs/exercise-psychology/Library/pubs/McAuley_Brain_Behavior_Immunity_2004.pdf>.

McAuliffe, Kathleen. 2008. "Curing the Wounds of Iraq with Virtual Therapy." <http://discovermagazine.com/2008/oct/17-curing-the-wounds-of-iraq-with-virtual-therapy#.UQ6uZfLDpM4>.

McCracken, L.; J. Gauntlett-Gilbert; & K. Vowles. 2007. "The Role of Mindfulness in a Contextual Cognitive-Behavioral Analysis of Chronic Pain-Related Suffering and Disability." *Pain*, 131 (1): 63–69. <http://www.painjournalonline.com/article/S0304-3959%2806%2900688-9/abstract>.

McGue, Matt; Steve Bacon; & David Lykken. 1993. "Personality Stability and Change in Early Adulthood: A Behavioral Genetic Analysis." *Developmental Psychology*, 29 (1): 96–109.

McNeely, Brent E. 2013. "The Miraj of Muhammad in an Ascension Typology." <http://www.bhporter.com/Porter%20PDF%20Files/The%20Miraj%20of%20

Muhammad%20in%20an%20Asceneion%20Typology.pdf>.

McWhinney, I. R. 1987. "Health and Disease: Problems of Definition." *CMAJ*, 136 (8): 815. <http://www.ncbi.nlm.nih.gov/pmc/articles/PMC1492121/>.

Medicinenet.com (MEDI). 2012. "Child Abuse Symptoms, Causes, Treatment—How Can Child Abuse be Prevented?." <http://www.medicinenet.com/child_abuse/page8.htm#how_can_child_abuse_be_prevented>.

Meerburg, B. G., G. Singleton; & A. Kijlstra. 2009. "Rodent-Borne Diseases and their Risks for Public Health." *Crit Rev Microbiol*, 35 (3): 221–70. <http://informahealthcare.com/doi/abs/10.1080/10408410902989837?journal Code=mby>.

Melton, J. G. 1996. "Astral Projection." Farmington Hills, MI: Thomson Gale.

Merriam-Webster's Collegiate Dictionary Online (MWD). 2013. "Health Care" (January 28). <http://www.m-w.com/dictionary/health_care>.

_____.2013a. "Mind" (January 28). <http://www.m-w.com/dictionary/mind>.

_____.2013b. "Body" (January 28). <http://www.m-w.com/dictionary/body>.

_____.2007. "Agency" (March 20). <http://www.m-w.com/dictionary/agency>.

Messman-Moore, Terri L.; & Patricia Long. 2000. "Child Sexual Abuse and Revictimization in the Form of Adult Sexual Abuse, Adult Physical Abuse, and Adult Psychological Maltreatment." *Journal of Interpersonal Violence*, 15 (5): 489–502. <http://jiv.sagepub.com/content/15/5/489.abstract>.

Meszaros, Istvan. 1995. *Beyond Capital*. London, MA: Merlin Press.

Milner, J. S.; & C. Dopke. 2008. "Paraphilia Not Otherwise Specified: Psychopathology and Theory." *Sexual Deviance, Second Edition: Theory, Assessment, and Treatment*. D. Laws & W. O'Donohue, eds. New York: The Guilford Press.

Milrod, B.; A. Leon; F. Busch; M. Rudden; M. Schwalberg; J. Clarkin; A. Aronson; M. Singer; W. Turchin; E. Klass; E. Graf; J. Teres; & M. Shear. 2007. "A Randomized Controlled Clinical Trial of Psychoanalytic Psychotherapy for Panic Disorder." *American Journal of Psychiatry*, 164: 265-272.

Mindfulness and Integrative Psychotherapy (MIND). 2013. "Mindfulness is an Approach to Freeing Oneself from Suffering" (February 04). <http://mindfulnessandpsychotherapy.co.uk/mindfulness/>.

Money, John. 1988. *Lovemaps: Clinical Concepts of Sexual/Erotic Health and Pathology, Paraphilia, and Gender Transposition in Childhood, Adolescence, and Maturity*. Buffalo, N.Y: Prometheus Books.

Monroe, Robert. 1977. *Journeys Out of the Body*. NY: Anchor Press.

Moore, Charles. 2010. "Inequality is Not a Social Illness to be 'Cured'" (February 9). <http://www.telegraph.co.uk/comment/columnists/charlesmoore/7193991/Inequality-is-not-a-social-illness-to-be-cured.html>.

Morad, Y., T. Wygnansky-Jaffe; & A. Levin. 2010. "Retinal Haemorrhage in Abusive Head Trauma." *Clin Exp Ophthalmol*, 38:514–520.

Morgan, Scott. 2008, "Rule #1 of Drug Legalization is Don't Talk About Drug Legalization." Drug Reform Coordination Network. <http://stopthedrugwar.org/speakeasy/2008/feb/18/rule_1_drug_legalization_dont_ta>.

Morris, J. N., J. Heady, P. Raffle; C. Roberts; & J. Parks. 1953. "Coronary Heart-Disease and Physical Activity of Work." *Lancet*, 265 (6795): 1053–7. <http://www.ncbi.nlm.nih.gov/pubmed/13110049>.

Muldoon, Sylvan Joseph; & Hereward Carrington. 1961. The Projection of the Astral Body. London: Rider.

Murphy, J. M.; M. Jellinek; D. Quinn; G. Smith; F. Poitrast; & M. Goshko. 1991. "Substance Abuse and Serious Child Mistreatment: Prevalence, Risk, and Outcome in a court Sample." *Child Abuse & Neglect*, 15 (3): 197–211. <http://www.sciencedirect.com/science/article/pii/014521349190065L>.

National Center for Biotechnology Information (NCBI). 2010. "The Miracle Drug" (May). *Can Fam Physician*, 56 (5): 407. <http://www.ncbi.nlm.nih.gov/pmc/articles/PMC2868602/>.

National Center for Complementary and Alternative Medicine (NCCAM). 2005. "What is Complementary and Alternative Medicine (CAM)?." <http://nccam.nih.gov/health/whatiscam>.

National Center on Domestic and Sexual Violence (NAT). 2011. "Power and Control Wheel." <http://www.ncdsv.org/images/Power_and_Control_wheel_NCDSV.pdf>.

National Committee to Prevent Child Abuse (NCPCA). 1998. "Child Abuse and Neglect Statistics." <http://web.archive.org/web/19980515052303/http://childabuse.org/facts97.html>.

National Defense Intelligence College (NDIC). 2006. "Educing Information: Interrogation: Science and Art—Foundations for the Future." .<http://www.fas.org/irp/dni/educing.pdf>.

National Health Service (NHS). 2013. "Computerised Cognitive Behaviour Therapy for Depression and Anxiety (Review of Technology Appraisal 51)." <http://www.nice.org.uk/guidance/TA97>.

National Science Foundation (NSF). 2002. "Science and Technology: Public Attitudes and Public Understanding Science Fiction and Pseudoscience—Belief in Alternative Medicine." <http://www.nsf.gov/statistics/seind02/c7/c7s5.htm>.

Neapolitana, Jerome L. 1999. "A Comparative Analysis of Nations with Low and High Levels of Violent Crime." *Journal of Criminal Justice,* 27 (3): 260. <http://www.sciencedirect.com/science/article/pii/S0047235298000646>.

Needham, J; & G. Lu. 2002. *Celestial Lancets: A History and Rationale of Acupuncture and Moxa*. NY: Routledge.

New Scientist (NEWS). 2006. "Ecstasy as a Brain Booster for Parkinson's?" (October). <http://www.newscientist.com/article/mg19225754.800-ecstasy-as-a-brain-booster-for-parkinsons.html>.

Nied, Robert; & B. Franklin. 2002. "Promoting and Prescribing Exercise for the Elderly." *Am Fam Physician.*, 65 (3): 419-427.

Noh Anh, Helen. 1994. "Cultural Diversity and the Definition of Child Abuse." *Child Welfare Research Review*. R. Barth, et al., eds. NY: Columbia University Press.

Norton, M. I.; E. Dunn; & L. Aknin. 2009. "From Wealth to Well-Being: Spending Money on Others Promotes Happiness." Invited talk at the Society for Personality and Social Psychology, Tampa, FL.

Nova Online (NO). 2000. "Time Can Vary." <http://www.pbs.org/wgbh/nova/time/thinktime.html>.

NSW Bureau of Crime Statistics and Research (NSW). 2010. "Does Prohibition Deter Cannabis Use." <http://www.lawlink.nsw.gov.au/lawlink/bocsar/ll_bocsar.nsf/vwFiles/mr_cjb58.pdf/$file/mr_cjb58.pdf>.

Nutt, David; Leslie A King; William Saulsbury; & Colin Blakemore. 2007. "Development of a Rational Scale to Assess the Harm of Drugs of Potential Misuse." *The Lancet*. <http://www.mapinc.org/drugnews/v07/n366/a01.html>.

O'Connor, D.; M. Crowe; & W. Spinks. 2005. "Effects of Static Stretching on Leg Capacity during Cycling." *Turin*, 46(1), 52–56.

Office on Violence Against Women (OVW). 2007. "About Domestic Violence." <http://www.ovw.usdoj.gov/domviolence.htm>.

Okun, M. A.; W. Stock; M. Haring; & R. Witter. 1984. "Health and Subjective Well-Being: A Meta-Analysis." *The International Journal of Aging & Human Development,* 19 (2): 111–132.

Oregon Department of Human Services (ODHS). 2002. "Hemorrhagic Escherichiosis from a County Fair." CD <http://www.oregon.gov/DHS/ph/cdsumMarchy/2002/ohd5119.pdf%29.&#32>.

Oswego City School District Regents Exam Prep Center (OCSD). 2012. "Regents Prep: Living Environment: Homeostasis." <http://regentsprep.org/regents/biology/units/homeostasis/index.cfm>.

Pagel, Walter. 1967. *William Harvey's Biological Ideas*. New York: Hafner.

Parker-Pope, T. 2001. "For a Healthy Brain You Really Need to Use Your Head—Physical and Mental Exercise Can Stave Off Mental Decline" (November 26). *The Wall Street Journal Europe*.

Patient Safety and Quality Healthcare (PSQH). 2013. "Barriers to Telemedicine Limit Patient Access to Quality Care" (February 03). <http://www.psqh.com/barriers-to-telemedicine-limit-patient-access-to-quality-care.html>.

Patrick, C. J. 2008. "Psychophysiological Correlates of Aggression and Violence:

An Integrative Review." *Philosophical Transactions of the Royal Society B: Biological Sciences*, 363 (1503): 2543–2555. <http://www.ncbi.nlm.nih.gov/pmc/articles/PMC2606710/>.

Pekkanen, Sarah. 1992. "Experts Tell FDA Some Hallucinogens May Aid Alcoholics, Terminally Ill and Psychiatric Patients." Newsletter of the Multidisciplinary Association for Psychedelic Studies. <http://www.maps.org/news-letters/v03n3/03324sfe.html>.

Peters, Edward. 1985. *Torture*. New York: Basil Blackwell Inc.

Piketty, Thomas; & Emmanuel Saez. 2003. "Income Inequality in the United States, 1913-1998." *Quarterly Journal of Economics*.

Pinker, Steven. 2002. *The Blank Slate: The Modern Denial of Human Nature*. New York, N.Y: Viking.

Pittman, Frank.1994. "A Buyer's Guide to Psychotherapy." *Psychology Today* (January 1). <http://www.psychologytoday.com/articles/199401/buyers-guide-psychotherapy>.

Pitts, Leonard. 2009. "Commentary: Why do we Tolerate Torture?" McClatchy's. <http://www.mcclatchydc.com/2009/05/07/67612/commentary-why-do-we-tolerate.html>.

Plante, Thomas G.; Laura Coscarelli; & Marie Ford. 2001. "Does Exercising with Another Enhance the Stress-Reducing Benefits of Exercise." *International Journal of Stress Management*, 8 (3): 201–213. <http://www.esf.edu/for/schuster/FOR%20475/exercise%20with%20another.pdf>.

Plotkin, Henry. 2004 *Evolutionary Thought in Psychology: A Brief History*. Hoboken, NJ: Blackwell.

Powell, Arthur A. 2008. *The Astral Body and Other Astral Phenomena*. London, UK: The Theosophical Publishing House. <http://hpb.narod.ru/AstralBody ByPowell-A.htm>.

Psychology Today (PSY). 1994. "Virtual Therapy" (November 01). <http://www.psychologytoday.com/articles/199411/virtual-therapy>.

Putnam, Robert. 2000. *Bowling Alone: The Collapse and Revival of American Community*. New York: Simon & Schuster.

_____.1993. *Making Democracy Work: Civic Traditions in Modern Italy*. Princeton, NJ: Princeton University Press.

Raman, Shankar. 1997. Lectures on Literary Theory. Cambridge, MA: MIT (spring).

Rath J. F.; D. Langenbahn; D. Simon; R. Sherr; J. Fletcher; & L. Diller. 2004. "The Construct of Problem Solving in Higher Level Neuropsychological Assessment and Rehabilitation." *Archives of Clinical Neuropsychology*, 19: 613-635.

Raub, J. 2002. "Psychophysiologic Effects of Hatha Yoga on Musculoskeletal and Cardiopulmonary Function: A Literature Review." The Journal of Alternative and Complementary Medicine, 8(6): 797-812.

Ray, Oakley Stern, ed. 2002. *Drugs, Society, and Human Behavior*. Boston, MA: McGraw-Hill.

Reader's Digest (READ). 1990. "Did You Know? New Insights Into A World That Is Full of Astonishing Stories and Astounding Facts." <http://books.google.ca/books?id=4tgqsTknBcUC>.

Reeves, Richard. 2009. "In Search of the Truth about Equality in Britain." *The Guardian* (London). <http://www.guardian.co.uk/books/2009/apr/05/spirit-level-richard-wilkinson>.

Rejali, Darius. 2007. "Torture, American Style" (December 16). *Boston.com*. <http://www.boston.com/bostonglobe/ideas/articles/2007/12/16/torture_american_style/?page=1>.

Renzetti, C. M.; & C. H. Miley. 1996. *Violence in Gay and Lesbian Domestic Partnerships*. PA: Haworth Press.

Ridgecrest Regional Hospital (RRH). 2013. "Barriers to the Up-Take of Telemedicine in Australia—A View from Providers." <http://www.rrh.org.au/publishedarticles/article_print_1581.pdf>.

Roach, J. 2011. "Evolution and the Prevention of Violent Crime." *Psychology*, 02 (4): 393.

Robertson, S. Ian. 2001. *Problem Solving*. UK: Psychology Press.

Rodriguez, Christina M.; & Ryan Henderson. 2010. "Who Spares the Rod? Religious Orientation, Social Conformity, and Child Abuse Potential." *Child Abuse & Neglect*, 34 (2): 84–94. <http://www.sciencedirect.com/science/article/pii/S0145213410000049>.

Roosa, M. W.; C. Reinholtz; & P. Angelini. 1999. "The Relation of Child Sexual Abuse and Depression in Young Women: Comparisons across Four Ethnic Groups." *Journal of Abnormal Child Psychology*, 27 (1): 65–76.

Rosch, Eleanor. 2007. "More than Mindfulness: When You Have a Tiger by the Tail, Let it Eat You." *Psychological Inquiry*, 18 (4): 258–264. <http://www.tandfonline.com/doi/abs/10.1080/10478400701598371>.

Rose, David. 2008. "Reckoning" (December 16). *Vanity Fair*. <http://www.vanityfair.com/magazine/2008/12/torture200812?currentPage=4>.

Ross, J. S.; J. Lackner; P. Lurie; C. Gross; S. Wolfe; & H. Krumholz. 2007. "Pharmaceutical Company Payments to Physicians: Early Experiences with Disclosure Laws in Vermont and Minnesota." *JAMA*, 297 (11): 1216–23. <http://jama.jamanetwork.com/article.aspx?articleid=206127>.

Ross, S. 1996. "Risk of Physical Abuse to Children of Spouse Abusing Parents."

Child Abuse & Neglect, 20 (7): 589. <http://www.sciencedirect.com/science/article/pii/0145213496000464>.

Roukema, Richard W. 2003. *What Every Patient, Family, Friend, and Caregiver Needs to Know About Psychiatry*. Washington, DC: American Psychiatric Pub.

Roth, Melinda. 1991. "All Opposed, Say Neigh" (December 15). *Riverfront Times*. <http://www.riverfronttimes.com/1999-12-15/news/all-opposed-say-neigh/>.

Rubin, Paul H. 2003, "Folk Economics." *Southern Economic Journal*, 70: 157–171.

Rumbold, G. 1999. *Ethics in Nursing Practice*. London, UK: Balliere Tindall.

Ryan, C. J. 2010. "Ethical Issues, Part 2: Ethics, Psychiatry, and End-of-Life Issues." *Psychiatr Times*, 27 (6): 26-27.

Sachpazidis, Ilias. 2008. "Image and Medical Data Communication Protocols for Telemedicine and Teleradiology (dissertation)." Department of Computer Science, Technical University of Darmstadt, Germany.

Sampson, W. 1995. "Antiscience Trends in the Rise of the 'Alternative Medicine'Movement.'" *Annals of the New York Academy of Sciences*, 775: 188–197. <http://onlinelibrary.wiley.com/doi/10.1111/j.1749-6632.1996.tb23138.x/abstract;jsessionid=B6F4CB73E08F8057A4FA555637631854.d04t01>.

Samsa, M. 2010. "The Cinderella Effect: Just a Fairytale?." <http://www.rationalskepticism.org/psychology/the-cinderella-effect-just-a-fairytale-t17731.html>.

Saper, R. B.; R. Phillips, et al. 2008. "Lead, Mercury, and Arsenic in US- and Indian-Manufactured Ayurvedic Medicines Sold via the Internet." *Journal of the American Medical Association*, 300 (8): 915–923. <http://www.ncbi.nlm.nih.gov/pmc/articles/PMC2755247/>.

Sarris, J.; & J. Wardle. 2010. *Clinical Naturopathy: An Evidence-Based Guide to Practice*. Australia: Elsevier.

Schechter, D. S.; S. Coates; T. Kaminer; T. Coots; C. Zeanah; M. Davies; I. Schonfield; R. Marshall; M. Liebowitz; K. Trabka; J. McCaw; M. Myers. 2008. "Distorted Maternal Mental Representations and Atypical Behavior in a Clinical Sample of Violence-Exposed Mothers and their Toddlers." *Journal of Trauma and Dissociation*, 9 (2): 123–149. <http://www.ncbi.nlm.nih.gov/pmc/articles/PMC2577290/>.

_____; & S. W. Coates. 2006. "Relationally and Developmentally Focused Interventions with Young Children and Their Caregivers Affected by the Events of 9/11". *September 11, 2001: Treatment, Research and Public Mental Health in the Wake of a Terrorist Attack*. Y. Neria, R. Gross, R. Marshall, and E. Susser, eds. New York: Cambridge University Press.

Scherman, Nosson, ed. 2011. *The ArtScroll English Tanach*. Brooklyn, NY:

Mesorah Publications, Ltd..

Schmidt, J. D.; & L. Sherman. 1993. "Does Arrest Deter Domestic Violence." *American Behavioral Scientist*, 36 (5): 601. <http://abs.sagepub.com/content/36/5/601>.

Schneider, K. 2011. "Toward a Humanistic Positive Psychology." *Existential Analysis: Journal Of The Society For Existential Analysis*, 22 (1): 32-38.

Schreiber, Mark. 2001. *The Dark Side: Infamous Japanese Crimes and Criminals*. Japan: Kodansha International.

Seligman, Martin E.P.; & Mihaly Csikszentmihalyi. 2000. "Positive Psychology: An Introduction." *American Psychologist*, 55 (1): 5–14.

Seltzer, Judith A.; & Debra Kalmuss. 1988. "Socialization and Stress Explanations for Spouse Abuse." *Social Forces*, 67 (2): 473–91. <http://www.jstor.org/discover/10.2307/2579191?uid=3738800&uid=2&uid=4&sid=21101664854423>.

Seto, M. C.; & H. Barbaree. 2000. "Paraphilias." *Aggression and Violence: An Introductory Text*. M. Hersen & V. Van Hasselt. Boston, MA: Allyn & Bacon.

Sexuality.about.com (SEX). 2013. "Zoophilia" (February 01) <http://sexuality.about.com/od/glossary/g/zoophilia.htm>.

Sheehan, Neil. 1988. *A Bright Shining Lie: John Paul Vann and America in Vietnam*. NY: Random House.

Sherwood, Lauralee. 2011. *Fundamentals of Human Physiology*. Belmont, CA: Brooks/Cole Cengage Learning.

Shlain, Leonard. 1991. *Art and Physics: Parallel Visions in Space,Time, and Light*. New York: William Morrow and Co., Inc.

Shorey, R. C., T. Cornelius; & K. Bell. 2008. "Behavioral Theory and Dating Violence: A Framework for Prevention Programming." *Journal of Behavior Analysis of Offender and Victim: Treatment and Prevention*, 1 (4): 298–311.

Shroder, Tom. 2007. "The Peace Drug" (November). *Washington Post*. <http://www.washingtonpost.com/wp-dyn/content/article/2007/11/20/AR2007112001777.html?referrer=emailarticle>.

Shukla, R.; R. Slack; A. George; T. Cheasty; B. Rowe; & J. Scutter. 1995. "Escherichia Coli O157 Infection Associated with a Farm Visitor Center." *Communicable Disease Report*, 5 (6): R86–R90. <http://www.ncbi.nlm.nih.gov/pubmed/7606276>.

Shumba, A., & O. Abosi. 2011. "The Nature, Extent and Causes of Abuse of Children with Disabilities in Schools in Botswana." *International Journal Of Disability, Development & Education*, 58(4), 373-388.

Siemieniuk, R. A. C.; H. Krentz; J. Gish; & M. Gill. 2010. "Domestic Violence Screening: Prevalence and Outcomes in a Canadian HIV Population." *AIDS*

Patient Care and STDs, 24 (12): 763–770. <http://online.liebertpub.com/doi/abs/10.1089/apc.2010.0235>.

Slade, Joseph W. 2001. *Pornography and Sexual Representation: A Reference Guide*, Volume 3. Westport, CT: Greenwood Press.

Sparling, P. B.; A. Giuffrida; D. Piomelli; L. Rosskopf; & A. Dietrich. 2003. "Exercise Activates the Endocannabinoid System." *NeuroReport*, 14 (17): 2209–11. <http://journals.lww.com/neuroreport/Abstract/2003/12020/Exercise_activates_the_endocannabinoid_system.15.aspx>.

Stampfer, M. J.; F. Hu; J. Manson; E. Rimm; & W. Willett. 2000. "Primary Prevention of Coronary Heart Disease in Women through Diet and Lifestyle." *New England Journal of Medicine*, 343 (1): 16–22. <http://www.nejm.org/doi/full/10.1056/NEJM200007063430103>.

Steel, Piers; Joseph Schmidt; & Jonas Shultz. 2008. "Refining the Relationship between Personality and Subjective Well-Being." *Psychological Bulletin*, 134 (1): 138–161.

Stevenson, Reed. 2009. "Dutch among Lowest Cannabis Users in Europe." *Reuters*. <http://www.reuters.com/article/2009/11/05/idUSL5730185>.

Stiglitz, J. E. 2012. *The Price of Inequality: How Today's Divided Society Endangers Our Future*. NY: W.W. Norton & Company.

Straus, Murray A. 2006. "Dominance and Symmetry in Partner Violence by Male and Female University Students in 32 Nations." *Trends In Intimate Violence Intervention*. <http://pubpages.unh.edu/~mas2/ID41E2.pdf>.

Strehle, E. M.; & N. Shabde. 2006. "One Hundred Years of Telemedicine: Does This New Technology have a Place in Paediatrics?" (December). *NIH*. <http://www.ncbi.nlm.nih.gov/pmc/articles/PMC2082971/>.

Suh, E. M.; & J. Koo. 2008. "Comparing Subjective Well-Being across Cultures and Nations: The 'What' and 'Why' Questions." *The Science of Subjective Well-Being*. Michael Eid & Randy J. Larsen, eds. New York: Guildford Press.

Sundberg, Norman. 2001. *Clinical Psychology: Evolving Theory, Practice, and Research*. Englewood Cliffs, NJ: Prentice Hall.

Swedlow, A.; G. Johnson; N. Smithline; & A. Milstein. 1992. "Increased Costs and Rates of Use in the California Workers' Compensation System as a Result of Self-Referral by Physicians." *N Engl J Med*, 327 (21): 1502–6. <http://www.nejm.org/doi/full/10.1056/NEJM199211193272107>.

Talayesva, Don C; & Leo Simmons. 1942. *Sun Chief: The Autobiography of a Hopi Indian*. CT: Yale University Press.

Taylor, L. H.; S. Latham; & M. Woolhouse. 2001. "Risk Factors for Human Disease Emergence." *Philosophical Transactions of the Royal Society B*, 356 (1411): 983-9. <http://www.ncbi.nlm.nih.gov/pubmed/11516376>.

Tax Justice Network (TAX). 2012. "Revealed: Global Super-Rich has at least $21

Trillion Hidden in Secret Tax Havens" (July 22). <http://www.taxjustice.net/cms/upload/pdf/The_Price_of_Offshore_Revisited_Presser_120722.pdf>.

Teasdale, John D. 1999. "Metacognition, Mindfulness and the Modification of Mood Disorders." *Psychiatric Journal: Clinical Psychology and Psychotherapy*. <http://www.mbcttrainingen.nl/Resources/Metacognition_mindfulness_m.pdf>.

Thaindian News (THAI). 2008. "Growth of Millionaires in India Fastest in World" (June 25). <http://www.thaindian.com/newsportal/world-news/growth-of-millionaires-in-india-fastest-in-world_10064367.html>.

Thase, Michael. 2007. "Endorphin Power: Fight Depression With Exercise." <http://www.everydayhealth.com/depression/specialists/endorphin-power-fight-depression-with-exercise.aspx>.

Theoklitou, D.; N. Kabitisis; & A. Kabitsi. 2011. "Physical and Emotional Abuse of Primary School Children by Teachers." *Child Abuse & Neglect*, 36: 64-70.

Thich Nhat Hanh. 1975. *The Miracle of Mindfulness*. NY: Beacon Books.

ThinkExist.com (TE). 2013. "Unknown" (February 19). <http://en.thinkexist.com/search/searchquotation.asp?search=physical%20health&page=3>.

Thomas-MacLean, R., et al. 2011. "No Cookie-Cutter Response: Conceptualizing Primary Health Care" (June 24). <http://www.uwo.ca/fammed/csfm/tutor-phc/pdf/TUTOR%20Definition%20of%20primary%20health%20care.pdf>.

Thornicroft, G. 2007. "What is Mental Health?." *The Lancet*, 370 (3): 841–850.

Tooby, J.; & L. Cosmides. 2005. "Conceptual Foundations of Evolutionary Psychology." *The Handbook of Evolutionary Psychology*. D. M. Buss, ed. Hoboken, NJ: Wiley.

Trebach, Arnold S.; Kevin B. Zeese; & Milton Friedman. 1992. *Friedman and Szasz on Liberty and Drugs: Essays on the Free Market and Prohibition*. Drug Policy Foundation Press.

Tschudin, Verena. 2003. *Ethics in Nursing: The Caring Relationship*. Edinburgh, UK: Butterworth-Heinemann.

Twohey, Megan. 2009. "How Can Domestic Abuse be Stopped?." *Chicago Tribune*. <http://www.chicagotribune.com/news/local/chi-abusers-02-jan02,0,1147422.story?page=1>.

United Nations Convention against Torture (UNCT). 1984. "United Nations Convention against Torture and Other Cruel, Inhuman or Degrading Treatment or Punishment." <http://www.un.org/millennium/law/iv-9.htm>.

United Nations Research Institute for Social Development (UNRISD). 2011. "Tackling Ethnic and Regional Inequalities." <https://owlspace-ccm.rice.edu/access/content/group/HUMA-SOCI-280-001-F11/Course%20Readings/February%207/UNRISD%20CH.3%20total.pdf>.

United States Bureau of Labor Statistics (USBLS). 2010. "Highlights of Women's Earnings in 2009." Report 1025. <http://www.bls.gov/cps/cpswom2009.pdf>.

United States Department of Health and Human Services (USDHHS). 2011. "Child Maltreatment 2011." <http://www.acf.hhs.gov/programs/cb/resource/child-maltreatment-2011>.

United States Institute of Medicine (USIM). 2005. "Complementary and Alternative Medicine in the United States" (January 15). <http://iom.edu/Reports/2005/Complementary-and-Alternative-Medicine-in-the-United-States.aspx>.

Uslaner, Eric; & Mitchell Brown. 2002. "Inequality Trust and Political Engagement." <http://siteresources.worldbank.org/EXTECAREGTOPSOCDEV/Resources/Uslaner_Inequality_trust_political_engagement.pdf>.

Valiathan, M. S. 2006. "Ayurveda: Putting the House in Order." *Current Science* (Indian Academy of Sciences), 90 (1): 5–6.

van Praag, H.; G. Kempermann; F. Gage; G. Kempermann; & F. Gage. 1999. "Ontogeny Running Increases Cell Proliferation and Neurogenesis in the Adult Mouse Dentate Gyrus." *Nature Neuroscience*, 2 (3): 266–70. <http://www.nature.com/neuro/journal/v2/n3/full/nn0399_266.html>.

Vitanza, S.; L. Vogel; & L. Marshall. 1995. "Distress and Symptoms of Posttraumatic Stress Disorder in Abused Women." *Violence and Victims*, 10 (1): 23–34. <http://www.ncbi.nlm.nih.gov/pubmed/8555116>.

Voget, F. W. 1961. "Sex Life of the American Indians." *The Encyclopaedia of Sexual Behavior*. A. Ellis & A. Abarbanel, eds. London, England: W. Heinemann.

Vollmer, August. 1936. *The Police and Modern Society*. Berkeley, CA:University of California Press.

Wallace, B. Alan. 2006. *The Attention Revolution: Unlocking the Power of the Focused Mind*. Boston, MA: Wisdom Publications.

Wampold, Bruce E. 2001. *The Great Psychotherapy Debate*. Mahwah, NJ: L. Erlbaum Associates.

Wachob, Lucas. 2011. "Column: In defense of Chicken 'Lovers'" (February 28). *The Breeze*: <http://www.breezejmu.org/opinion/columnists/article_f08fbb0c-42ca-11e0-ab43-00127992bc8b.html>.

Walter, Jennifer K.; & Eran P. Klein, eds. 2003. *The Story of Bioethics: From Seminal Works to Contemporary Explorations*. Washington, DC: Georgetown University Press.

Warshaw, C. 1993. "Limitations of the Medical Model in the Care of Battered Women." *Violence Against Women: The Bloody Footprints*. P. Bart; & E. Moran. CA: Sage.

Weber, Max. 1930. *The Protestant Ethic and the Spirit of Capitalism*. Talcott

Parsons, tr. New York: Scribner.

Whishaw, Ian Q.; & Bryan Kolb. 2010. *An Introduction to Brain and Behavior*. New York: Worth Publishers.

Whitaker, D. J.; T. Haileyesus; M. Swahn; & L. Saltzman. 2007. "Differences in Frequency of Violence and Reported Injury Between Relationships with Reciprocal and Nonreciprocal Intimate Partner Violence." *American Journal of Public Health*, 97 (5): 941–947. <http://www.ncbi.nlm.nih.gov/pmc/articles/PMC1854883/>.

Wierzbicki, M.; & G. Pekarik. 1993. "A Meta-Analysis of Psychotherapy Dropout." *Professional Psychology: Research and Practice*, 24 (2): 190–195. <http://psycnet.apa.org/index.cfm?fa=search.displayRecord&uid=1993-30339-001>.

Wikipedia (WK). 2013. "Positive Psychology" (January 25). <http://en.wikipedia.org/wiki/Positive_psychology>.

_____.2013a. "Physical Exercise" (January 25). <http://en.wikipedia.org/wiki/Physical_exercise>.

_____.2013b. "Health Care" (January 28). <http://en.wikipedia.org/wiki/Health_care>.

_____.2013c. "Mental Health" (January 28). <http://en.wikipedia.org/wiki/Mental_health>.

_____.2013d. "Problem Solving" (January 28). <http://en.wikipedia.org/wiki/Problem_solving>.

_____.2013e. "Psychological Resilence" (January 28). <http://en.wikipedia.org/wiki/Psychological_resilience>.

_____.2013f. "Fitness" (January 28). <http://en.wikipedia.org/wiki/Fitness>.

_____.2013g. "Substance Abuse" (January 28). <http://en.wikipedia.org/wiki/Substance_abuse>.

_____.2013h. "Violence" (January 28). <http://en.wikipedia.org/wiki/Violence>.

_____.2013i. "Disease" (January 28). <http://en.wikipedia.org/wiki/Disease>.

_____.2013j. "Mind" (January 28). <http://en.wikipedia.org/wiki/Mind>.

_____.2013k. "Soul" (January 28). <http://en.wikipedia.org/wiki/Soul>.

_____.2013l. "Psychotherapy" (January 28). <http://en.wikipedia.org/wiki/Psychotherapy>.

_____.2013m. "Evolutionary Psychology" (January 29). <http://en.wikipedia.org/wiki/Evolutionary_psychology>.

_____.2013n. "Zoonosis" (January 29). <http://en.wikipedia.org/wiki/ Zoonosis>.

_____.2013o. "The Spirit Level: Why More Equal Societies Almost Always Do Better" (January 29). <http://en.wikipedia.org/wiki/The_Spirit_Level:_Why_More_Equal_Societies_Almost_Always_Do_Better>.

_____.2013p. "Arguments for and against Drug Prohibition" (January 29). <http://en.wikipedia.org/wiki/Arguments_for_and_against_drug_prohibition>.

_____.2013q. "Alternative Medicine" (January 29). <http://en.wikipedia.org/wiki/Alternative_medicine>.

_____.2013r. "Torture" (January 29). <http://en.wikipedia.org/wiki/Torture>.

_____.2013s. "Private Healthcare" (January 31). <http://en.wikipedia.org/wiki/Private_healthcare>.

_____.2013t. "Public Health" (January 31). <http://en.wikipedia.org/wiki/Public_health>.

_____.2013u. "Subjective Well Being" (January 31). <http://en.wikipedia.org/wiki/Subjective_well_being>.

_____.2013v. "Zoophilia" (February 01). <http://en.wikipedia.org/ wiki/Zoophilia>.

_____.2013w. "Income Inequality" (February 02). <http://en.wikipedia.org/ wiki/Income_inequality>.

_____.2013x. "Technology and Mental Health Issues" (February 02). <http://en.wikipedia.org/wiki/Technology_and_mental_health_issues>.

_____.2013y. "Virtual Reality Therapy" (February 03). <http://en.wikipedia.org/wiki/Virtual_reality_therapy>.

_____.2013z. "Telemedicine" (February 03). <http://en.wikipedia.org/wiki/Telemedicine>.

_____.2013aa. "Traditional Chinese Medicine" (February 04). <http://en.wikipedia.org/wiki/Traditional_Chinese_medicine>.

_____.2013bb. "Mindfulness (Psychology)" (February 04). <http://en.wikipedia.org/wiki/Mindfulness_(psychology)>.

_____.2013cc. "Mindfulness" (February 04). <http://en.wikipedia.org/wiki/Mindfulness>.

_____.2013dd. "Natural Killer Cell" (February 13). <http://en.wikipedia.org/wiki/Natural_killer_cell>.

_____.2013ee. "Child Abuse" (February 14). <http://en.wikipedia.org/wiki/Child_abuse>.

_____.2013ff. "Cinderella Effect" (February 14). <http://en.wikipedia.org/wiki/Cinderella_effect>.

_____.2013gg. "Astral Projection" (February 15). <http://en.wikipedia.org/wiki/Astral_projection>.

_____.2013hh. "Conservation Medicine" (February 15). <http://en.wikipedia.org/wiki/Conservation_medicine>.

_____.2013ii. "HIV" (February 15). <http://en.wikipedia.org/wiki/HIV>.

_____.2013jj. "Prevention of HIV/AIDS" (February 15). <http://en.wikipedia.org/wiki/Prevention_of_HIV/AIDS>.

_____.2013kk. "Domestic Violence" (February 17). <http://en.wikipedia.org/wiki/Domestic_violence>.

_____.2013ll. "Borderline Personality Disorder" (February 17). <http://en.wikipedia.org/ wiki/Borderline_personality_disorder>.

_____.2013mm. "List of Torture Methods and Devices" (February 18). <http://en.wikipedia.org/wiki/List_of_torture_methods_and_devices>.

_____.2013nn. "Medical Ethics" (February 19). <http://en.wikipedia.org/wiki/Medical_ethics>.

_____.2013oo. "Nursing Ethics" (February 19). <http://en.wikipedia.org/wiki/Nursing_ethics>.

_____.2011nn. "Design Elements and Principles" (September 30). <http://en.wikipedia.org/wiki/Design_elements_and_principles>.

_____.2011oo. "Interpretation (Logic)" (April 13). <http://en.wikipedia.org/wiki/Interpretation_(Logic)>.

_____.2011pp. "Unsolved Problems in Linguistics" (February 20). <http://en.wikipedia.org/wiki/Unsolved_problems_in_linguistics>.

_____.2008. "Posthumanism" (October 20). <http://en.wikipedia.org/wiki/Posthumanism>.

_____.2008a. "Transhumanism" (October 20). <http://en.wikipedia.org/wiki/Transhumanism>.

_____.2008b. "Lowest Common Denominator" (March 26). <http://en.wikipedia.org/ wiki/Least_common_denominator>.

_____.2008c. "Infinity" (November 11). <http://en.wikipedia.org/wiki/Infinity>.

_____.2008d. "Transfinite Number" (November 10). <http://en.wikipedia.org/wiki/Transfinite_ number>.

_____.2008e. "Quantum Mechanics" (November 26). <http://en.wikipedia.org/wiki/Quantum_mechanics>.

_____.2008f. "Copenhagen Interpretation" (November 26). <http://en.wikipedia.org/wiki/Copenhagen_interpretation >.

_____.2008g. "Many Worlds Interpretation" (November 26). <http://en.wikipedia.org/wiki/Many_Worlds_Interpretation>.

_____.2008h. "Hyperspace (Science Fiction)" (November 23). <http://en.wikipedia.org/wiki/Hyperspace_(science_fiction)>.

_____.2008i. "Time Travel" (November 26). <http://en.wikipedia.org/wiki/Time_travel#Time_dilation>.

_____.2008j. "Wormhole" (November 25). <http://en.wikipedia.org/wiki/Wormhole>.

_____.2007. "Linguistics" (March 04). <http://en.wikipedia.org/wiki/Linguistics>.

Wikiversity (WKV). 2008. "Why 10 Dimensions" (November 23). <ttp://en.wikiversity.org/wiki/Why_10_dimensions>.

Wilkinson, Richard G.; & Kate Pickett. 2009. *The Spirit Level: Why More Equal Societies Almost Always Do Better*. London, UK: Allen Lane.

Williams, George C. 1996. *Adaptation and Natural Selection*. Princeton, NJ: Princeton University Press.

Williams, J. M. G.; D. Duggan; C. Crane; & M. Fennell. 2006. "Mindfulness-Based Cognitive Therapy for Prevention of Recurrence of Suicidal Behavior." *J Clin Psychol*, 62 (2): 201–210.

Wilmore, J.; & H. Knuttgen. 2003. "Aerobic Exercise and Endurance Improving Fitness for Health Benefits." *The Physician and Sportsmedicine*, 31 (5): 45.

Widom, C. S. 1999. "Post-Traumatic Stress Disorder in Abused and Neglected Children Grown up." *American Journal of Psychiatry*, 156 (8): 1223–1229. <http://ajp.psychiatryonline.org/article.aspx?articleid=173639>.

Wilhelm, Richard; & Cary F. Baines. 1930. *The Secret of the Golden Flower*. London, UK: RKP.

Winnett, Robert. 2005. "Foreign Office Faces Probe into 'Manipulation'" (March 20). *The Sunday Times*. <http://www.thetimes.co.uk/tto/news/>.

Wittgenstein, Ludwig.1953. *Philosophical Investigations*. G. E. M. Anscombe and R. Rhees, eds. G.E.M. Anscombe, tr. Oxford: Blackwell.

Woolger, Roger. 2008. "Beyond Death: Transition and the Afterlife." <http://www.rcpsych.ac.uk/PDF/RWoolgerTransition.pdf>.

Worell, Judith. 2001. *Encyclopedia of Women and Gender: Sex Similarities and Differences and the Impact of Society on Gender*. San Diego, CA: Academic Press.

World Health Organization (WHO). 2013. "Health Systems" (January 28). <http://www.who.int/topics/health_systems/en/>.

_____.2008. "Global Burden of Disease." <http://www.who.int/topics/global_burden_of_disease/en/>.

_____.2008a. "WHO: Obesity and Overweight" (December 18). <http://web.archive.org/web/20081218104805/http://www.who.int/dietphysicalactivity/publications/facts/obesity/en/>.

_____.2002. "World Report on Violence and Health." <http://www.who.int/violence_injury_prevention/violence/world_report/en/>.

_____.1986. "The Health Hazards of Organized Violence. Report on a WHO Meeting." Veldhoven 22–25.

World Medical Association (WMA). 1975. "Declaration of Tokyo." <http://www.wma.net/en/30publications/10policies/c18/index.html>.

Wright, Robert C. M. 1995. *The Moral Animal: Evolutionary Psychology and Everyday Life*. New York: Vintage Books.

Wynn, Charles M.; Arthur W. Wiggins; & Sidney Harris. 2001. *Quantum Leaps in the Wrong Direction: Where Real Science Ends—and Pseudoscience Begins.* Joseph Henry Press.

Yamey, Gavin. 2011. "Torture: European Instruments of Torture and Capital Punishment from the Middle Ages to Present." *British Medical Journal*, 323: 346.

Yang, Erzeng. 2007. *The Story of Han Xiangzi.* WA: University of Washington Press.

Yogananda, Paramahansa. 1946. *Autobiography of a Yogi.* New York: The Philosophical library.

YouTube (YOUT). 2013. "Introduction to Second Life (Historical View)" (February 03). <http://www.youtube.com/watch?v=b72CvvMuD6Q>.

_____.2013a. "Jeopardy Virtual Iraq-Afghanistan PTSD Exposure Therapy Question" (February 03). <http://www.youtube.com/watch?v=OKOy jutfn04>.

Youngstedt, S. D. 2005. "Effects of Exercise on Sleep." *Clin Sports Med.*, 24(2): 355–65. <http://www.svl.ch/Sport+Schlaf/3.pdf>.

Zimmermann, Bernd. 2013. "On Mathematical Problem Solving Processes and History of Mathematics." <http://www.icme-organisers.dk/tsg18/S12Bernd Zimmermann.pdf>.

INDEX

•A•

•B•

•C•

•D•

•E•

•F•

•G•

•H•

•I•

•J•

•K•

•L•

•N•

•O•

•P•

•Q•

•R•

•S•

•U•

•V•

•W•

•X•

•Y•

•Z•